Varicose Veins and Telangiectasias

Diagnosis and Treatment

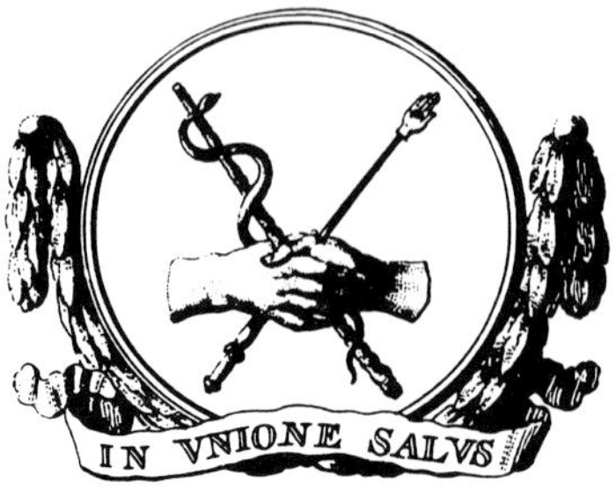

Emblem of Hunczovsky*

This graphic symbol with its caption, "In Union Health," depicts the age-old emblems of medicine: the Aesculapian rod with a serpent and another rod showing a hand with an eye in its palm. Bringing these two emblems together in this way represents a unification of the disciplines of medicine and surgery to form a combined medical practice. In 1787 such a unification was hoped to be successful in improving total patient care and offering an advantage to all who were sick.

The occasion for the development of this symbol was the second anniversary of the opening of the 2000-bed Vienna General Hospital and its merger with the 1200-bed Academia Medico-Chirurgica "Iosephina." These two institutions were combined to provide the best possible care with the best equipment available. The new institution was founded by Emperor Joseph II, who had traveled throughout Europe and learned of the improvements in education of military surgeons in France and the elevation of surgeons to academic rank by King Louis XV.

The great Vienna General Hospital eventually became the site of a massive collection of precious medical books, surgical instruments, and the historical anatomic wax museum. It was also the location of the military medical school known as the Josephinum. In the twentieth century the symbol of the Vienna General Hospital became the signet of the Austrian Society of Surgeons as a reminder of the original attempt to create modern surgery approximately 200 years earlier.

In its original form, this emblem was chosen by the Working Group for Phlebology of the Austrian Society of Dermatology. This choice was appropriate because the rod of Aesculapius represents academic theoretical traditions of medicine and conservative nonsurgical care. The seeing hand, which "sees" what the hand does, is the symbol for both experience in medicine and the manual dexterity associated with surgical skill.

To physicians dedicated to the care of patients with varicose veins and telangiectasias, the symbol is a reminder of the union of surgery and sclerotherapy, an alliance that is necessary for optimum care of the venous insufficiency produced by microphlebectasias and macrophlebectasias. Chosen to be the logo for the Fifth European-American Venous Symposium in Vienna, this symbol is an appropriate frontispiece for this book.

*Modified from Holubar H. "In Unione Salus": A short historical perspective on the development of surgical education in Austria in the 18th century. Vasa 20:10-11, 1991.

Varicose Veins and Telangiectasias

Diagnosis and Treatment

EDITED BY

John J. Bergan, M.D., Hon. F.R.C.S. (Engl.)

Clinical Professor of Surgery, University of California, San Diego, San Diego, California; Clinical Professor of Surgery, Uniformed Services University of the Health Sciences, Bethesda, Maryland; Attending Surgeon, Scripps Memorial Hospital, La Jolla, California

Mitchel P. Goldman, M.D.

Assistant Clinical Professor of Dermatology/Medicine, University of California, San Diego, San Diego, California

with 265 *illustrations, including* 100 *in color*

QMP

QUALITY MEDICAL PUBLISHING, INC

ST. LOUIS, MISSOURI 1993

Every effort has been made to ensure the accuracy of the drug dosages listed in this book; however, the health care professional is legally responsible for verifying the indications and dosage requirements with the manufacturers' package inserts and is thus advised.

Printed in the United States of America.

PUBLISHER Karen Berger
EDITOR Beth Campbell
PROJECT MANAGER Carlotta Seely
PRODUCTION Shelley Zinselmeier
BOOK DESIGN Susan Trail
COVER DESIGN Diane M. Beasley

Quality Medical Publishing, Inc.
11970 Borman, Suite 222
St. Louis, Missouri 63146

LIBRARY OF CONGRESS CATALOGING-IN-PUBLICATION DATA

Varicose veins and telangiectasias: diagnosis and treatment / edited by
John J. Bergan, Mitchel P. Goldman.
p. cm.
Includes bibliographical references and index.
ISBN 0-942219-44-9 (casebound)
1. Varicose veins. 2. Telangiectasia. I. Bergan, John J., 1927-
II. Goldman, Mitchel P.
[DNLM: 1. Telangiectasia—diagnosis. 2. Telangiectasia—therapy.
3. Varicose Veins—diagnosis. 4. Varicose Veins—therapy. WG620
V299]
RC695.V35 1993
616.1'43—dc20
DNLM/DLC
for Library of Congress 92-48328
CIP

VT/WW/WW
5 4 3 2 1

Contributors

John J. Bergan, M.D., Hon. F.R.C.S. (Engl.)
Clinical Professor of Surgery, University of California, San Diego, San Diego, California; Clinical Professor of Surgery, Uniformed Services University of the Health Sciences, Bethesda, Maryland; Attending Surgeon, Scripps Memorial Hospital, La Jolla, California

Pierre Boivin, M.D.
Co-Director of Phlebology Courses, University of Paris VI; Vascular Surgery Service, Salpetrière Hospital; Vascular Medicine Service, Broussais Hospital, Paris, France

Philip D. Coleridge Smith, M.A., F.R.C.S.
Senior Lecturer and Consultant Surgeon, Department of Surgery, University College and Middlesex School of Medicine, London, England

André Cornu-Thenard, M.D.
Co-Director of Phlebology Training, Cardiology and Surgery Services, St. Antoine Hospital, University Hospital Center, Paris, France

Ralph G. DePalma, M.D.
Lewis Saltz Professor, Department of Surgery, George Washington University, Washington, D.C.

David M. Duffy, M.D.
Assistant Clinical Professor of Medicine (Dermatology), University of California, Los Angeles, Los Angeles, California

Mitchel P. Goldman, M.D.
Assistant Clinical Professor of Dermatology/ Medicine, University of California, San Diego, San Diego, California

Abraham Lechter, M.D.
Professor of Surgery and Chief, Department of Surgery, Escuela Militar de Medicina y Hospital Militar Central, Bogota, Colombia, South America

Gregory L. Moneta, M.D.
Associate Professor of Surgery, Department of Surgery, Division of Vascular Surgery, Oregon Health Sciences University, Portland, Oregon

Peter Neglén, M.D., Ph.D.
Associate Professor, Department of Surgery, Faculty of Medicine and Health Sciences, United Arab Emirates University, Al-Ain, Abu Ohabi, United Arab Emirates

H.A. Martino Neumann, M.D.
Professor of Dermatology, Department of Dermatology, University Hospital Maastricht, Maastricht, The Netherlands

John M. Porter, M.D.
Professor of Surgery, Department of Vascular Surgery, Oregon Health Sciences University, Portland, Oregon

Pauline Raymond-Martimbeau, M.D.
Director, Dallas Noninvasive Vascular Laboratory, Dallas, Texas

John D.S. Reid, M.D., F.R.C.S.(C), F.A.C.S.
Clinical Assistant Professor, Department of Surgery, Division of Vascular Surgery, University of British Columbia, Vancouver, British Columbia, Canada

Sidney S. Rose, F.R.C.S. (Engl.)
Consultant Vascular Surgeon, Department of Surgery, University Hospital of South Manchester, Manchester, England

Ulrich Schultz-Ehrenburg, M.D.
Professor of Dermatology, Department of Dermatology, St. Josef Hospital, Ruhr-University of Bochum, Bochum, Germany

John H. Scurr, B.Sc., M.B.B.S., F.R.C.S.
Consultant Surgeon and Senior Lecturer, Department of Surgery, Middlesex and University College Hospitals, University of London, London, England

Joseph G. Sladen, M.D., F.R.C.S.(C)
Clinical Professor of Surgery, Department of Vascular Surgery, St. Paul's Hospital, University of British Columbia, Vancouver, British Columbia, Canada

David S. Sumner, M.D.
Professor, Department of Surgery, and Chief, Section of Peripheral Vascular Surgery, Department of Surgery, Southern Illinois University School of Medicine, Springfield, Illinois

Dig. J. Tazelaar, M.D.
Department of Dermatology, De Tjongerschans, Algemeen, Ziekenhuis Heerenveen, Thialfweg, Heerenveen, The Netherlands

Paul K. Thibault, M.D.
Director, Newcastle Laser Center, Newcastle, New South Wales, Australia

Olav Thulesius, M.D., Ph.D.
Professor, Department of Clinical Physiology, Faculty of Health Sciences, University of Linkoping, Linkoping, Sweden

Paul S. van Bemmelen, M.D., Ph.D.
Fellow in Vascular Surgery, Department of Vascular Surgery, Southern Illinois University, Springfield, Illinois

J. Leonel Villavicencio, M.D., F.A.C.S.
Professor of Surgery, Department of Surgery, Uniformed Services University of the Health Sciences, Bethesda, Maryland

Margaret A. Weiss, M.D.
Instructor, Department of Dermatology, Johns Hopkins University School of Medicine, Baltimore, Maryland

Robert A. Weiss, M.D.
Assistant Professor, Department of Dermatology, Johns Hopkins University School of Medicine, Baltimore, Maryland

To my lovely wife

Elisabeth

J.J.B.

To my beautiful family

Hedy, Risa, and **Melissa**

M.P.G.

Foreword

Although venous disease has been documented as afflicting mankind since antiquity, in recent years it has undergone a rapid and exciting revolution. Operations for varicose veins rarely appear on schedules in major centers; when they do, it is usually as ambulatory surgery. The saphenous vein is almost sacrosanct, being preserved whenever possible for heart and lower extremity bypass surgery.

Many of the changes in this field of surgery have been stimulated by better understanding of venous anatomy and functional physiology achieved through the use of newer and more sophisticated instrumentation. Unfortunately, much of this advancement has not yet reached the practicing physician or the medical student.

The American Venous Forum and the North American Society of Phlebology are newly created organizations founded to stimulate research and disseminate information among physicians interested in venous disease. Early interest in these organizations has been most encouraging. Through these organizations markedly divergent groups of physicians from all over the world can exchange information regarding conditions of mutual interest. Colleagues in internal medicine, dermatology, surgery, family practice, and all other branches of medicine have been encouraged to become aware of current advances in the treatment of venous conditions.

In this book Drs. Bergan and Goldman stress the fact that varicose veins and telangiectasias are derived from the same fundamental pathophysiology. Correctly, they highlight the fact that accurate diagnosis precedes precise intervention and care. The chapters included in this volume explain the similarities and the differences between varicose veins and telangiectasias, describe the history of current methods of intervention, and provide a background for further evaluation of clinical results of both surgical care and sclerotherapy.

I am happy to join the editors of this book in hoping that this volume and its teaching will go forward to improve the care of patients with venous problems.

George Johnson, Jr., M.D., F.A.C.S.

President, American Venous Forum
Chapel Hill, North Carolina

Preface

The purpose of this volume is to bring together observations, facts, and theories that can guide physicians in the care of patients with varicose veins and telangiectasias. In the past, medical literature on this subject has focused on elements of the problem without providing unifying explanations of etiology and pathogenesis to guide specific treatments. Furthermore, an emphasis on the etiology of venous stasis in general and a focus on the causes of venous stasis ulcerations in particular have produced confusion in the treatment of simple varicosities and telangiectasias.

Treatment has been further obscured by the rise and fall of alternative techniques in care. In addition, a decreasing interest in the treatment of venous problems by cardiovascular surgeons has hampered the teaching of diagnosis and care of varicose veins and telangiectasias in academic environments. It is paradoxical that those individuals who should have the greatest interest in treating venous stasis in its various manifestations have a vested interest in preservation of the saphenous vein as a conduit in coronary revascularization and peripheral bypass. For these reasons we thought that it was time to bring this volume through the arduous process of publication.

The thoughtful reader of this book will quickly note the differing methods of diagnosis, disagreements in explanation of phenomena, alternative indications for intervention, and even completely different techniques that appear in the chapters that follow. Students of this field will recognize that rapid developments in knowledge of venous phenomena and their treatment reach disparate medical centers in a nonsimultaneous fashion. Further, in a field of endeavor characterized by few absolutes, there is room for alternative views and explanations.

Not long ago, an editorial in *Lancet* stated: "Varicose veins is probably the commonest as well as the worst treated disorder presenting to general surgeons" (Lancet 1:333, 1975). In response, the respected vascular surgeon Adrian Marston wrote: "To call a condition which is found in 50% of the adult European population a disorder is scarcely logical." Mr. Marston said further that "a sizable minority, perhaps a third of people attending varicose vein clinics, require no treatment at all." He correctly indicated that "most come simply because they do not like the appearance of their legs" (Marston A. Lancet 1:453, 1975). It is precisely those individuals with cosmetic complaints who see advertisements in newspapers and then attend the clinics that advertise sclerotherapy for varicose veins. Neither the patients nor the physicians realize that optimum care is achieved through precise diagnosis and utilization of all, not just one, of the various modalities available for care.

This issue was summarized in a wise editorial in the *British Journal of Surgery* by a well-known general/vascular surgeon and phlebologist, Bo Eklof. In citing the Latin phrase *ad utrumque paratus,* from the seal of the University of Lund in Sweden, he pointed out that this phrase, which means "to be prepared for both the sword as well as the book," could be "transcribed for the modern treatment of varicose veins: use the knife as well as the syringe." Eklof noted that simple physical examination supplemented by nondirectional Doppler ultrasound could be used routinely. With this approach, evaluation for obstruction, patency, or reflux in both the superficial and the deep venous system could be accomplished. Further, Eklof stated that the vascular laboratory and phlebography would be necessary in the few cases in which symptoms and clinical findings correlate poorly, when a problem of deep venous insufficiency is involved, or for patients with congenital angiodysplasia.

In this volume an analogy is drawn between the anatomic aspects of telangiectasias and varicose veins. Both are collections of elongated, dilated, tortuous venous vessels with incompetent valves. The thoughtful reader will see that treatment of the gross anatomic abnormality is best achieved by surgical removal and that treatment of the almost microscopic pathologic vessels is best achieved by obliteration through sclerotherapy. Since patients will present to the interested physician with both forms of phlebectasia, a treatment plan guided by accurate diagnosis will be recognized as essential.

Attention must be given to socioeconomic considerations in the diagnosis and treatment of varicose veins and telangiectasias. Since both conditions are very common, it is incumbent on the medical profession to decrease the costs of care for society without compromising the quality of care to the individual. This balance can be achieved by eliminating the hospital stay and employing ambulatory surgery. Correct selection of compression sclerotherapy will further reduce cost. In fact, it has been calculated that 20% of patients can be treated with compression sclerotherapy as an alternative to surgery. This approach could reduce the total cost of treatment of varicose veins by at least one third in comparison with the sole use of inpatient surgery (Eklof B. Br J Surg 75:297, 1988).

The chapters that follow will attempt to shed light on the obscure problems that comprise the diagnosis and treatment of varicose veins and telangiectasias. Some of the confusion in current practice is related to the history of diagnosis and treatment of the condition. Without returning to the fascinating investigations of the ancients, one can learn much from events that occurred after 1900. In 1916 Homans described the postphlebitic limb and discussed the effects of deep vein thrombosis. Although the clarification of these effects and Homans's notation that incompetence of perforating veins of the calf and ankle occurred in "venous disease" were important advances, his use of the terms "varicose ulcers" and "venous ulcers" did not help to explain the situation. Now, in looking back on the observations of Homans, we can say that cure of advanced manifestations of venous stasis can be achieved through complete elimination of superficial reflux. On the other hand, palliation is the only thing that can be achieved in the treatment of patients with severe deep venous insufficiency. Homans's emphasis on the importance of valve incompetence has been reinforced by subsequent investigations (Homans J. Surg Gynecol Obstet 22:143, 1916).

It was not until 1953 that Cockett described the three constant perforating veins in the medial aspect of the lower third of the leg. The importance of this observation has been obscured by recent investigations. However, the truth of Cockett's thesis remains: perforating vein incompetence results in high pressure transmitted from the calf pump during exercise directly to the unsupported veins superficial to the membranous fascia and the intradermal vessels of the skin. The result of this high pressure "leak" is elongation, tortuosity, dilation, and valve incompetence in the affected vessels (Cockett FB, Jones DEE. Lancet 1:17, 1953).

Another important observation that seems to have gone unrecognized by subsequent physicians is that perforator incompetence can exist without complete incompetence of the deep veins of the leg (Dodd H, Cockett FB. The Pathology and Surgery of the Veins of the Lower Limb. Edinburgh: Churchill Livingstone, 1976). This fact supports the hypothesis that treatment of superficial incompetence can cure a patient whereas treatment of incompetence associated with deep venous insufficiency is merely palliative.

Another confusing factor in treating varicose veins is that some workers believe that no venous ulcer can exist without perforator incompetence (Burnand et al. Surgery 82:9, 1977). Others have pointed out that cutaneous ulceration has been demonstrated in patients with only saphenous insufficiency (Wright DDI, et al. Br J Surg 75:395, 1988). Even the marvelously executed studies of Bjordal in the early 1970s led to some confusion. It has been understood by many that Bjordal demonstrated that incompetent perforating veins contributed little to increased pressure in the superficial system. In fact, Bjordal's studies clearly show that flow through perforating veins in the patients he studied was bidirectional, both inward and outward (Bjordal RI. Acta Chir Scand 138:251, 1972). The fact that Bjordal concluded that most of the flow was directed inward does not detract from the other part of his observation, that outward flow was, indeed, present. Such outward directed flow conforms to the observations of Cockett that high exercising pressure is transmitted directly to the most poorly supported venules of the skin and subcutaneous veins.

Another concept related to the etiology of varicosities has added to the confusion. This matter is the observation of arteriovenous anastomoses in association with varicose veins and the increased oxygen content of such veins (Haimovici H, et al. Ann Surg 164:990, 1966; Schalin L. In Eklof B, et al., eds. Controversies in the Management of Venous Disorders. London: Butterworth, 1989, p 182). Although many have criticized the interpretation of those observations, not many have questioned the observations themselves. Because of respect for the wisdom of Browse, the criticism leveled by him in a commentary on the work of Schalin has been cited. Browse argued that demonstrating a fistula requires physiologic techniques, and he pointed out that radiologic results are also open to subjective interpretation. Nevertheless, there is direct evidence of pathologic fistula development in limbs with venous disease. This evidence comes from the work of Gius, who described the existence of arteriovenous anastomoses at operation through the use of a dissecting microscope. Gius noted that the histology of these vessels showed a uniformly hypertrophied muscle coat (Haimovici H, et al. Radiology 87:696, 1966). Further work has shown that these anastomoses are of capillary caliber and are thought to open in response to alterations in temperature or pressure (Ryan TJ, Copeman PWM. Br J Dermatol 81:563, 1969). This last observation lends credence to the importance of arteriovenous anastomoses in the development of varicose veins and telangiectasias. A unifying hypothesis of increased hydrostatic and hydrodynamic pressure being transmitted to the veins and venules of the lower extremity could very well lead to a breakdown in the capillary barrier and to the development of direct arteriovenous connections.

In the preparation of this volume, it became clear that a review of the vast literature on the subject of venous disease suggests that many old theories are founded on signs whereas others are based on conjecture. As will be shown in this book, a great degree of understanding about venous stasis and venous ulceration was achieved even in ancient times. On the other hand, throughout the ages there have been many misconceptions about venous disease, some of which have been transmitted directly to us today. Like Eklof, we can only hope that increased international awareness of the problem of venous disease, venous stasis, and telangiectasias will produce an increased level of scientific inquiry and activity. Ultimately, if this book contributes to improved management of the common, if not lethal, disorder of venous stasis, then we will feel rewarded indeed.

John J. Bergan
Mitchel P. Goldman

Contents

PART ONE

Fundamental Considerations

Chapter 1

Physiologic Observations on Causes of Varicose Veins

Olav Thulesius

VARICOSE VEINS AND VENOUS INSUFFICIENCY

Venous insufficiency is defined as any abnormality of the peripheral venous system that reduces or impedes venous return. It includes not only the veins themselves and their patency, wall properties, and valves but also the important extravascular factors that largely determine venous return from the extremities, such as the muscle pumps of the foot, calf, and thigh, which, in turn, are dependent on proper neuromuscular function and the mobility of joints (especially the ankle) and connective tissue support by fascia.

Varicose veins per se may or may not be an integral part of the full-blown picture of venous insufficiency, characterized by venous hypertension, edema, and leg ulcers. The spectrum of varicose veins is great: they can be an early sign of venous insufficiency, which should be treated to prevent disease progression, or they may be a late sign, appearing as dilated collaterals.

Varicose veins are dilated, tortuous veins exhibiting reflux because of valvular insufficiency. Dilatation of the veins may be primary, initiated by an unknown process, or it may be the result of postthrombotic changes, arteriovenous fistula, or diverted flow (collateral flow) resulting from blockage of deep veins. The question, however, arises about the site and mechanism of the initial fault in primary varicose veins, which initiated the disease process. The most likely candidates are defective venous valves that are unable to close properly or weakness of the venous wall that leads to distention and reflux.

Venous Valves

A functional evaluation of venous valves can be made by determining the pressure at which leakage occurs after retrograde filling of isolated veins. A study of saphenous veins of the thigh from 20 healthy controls and 20 patients with distal varicose veins revealed a significantly lower leak pressure in long saphenous varicose veins (79 mm Hg) as compared to that of normal veins (197 mm Hg).[1] Surprisingly, however, there were five cases without immediate leakage in controls and three cases with normal leak pressure (200 to 300 mm Hg) in patients with varicose veins. These results are not consistent with the concept of a generalized tendency toward leaky valves in cases of primary venous insufficiency; moreover, even individuals without venous disease can have incompetent valves.

Venous Wall

Most evidence about varicose veins suggests that they are caused by a primary abnormality of the venous wall that results in increased distention. The wall elements responsible for distensibility characteristics are connective tissue and smooth muscle. These elements, which reside in the media, may be affected by the disease process. Since alterations of venous wall viscoelastic properties are important in regard to the development of varicose veins, the fundamental principles are discussed here.

The venous viscoelastic properties can be viewed as a three-component mechanical model (Figure 1-1). The model is composed of smooth muscle (internal elastic element and a viscous dashpot) and connective tissue (parallel elastic element). The latter can be recruited in the relaxed state or at maximal distention. When stretch is applied to this model, elongation (length) and stress (tension) can be measured. This action is best depicted in a length-tension diagram (Figure 1-2). The slope of the length-tension relationship is an expression of the elastance (stiffness) of the stretched wall elements. When smooth muscle is contracted, stretch elongates the internal elastic elements and the dashpot. This change is reflected in a slight slope of the length-tension curve, which indicates low elastance. In a dilated vein, with relaxed smooth muscle, the length-tension curve initially has a flat slope

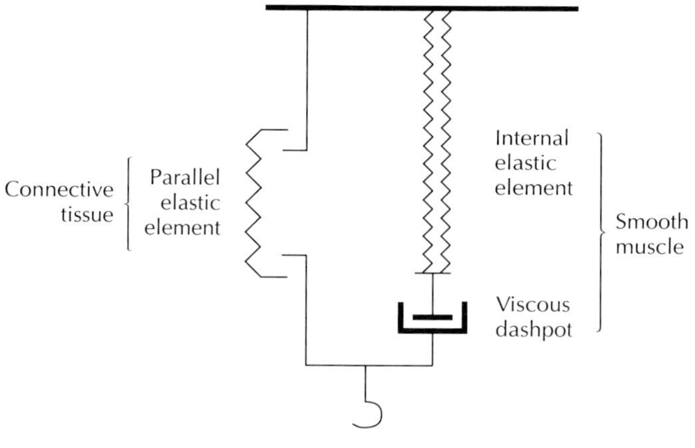

FIGURE 1-1. Three-component mechanical model characterizing the viscoelastic properties of a normal vein with two parallel elastic elements, one inside the contractile portion of smooth muscle and the other in the connective tissue. The latter is recruited only in fully dilated veins. The viscous dashpot element is also part of the smooth muscle.

because of filling from the partially collapsed state to the filled round transection. Thereafter the wall elements become stretched, demonstrating a steeper slope than that of the contracted state. In this stretched state, the parallel elastic elements of connective tissue become weight-bearing and are responsible for measured elastance. Therefore stiffness is higher in relaxed veins.

Connective tissue and lysosomal enzymes. In primary varicose veins, the initial interest was focused largely on the weakness of connective tissue elements and the possibility of a destructive process initiated by the local release of lysosomal enzymes. Niebes[2] demonstrated elevated serum levels of beta-glucoronidase and N-acetyl-beta-glucaminidase in cases involving primary varicose veins. We were able to confirm these findings, but we later found that this abnormality was not confined to patients with primary varicose veins but also could be demonstrated in postthrombotic states.[3] Therefore it is likely that lysosomal enzymes and tissue damage may be involved in the fully developed disease process of venous insufficiency but not in the initial state. A loosening of connective tissue, however, may be considered a result of hormonal changes associated with varicosis of pregnancy.

The concept of lysosomal enzymes and cytokines has recently received renewed attention in patients with leg ulcers. Coleridge Smith et al.[4] presented evidence that trapped white blood cells release enzymes that damage wall elements, induce increased capillary permeability, and promote thrombus formation.

Smooth muscle. Evidence is accumulating to implicate a deficient contractile function as a cause of varicose veins. In lower extremity veins, the amount of smooth muscle increases from proximal to distal, with a thicker muscle coat in foot veins compared to thigh veins. This increase can be viewed as an adaptive process that enables distal veins to withstand hydrostatic pressure better than proximal veins do. Therefore smooth muscle must play an important role in the physiologic function of lower extremity veins. This role involves serving as a local control mechanism rather than maintaining centrally governed vasomotor control through the sympathetic nervous system.

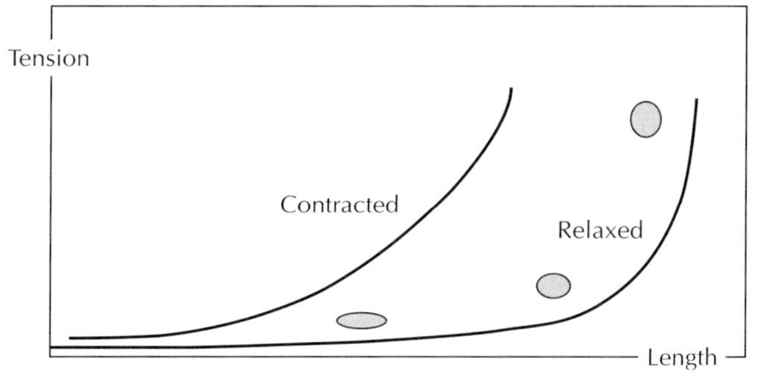

FIGURE 1-2. Length-tension diagram showing the action of a vein when contracted and relaxed during the process of filling and stretching. Steepness of the slope indicates the elastance (stiffness of wall). Characteristics of the wall are evident only in filled veins. Low initial slope of the relaxed (dilated) vein is only an indication of the expansion of the partially collapsed vein.

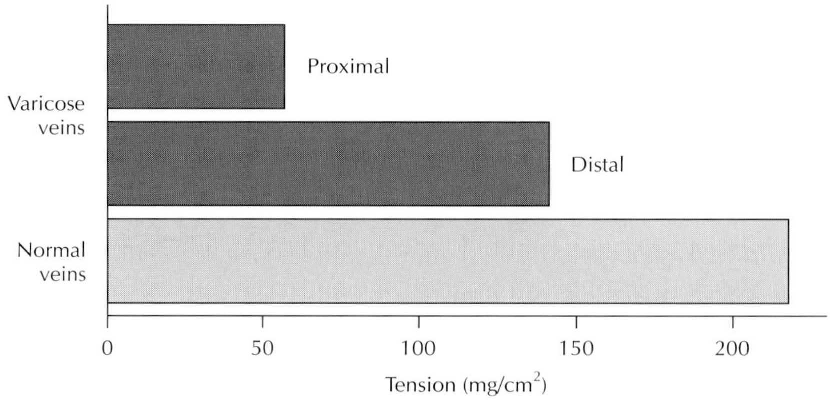

FIGURE 1-3. In vitro contractile responses of isolated preparations of the long saphenous vein in patients with varicose veins and in controls.

The in vitro measured maximal contractile force of varicose saphenous vein preparations to norepinephrine was shown to be lower than that of controls[5] (Figure 1-3). Recently, it has been shown that alpha-adrenergic responsiveness of superficial hand veins in patients with varicose veins was lower than that of healthy controls.[6]

Another important parameter of smooth muscle function not related to shortening or generation of tension is associated with viscoelastic wall properties. Contrary to what one would expect, resistance to deformation is lower in contracted (vs. relaxed) vascular preparations.[7] We have been able to show that foot veins in patients with venous insufficiency display a reduced compliance (increased stiffness) and a higher elasticity modulus, a finding that is in agreement with the assumption of damaged smooth muscle in varicose veins.[8] Another indication of smooth muscle derangement is the loss of or reduction in stress relaxation and stress-release contraction in varicosis[9] (Figure 1-4). Stress relaxation in leg veins implies that the increase in venous volume that takes place with distal translocation of blood volume in a change from the supine to the upright position or with temporary outflow impediment is balanced and retarded. Alternatively, emptying of a normal vein is followed by venous contraction, as happens after venous emptying during exercise; that is, the reduction in volume is retarded because of smooth muscle hysteresis.

Superficial veins are involved in thermoregulation since venous blood flow favors dissipation of heat. Therefore a rise in local and overall body temperature results in venodilatation. Venoconstriction favors preservation of body heat since it diverts surface blood flow to deep veins surrounding arteries and promotes countercurrent heat exchange with precooling of arterial blood directed to acral regions. Normal superficial veins are sensitive to cooling, with vasoconstriction elicited by a very effective mechanism that is independent of sympathetic vasoconstrictor nerves but based on the blockade of the NA^+,K^+-ATPase (sodium pump).[10] This mechanism is not operative in varicose veins (Figure 1-5).

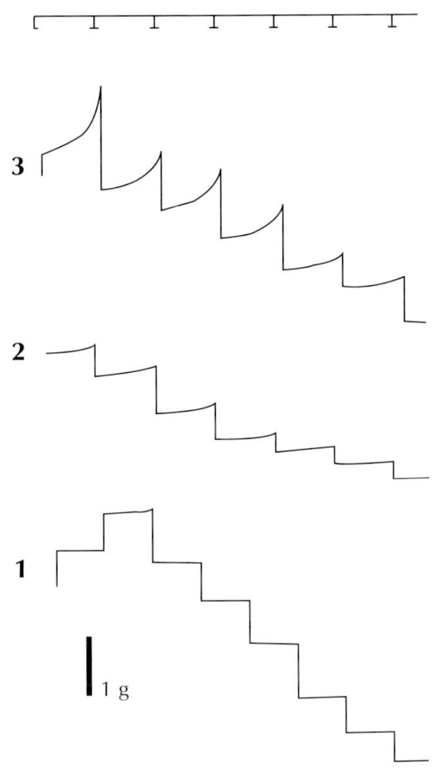

FIGURE 1-4. Recording of passive tension of a piece of latex (*1*), a venous preparation from a varicose vein (*2*), and a normal vein (*3*). Stress relaxation (slow decrease of tension) is clearly seen in the normal vein. Curves were obtained by stepwise stretch of 0.2 mm of a preparation measuring 10 × 4 mm. Time marking: 1 minute at top (*Note:* Record should be read from right to left). (From Thulesius O, Gjöres JE. Reactions of venous smooth muscle in normal men and patients with varicose veins. Angiology 25:145-154, 1974.)

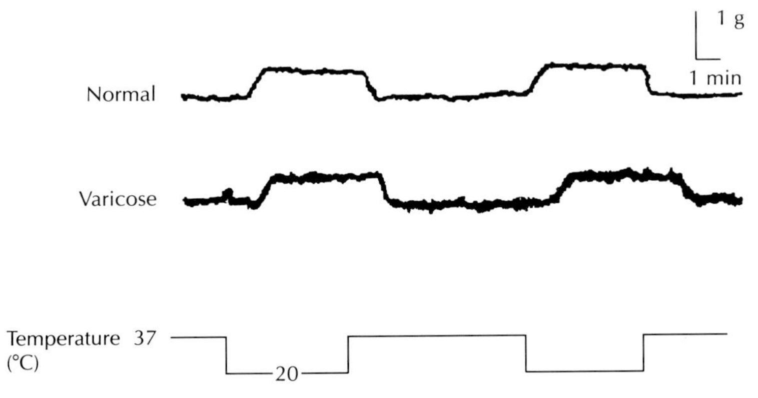

FIGURE 1-5. Effect of cooling on the tension of the human great saphenous vein. Note that cooling from 37° to 20° C in the normal vein induces contraction and dilatation in the varicose vein. (Recordings indicate tension of strips from isolated human great saphenous veins in a thermostated organ bath. Top: Normal preparation; middle: varicose vein; bottom: record of temperature.)

Recently Raju et al.[11] presented evidence to show that the degree of deep venous insufficiency is related to changes in venous wall compliance.

Endothelium

The role of endothelium in controlling local vasomotor function has been clearly established. The existence of an endothelium-derived relaxing factor has been consistently demonstrated in arteries. The situation on the venous side is the opposite of that of the arterial side: saphenous vein endothelium has a contraction-facilitating effect in response to stimulation with norepinephrine. In varicose veins, however, endothelium-mediated enhancement of vasoconstriction induced by norepinephrine is reduced as a result of endothelial damage. This effect also has been documented by ultrastructural studies.[12] Therefore local dilatation of veins with the development of varicose veins can be initiated by endothelial damage.

DEVELOPMENT OF VARICOSE VEINS

The pathophysiologic process of the development of varicose veins is presented in Figure 1-6. This concept takes into account the development of both primary and secondary (postthrombotic) varicose veins. In the primary category, knowledge is accumulating to show that the initial abnormality resides in the smooth muscle coat of the media of veins and is caused by hereditary weakness, hormonal influences during pregnancy, or endothelial damage. (In the case of hormonal influences during pregnancy, a loosening of connective tissue elements also may occur.) The primary abnormality induces venous distention with secondary valvular insufficiency, reflux, and venous hypertension.

In secondary, or postthrombotic, varicose veins, the scenario is different. The condition begins with the inflammatory process of recanalization (phlebitis), which can damage the delicate valve leaflets and lead to valvular insufficiency and reflux. Other aspects of the postthrombotic state are characterized by incomplete recanalization and phlebofibrosis (Figure 1-7).

Perforator Veins

The superficial and deep veins of the lower extremity are connected by short perforator veins that transverse the deep fascia, usually at an oblique angle. The function of perforator veins is to drain blood from the superficial to the deep venous system, except in the foot where drainage is from inside to outside. The normal direction of blood flow in perforator veins is guided by two factors: the presence of valves and the moving fascia, both of which direct blood flow from outside to inside on the thigh and calf. Since there are approximately 30 perforator veins on the thigh and 40 on the calf and the foot, when the surface area of the various parts is considered, it can be seen that the density of perforators increases distally.

As a consequence of thrombotic injury to valves or flow-induced dilatation and

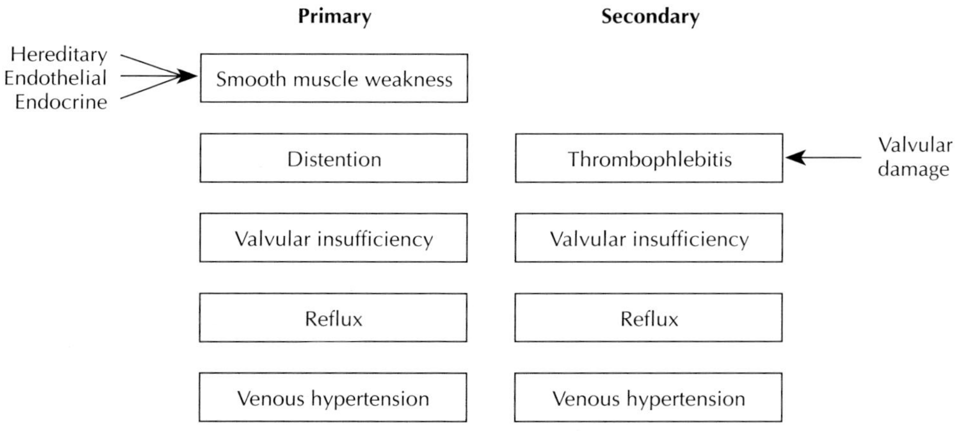

FIGURE 1-6. Pathophysiology of varicose veins in primary and secondary (postthrombotic) varicose veins.

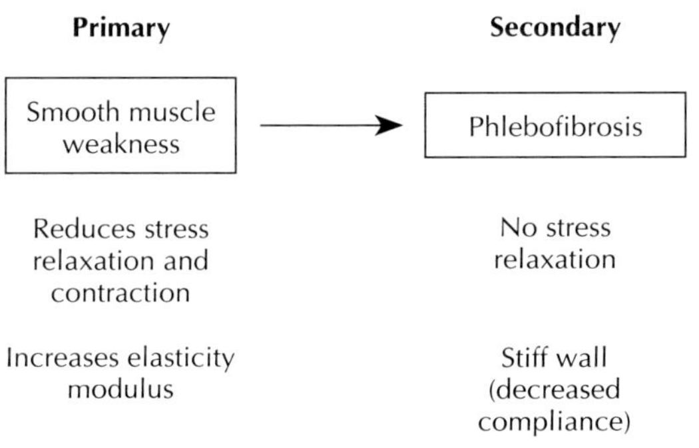

FIGURE 1-7. Abnormalities characterizing the venous wall in primary and secondary (postthrombotic) varicose veins.

valvular incompetence, the direction of venous blood flow may become inverted, with a "blowout" flow occurring during exercise. (The flow-induced dilatation of perforator veins usually takes place after long-standing superficial venous insufficiency in the long, or greater, saphenous vein.) Blowout flow in a single insufficient ankle perforator vein during dorsiflexion of the foot can be in excess of 100 ml/min and may be greater with weight-bearing exercise such as walking.[13]

Some clinically important perforators that drain the long saphenous vein are found on the medial aspect of the calf, 5 to 25 cm above the sole of the foot ("Cockett's perforators"), on the dorsal aspect of the calf, and (a few) on the thigh. The pathophysiologic importance of perforator insufficiency is related to recurrence of varicose veins and local venous hypertension.

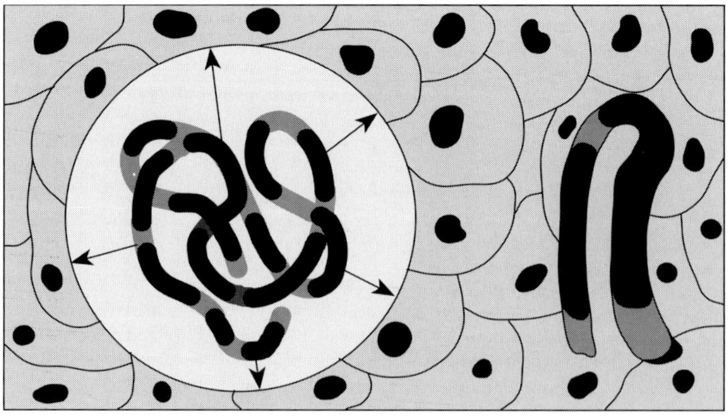

FIGURE 1-8. Schematic representation of a microvarix surrounded by a halo of edema. (From Bollinger A, Fagrell B. Clinical Capillaroscopy. Toronto: Hofgrefe & Huber, 1990, p 32.)

Microvarices

With superficial varicose veins, coiled and distended skin capillaries occur in a patchy distribution. With advanced deep venous insufficiency and venous hypertension, capillary distention leads to the development of microvarices, or glomerulus-like tortuous capillaries surrounded by a halo formation caused by local edema[14] (Figure 1-8).

Reticular varices are small ectatic cutaneous veins, probably dilated venules in the upper corium. Also called hyphen webs, they can be present together with large truncal varices of the saphena system or can occur in isolation. These varices usually have no functional consequences in themselves if they are not associated with other abnormalities.

REFERENCES

1. Thulesius O, Ekman L, Gjöres JE. Functional study of isolated venous valves, with special comments on the etiology of varicose veins. In American European Symposium on Venous Diseases. Montreux, 1974, pp 74-76.
2. Niebes P. Determination of enzymes and degradation products of glucosaminoglycan metabolism in the serums of healthy and varicose subjects. Clin Chim Acta 42:399-403, 1972.
3. Thulesius O, Gjöres JE, Eriksson O, Berlin E. Mechanical and biochemical factors in chronic venous insufficiency. Vasa 13:195-200, 1984.
4. Coleridge Smith PD, Thomas P, Scurr JH, Dormandy JA. Causes of venous ulceration: A new hypothesis. Br Med J 296:1726-1727, 1988.
5. Thulesius O, Ugaily-Thulesius L, Gjöres JE, Neglén P. The varicose saphenous vein, functional and ultrastructural studies, with special reference to smooth muscle. Phlebology 3:89-95, 1988.
6. Blöchl-Daum B, Schuller-Petrovic S, Woltz M, Korn A, Böhler K, Eichler H-G. Primary defect in alpha-adrenergic responsiveness in patients with varicose veins. Clin Pharmacol Ther 49:49-52, 1991.

7. Gow BS. The influence of vascular smooth muscle on the viscoelastic properties of blood vessels. In Bergel DH, ed. Cardiovascular Fluid Dynamics, vol 2. London: Academic Press, 1972, pp 65-110.
8. Norgren L, Thulesius O. Pressure-volume characteristics of foot veins in normal cases and patients with venous insufficiency. Blood Vessels 12:1-12, 1975.
9. Thulesius O, Gjöres JE. Reactions of venous smooth muscle in normal men and patients with varicose veins. Angiology 25:145-154, 1974.
10. Thulesius O, Yousif MH. Na^+, K^+-ATPase inhibition. A new mechanism for cold-induced vasoconstriction in cutaneous veins. Acta Physiol Scand 141:127-128, 1990.
11. Raju S, et al. Observations on the calf venous pump mechanism: Determinants of post-exercise pressure. American Venous Forum, Third Annual Meeting. Fort Lauderdale, Fla., Feb. 1991.
12. Thulesius O, et al. Endothelial-mediated enhancement of noradrenaline-induced vasoconstriction in normal and varicose veins. Clin Physiol 11:153-159, 1991.
13. Thulesius O, Gjöres JE, Berlin E, Grip A, Kristoffersen K. Blood flow in perforator veins of the calf. In May R, Partsch H, Stabesand J, eds. Perforating Veins. Munich: Urban & Schwarzenberg, 1981.
14. Bollinger A, Fagrell B. Clinical Capillaroscopy. Toronto: Hofgrefe & Huber, 1990.

Chapter 2

Anatomic Observations on Causes of Varicose Veins*

Sidney S. Rose

The idea of valvular venous incompetence that allows reversal of blood flow and resultant dilatation was first conceived by William Harvey in 1628.[1] It was the natural corollary to his theory of circulation of the blood. Before Harvey's studies the humoral theory had held sway for centuries. Blood in the veins was thought to be thickened by "gross and evil humours" that distended the veins by viscosity. Bandaging the limb was contraindicated because it would drive these humors back into the body.

Harvey's theory was developed after he became interested in studying venous valves while in Padua at the Anatomy School of Fabricius.[2] Harvey made two fundamental observations: (1) the direction of the valve was such that blood could only flow toward the heart, and (2) the heart was a pump, not merely a receptacle (as was formerly thought). It is ironic that the final and third link in the circulatory chain—the capillaries—was described by Malpighi[3] only 8 years after Harvey's death.

The theory of valvular incompetence proposed by Harvey was the subject of heated debate for the next 20 years. It was finally accepted, along with the theory of primary valvular incompetence, as the cause of varicose veins. This mechanical theory, as it has become known, has been propagated in most surgical texts since the time of Harvey, and surgical treatment of varicose veins has been governed by this theory. This approach has stimulated various forms of proximal ligation of incompetent veins to replace incompetent valves.

Since the results of such surgery have not been universally successful, many generations of surgeons have been motivated to vary their techniques. As a result,

*Modified from Hobbs J, Nicolaides AN, Yao JST, eds. Investigation of Chronic Venous Insufficiency. London: Med-Orion Publishing, 1993.

THEORETICAL CAUSES OF VARICOSE VEINS

- Heredity
- Race
- Gender
- Posture
- Gravitational back pressure
- Pregnancy
- Hormonal influence
- Weight
- Primary valvular incompetence
  - Decreased number of valves
  - Aging
- Incompetent perforating veins
- Arteriovenous communications
- Vein wall weakness
- Vein wall abnormality
- Secondary valvular incompetence
  - Phlebitis
  - Deep vein thrombosis

various additions and modifications to the operative treatment have been developed. Ultimately, even Harvey's theory was called into question. Additional theories have included vein wall weakness and perforating vein incompetence. Other less popular theories have been advanced, and they are discussed here (see box).

GENERAL FACTORS AFFECTING VEIN WALL

The common element in the cause of varicose veins is a basic genetic defect. Gender, pregnancy, hormones, enzymes, and other humoral factors all are superimposed on this genetic element. Gravitational back pressure also plays a role. Whether such pressure is primary or secondary is debatable. The debate involves consideration of the contribution of each of these factors individually and as a whole. It is important to remember that the total effect may be greater than the sum of its parts.

Heredity

No doubt exists that an inherited genetic defect is present in patients with varicose veins. There is also a familial tendency. Whole families may be affected, and it is common for a mother and a daughter to have the same pattern of varicosities. Sometimes a generation is skipped. Occasionally the link is established only through maternal or paternal aunts. Congenital anatomic abnormalities of veins have been suggested as a cause of varicosities, but this theory has never been verified. The congenital view is contested by Nicholson,[4] who reported that 68% of cases do not develop until an individual reaches the age of 18 years, with the main incidence occurring between the ages of 18 and 35 years.

Race

Inbred racial differences have been observed that support the theory of genetic influence. Varicosity is common in the Western world. However, surgery for varicose veins in East Africa is an extremely rare event. In the Caribbean, where there are people of mixed race who tend to have many pregnancies, varicose veins are present in a high proportion of women. The mass deportations to the Caribbean Islands that occurred during Oliver Cromwell's occupation of Ireland in the seventeenth century led to the introduction of Irish blood, which probably has had a considerable effect on the prevalence of varicose veins.

Gender

Varicose veins occur predominantly in females, with the female : male ratio ranging from 4 : 1 to 8 : 1 in North America and Europe. The incidence of varicose veins in these areas is reported to be 2% of the adult population.

Posture

Upright posture has a detrimental effect on varicose veins. Although such posture causes the symptoms, it probably is not the primary cause of varicosity. However, once the vein has become incompetent, it will be affected by gravitational back pressure.

In comparing the habits of races in which varicose veins are rare, one striking postural difference is a natural adoption of the squatting position during defecation and parturition by Africans. In this position, strain is transmitted into the pelvis rather than the groin, as occurs with these acts in Western nations. In the groin, pressure is transmitted to the femoral and saphenous veins. It is interesting to note that the incidence of varicose veins increases among blacks who have moved from Africa to a Western environment, as has been shown in studies in cities in the United States.

Gravitational Back Pressure

Gravitational back pressure is not entirely responsible for vein dilatation; if this were the case, the vein wall would respond uniformly. Such pressure would not explain the localized development of lateral, saccular, and irregular blowouts, as described earlier.

Gravitational back pressure is the main cause of symptoms, however, and therefore it has been held responsible for causation of varicose veins. The patient's complaint of chronic aching pain is the result of stasis that develops gradually over time. Symptoms may be absent or minimal; however, as dilatation continues to extend the affected vein, incompetence of a protecting valve that is located either proximally or in a perforating vein can develop gradually or suddenly. When this occurrence is sudden, such valve incompetence causes rapid development or exacerbation of a varicosity. This action produces localized discomfort in a vein that was previously asymptomatic or not apparent. Pain is caused by reflux and may be quite sharp initially. The pain soon decreases to an ache as the affected vein wall adjusts.

The physiologic response to increased pressure in a normal vein is hypertrophy, not dilatation. This fact is demonstrated in the reversed normal saphenous vein when used as an arterial bypass. In this situation it is able to cope with arterial blood pressure. Similarly when an in situ vein graft is performed, the vein, with all its valves destroyed, responds to the raised internal pressure by hypertrophy, not dilatation.

Finally, if hydrostatic pressure is the major cause of varicosities, they should develop at the point of greatest dependency and become larger from below in an upward direction. However, this is not the case. The largest varicose clusters are often found just below the knee. Increased hydrostatic pressure resulting from occupational strain, exemplified in operatic tenors and weight lifters, has been invoked as the cause of varicosity, but it is doubtful whether this change occurs in the absence of a genetic factor. On the other hand, if competent valves are present proximal to a venous blowout, they will become distended by the accumulation of venous blood arriving from the periphery until there is sufficient pressure to empty them. The symptoms therefore are caused by stasis rather than back pressure. Both these factors may coexist.

Pregnancy

Further etiologic clues are found from the study of varicose veins that develop during pregnancy. In this physiologic model, varicose veins not only develop but also subsequently disappear. The development of varicose veins during pregnancy sheds some light on vein wall and vein valve theories. Varicose veins of pregnancy appear early and gradually increase during pregnancy; many veins disappear shortly after delivery. This phenomenon demonstrates that the formation of varicose veins is reversible under special circumstances. It also means that any valves that became incompetent were able to regain competence. These valves must not have undergone any basic structural change during pregnancy. Every valid etiologic theory of varicose veins must explain how this happens because varicosities of pregnancy are macroscopically and microscopically indistinguishable from varicose veins that develop independently of pregnancy. For further discussion of the effects of pregnancy and the menstrual cycle, see Chapter 3.

Hormonal Influence

In the past it was thought that uterine pressure was the cause of varicose veins of pregnancy. Actually these varicosities begin to appear long before the uterus is large enough to cause increased back pressure. Now it is accepted that venous dilatation is the result of hormonal influences rather than pressure alone. As the hormonal changes begin with the onset of pregnancy, the varicose process begins immediately. Nevertheless, the veins do not become visible until the dilatation has had time to develop at about the sixth week. Sometimes they appear earlier.

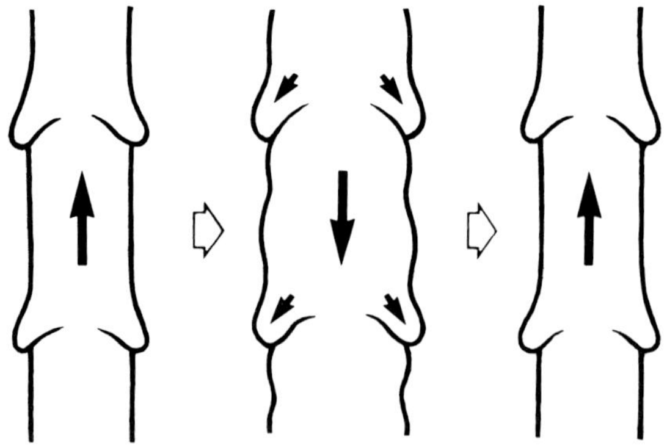

FIGURE 2-1. Diagrammatic representation of development and removal of varicose veins of pregnancy.

It has been suggested that estrogens and/or progesterones are responsible for venous dilatation of pregnancy. These hormones cause loss of vein wall tone through an effect on genetically susceptible smooth muscle cells and supporting tissues. When the vein becomes dilated, the valve ring expands until the commissure separates and the cusps are unable to meet. Dilatation of the vein wall and valve ring therefore produces secondary valvular incompetence (Figure 2-1).

After pregnancy ends, the circulating hormones return to normal and the situation is reversed. Muscle cells that were marginally affected are able to recover, and veins that were minimally affected regain much of their tone. The valve ring contracts and valves are able to close. Thus valvular competence is restored. In a first pregnancy some veins may not be sufficiently dilated to become clinically obvious, and they appear only with the second pregnancy. Only those veins that have been dilated beyond repair become permanently varicose. This fact explains the aggravation of symptoms that normally occurs during the first day or two of menstruation.

When combined with an underlying genetic defect, pregnancy may cause a female : male predominance of varicosity of 8 : 1. However, even in the nullipara, the ratio of varicosities is still 5 : 1. Although genetic background must be the same in both sexes, the added influence of female sex hormones explains why varicose veins occur more frequently in women, even in the absence of pregnancy. On the other hand, varicose veins in men are often much larger, though less symptomatic, than those in women.

Weight

No specific relationship has been established between obesity and truncal varicosities. However, in susceptible individuals there appears to be an increase in the number and irregularity of visible reticular veins in limbs with excessive subcutaneous fat. This condition often is associated with a profusion of intradermal telangiectasias.

Primary Valvular Incompetence

The theory of primary valvular incompetence is based on Harvey's mechanical theory. It has been postulated that an individual with varicose tendency is either born with fewer than normal valves or suffers from atrophy of the valves with advancing age. A combination of the two factors also has been suggested. To this genetic concept of primary valve failure is added the theory of sequential descending valvular incompetence.[5] It has been postulated that the first valve to become incompetent is the uppermost. This valve may be the one at the saphenofemoral junction or the valve in the middle third of the thigh at the adductor canal. It has been suggested that incompetence proceeds peripherally as each successive valve succumbs to increasing back pressure from above. The entire vein and valve complex then responds by venous dilatation.

Although this theory is conceptually attractive, it is not in accord with clinical findings. Furthermore, pathologic changes that occur in the valve have been described only incompletely. The most detailed description of valve pathology comes from Gottlob and May,[6] who investigated changes in valves resulting from phlebitis. In such cases the valve is damaged acutely by blood clot and chronically by fibrosis and atrophy. These facts are not relevant to development of valve failure in primary varicose veins. In primary venous insufficiency it is rare to find any inflammatory reaction unless phlebitis or local trauma has occurred.

The question that arises is whether the valve can lose its tension or can atrophy spontaneously. If so, why and how? Functionally the normal valve is extremely strong. Attempts to rupture it experimentally by increasing intraluminal pressure have shown that valves withstand pressures well over 300 mm Hg.[7,8] The valve ring is the strongest and least distensible part of the vein wall. The ring is seen as a beaded shadow on venograms.

Informative descriptions of normal venous valves are few. Long ago the best description was given by Franklin[9] in his historical monograph.

VENOUS VALVE

The anatomy of the normal venous valve reveals several interesting structural features (Figure 2-2). The facts presented here are from a study of valves obtained during vein surgery and from cadavers.[10,11] In the past, the valve was thought to be an inert flap of connective tissue covered on each aspect by a layer of endothelium. Actually the structure is much more complex. The constituent parts are agger, sinus, cusps, cornua, and commissure (Figure 2-3). In some larger valves a central nodule is found on the free border of the cusp. The valves, other than those at major junctions, often are not easy to identify or isolate. This situation often has made it difficult to obtain a meaningful section through the correct plane.

Histology: Light Microscopy

The normal valve leaflet is connected to the venous wall by a complex fibromuscular structure forming a humplike mass originating from the media and

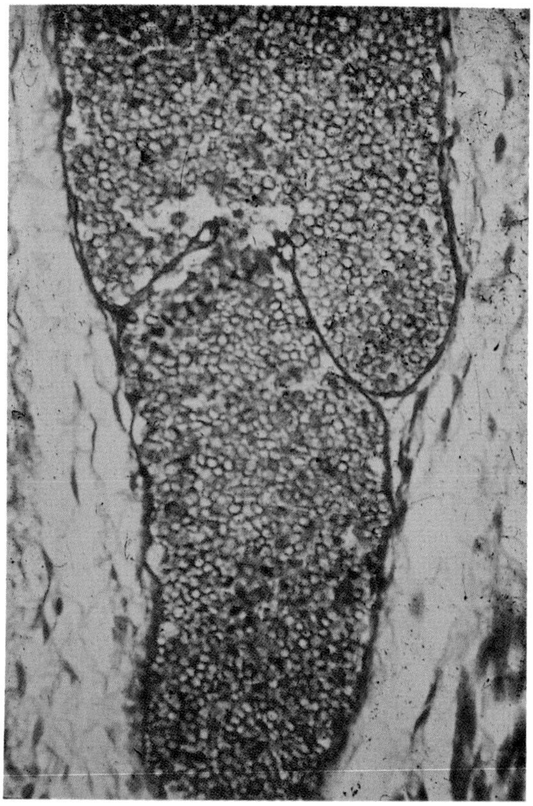

FIGURE 2-2. Macroscopic view of venous valve.

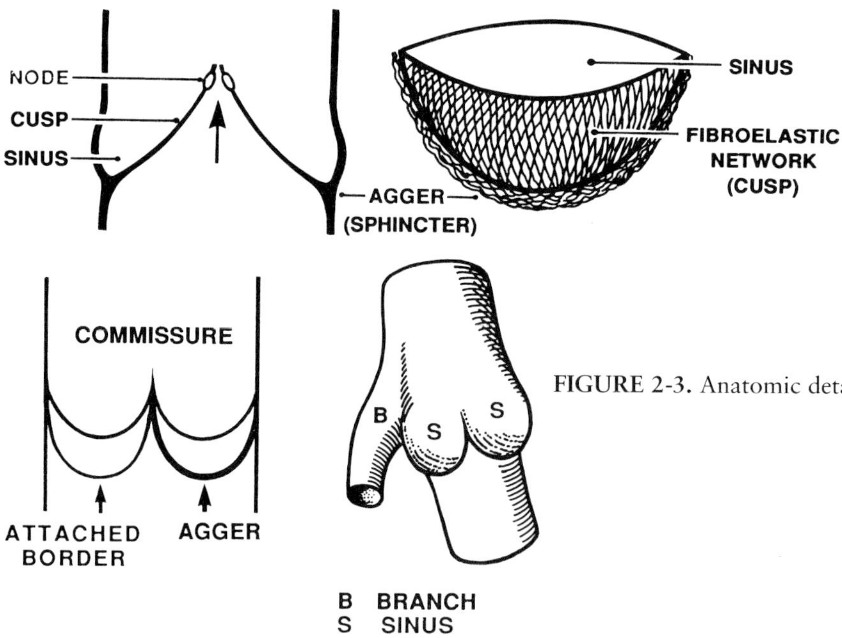

FIGURE 2-3. Anatomic detail of venous valve.

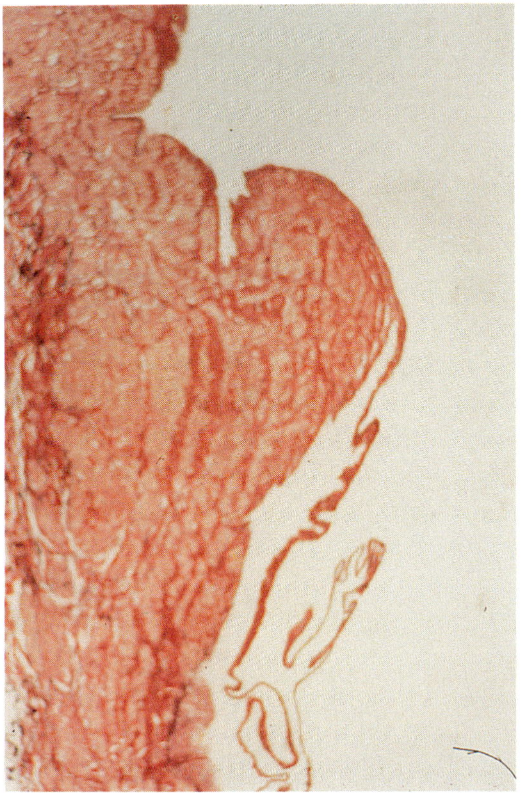

FIGURE 2-4. Valve leaflet is connected to venous wall by a complex fibromuscular structure. This structure forms a humplike mass that originates from the media and extends into the base of the cusp (elastic van Gieson stain: collagen, red; muscle, pale; elastic tissue, blue/black).

extending into the base of the cusp. This mass contains well-identified groups of muscle fibers supported by a collagen matrix (Figure 2-4). According to most authorities, the muscle extends into the base of the cusp and no further. Franklin,[9] however, described the presence of muscle cells in the cusp, stating that: "They [muscle cells] are said to lie transverse to the long axis of the vein, especially near the free border, to occur in some valves, but not in others, and more often in the larger valves." My colleagues and I have not confirmed this, but we have identified a number of scattered fibromyoblasts that may have been the cells to which Franklin referred. The aggregation of circular muscle fibers at the base of the valve that Franklin describes has every appearance of being a localized sphincter. Franklin also agreed with Sappey,[12] who was unable to find any nerve supply. Absence of a nerve supply subsequently has been confirmed by electron microscopy and immunohistochemical techniques not available to Franklin or Sappey.

The internal elastic lamina of the vein wall continues from the subendothelium of the vein in a linear fashion under the luminal surface of the cusp throughout its length. The lamina divides the cusp into two portions, one facing the sinus and the

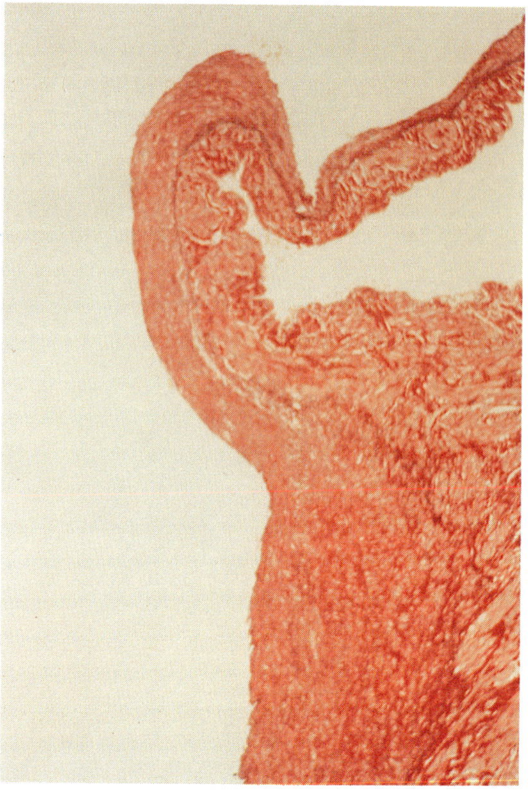

FIGURE 2-5. Venous valve seen through light microscopy on high power. Van Gieson's stain: collagen, red; muscle, pale; elastic tissue, dark. Luminal surface of valve cusp is smooth and continuous with luminal endothelium seen in upper part of section. Endothelium that lines sinus is folded and produces an irregular surface. Elastic tissue is continued into valve cusp, where it divides into two portions longitudinally.

other facing the lumen. The endothelium on the sinus side runs transversely and presents a pitted appearance. The endothelium on the luminal aspect runs longitudinally in common with the rest of the luminal endothelium (Figure 2-5). The result is a much smoother surface. Elastic tissue in the cusp generally extends to the free border, where it fans out, but in some specimens it ends in a nodule consisting of a concentration of elastic fibers lying in whorls of collagen (Figure 2-6). In the cusps of the valve, scattered pale-staining cells that appear to be fibromyoblasts are seen.

The complexity of the whole valve structure—the muscle hump, the arrangement of muscle cells, and the peculiarity of the terminal nodule—suggests that the valve may be more than a passive structure. The valve may be able to open and close actively in response to circulatory demands. Transmission electron microscopy reveals that the total length of the cusps is greater than the diameter of the vein (Figure 2-7, *A*). This is thought to allow expansion of the valve ring during dilatation. The peculiar construction of the cusp suggests that it possesses the ability to "ruche up" when the vein contracts. It is possible that movement begins in the muscle hump and

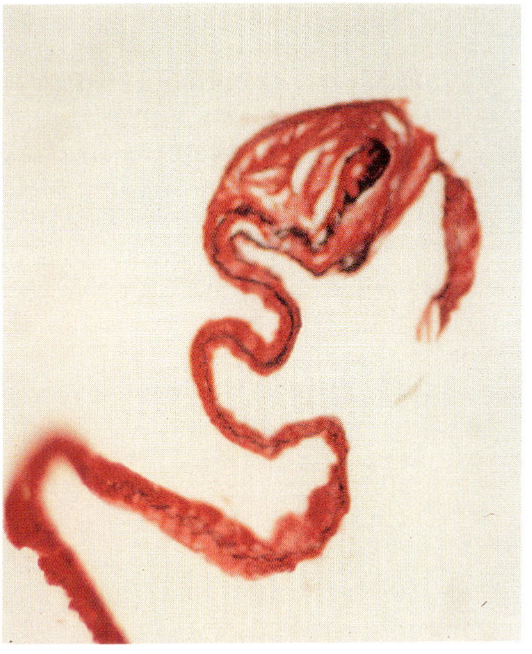

FIGURE 2-6. "Nodule" seen through light microscopy on high power. Van Gieson's stain: collagen, red; elastic tissue, dark (traced through cusp and terminating in nodule).

A

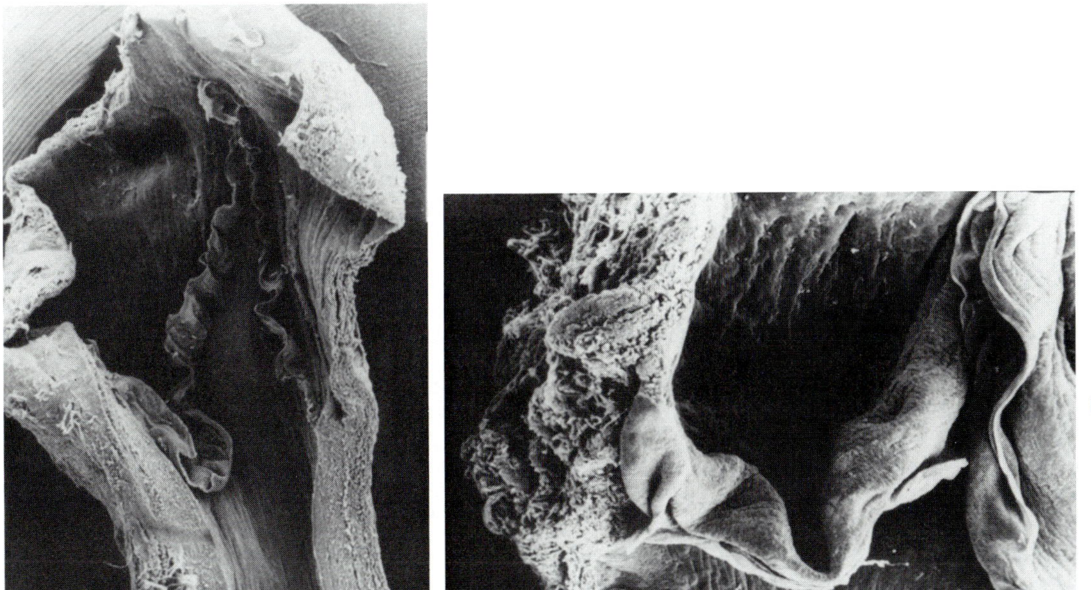

B

FIGURE 2-7. Transmission electron microscopy of venous valve. (Courtesy Dr. Aron Mashiah and Kaplan Hospital, Rehovot, Israel.)

runs out through the leaflet, which elongates and contracts according to intraluminal pressure and flow. This process produces an elongation and contraction of the opposing leaflets to ensure contact and competence in all phases of venous activity. The specialized nodules at the free edge may signal when the leaflets come into contact with each other. Distribution of elastic tissue suggests that this action can be activated from the basal muscle aggregation. Because of the valve length, it is conceivable that some degree of prolapse may occur under normal conditions and may be regarded as physiologic. Further, it may be that the floppy valve syndrome of Kistner[13] is a pathologic version of the same phenomenon. However, this possibility is a matter for further research.

Finally, it is noteworthy that the electron microscope scan shows that the endothelium is disposed longitudinally on the luminal aspect of the valve cusp in continuity with the endothelium lining the lumen of the vein while it runs transversely on the sinus aspect of the valve (Figure 2-7, *B*).

Venous Valve in Varicose Veins

In general, the venous valve in varicose veins shows no pathologic change in the absence of previous phlebitis.[14,15] Examination of varicose and normal valves shows no histologic difference between functionally competent and incompetent valves. In contrast, valves that have been involved in phlebitis show fibrosis, cystic degeneration, and adhesions. Such changes render them incompetent, but this type of lesion is not seen in uncomplicated varicose veins.

In long-standing cases of valvular incompetence, disuse atrophy may occur. This condition is as likely to be secondary as primary. Senile valvular atrophy also has been described in anatomic dissections, but it was not associated with varicose veins.[16]

On balance, evidence supporting the theory of primary valvular insufficiency as a cause of varicose veins is presumptive rather than proven. There is a good deal of argument against it. For example, if valve incompetence were a precipitating factor in causing varicose veins, the involved valve should be the first to show changes; however, what might be described as an early change has never been reported. Instead, Eger and Casper[17] presented anatomic evidence that the valvular defect in primary varicose veins was not the result of damage to the cusps but was caused by dilatation of the valve ring. Also, Leu[14] found that there was no reduction in number of valves with increasing age. The theory of sequential descending incompetence also is questionable. Further, it is difficult to explain the absence of varicosities in reported cases of senile atrophy of saphenous valves.[16] In addition, varicosity may develop in a circumscribed group of veins that communicate with veins of normal caliber, as described by King,[18] who showed that varicose veins could develop equally in an upward or downward direction.

Ludbrook[19] and others have demonstrated that some valves that are competent with the patient in a supine position become incompetent when the subject is erect. This finding focuses attention on the valve ring. Perhaps a weakened valve ring dilates when the patient is in the upright position. This dilatation occurs despite the reflex vasoconstriction that occurs in the erect position. Ludbrook attempted to verify the theory of sequential descending valvular incompetence but was unable to do so. Finally, if the absence of competent valves is the cause of varicose veins, a reversed or in situ saphenous arterial bypass should become varicose because all the valves are inactivated or destroyed. In fact, the opposite occurs. The vein wall follows established physiologic principles and hypertrophies in response to the extra pressure.

INCOMPETENT PERFORATING VEINS

The presence of incompetent valves in perforating veins is believed by many to be a primary cause of varicosity. Early anatomists were aware of the communicating veins between the deep and the superficial venous systems. In particular, surgeons of the French anatomic-pathologic school of the early nineteenth century first described these communicating veins with particular reference to varicose veins. Studies of Bordeu[20] in 1775 and Briquet[21] in 1824 were confirmed by their British counterparts later in the nineteenth century, including Colles (1844),[22] Brodie (1846),[23] and Gay (1868).[24] Further descriptions were offered in the twentieth century with anatomic reports of Kosinski (1926)[25] and Franklin (1927).[9] It was Turner-Warwick[26] and Linton[27] who again drew attention to the perforating veins from a clinical point of view.

In 1947, Myers[28] reintroduced stripping of the internal saphenous vein with a new and improved stripper that he thought would deal with incompetent tributaries including perforators. However, early optimism evaporated as it became apparent that Myers's results were still imperfect.

In 1956, Dodd and Cockett[29] attempted to explain the occurrence of varicosities below a competent valve. They emphasized that failures associated with stripping were caused by uncorrected valvular incompetence in perforating veins. They believed that incompetent perforating veins also played an important part in the causation of varicose veins and that this fact justified a major change in operative technique. This concept was well received, and subsequent surgical treatment was based on this theory. Perforator ligation, alone or in conjunction with stripping, was performed enthusiastically with some improvement in results. The degree of improvement, however, was not commensurate with the increased technical difficulties of the procedure. The operation became increasingly time-consuming. These procedures are still widely practiced, but experience has raised doubts about the importance of the incompetent perforator.

Varicosities often appear in localized clusters that seem isolated; when dissected, they show no obvious connection to incompetent truncal or perforating veins. After numerous dissections, Linton showed that normal perforating veins are <2 mm in diameter, and he regarded only those >4.4 mm as pathologic. Linton was surprised to find that in cases of varicose veins 79% of those examined were <2.4 mm. In a more recent report by Schalin,[30] only 21% of perforators were ≥ 2.5 mm in diameter. Only 8 of 74 perforators were >4 mm. Schalin summarized: "The absence of perforating veins in 47 per cent of varicose veins operated on and no more than eight subfascial branches being equal to or larger than 4 mm out of a total of 131 branches examined, in the 53 per cent of varicose veins in which

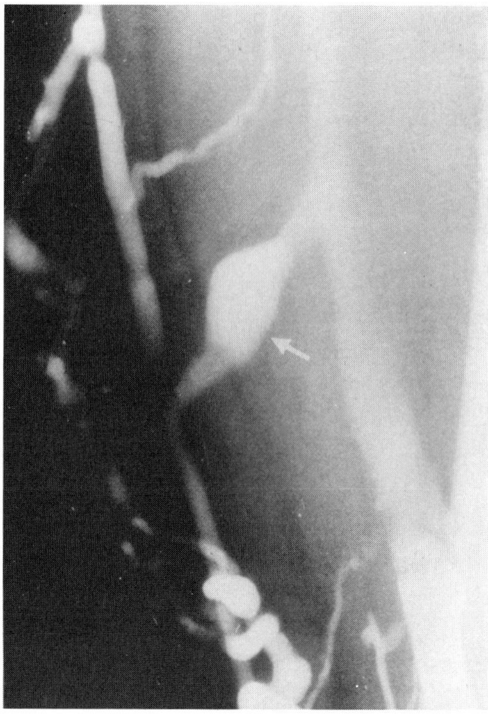

FIGURE 2-8. Phlebogram of localized (arrow) varicose deep perforator. (From Browse NL, Burnand KG, Lea Thomas M, eds. Diseases of the Veins: Pathology, Diagnosis, and Treatment. London: Edward Arnold, 1988, p 231.)

perforators were found, constitutes a very impressive discrepancy between expectation and observation."

Difficulty in localizing perforating veins in relation to the varicosities has been emphasized by Haeger.[31] By thermography, he counted "hot spots" that were thought to overlie incompetent perforators. When these spots were checked by phlebography, perforators were completely absent in 74 (47%) of 157. Actually, those that were found (83 of 157) were smaller than expected and did not correlate well with thermographic hot spots.

Pflug and Daintree Johnson[32] used perioperative microscopy to reveal that most suspect incompetent perforating veins divide subfascially into two or more normal-looking branches that diverge into the muscle. Instead of increasing in size when dissected inward, they become narrower. In this situation the subcutaneous part of connecting veins shows a greater dilatation that gradually decreases in a centrifugal direction, the opposite of what would be expected. Single dilated incompetent perforators were recorded in both of these reports, but the number is disproportionately small compared with the number of varicosities described.

The direction of flow in perforating veins has been thought to be from superficial to deep, but this flow was reversed when perforators became incompetent. Bjordal[33] used a square-wave flowmeter to show that the net flow in incompetent perforating veins was mainly directed inward. He noted that there was an outward flow, but this flow was more than compensated for by the inward flow. This finding conflicts with current acceptance of the venous refill time after emptying as a standard measure of incompetence. Such testing assumes that reflux occurs entirely through incompetent perforators. In fact, there are at least two perforating veins in the foot that are valveless and that allow open communication between the superficial and the deep venous system. Incompetent perforators also may be present as a secondary rather than a primary phenomenon, for example, perforators involved in the varicose process (Figure 2-8). The theory of primary varicosity of deep perforators as the cause of varicose veins therefore has lost many of its advocates.

ARTERIOVENOUS COMMUNICATIONS

Observations by some workers while treating varicose veins have led them to give support to arteriovenous (AV) communications as a theory of causation. These observations may be summed up as follows: blood in varicose veins is often as red as arterial blood. Pigeaux[34] noted this fact as long ago as 1843. He attributed the finding to widening of the capillary bed with increased arterial flow.

Some varicosities may occasionally pulsate,[35] and Blalock[36] found oxygen tension to be increased in blood taken from the internal saphenous vein in a patient with varicose veins. Also, varices are found in association with known AV fistulas. When the fistulas are closed, the varicosities disappear.

The main proponents of the AV fistula causation theory, Wolf,[35] Haimovici,[37] and Schalin,[30] have shown what they believe to be small AV communications exposed at operation. Because these investigators are experienced observers, it is necessary to evaluate the arguments that they have advanced. Blalock's report[36] of raised oxygen levels in blood taken from the saphenous vein has been the source of considerable controversy. His observations have been confirmed by some workers, but they have not been consistently reproduced. The AV connection theory was strongly disputed by de Takats et al.[38]

Venous pulsation in a varicosity is usually transmitted from an adjacent artery. Such pulsation is significant only if it is associated with a known AV fistula or if it occurs in a dilated venous capillary. Varicose veins are associated with peripheral vasodilatation, and venous capillaries are often dilated as part of the process. If the capillary bed is opened in this way, a functional AV short circuit may develop and act as a shunt. This occurrence would explain the "arterialization" of varicose vein blood and the pulsatile flow transmitted from the dilated arterial capillary into the dilated venous capillary. It may be that this action is what has been called an AV communication.

Detection of the capillary changes that are necessary to explain the presence of AV communications is difficult. Such changes that occur in the vascular bed vary in accordance with circulatory demands. This fact may explain why such connections are not found more frequently and why the theory has not gained much support. Haeger[39] claimed that if arterialization of venous blood occurs, it is probably the result of, and not the cause of, varicosity.

It is interesting to note that in the seventeenth century it was thought that the prime cause of varicose veins was an excessive volume of blood being propelled through venous capillaries. This action was said to have a dilating effect on the vein wall. This theory leads us to consideration of the weak vein wall theory, which has gained support in recent years.

VEIN WALL WEAKNESS

The most obvious clinical abnormality in varicose veins is the dilated vein and therefore the vein wall. Traditionally, a weak vein wall has been the main alternative theory to primary valvular incompetence. Although the latter generally has been preferred, the weak vein wall theory has had many followers.[15] The mechanical theory of varicose dilatation states that a weak vein wall is a secondary manifestation of valvular incompetence caused by exposure of the vein wall to pressures it cannot withstand. Examination of this pronouncement, however, raises many questions. For example, what is the reaction of a normal vein to an increase in pressure? The average standing hydrostatic head of pressure from the right atrium to the ankle in the upright position is 85 mm Hg. This pressure may be raised by coughing, breathing against resistance (Valsalva), or straining. Adjustments of the degree of venous wall tone are responsible for maintaining this pressure within normal limits. The degree of tonicity present in a normal saphenous vein is most apparent to vascular surgeons at operation. The vein contracts markedly on handling in preparation for a vein bypass. Even a varicose vein contracts on handling—however, to a limited degree in which the response is not uniform. The surgeon can determine the strength of the venous wall by the pressure required to distend the vein in order to enlarge its lumen. Ackroyd et al.[7] demonstrated that a normal vein wall is capable of withstanding pressures in excess of anything it may be called on to endure.

Several frequently encountered circumstances are not explained by valve incompetence but are explained by weakness of the vein wall. For example, a saphena varicosity is often a saccular dilatation occurring laterally as a blowout (Figure 2-9). The vein wall is involved locally only at the base of the blowout. Furthermore, a varicose vein often consists of a string of dilatations interspersed throughout areas of comparative normality. If dilatation were a result of back pressure alone, the whole venous wall should be affected evenly. Lateral and fusiform blowouts are caused by localized areas of weakness in the vein wall, resulting in an irregular pattern of dilatation of the vein.

Nylander[40] has described this phenomenon as the meandering syndrome (Figure 2-10). He compared the tortuous appearance of a varicose vein to a meandering river and attributed this effect to the same mechanism that produces tortuosity in a hose when the water is turned on. However, this picturesque analogy is misleading because tortuosity occurs only when the water is at jet pressure, not at flow levels comparable to those encountered in venous flow.

Tortuosity of a varicose vein is caused by a combination of factors. First is the irregular distribution of involved areas. Second, the varicosity assumes a tortuous course when the vein elongates between two fixed points. Elongation is caused by

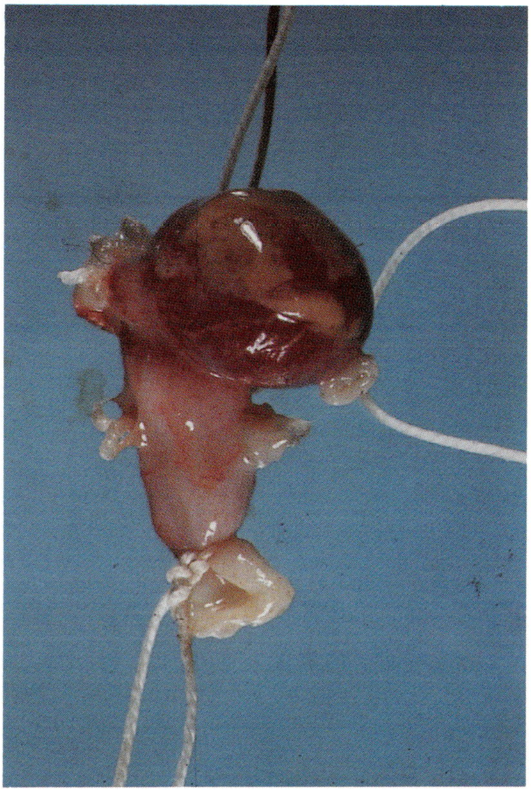

FIGURE 2-9. Localized saphenous varicosity. Main tributaries have been ligated.

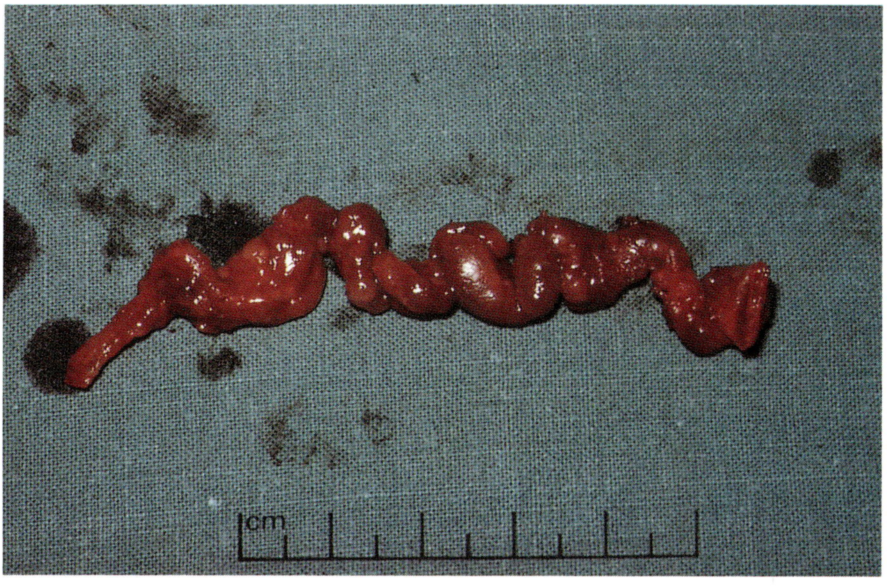

FIGURE 2-10. Tortuous varicosity known as meandering syndrome.

involvement of longitudinal muscle. Third, vein valve cusps are arranged so that each successive pair is at right angles to the last. This situation tends to produce a degree of torsion in the long axis of the vein that will act in combination with the other changes. Varicosities also can develop below and in between competent valves (Figure 2-11). This occurrence is commonly seen and was fully described by Cotton[41] in 1961. It can be argued that the reason for dilatation below a competent valve is incompetence of an associated perforator, which produces back pressure in the superficial vein. However, pressure in the superficial vein can rise only briefly in response to a rise in deep venous pressure if there is no obstruction to the flow of blood above and below the involved perforator. If there is deep venous obstruction, venous hypertension will develop that should be evenly distributed between the superficial and the deep system.

The response of a normal vein wall to a rise of internal pressure will be a contraction to expel the excess blood. On the other hand, if an inherent weakness of the vein wall is present, pooling of blood in the superficial vein will occur because it cannot contract properly in response to the pressure change. If the valve ring above dilates as a consequence of a weakened vein wall and incompetence develops, gravitational back pressure will cause an exacerbation of symptoms.

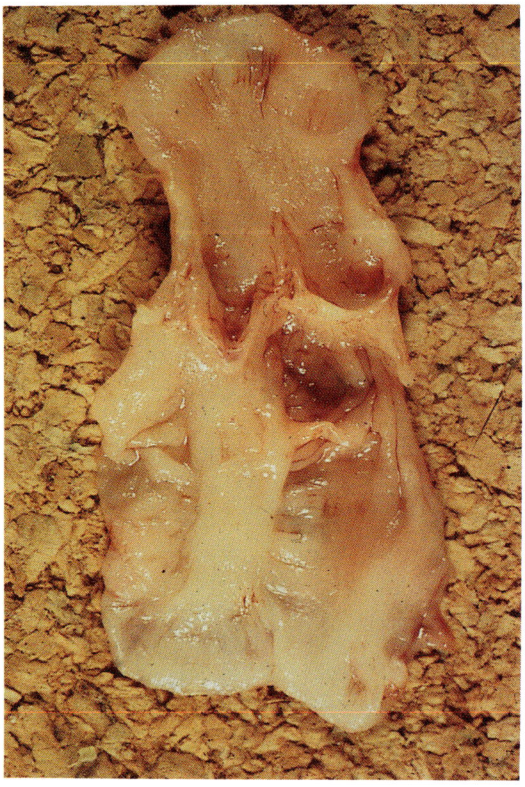

FIGURE 2-11. Localized weakness of vein wall below competent valves.

VEIN WALL ABNORMALITY

Veins have been regarded purely as valved conduits through which blood is returned to the heart, with little attention paid to vein wall function. However, changes in the venous reservoir can occur during shock and hemorrhage. The reservoir changes are caused by a balance of vasoconstriction and vasodilatation that affects veins as well as arteries. Indeed, changes in venous caliber are much greater than those in arteries and involve extremes of tonal adjustment. It has been suggested that minor variations in tone assist venous return by an effect on the vis a tergo at night when the other mechanisms of venous return are at a low ebb.[15]

The main constituents of the vein wall are muscle layers, collagenous matrix, and elastic tissue, which all interact to maintain tone. Collagen provides strength and prevents overdistention. Muscle provides contractility, and the interaction of elastic tissue with muscle and collagen provides compliance. The degree of venous tone mainly depends on the state of reactivity of the muscle layer. Loss of tone, therefore, must be in this layer. However, the matrix in which the muscle functions is inseparable from it. The whole structure, together with the venous valve, must act in concert. All vein wall constituents require close scrutiny.

LIGHT MICROSCOPY

Normal Vein

Examination of the normal vein wall reveals the medial coat as the most prominent feature (Figure 2-12). The medial coat consists of a well-developed circu-

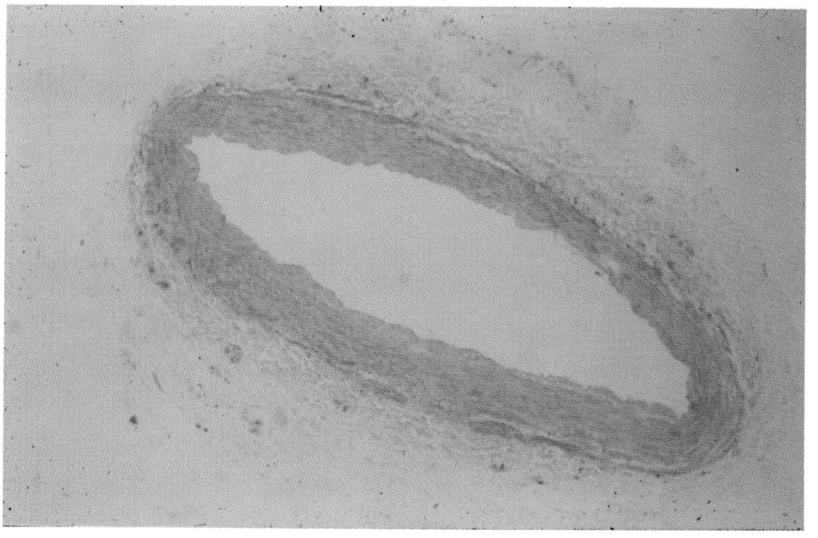

FIGURE 2-12. Normal vein seen through light microscopy on low power. Hematoxylin and eosin stain used. Regularity of muscle pattern is noted in media.

lar muscle layer arranged in regular whorls that are supported on the scaffold of a tightly packed collagenous matrix. Immediately internal to the medial coat is a thin inner layer of longitudinal cells lying in a matrix of loose subendothelial connective tissue. This layer is separated from the endothelium by a distinct elastic lamina. Other elastic fibers are scattered sparsely throughout the vein wall. Surrounding the medial coat there is an outer longitudinal muscle layer arranged loosely in bundles that merge into the adventitia. The adventitia forms the outer coat in which connective tissue again becomes predominant. It contains numerous vasa vasorum, nerve filaments, and occasional nerve endplates. However, the structure of veins taken from different sites demonstrates a wide variation in wall thickness, muscle content, and number of valves. Changes are related to the site of the vein and the function it serves.

Varicose Vein

In the varicose vein the most striking change is a marked increase of collagenous tissue that appears to invade muscle layers and causes a breakup of the regular cellular pattern, with separation and interruption of muscle cells (Figure 2-13). The intima is intact in early cases, but in long-standing varicosities there is a tendency for some loss of endothelial cover. Desquamation of surface cells exceeds the rate of replacement. There is no evidence of an inflammatory reaction. In addition to an increase in interstitial collagen, in advanced cases subintimal deposits of collagenous tissue are present that superficially resemble arteriosclerotic plaques (Figure 2-14).

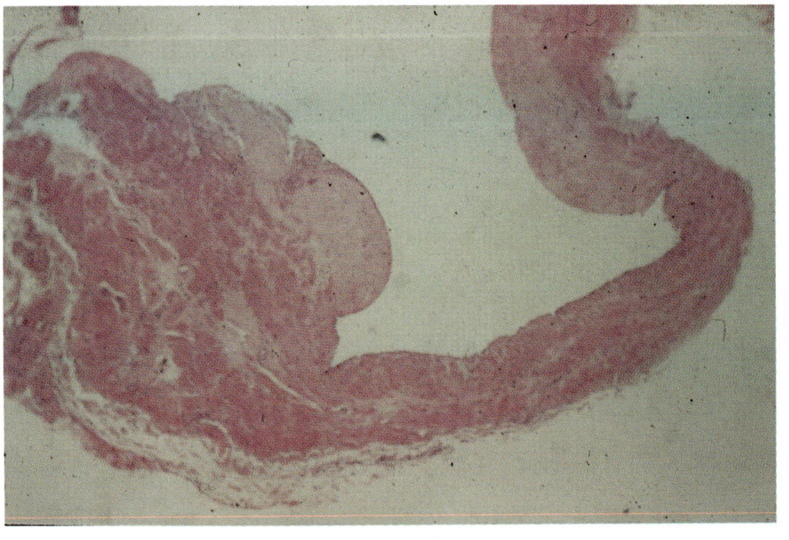

FIGURE 2-13. Varicose vein seen through light microscopy. Hematoxylin and eosin stain used. Shows breakup of muscle pattern and development of callenous infiltration with subendothelial plaque formation.

Typically the muscle cell pattern is grossly distorted in affected areas. These areas are scattered in a patchy distribution, with parts of the wall still retaining a normal pattern. This situation has led to differences in histologic description of varicose veins. In localized blowouts, the muscle layer disappears completely and the thinned wall consists mainly of collagen and elastic tissue (Figure 2-15).

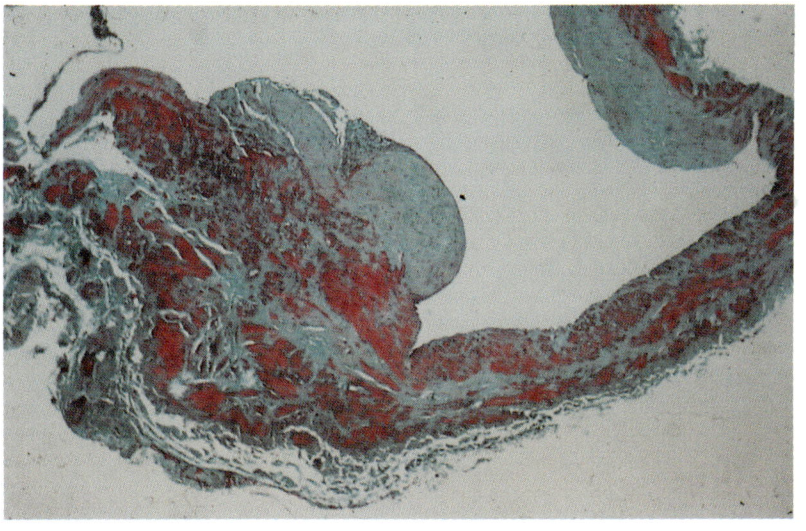

FIGURE 2-14. Same specimen as Figure 2-13 shown with Masson's stain. Collagen, blue; muscle, red.

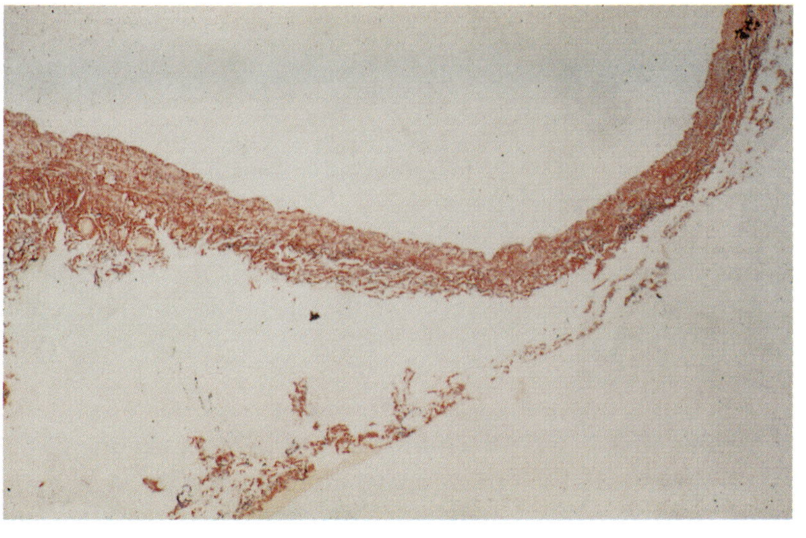

FIGURE 2-15. Varicose blowout seen through light microscopy. Van Gieson's stain: collagen, red; muscle, pale; elastic tissue, dark.

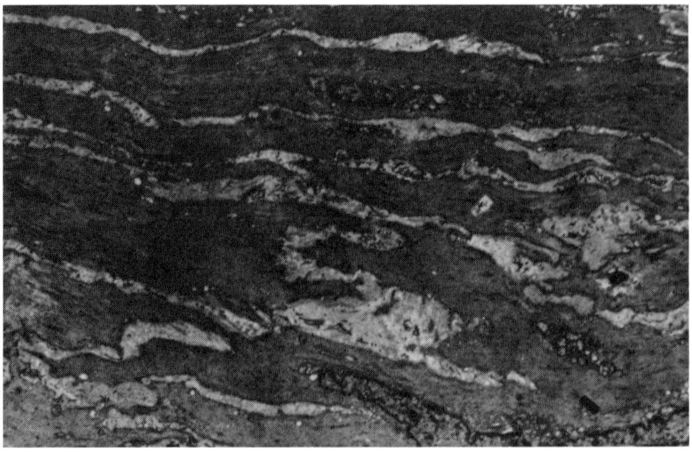

FIGURE 2-16. Transmission electron microscopy of normal vein shows regular pattern of muscle cells lying in close relationship to one another.

TRANSMISSION ELECTRON MICROSCOPY

Normal Vein

In the normal vein, muscle cells show well-marked nuclei with a clearly defined chromatin network (Figure 2-16). Cells lie in close proximity to one another and are surrounded by a fine layer of amorphous fibrous tissue. Muscle cells are supported by regularly arranged collagen fiber bundles in vertical and horizontal disposition. The cell cytoplasm contains occasional vacuoles, some of which contain granular material, which suggests secretory activity.

Varicose Vein

In the varicose vein a completely different picture is seen. Muscle cells become separated because of a marked increase in collagenous matrix (Figure 2-17). In areas most affected, collagen fibers become packed in an irregular manner between muscle cells. Many elastic fibers are scattered throughout these areas. The fibers are not part of the internal elastic lamina, which is often fragmented.

The increasing infiltration of collagen continues as the condition deteriorates. Muscle cells become further separated. Eventually, in blowout areas the wall consists entirely of collagen bundles lined by endothelium, with the muscle fibers having completely disappeared (Figure 2-18).

At higher magnifications a marked difference in the cell nucleus is noted. Both normal and varicose cells have a well-differentiated chromatin skein, but the varicose cell shows numerous apparent erosions along its length. In the cytoplasm an increase in "vacuole" formation is present. Some of the vacuoles contain granules and others appear to be empty. A pericellular halo of amorphous fibrous tissue is present that seems to have been secreted by the muscle cell itself, probably as a result

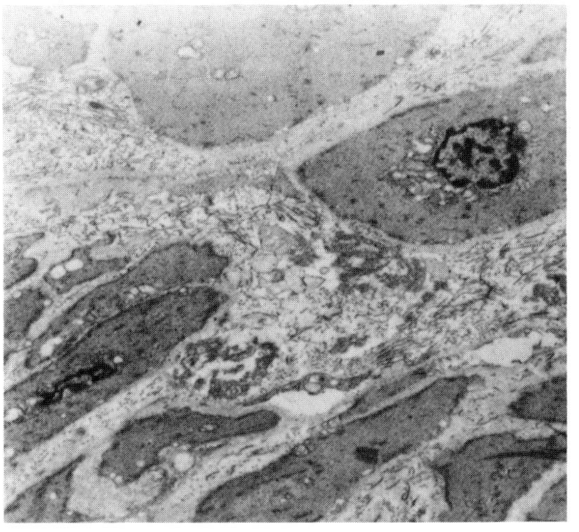

FIGURE 2-17. Transmission electron microscopy of varicose vein. Muscle cells are separated by collagen fibrils and show evidence of vacuolar activity.

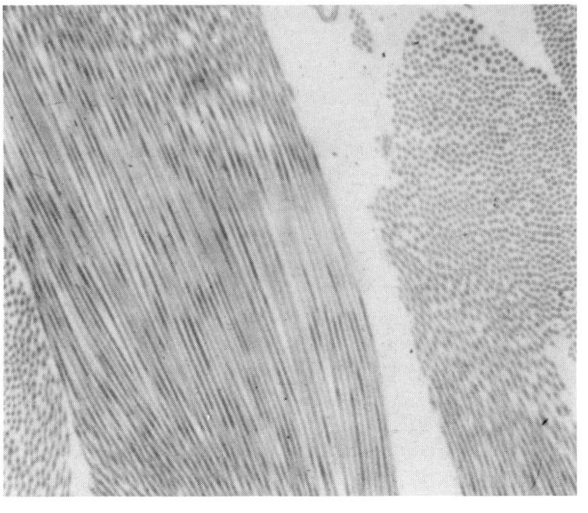

FIGURE 2-18. Transmission electron microscopy of venous blowout. Muscle cells are completely replaced by collagen fibrils, which appear to be normal.

of increased secretory activity. The cytoplasm of the abnormal cell presents a more disordered appearance than that of its normal counterpart. Both cells possess hemidesmosomes that appear as small, intermittent dark areas situated at the margin of the cell membrane. Figure 2-19 shows a varicose muscle cell; at a magnification of $\times 30{,}000$, it is interesting to find that the muscle cell is capable of phagocytosis. Some collagen fibers appear to have been ingested by the muscle cell. The characteristic banding is still distinguishable.

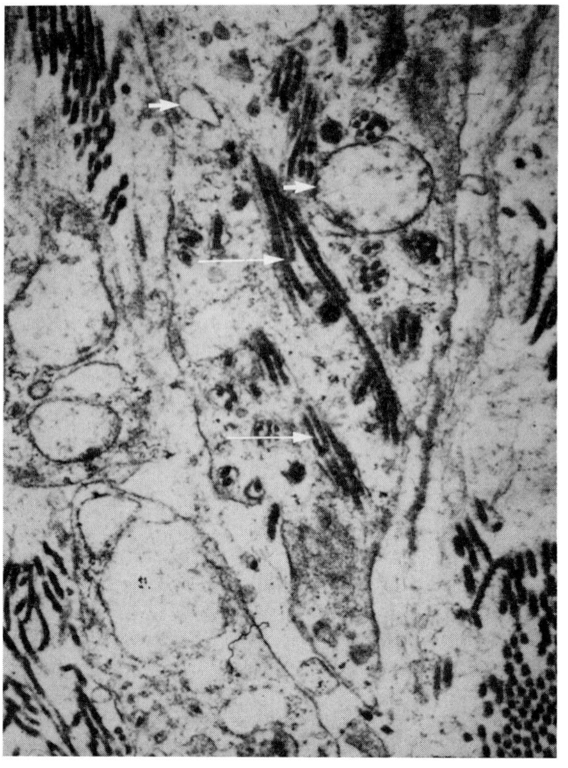

FIGURE 2-19. Transmission electron microscopy of varicose vein (×30,000). Muscle cell contains many vacuoles (short arrows) and shows evidence of phagocytosis of collagen fibrils (long arrows).

PROCESS OF VARICOSITY

The main pathologic feature of the process of varicosity is separation of muscle cells by collagen. This characteristic has been described by many authors.[42-46] Since collagen fibers appear to have a normal structure and muscle cells are markedly deranged, it is logical to assume that the latter are responsible for the changes of varicosity. Biologic assay and tissue culture may produce a more definitive answer.

Separation of the muscle cells results in widening of the functional gap between them. This gap needs to be bridged if the contractile state of one muscle cell is to be transmitted to another. When adjustments in venous tone occur, the muscle layer of the vein wall must act as a coordinated whole; this action must occur during the more active process of constriction, as well as during the less active process of dilatation. Communication between muscle cells must be instantaneous. Hemidesmosomes are thought to be involved in this process. These structures are seen as darker areas in cell membranes situated at intervals along their length. It is through these bodies that coordination of muscle cell contraction occurs. This action occurs through a combination of physical, chemical, and electrical stimuli. Hemidesmosomes may be involved in two ways. Small lacunae in the cell membrane in relation to hemidesmosomes may allow protoplasmic fibrils to pass between muscle cells to connect cytoplasms. Glycoproteins such as fibronectin and laminin help to bind muscle cells to the matrix through a network of fibrils attached to a cell wall endplate. The precise area of attachment has not been identified, but it is thought to be related to the hemidesmosome. Both mechanisms enable cells to function as a unified unit. Therefore if the cells become separated, collective action becomes impossible. There is probably an optimum gap between muscle cells that allows their unified function. This gap has been estimated at 0.04 mmu.

Finally, contact between muscle cells and matrix also may occur by chemical or electrical means to enable continuing function during the early stage of separation. As the varicose condition develops, muscle cells undergo changes in form. The cells become larger, irregular, and hypersecretory. They are paler, with many cells appearing shadowy in outline and substance. In short, they show evidence of a severe metabolic disturbance.

FUNCTION OF MUSCLE CELL

The following account of normal cell function is from the work of Vanhoutte and Shepherd.[47] Muscle cells have the basic structure and functional characteristics of vascular smooth muscle cells in general. They contain contractile tissue controlled by contractile proteins that are triggered by an increase in the level of cytoplasmic calcium. The contraction of muscle cells depends on cell length at the moment of stimulation. Longer cells have a more complete contraction. When venous smooth muscle is activated, the constrictor response is determined mainly by local conditions. Intraluminal pressure is the main stimulus brought about by variations in the blood content. It causes mobilization or pooling of blood that adjusts the degree and direction of muscle response. In limb veins contraction of smooth muscle is stimulated by local liberation of cellular neurohumoral mediators. Among these mediators, norepinephrine causes contraction of venous smooth muscle by activation of adrenoceptors on the cell membrane. It is by this means that venous tone is maintained.

In abnormal muscle cells an abnormal metabolic process that interferes with the normal mechanism of contraction is probably taking place. Therefore involved muscle cells may lose their power to contract, at first individually and then collectively as they separate, or even before separating. Weakened muscle cells separate, lose contact, and the muscular grid sags. Simultaneously there is invasion of the intercellular space by collagen together with some elastic tissue. The primary lesion that develops in the muscle cell must be considered to be due to a genetic defect which orchestrates the interplay of factors involved in producing a "varicose" cell.

PHYSICOCHEMICAL FACTORS AFFECTING VEIN WALL

Increased venous wall distensibility found in varicose veins is attributable to a lesion in the muscle layer. Yet since muscle cells, collagen, and elastic fibers must all act in concert, how are other tissues affected? It could be argued that the basic lesion is present in collagen tissue, which, by its overgrowth, engulfs muscle cells and impedes their function. Alternatively, the muscle cell appears to be deranged, whereas collagen and elastic fibers appear to be normal.

Many enzymes have been considered to play a primary role in venous distention, but none has been clearly implicated. Collagenase, increased lysosomal activity,[48] elastase and alteration in collagen, and elastin and adenosine triphosphate content in the vein wall all have been reported as possible causative factors. Plasminogen activator and fibrinolysin levels are reduced, with possible effects on the blood clotting mechanism. The hexosamine content is consistently raised.[44] The effect of estrogens on enzyme activity also is under examination.[49] In addition, circulating noradrenaline has aroused interest as a cause of local vasodilatation.[47,50] The effect of noradrenaline on the vein wall is somewhat paradoxical. It acts as a vasodilator intraluminally and therefore may contribute to turbulence, but it also serves as a contractile stimulant to the muscle fibers in the vein wall. Therefore a distinction must be made between the last two factors. Noradrenaline may be advanced as a primary factor because it is considered to have its vasodilator effect on a normal vein wall, whereas turbulence, even without the mediation of noradrenaline, would presumably be effective on a vein wall that has already undergone pathologic change. The total noradrenaline effect provides a composite stimulus that produces a response in accordance with local needs. Kline and Byrne[51] have suggested turbulence as a physical cause of varicosity because of the relationship of early dilatation to a valve either immediately proximal to or distal to dilatation where turbulence is most pronounced. Turbulence may act physically or through local production of noradrenaline. These factors must be considered, but their relevance to the development of varicose veins has not yet been accurately identified.

Evidence suggests that the basic lesion is located in the muscle cell in the vein wall, but further investigation is necessary, particularly into the activity of various types of collagen, collagenase, elastin, elastase, and the relationship of these substances to the sex hormones.

SUMMARY

The common point of physical, hormonal, and enzyme changes described here is loss of vein wall tone followed by increased distensibility.[8] The vein then begins to dilate locally. The dilatation may remain as a local blowout, but if it extends to valve sphincter level, the vein commissure separates. When this change takes place, secondary valvular incompetence develops. When the valve allows reflux to occur, the already weakened vein distends further and the varicose vein either enlarges or appears clinically for the first time. Eventually, a functionless valve may undergo disuse atrophy, but it is capable of persisting for a long time.

The valve–vein wall argument is summarized by a diagram produced by Edwards and Edwards[52] in 1940. This diagram often has been reproduced without the full caption and used incorrectly to illustrate primary valvular failure as the cause of varicose veins. In fact, the full caption shows it was intended to convey the opposite. Dilatation of the valve ring, not valvular atrophy, is clearly identified as the cause of valvular incompetence (Figure 2-20).

A

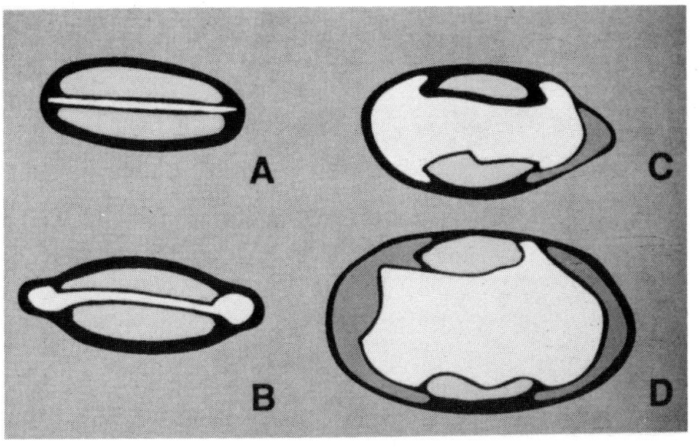

B

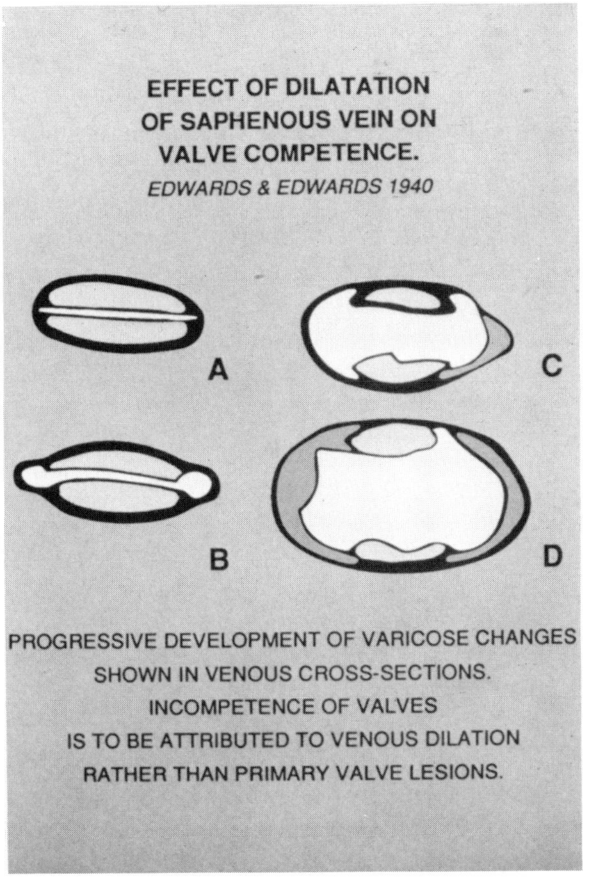

FIGURE 2-20. A, This diagram is often reproduced without its caption, as shown here. Without its caption, the diagram suggests support of the primary valve failure theory. **B,** Full caption shows that the diagram was intended to convey the opposite—that dilatation of the valve ring, *not* valve atrophy, should be identified as the cause of valvular incompetence.

It seems that the solution to this basic problem lies in a study of normal and abnormal metabolic activity of the enzyme-hormone complex in the muscle cell of the vein wall. If this activity is understood, it may be possible to control the tendency to varicosities in susceptible individuals and either limit the extension of the condition or minimize postoperative recurrence. The widespread occurrence of varicose veins and their potential to cause disability justify investigations or modifications of treatment that may contribute to their prevention.

■ ■ ■

Secondary varicose veins are those that follow an attack of phlebitis. In an attack of moderate severity, the affected portion of vein wall and any contained valve are involved in a process of occlusion by thrombosis, fibrosis with organization of the clot, and recanalization, resulting in venous dilatation in all but the smallest veins. If the affected vein is superficial, it is clinically obvious, but if it is deep, the degree of superficial varicosity that follows depends on the degree of deep venous reflux or persisting obstruction. When the wall of a deep perforating vein is involved in the process and its protecting valve is destroyed, a superficial varicosity may result. The majority of varicose veins, however, occur in the absence of a history of deep phlebitis, and less than half the cases of deep phlebitis develop superficial varicosities. Possibly this is because the presence of genetic factors also is required. Therefore it is possible that primary and secondary varicose veins have something in common if it is postulated that varicose veins that develop after deep phlebitis do so only in the presence of genetic factors.

REFERENCES

1. Harvey W. De Motu Cordis, 1628.
2. Fabricius H. De Venarum Ostiolis, 1603.
3. Malpighi M. Opera Omnia [1687]. Bethesda, Md.: National Library of Medicine.
4. Nicholson BB. Varicose veins: Etiology and treatment. Arch Surg 15:351-376, 1927.
5. Zancani A. Über die Varicen der unteren Extremitäten: Experimentelle und klinische Untersuchungen. Arch Klin Chir 96:91, 1911.
6. Gottlob R, May R. The Venous Valve. Berlin: Springer Verlag, 1988.
7. Ackroyd JS, Pattison M, Browse NL. A study of the mechanical properties of fresh and preserved human femoral vein wall and valve cusps. Br J Surg 72:117-119, 1985.
8. Thulesius O, Gjöres JE. Valvular function and venous distensibility. In Negus D, Jantet G, eds. Phlebology 85. London: John Libbey, 1986, pp 26-28.
9. Franklin KJ. The valves in veins. An historical survey. Proc R Soc Med 21:1-33, 1927.
10. Butterworth DM, Rose SS, Clark P, et al. Light microscopy, immunohistochemistry, and electron microscopy of the valves of lower-limb veins and jugular veins. Phlebology 7:27-30, 1992.
11. Rose SS, Mashiah A. The scanning electron microscope in the pathology of varicose veins. Isr J Med Sci 27:202-205, 1991.
12. Sappey R. Traite d'Anatomie, 1869.
13. Kistner RL. Primary venous valve incompetence in the leg. Am J Surg 140:218-224, 1980.
14. Leu HJ. Morphological alteration of non-varicose and varicose veins. A morphological contribution to the discussion on the pathogenesis of varicose vein. Basic Res Cardiol 4:435-444, 1979.
15. Rose SS, Ahmed A. Some new thoughts on the aetiology of varicose veins. Int J Cardiovasc Surg 27:584-593, 1985.

16. Klotz K. Destruction of valves in senile patient without development of varicosities. Arch Anat Physiol Leipzig 1:159, 1888.
17. Eger SA, Casper SL. Aetiology of varicose veins from an anatomic aspect based on dissections of 38 adult cadavers. JAMA 123:148, 1943.
18. King ESJ. Genesis of varicose veins. Aust N Z J Surg 20:126, 1950.
19. Ludbrook J. Valvular defect in primary varicose veins—Cause or effect. Lancet 2:1289, 1963.
20. Bordeu M. Recherches sur les Maladies Chronique. Paris: Presse Medicale, 1775.
21. Briquet P. Trunk, tributaries, tertiaries and telangiectases. Paris: These de Paris, 1824.
22. Colles A. Lectures on the Theory and Practice of Surgery, 1844.
23. Brodie B. Lectures on Pathology and Surgery. London, 1846.
24. Gay J. On Varicose Disease of the Lower Extremities. The Lettsomian Lectures of 1867. London: Churchill, 1868.
25. Kosinski CJ. Observations on the superficial venous system of the lower extremity. J Anat 60:131, 1926.
26. Turner-Warwick W. The Rational Treatment of Varicose Veins and Varicocoele. London: Faber & Faber, 1931.
27. Linton RR. The communicating veins of the lower leg and the operative technique for their ligation. Ann Surg 107:582, 1938.
28. Myers TT, Cooley JC. Varicose vein surgery in the management of the postthrombotic limb. Surg Gynecol Obstet 99:733, 1954.
29. Dodd HJ, Cockett FB. The Pathology and Surgery of the Veins of the Lower Limb, 2nd ed. Edinburgh: Churchill Livingstone, 1976.
30. Schalin L. Arteriovenous communications to varicose veins in the lower extremities studied by dynamic radiography. Acta Chir Scand 146:397-406, 1980.
31. Haeger K. Practical anatomy. In Haeger K, ed. Venous and Lymphatic Disorders of the Leg. Lund: Scandinavian University Books, 1966.
32. Pflug J, Daintree Johnson H. In Proceedings of American-European Symposium on Venous Diseases, pp 56-57. Foundation for International Cooperation in Medical Sciences, 1974.
33. Bjordal R. Circulation patterns in incompetent perforating veins in the calf and in the saphenous system in primary varicose veins. Acta Chir Scand 138:251, 1972.
34. Pigeaux. Maladies des Vaisseaux. A Treatise. Paris, 1843.
35. Wolf G. Praxis 36:41, 1941.
36. Blalock A. Oxygen content of blood in patients with varicose veins. Arch Surg 19:898-905, 1929.
37. Haimovici H. Arteriovenous shunting in varicose veins. J Vasc Surg 2:684, 1985.
38. de Takats G, Quint H, Tillotson BI, Crittenden PJ. Carbon dioxide and oxygen levels in varicose veins. Arch Surg 18:671, 1929.
39. Haeger K. Hot spots, perforating veins and thermography. Triangle 8:18, 1967.
40. Nylander G. Meanders of the great saphenous vein. Angiology 20:587-592, 1969.
41. Cotton LT. Gross anatomy and development of varicose veins. Br J Surg 48:589, 1961.
42. Zwillenberg LO, Lanzt L, Zwillenberg H. Possible influence of smooth muscle on collagen. Angiologia 8:318-346, 1971.
43. Svejcar J, Prerovsky I, Linhart J, Kruml J. Content of collagen, elastin and water in walls of the internal saphenous vein. Clin Res 1:296, 1962.
44. Svejcar J, Prerovsky I, Linhart J, Kruml J. Collagen, elastin and hexosamine in primary varicose veins. Clin Sci 24:325, 1963.
45. Jurukova Z, Milenkov C. Ultrastructural evidence for collagen degradation in the walls of varicose veins. Exp Mol Pathol 37:37-47, 1982.
46. Staubesand J. Intracellular collagen in smooth muscle. Beitr Pathol 1:187-193, 1977.
47. Vanhoutte PM, Shepherd JT. Adrenergic pharmacology of human and canine peripheral veins. Fed Proc 44:37, 1985.
48. Niebes P, Berson I. Determination of Enzymes and Degradation. London: Churchill Livingstone, 1976, p 35.

49. Woolley DE. On the sequential changes in the level of estradiol and progesterone during pregnancy and parturition and collagenolytic activity. In Piez KA, Reddi AH, eds. Extracellular Matrix Biochemistry. New York: Elsevier Science Publishing, 1984, p 138.
50. Crotty TP. Noradrenalin as an inducer of varicosities in the dog vein. J Med Sci 157:166, 1988.
51. Kline AL, Byrne P. Turbulence as a factor in the aetiology of varicose veins. Br J Surg 59:915, 1972.
52. Edwards JE, Edwards EA. The saphenous valves in varicose veins. Am Heart J 19:338, 1940.

Chapter 3

Pathogenesis of Varicose Veins and Chronic Venous Insufficiency

Philip D. Coleridge Smith and John H. Scurr

Venous disease has been recognized since the time of Papyrus of Ebers (c. 3500 BC), and yet the pathogenesis of its most common manifestation, varicose veins, and its most tiresome complication, venous ulceration, are still incompletely understood. A number of hypotheses have been advanced to explain the mechanism by which varicose veins develop. These theories have been based largely on anatomic and pathologic studies of excised varicose veins or investigations of anatomic structures in cadavers. Relatively few studies focusing on the development of varicose veins have involved the use of functional methods of investigation because until recently this approach necessitated phlebography, an excessively invasive method for studying a relatively benign condition. Recently, however, histologic and immunohistologic methods have been used to investigate changes in varicose vein wall structure, including metabolic processes involved in their development.

DEVELOPMENT OF VARICOSE VEINS

It has been suggested that varicose veins develop from a failure of venous valves that is caused by increased venous pressure resulting from the lack of valves above the saphenofemoral junction.[1] The upright posture of humans has been suggested as the principal cause of increased pressure that results in valve failure.[2] Some authors have concluded that the primary problem is a failure of more proximal valves, which is succeeded, in turn, by incompetence of more distal valves. Others have suggested that the reverse process takes place, with valvular incompetence developing distally and moving proximally.[3]

Trendelenburg[4] was the first to suggest that the failure of proximal valves resulted in incompetence more distally. He suggested that ligation of a proximal part of the vein would protect its distal segments. Unfortunately, studies of this procedure revealed a high rate of varicose vein recurrence.

Anatomic studies of the distribution of venous valves in the proximal, femoral, and iliac veins showed that in some subjects the valves are absent in the common and external iliac veins.[5,6] It was suggested that this lack may predispose the individual to subsequent development of varicose veins since the hydrostatic pressure of blood resting on the valves below the iliac segment would be increased. However, Basmajian,[7] in a series of 100 cadaveric dissections, demonstrated that, in one limb with varicosities of the long (greater) saphenous vein and in two limbs with varicosities of the short (lesser) saphenous vein, there were competent valves above the entry of these veins into the deep veins. In addition, no varices were found in 40 limbs in which no valve was present above the saphenofemoral junction. Therefore it is clear that the presence or absence of valves in the proximal venous system does not always influence the subsequent formation of distal varices.

One method of establishing whether or not the sequence of valve destruction occurs proximally to distally would be to compare patients with severe and mild varicose veins to determine whether or not long saphenous vein incompetence preceded incompetence and varicosity of its branches. Such a comparison was done by Ludbrook,[8] who used foot vein pressures to judge severity of venous incompetence. Ludbrook was able to show no difference between the severity of valvular incompetence in groups with mild and severe varicosity, and he concluded that long saphenous vein incompetence might well precede worsening varices in side branches. There are other possible interpretations of Ludbrook's data, and the matter has been investigated by other authors.

Folse[9] investigated a series of patients with varicose veins by using Doppler ultrasound. He demonstrated venous reflux in the common femoral vein in many of these patients and concluded that varices were likely to be a consequence of descending valve failure. In a few patients, Folse found competent proximal saphenous veins with varices arising from a midthigh perforating vein. He concluded that the theories of Fegan and Kline[3] on distal-to-proximal progression of varicosities were incorrect. Unfortunately, Folse's reliance on continuous-wave Doppler ultrasound means that he would not be certain that he was insonating the femoral vein. Therefore his conclusions must be regarded with caution. In contrast, Rose and Ahmed[10] used Doppler ultrasound and preoperative examination to investigate a series of 300 cases and found that 63% of long saphenous vein varicosities occurred below a competent saphenofemoral junction. This finding suggests that proximal events are irrelevant in the development of varices.

The suggestion by Fegan and Kline[3] that valvular incompetence may arise distally and progress proximally is based on an investigation of patients undergoing sclerotherapy for varicose veins. These authors theorized that varicosities appeared first in the branches of the distal long saphenous vein (i.e., in the calf) and then progressed more proximally. Fegan and Kline used both clinical examination and Doppler ultrasound imaging. They also suggested that appropriate management of distal varices, such as the use of injection sclerotherapy, might restore the competence of proximal valves as determined by measurements from a tourniquet test. Chant et al.[11] confirmed these findings by treating distal varices through the use of injection sclerotherapy. This approach resulted in a radiologically demonstrated reduction in diameter of the proximal long saphenous vein. Chant et al. concluded that saphenofemoral incompetence is a consequence of distal varicosities rather than the cause of the varicosities.

The study of Basmajian[7] suggests that it is unlikely that varicose veins are a consequence of an absence of proximal valves in the iliac or femoral veins. The observations of Fegan and Kline,[3] Rose and Ahmed,[10] and Chant et al.,[11] based on different methods of investigation, imply that distal disease may determine the severity of proximal venous incompetence. With duplex ultrasound imaging, it now should be possible to obtain substantially greater information about the competence or incompetence of distal veins and associated varices.

Calf Perforating Veins: Cause or Effect?

Cockett[12] described large perforating veins of the medial calf (Cockett's perforators) and their association with overlying varicosities and ulceration. He placed considerable emphasis on the treatment of venous ulcers by ligation of these vessels. Cockett complained that venous ulcers were not described in anatomy texts of the time. Our experience with duplex ultrasound imaging suggests that perforating veins tend to be of small diameter (1 to 2 mm) in the normal state but increase in size in patients with venous disease. Thus the causal association suggested by Cockett is not so obvious. Since the efficacy of perforator ligation in healing ulcers was not rigorously tested by him in a clinical trial, Cockett's assertions must be viewed with care. Subsequent investigations resulted in mixed findings, with some papers reporting efficacy[13] but objective studies showing no substantial benefit.[14,15] The authors of one study involving functional methods of assessment found it necessary to include both local deep vein incompetence and perforator incompetence in the calf in their model of pathogenesis.[16]

The precise role of perforating veins of the calf in the pathogenesis of varicose veins and venous ulceration remains to be fully elucidated. Our own work suggests that the direction of blood flow in these vessels is highly dependent on disease in other veins, with inward or outward flow occurring according to the perturbation of blood flow in other vessels.[17]

Varicose Veins: Vein Wall or Valve Problem?

An alternative explanation for the development of varicose veins is defective structure of the vein wall. In 1961, King[18] pointed out that in varicose veins early swelling is found distally, not proximally, to the valve so that hydrostatic pressure above the valve is unlikely to damage the vein wall. Although histologic examination of the vein wall in the early stages of varicosis shows hypertrophy of the muscle coat and increased vascularity of the adventitia, these observations could be attributed to local abnormality of blood flow induced by a chemical stimulus, possibly of a hormonal nature. Nevertheless, it is apparent that King's observations implied a disease affecting the vein wall that eventually results in loss of mechanical integrity and dilatation of the vessel with incompetence of its valves.

The question of whether or not vein wall distention precedes the development of varicosities or occurs as a consequence of valve failure is critical to the pathogenesis. This issue has been studied by Cotton,[19] who also investigated the relationship of varicosities and dilatations of the vein wall to the valves contained within the veins. He investigated veins that were removed at operation and venograms of patients with varicosities. Cotton demonstrated that varicosities usually occurred distally to the valve, which, in keeping with King's observations, suggests that a failure in the vein wall may precede disruption of the valve itself.

The nature of vein wall failure may be attributable to defective connective tissue regulation. Unfortunately, the biochemistry of connective tissue regulation is incompletely understood. The collagen, elastin, and hexosamine content of vein walls was investigated in 1962 by Svejcar et al.,[20] who found that collagen content was significantly lower in varicose veins and potential varicose veins as compared to normal veins. In addition, Svejcar et al. noted that varicose veins contain relatively more muscle than normal veins. The hexosamine content was significantly higher in actual and potential varicose veins than in normal veins, and there was a greater variation of water and hexosamine content in different segments of varicose veins compared to normal veins. These authors suggested that their investigation might indicate an inherited anomaly of collagen metabolism. The reliability of these data is open to question since the date of investigation precedes that of modern monoclonal antibodies. The analyses of Svejcar et al. were made by using biochemical assays. In addition, different types of collagen are now recognized that were not assessed separately in this study. However, further investigations by Andreotti et al.[21] suggest that there are reduced amounts of collagen and elastin in varicose veins as compared with those of controls.

Subsequently, Haardt[22] investigated vein wall metabolism by using monoclonal stains for lactate dehydrogenase, alkaline phosphatase, adenosine triphosphate, lysosomal enzymes, beta-D-glucuronidase, nonspecific esterase, and acid phosphatase. He found an increase in the amount of lysosomal enzyme activity in varicose veins as compared to normal veins, with the increase being greater in the media than in the intima. In general, Haardt was able to show a decline in enzyme activity responsible for energy metabolism in varicose veins, and he suggested that this might be accompanied by a decline in the contractility of the vein wall. Haardt thought that the increase in lysosomal enzymes would reflect the change in collagen with thickening and fibrillation of the individual fibers. However, it is unclear whether these changes are a cause or a consequence of the varicose process.

More recently, Obitsu et al.[23] examined normal and varicose veins with light and transmission electron microscopy. They concluded that valve failure began with depression of the valve commissure and involved subsequent expansion between valve cusps. In this study elongation of the cusps and bulbous thickening of the free edge cusp were noted. Hyperplasia of valve cusp collagen also was found, but this condition could be a secondary change in response to increased venous pressure.

Histologic Examination

The most prominent histologic change noted in varicose veins is an increase in the medial fibrous tissue, resulting in the separation of smooth muscle layers.

Collagen and fibrous tissue also accumulate in the subintima, and elastic fibers tend to spread throughout the vein wall instead of being restricted to the internal and external elastic laminae. These changes have a patchy distribution.[10] Electron microscopy of smooth muscle cells shows them to contain collagen fibers, which suggests that the smooth muscle cell has taken on phagocytic properties. The muscle cells are separated from one another by a considerable increase in fibrous tissue, which suggests that they are being replaced by fibrous tissue.

Immunohistochemical Study of Vein Wall Components

A detailed immunohistologic study of eight varicose saphenous vein samples and four normal controls was carried out in 1987, when a search for the infiltrating "immune competent" cells in the vessel wall was made.[24] Few infiltrating cells were found, but those present were tissue macrophages carrying the FCR1 receptor. The most surprising finding was the appearance of class II major histocompatibility antigens on the endothelium, macrophages, and smooth muscle cells of the thickened tunica media. Up-regulation of human lymphocyte antigen, class D and class D–related (HLA-D/DR) was present in all three cell types, but there was preferential up-regulation of HLA-D/DQ in the smooth muscle cells. The function of the class II locus is to present processed antigens to T cells that are induced by interferon gamma (IFN-gamma) and tumor necrosis factor alpha (TNFa). At this site, HLA-D/DQ is probably involved in the maintenance of a chronic inflammatory process. This activity is almost certainly secondary to the disease process, but the site of HLA-D/DQ expression within the thickened media of the vessel suggests a possible active role in the pathology of the disorder.

Chemical Changes in Vein Wall

Plasminogen activator is reduced in varicose veins in comparison with control subjects.[25,26] This reduction may represent a simple association with the inflammatory process in varicose veins or a relationship with the development of varicosities. It has been shown that fibrinolytic processes are down-regulated in varicose veins excised from limbs with lipodermatosclerotic skin.

Present research suggests that abnormalities are present in both the vein wall and the valve cusps. However, in which order these abnormalities occur is unclear. We suggest that early valve failure is characterized by a small-diameter, high-velocity jet of blood flowing through valve orifices. This has been observed in undilated veins. One possibility is that turbulent blood flow, which has a substantial effect on endothelial cells, may result in changes in the metabolism of endothelial cells, which produce tissue growth factors. Certainly, varicose veins may develop upstream from an arteriovenous fistula.[27] High-velocity retrograde flow through a valve results in turbulent flow, with the overlying vein being subjected to severe turbulence. This action may result in distention of the valve in the region of the turbulent flow.

Effects of Blood Flow

Gius[28] has suggested that arteriovenous communications contribute to the pathogenesis of varicose veins. This theory also has been supported by Piulachs and Vidal-Barraquer.[29] Gius based his findings on examination of vessels at operation combined with histologic evidence of proliferating vessels obtained from the skin in some patients and the visual evidence that bright blood issues from varices at operation. Through the use of radiologic criteria, Haimovici et al.[30] also have suggested that arteriovenous shunting is associated with the development of varicose veins. However, subsequent investigation has failed to confirm the presence of such communications.

Etiologic Factors

Varicose veins may develop as a consequence of many factors, including age, sex, race, weight, height, pregnancy, diet, bowel habits, occupation, heredity, alcohol intake, clothing, and posture. Varicose veins may occur at any age in adult life, but they appear to be more common with advancing years. A peak frequency between the ages of 50 and 60 years has been reported.[31] Large surveys have demonstrated that there is a female-to-male predominance of between 2 : 1 and 4 : 1.

Pregnancy. A number of studies have investigated the incidence of varicose veins developing during pregnancy. Such incidence varies between 8% and 20%, depending on the study, and appears to be more common in multiparous than in primiparous women.[32-34] The development of varicose veins during pregnancy may reflect the effect of estrogen and progesterone on the vein wall. Alternatively, it has been suggested that compression of the iliac veins by the uterus may result in increased pressure in the lower veins.

Race. Foote[35] stated that varicose veins were uncommon in Africans, and Dodd[36] found only three cases of varicose veins in 11,000 inpatient admissions in a tribal reserve in Zulu Lane. Burkitt has claimed that there may be a dietary link to this observation. He suggested that the high-fiber diets normally eaten by Africans resulted in relative ease of defecation and no rise in intra-abdominal pressure. Burkitt assumed this was an important factor in the development of varicose veins, but his theory now seems doubtful.

Height and weight. The static foot vein pressure measured by manometry is undoubtedly related to the height of the subject. Therefore it has been suggested that tall subjects may be at greater risk than shorter subjects. In a survey in Switzerland, Widmer[37] found no association between the presence of varicose veins and height or weight. Myers[38] and Ludbrook[39] found that patients with varicose veins were heavier than age- and sex-matched controls without varicose veins. This finding was not confirmed by Widmer in the Basel study.

Posture. The effect of posture on varicose veins has been investigated by a number of authors. In a study of department store employees, Lake et al.[40] noted that 74% of those who stood while working had varicose veins compared with 57% of those who sat. Santler et al.[41] reviewed 2854 patients with varicose disease and found that 6.3% were required to walk in their occupation, 29.2% spent their time sitting, and 64.5% stood still at work. These data tend to suggest that occupations involving standing carry an increased risk of varicose veins.

Heredity. A large number of patients presenting with varicose veins recall that many of their close relatives also had varicose veins. However, since the prevalence of varicosis is so high in Western countries, it is not surprising to find such a phenomenon. A number of studies have investigated the association between varicose veins in relatives. It has been shown that between 50% and 75% of the relatives of a person with varicose veins may be affected by varicosities. In 1963, a study by Gunderson and Hauge[42] found that 43% of the relatives of women and 19% of the relatives of men had varicose veins. This figure is far higher than would be expected from the prevalence of the disease determined during epidemiologic studies. However, it is somewhat less than what would be expected if the inheritance were of a truly dominant nature. Therefore we conclude that the inheritance of varicose veins is polygenic.

■ ■ ■

The preceding data show that the question of how varicose veins develop is still unanswered. It is unlikely that the cause of this problem is related to the anatomic distribution of valves in the proximal venous system, and pressure effects alone are not the explanation. Distention of the vein at or below the level of the cusp may lead to valvular incompetence, or the valvular incompetence may precede and initiate distal distention of the vein. Too little data are available to decide which is the case. Both inherited and environmental factors are important in the pathogenesis of varicose veins, although the contribution of each to the disease awaits a full understanding of the processes that result in varicosities. We are impressed with how little is known of the pathologic mechanisms in this disease.

CHRONIC VENOUS INSUFFICIENCY AND VENOUS ULCERATION

Venous ulceration occurs when the muscle pumping mechanisms of the leg are impaired because of disease in the superficial or deep venous systems.[43] This ulceration may simply be a consequence of varicose veins, which account for 20% to 50% of venous leg ulcers,[44,45] or it may result from incompetence of deep vein valves. Venous ulceration may arise from previous deep vein thrombosis or primary valve failure in a manner similar to that resulting in incompetence of superficial veins in patients with varicose veins.[46] The consequence of incompetent lower limb vein valves is that the pumping mechanism no longer reduces pressure in veins during walking. A cannula placed in the dorsal foot vein usually shows a reduction in the resting pressure from 80 to 100 mm Hg to 10 to 20 mm Hg in a physically fit person.

Patients with severe impairment of the calf muscle pump may not be able to reduce foot vein pressure below the resting level.[47] The presence of substantial venous reflux will result in rapid refilling of calf veins after exercise that is expressed as a rapid rise in foot vein pressure. These two components of foot venous pressure have been combined by some authors to facilitate analysis of the severity of venous impairment. A number of indexes of venous function have been described, which gives an indication of the magnitude of the problem.[48-50] However, some patients seem to tolerate severe muscle pump impairment without ulceration, yet others suffer ulcers of the leg with only moderate venous impairment.

Clearly, other factors are important in the pathogenesis of this disease, but what leads to increased or decreased susceptibility of certain patients to ulcers of the leg remains unclear. Hypotheses have been proposed since the Middle Ages, but recently they have revolved around the theory that ulceration is attributable to skin hypoxia.[51]

Mechanisms of Ulceration

Homans[52] has suggested that ulceration of the skin overlying large varicosities is caused by low oxygen levels in stagnant blood of the varicosities, which results in cutaneous hypoxia. Oxygenation of varicose vein blood also has been the subject of several studies by other authors.[53,54] It is clear that in supine patients the hemoglobin oxygen saturation of varicose veins is greater than that of veins in a normal state. With standing, no difference in this variable is noted between normal and varicose veins. Therefore, even if venous blood were responsible for cutaneous nutrition, there would be no difference in hemoglobin oxygen saturation between patients with varicose veins and normal subjects.[55] Elevated venous oxygen tension in patients with venous disease suggests that arteriovenous fistulas may be present, depriving the skin of oxygen.[56,57] Unfortunately, research involving the use of microspheres and macroaggregates has failed to demonstrate an increase in arteriovenous shunting in the skin of patients with venous disease.[58]

Fibrin cuff theory. In 1982, Browse and Burnand[59] proposed that oxygen diffusion into cutaneous tissues was restricted by a pericapillary fibrin cuff. They suggested that increased capillary pressure resulting from elevated venous pressure produces an increased loss of plasma proteins, including fibrinogen, through the capillary wall. Fibrinogen then polymerizes to produce the "fibrin cuff" that surrounds cutaneous capillaries. Measurements of capillary protein loss by Browse and Burnand showed that fibrinogen was quantitatively the most important plasma protein leaking into tissues in patients with venous disease. Subsequent measurements of fibrinolysis have shown that patients with venous disease have reduced venous fibrinolytic activity, which might explain why the fibrin cuff persists.[60]

The fibrin cuff theory has tended to perpetuate the suggestions of previous authors that the nature of venous ulceration is closely related to the deprivation of oxygen in tissue. However, it is difficult to find satisfactory evidence that cutaneous and subcutaneous tissues are hypoxic in liposclerotic skin. There is no published evidence to prove that fibrin provides a barrier to oxygen diffusion. It seems probable from the composition of other human connective tissue that such a fibrin gel would comprise much water with a small amount of fibrin. Small molecules diffusing through such a cuff might be expected to have no greater difficulty than when diffusing through water in other human tissue. If the assumption is made that the fibrin layer contains 0.5% fibrin (similar to that of a fibrin blood clot), calculations reveal no impairment of tissue oxygen delivery. Even a cuff consisting of 100 times more fibrin than this would result in a reduction of oxygen delivery of only 50%.[61] However, the results of these calculations have not been confirmed by measurement. Browse and Burnand[59] employed a piece of commercial bovine fibrin from a suture manufacturer in order to assess the permeability of fibrin. They found that this material significantly impeded the passage of oxygen. Yet it is unlikely that fibrin cuffs seen in humans are of the same composition.

The evidence advanced to support the assertion that skin is hypoxic comes from data obtained by transcutaneous oximetry.[62,63] A Clark-type electrode equipped with an integral heater is applied to the skin in order to register the oxygen availability at the skin surface. Such a device was originally devised for neonatal monitoring, in which skin heating was used so that the resulting vasodilation would ensure that measurements accurately reflected arterial oxygen tension. In venous disease different findings have been obtained, depending on whether the transducer is heated to 43° or 37° C. At higher temperatures used by most authors, it has been found that patients with venous disease tend to have lower transcutaneous oxygen tension readings than normal subjects.[62,63] Measurements made with an electrode temperature of 37° C are even more paradoxical.[64] Under these circumstances, cutaneous oxygenation is *greater* in patients with venous disease than in normal subjects. Obviously, not only does the technique have a number of limitations, but transcutaneous oxygen tension may be influenced by many factors other than cutaneous oxygenation.

Direct measurement of cutaneous oxygen tension would be the most satisfactory method of investigation if it were not fraught with technical difficulties. For example, it would be necessary to advance a microelectrode through the skin and measure oxygen tension by polarography or one of the more recent fiberoptic methods that involve the use of dye phosphorescence quenching. It is debatable whether this approach could be considered a reasonable investigation in skin that is prone to ulceration, but it is certainly within the capabilities of modern technology.

Some authors have tried to assess gas exchange in cutaneous microcirculation by alternative methods. Hopkins et al.[65] used positron emission tomography techniques to assess cutaneous blood flow and oxygen extraction in cutaneous and subcutaneous tissues of patients with venous disease. They noted a reduction in the oxygen extraction ratio in such tissues but also a substantial increase in cutaneous blood flow. Thus it is unclear whether oxygen delivery actually was increased or decreased.

We have measured the clearance of xenon 133 from skin to assess the efficiency of microcirculation in handling a molecule similar in size to oxygen. This gas has a molecular weight four times that of oxygen; therefore the diffusion rate would be half that of oxygen, if it is assumed that there is similar solubility for oxygen and xenon in body fluids (water). We used Sjerson's technique,[66] in which xenon gas is applied topically to the skin and diffuses readily into the dermis and subcutaneous fat. This method avoids direct injection of solutions of xenon, which might alter cutaneous blood flow. Measurements were made in the liposclerotic skin of patients with venous disease and compared to those of control subjects under conditions of reactive hyperemia after 5 minutes of arterial cuff occlusion to the leg. No difference in xenon clearance was found between patients with venous disease and control subjects.[67] This finding was a surprise and led us to assess further methods of measurements of cutaneous gas exchange.

The rate of transcutaneous oxygen tension recovery after a period in which arterial blood supply has been interrupted is another measurement that may be used to determine whether a diffusion barrier for oxygen exists. We measured the time taken for cutaneous reoxygenation after a period of ischemia that was produced by inflating a leg cuff above systolic arterial pressure for 5 minutes. No difference was found between the control group and the venous disease group.[68] These results led us to conclude that, in patients with chronic venous insufficiency, it is unlikely that there is a substantial abnormality in the delivery of oxygen to tissues. Unfortunately, until a satisfactory method for measuring skin oxygenation is developed, it will not be possible to answer this question completely. The possibility remains that some elements in the skin may receive insufficient nutrition, which renders them susceptible to injury by mechanical or other factors.

White cell trapping theory. The search for additional or alternative mechanisms of skin damage in venous disease has resulted in a focus on the blood itself. Moyses et al.[69] studied the limbs of normal subjects in response to increased venous pressure. They measured hematologic parameters as an index of the effect of the venous hypertension. Their subjects sat on a bicycle saddle without moving and with their limbs dependent for a period of 40 minutes. Blood samples were taken from the long saphenous vein at the ankle. Moyses et al. found that the hematocrit level and red cell count increased in parallel, as would be expected. The white cell count remained unchanged despite an increased hematocrit level. White cells were being "lost" from the circulation, and after 40 minutes, this loss accounted for a 25% difference.

Thomas et al.[70] performed a similar study comparing patients with normal lower limbs with patients having venous disease that resulted in lipodermatosclerosis and ulceration. Their patients were permitted to sit with their legs dependent, a less stringent requirement than that of Moyses. Blood sampling was again done from the long saphenous vein at the ankle. After 60 minutes, patients with venous disease were "trapping" 30% of white blood cells and control subjects were trapping 7%. This led us to examine cutaneous microcirculation by using capillary microscopy. We found that venous hypertension appeared to reduce the number of visible capillary loops in patients with venous disease but not in control subjects, which suggested that capillary damage may be occurring during venous hypertension.[71]

Bollinger et al.[72] investigated events in venous disease using fluorescence capillary videomicroscopy. They measured the rate of diffusion of fluorescein out of capillaries after an intravenous injection. Bollinger et al. were able to show that capillaries in patients with venous disease are much more permeable to this molecule than are normal veins, contrary to the suggestions made in the fibrin cuff hypothesis. Using simultaneous fluorescence and light capillary microscopy, Franzeck et al.[73] described the appearance of capillary loops that are filled with red blood cells but do not appear to be perfused. They suggested that this appearance may be due to capillary "thrombosis."

White blood cell margination normally occurs in arterioles, capillaries, and venules. This phenomenon is thought to cause tissue injury following ischemia. White blood cells are substantially larger than red blood cells and are responsible for many of the rheologic properties of blood. White blood cells take 1000 times longer than red blood cells to deform on entering a capillary bed and are responsible for approximately half of the peripheral vascular resistance in the circulation despite their small numbers.[74] In myocardial infarction, white blood cells cause capillary occlusion, which can be prevented in experimental animals by producing leukopenia.[75,76]

White blood cells have been implicated as the mediators of ischemia in many types of tissue, including myocardium, brain, lung, and kidney.[77-80] Polymorphonuclear leukocytes, particularly those attached to capillary endothelium, may become "activated" when cytoplasmic granules containing proteolytic enzymes are released.[81] In addition, a nonmitochondrial "respiratory burst" permits these cells to release free radicals, most notably superoxide radicals, which have nonspecific destructive effects on lipid membranes, proteins, and connective tissue compounds.[82] Leukocytotactic factors also are released, attracting polymorphonuclear cells.

We published a hypothesis suggesting that white blood cell trapping resulted in the triggering of such processes, causing degradation of tissues[83] (Figure 3-1). We proposed that white blood cells might cause occlusion of capillaries, a suggestion originally made by Moyses.[69] If some capillaries were occluded, heterogenous perfusion might result, causing tissue hypoxia and ischemia. From these data it can be

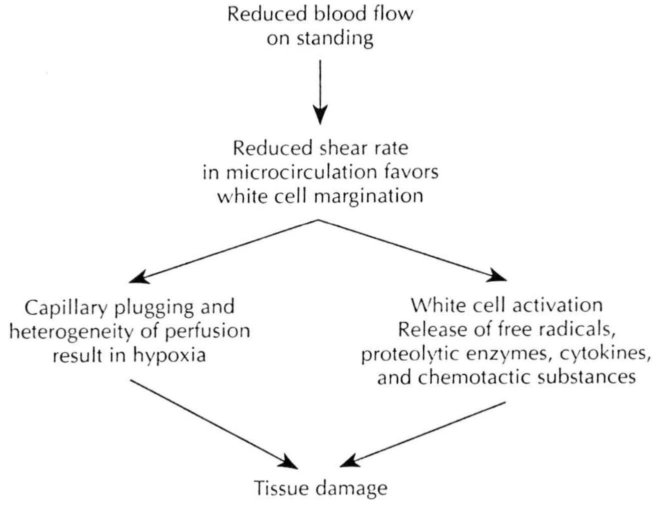

FIGURE 3-1. White cell "trapping" hypothesis. (Modified from Coleridge Smith PD, Thomas P, Scurr JH, Dormandy JA. Causes of venous ulceration: A new hypothesis. Br Med J 296:1726-1727, 1988.)

seen that we have not been able to support the assertion that venous ulceration is caused by tissue hypoxia. In fact, we specifically investigated the microcirculation to determine whether the response to venous hypertension results in its degradation. Although we used laser Doppler fluxmetry and transcutaneous oximetry, we were unable to show vascular deficits in patients with venous disease when they sat still with lower limbs dependent for 30 minutes.[71] Subsequently, we applied a more severe venous hypertensive insult to the normal circulation by placing a cuff around the leg and inflating it to 80 mm Hg for 15 minutes and measuring the hyperemic response. We were able to show a small reduction in microcirculatory function by this means, which suggests that microcirculatory injury may be produced in the short term (15 minutes) by an increased venous pressure in the leg.[84]

The second part of this theory suggested that white blood cell activation releases proteolytic enzymes, superoxide radicals, and chemotactic substances. All classes of white blood cells appear to become trapped, and so a wide range of phenomena is possible. Monocytes might become activated, releasing interleukin-1 (IL-1) and TNFa.[85] These agents may produce endothelial cell activation to permit the passage of much larger than normal molecules.[86] Decreased fibrinolysis observed in patients with venous disease may be a result of the effects of IL-1.[87] IL-1 acts on endothelial cells to stimulate production of the fibrinolytic inhibitor plasminogen activator inhibitor-1 (PAI-1) and decrease the production of tissue plasminogen activator (t-PA), producing a reduction in fibrinolysis.

To what extent are white blood cells implicated in venous disease? Although the inflammatory cells have been described in dermatology texts in discussion of venous disease, they have not previously been implicated in the ulcer process. Therefore we performed biopsies on supramalleolar skin in patients undergoing varicose vein surgery.[88] Three distinct groups of patients were studied. The first group included patients with no evidence of skin changes as a consequence of their venous disease. The next group exhibited lipodermatosclerosis without ulceration of the limb. The final group had ulceration with lipodermatosclerosis. Patients with normal skin had a low number of white blood cells ($4/mm^2$) in the upper 0.5 mm of the skin. There were 8 times as many in patients with liposclerotic skin, and 43 times as many in patients with healed venous ulcers. The majority of white blood cells are macrophages with a T-lymphocyte component but without an excess of neutrophils in comparison to normal limbs. Thus this infiltrate is a reflection of a chronic inflammation, which suggests that an investigation of leukocyte products might elucidate mechanisms involved in venous ulceration. We also have identified IL-1 as an inflammatory mediator in this process.

Free radical injury and white blood cell activation are widely invoked as the mechanisms of injury during ischemia. There is little doubt that the process of ischemia destroys tissue. It is now recognized that ischemia is clearly an active process of tissue destruction rather than a passive one of cellular death due to hypoxia alone. We suspect that the same is true for lipodermatosclerosis and venous ulceration, but we have only circumstantial evidence to support this suggestion. Recently, McCollum[89] has been able to demonstrate up-regulation of neutrophil production of free oxygen radicals and increased production of thromboxane A_2 in response to elevated venous pressure in leg veins of patients with chronic venous insufficiency.

Associated Changes

Although abnormalities of the microcirculation are important in venous disease, other skin structures become damaged in patients with chronic venous insufficiency. The regulation of the microcirculation is dependent on intact innervation. The vasoconstrictor response of microcirculation is impaired in the leg skin of patients with venous disease.

We have recently assessed the presence of neuropathy in patients with venous disease to determine whether there is an associated nerve injury. We found normal thresholds of sensation in the foot related to vibration (A_α fiber) and cooling (A_β fiber) but substantially increased thresholds for skin warming (C fiber) (patient median: 3.4° C with interquartile range of 2.4 to 5.8; control median: 1.2° C with interquartile range of 2.1 to 1.1). These data suggest that this nerve fiber type is particularly susceptible to injury in patients with venous disease. The consequence of this finding for microcirculation is unclear, but it implies a loss of external regulation. We have measured vasomotion (cyclical fluctuations in flow assessed by laser Doppler fluxmetry) and have performed frequency analysis by Fourier transform analysis.[90] These methods revealed that the main vasomotion component was increased in magnitude and frequency in patients with liposclerotic skin compared with that of control subjects. This finding also may suggest a loss in neuronal regulation of the microcirculation.

Bollinger et al.[91] have elegantly demonstrated that cutaneous lymphatic capillaries are abnormal and damaged in venous disease, with dilatation and incompetence of their valves noted. Eventually, lymphatic vessels become destroyed and cannot be found in the most severely affected skin. This destruction can result in impairment of lymphatic drainage, which may account for some features of chronic venous insufficiency. It seems probable that the changes reported by Bollinger are a consequence of the inflammation described here. However, the precise relationship of the lymphatic abnormality to the ulceration process is unclear and warrants further elucidation.

Pharmacologic Treatment

Although bandaging and stockings have been used effectively for years in the treatment of chronic venous insufficiency, modern pharmacologic science may provide assistance in healing venous ulcers. Enhancing fibrinolysis has been used in an attempt to promote removal of the fibrin cuff.[92] Unfortunately, this treatment approach did not result in any improved ulcer healing. Drugs that reduce white blood cell activation may be useful in healing venous ulcers. Pentoxifylline (Trental, Hoechst-Roussel, Somerville, N.J.) reduces the likelihood of white blood cell activation by an effect that appears to be dependent of other known activators of neutrophils (e.g., TNFa), resulting in a lower likelihood of endothelial adhesion.[93] In a multicenter study of 82 patients, the use of pentoxifylline was shown to result in better healing rates for ulcers than did placebo.[94] It has been recommended that this drug may be useful for the treatment of resistant ulcers.[95] Prostaglandin E_1 inhibits the respiratory burst of neutrophils, preventing the release of superoxide radicals. A preliminary study suggested that this, too, is effective in healing venous ulcers.[96] Other pharmacologic treatment strategies are possible and await evaluation. Adjuvant pharmacologic treatment eventually may become commonplace in the management of venous ulceration.

■ ■ ■

The precise mechanisms through which venous hypertension causes ulceration remain unclear. Abnormalities in several structures have been identified. It is difficult to identify which are "participants" and which are "spectators." A better understanding of the initiating processes of this problem may lead to improvement in the management of patients with venous ulceration.

ACKNOWLEDGMENTS

We offer heartfelt thanks to the following members of the Department of Surgery of University College and Middlesex School of Medicine in London who have undertaken much of the work described in this chapter and have made substantial intellectual contributions to our understanding of venous disease: Mr. T.R. Cheatle, Dr. S. Chittenden, Mr. J. Farrah, Ms. G.M. McMullin, Mr. S. Sarin, Mr. H.J. Scott, Mr. S. Shami, and Mr. D. Shields. We are grateful to Miss L. Wilkinson for kindly summarizing the findings related to inflammatory changes in varicose veins that were described in her M. Phil. thesis.

REFERENCES

1. Friedrich N. Uber das Verhalten der Klappen in den Cruralvenen, sowie uber das Verkommen von Klappen in den grossen Venanstaemmen des Unterleibes. Morph Johrb 7:323-325, 1882.
2. Barber RF, Shatara FI. The varicose disease. NY State J Med 25:162-166, 1925.
3. Fegan WG, Kline AL. The cause of varicosity in the superficial veins of the lower limb. Br J Surg 59:798-801, 1972.
4. Trendelenburg F. Über die Unterbindung der vena saphena magna bei unterschenkelvarizen. Beitr Klin Chir 7:195-210, 1891.
5. Eger SA, Casper SL. Etiology of varicose veins from an anatomic aspect based on a dissection of 38 adult cadavers. JAMA 123:148-149, 1943.
6. Eger SA, Wagner FB. Etiology of varicose veins. Postgrad Med 6:234-238, 1949.
7. Basmajian JV. The distribution of valves in the femoral, external iliac, and common iliac veins and their relationship to varicose veins. Surg Gynecol Obstet 95:537-542, 1952.
8. Ludbrook J. Valvular defect in varicose veins. Cause or effect? Lancet 2:1289-1292, 1963.
9. Folse R. The influence of femoral vein dynamics on the development of varicose veins. Surgery 68:974-979, 1970.
10. Rose SS, Ahmed A. Some thoughts on the aetiology of varicose veins. J Cardiovasc Surg 27:534-543, 1986.
11. Chant ADB, Jones HO, Townsend JCF, Edmund Williams J. Radiological demonstration of the relationship between calf varices and saphenofemoral incompetence. Clin Radiol 23:519-523, 1972.
12. Cockett FB, Elgan Jones DE. The ankle blow-out syndrome—A new approach to the varicose ulcer problem. Lancet 2:17-23, 1953.

13. Negus D. Prevention and treatment of venous ulceration. Ann Roy Coll Surg 67:144-148, 1985.
14. Burnand KG, Lea Thomas M, O'Donnell T, Browse NL. The relative importance of incompetent communicating veins in the production of varicose veins and venous ulcers. Surgery 82:9-14, 1977.
15. Burnand KG, Lea Thomas M, O'Donnell T, Browse NL. Relation between postphlebitic changes in deep veins and results of surgical treatment of venous ulcers. Lancet 1:936-938, 1976.
16. Zukowski AJ, Nicolaides AN, Szendro G, et al. Haemodynamic significance of incompetent calf perforating veins. Br J Surg 78:625-629, 1991.
17. McMullin GM, Coleridge Smith PD, Scurr JH. Which way does blood flow in the perforating veins of the leg? Phlebology 6:127-132, 1991.
18. King ESJ. The genesis of varicose veins. Aust N Z J Surg 48:589-598, 1961.
19. Cotton LT. Varicose veins: Gross anatomy and development. Br J Surg 48:589-598, 1961.
20. Svejcar J, Prerovsky I, Linhart J, Kruml J. Content of collagen, elastin, and water in walls of the internal saphenous vein in man. Circ Res 11:296-300, 1962.
21. Andreotti L, Cammelli D, Banchi G, Guarnieri M, Serantoni C. Collagen, elastin, and sugar content in primary varicose veins. Ric Clin Lab 8:273-285, 1978.
22. Haardt B. Histochemistry of normal and varicose veins. Phlebology 2:135-158, 1987.
23. Obitsu Y, Ishimaru S, Furukawa K, Yoshihama I. Histopathological studies of varicose veins. Phlebology 5:245-254, 1990.
24. Wilkinson L. The presence of immune cells in vascular disease [M. Phil. thesis]. London: University College London, 1987.
25. Layer GY, Pattison M, Evans B, Davies DR, Burnand KG. Tissue fibrinolytic activity is reduced in varicose veins. In Negus D, Jantet G, eds. Phlebology '85. London: John Libbey, 1986, pp 10-13.
26. Wolfe JHN, Morland M, Browse NL. The fibrinolytic activity of varicose veins. Br J Surg 66:185-187, 1979.
27. Holman EF. Development of arterial aneurysms. Surg Gynecol Obstet 100:599-611, 1955.
28. Gius JA. Arteriovenous anastomoses and varicose veins. Arch Surg 81:299-310, 1960.
29. Piulachs P, Vidal-Barraquer E. Pathogenic study of varicose veins. Angiology 4:59-100, 1953.
30. Haimovici H, Steinman C, Caplan LH. Role of arteriovenous anastomoses in vascular diseases of the lower extremity. Ann Surg 164:990-1002, 1966.
31. DeSilva A, Widmer LK, Martin H, et al. Varicose veins and chronic venous insufficiency. Vasa 3:118, 1974.
32. Dodd HJ, Wright HP. Vulval varices in pregnancy. Br Med J 1:831-832, 1959.
33. Kilbourne NJ. Varicose veins in pregnancy. Am J Obstet Gynecol 25:104-112, 1933.
34. Nabatoff RA. Varicose veins in pregnancy. JAMA 174:1712-1716, 1960.
35. Foote RR. Varicose veins. London: Butterworth, 1955.
36. Dodd HJ. The cause, prevention, and arrest of varicose veins. Lancet 2:809-811, 1964.
37. Widmer LK. Peripheral venous disorders. Prevalence and sociomedical importance. Observations in 4,529 healthy persons. Basel III study. Berne: Hans Huber, 1978.
38. Myers TT. Varicose veins. In Barker NW, Hines EA, eds. Barker and Hines Vascular Disease, 3rd ed. Philadelphia: WB Saunders, 1962.
39. Ludbrook J. Obesity and varicose veins. Surg Gynecol Obstet 118:843-844, 1964.
40. Lake M, Pratt GH, Wright IS. Arteriosclerosis and varicose veins: Occupational and other factors. JAMA 119:696-701, 1942.
41. Santler R, Ernst G, Weiel B. Statistisches über der varikosen Symptomenkomplex. Hautarzt 10:460-463, 1956.
42. Gunderson J, Hauge M. Hereditary factors in venous insufficiency. Angiology 20:346-355, 1969.
43. Nicolaides AN, Zukowski A, Lewis R, Kyprianou P, Malouf GM. Venous pressure measurements in venous problems. In Bergan JJ, Yao JST, eds. Surgery of the Veins. Orlando, Fla.: Grune & Stratton, 1985, pp 111-118.
44. Dodd H, Cockett FB. The pathology and surgery of the veins of the lower limb. Edinburgh: Churchill Livingstone, 1976.
45. Hoare MC, Nicolaides AN, Miles CR, et al. The role of primary varicose veins in venous ulceration. Surgery 92:450-453, 1982.

46. Kistner RL. Primary venous valve incompetence of the leg. Am J Surg 140:218-224, 1980.
47. Pollack AA, Taylor BE, Myers TT, Wood EH. The effect of exercise and body position on the venous pressure at the ankle in patients having venous valvular defects. J Clin Invest 28:559-563, 1949.
48. Schanzer H, Converse Pierce E. Pathophysiologic evaluation of chronic venous stasis with ambulatory venous pressure studies. Angiology 33:183-191, 1982.
49. Psathakis ND, Psathakis DN. Investigation of the venous haemodynamics of the lower limb by venous pressure models. Angiology 37:499-507, 1986.
50. Christopoulos D, Nicolaides AN, Szendro G. Venous reflux, quantification, and correlation with the clinical severity of chronic venous disease. Br J Surg 75:352-356, 1988.
51. Browse NL. Venous ulceration. Br Med J 286:1920-1922, 1984.
52. Homans J. The aetiology and treatment of varicose ulcers of the leg. Surg Gynecol Obstet 24:300-311, 1917.
53. Fontaine R. Remarks concerning venous thrombosis and sequelae. Surgery 41:6-24, 1957.
54. Blumhoff RL, Johnson G. Saphenous vein Po_2 in patients with varicose veins. J Surg Res 23:35-36, 1977.
55. Scott HJ, Cheatle TR, McMullin GM, et al. A reappraisal of the oxygenation of the venous blood of varicose veins. Br J Surg 77:934-936, 1990.
56. Pratt GH. Arterial varices. A syndrome. Am J Surg 77:456-460, 1949.
57. Brewer AC. Arteriovenous shunts. Br Med J 2:270, 1950.
58. Lindmayer W, Lofferer O, Mostbeck A, Partsch H. Arteriovenous shunts in primary varicosis: A critical essay. Vasc Surg 6:9-14, 1972.
59. Browse NL, Burnand GJ. The cause of venous ulceration. Lancet 2:243-245, 1982.
60. Browse NL, Gray L, Jarrett PEM, Morland M. Blood and vein wall fibrinolytic activity in health and vascular disease. Br Med J 2:478-481, 1977.
61. Michel CC. Oxygen diffusion in edematous tissue and through pericapillary cuffs. Phlebology 5:223-230, 1990.
62. Stacey MC, Burnand KG, Layer GT, Pattison M. Transcutaneous oxygen tension as a prognostic indicator and measure of treatment of recurrent ulceration. Br J Surg 74:545, 1987.
63. Clyne CAC, Ramsden WH, Chant ADB, Wenster JHH. Oxygen tension in the skin of the gaiter area of limbs with venous ulceration. Br J Surg 72:644-647, 1985.
64. Dodd HJ, Gaylarde PM, Sarkany I. Skin oxygen tension in venous insufficiency of the lower leg. J Roy Soc Med 78:373-376, 1985.
65. Hopkins NFG, Spinks TJ, Rhodes CG, Ranicar ASOA, Jamieson CW. Positron emission tomography in venous ulceration and liposclerosis. Br Med J 286:333-336, 1982.
66. Sjerson P. Blood flow in cutaneous tissue in man studied by washout of radioactive xenon. Circ Res 25:215-229, 1969.
67. Cheatle TR, McMullin GM, Farrah J, et al. Three tests of microcirculatory function in the evaluation of treatment for chronic venous insufficiency. Phlebology 5:165-172, 1990.
68. Stibe ECL, Cheatle TR, Coleridge Smith PD, Scurr JH. Liposclerotic skin: A diffusion block or a perfusion problem? Phlebology 5:231-236, 1990.
69. Moyses C, Cederholm-Williams SA, Michell CC. Hemoconcentration and the accumulation of white cells in the feet during venous statis. Int J Microcirc Clin Exp 5:311-320, 1987.
70. Thomas PRS, Nash GB, Dormandy JA. White cell accumulation in the dependent legs of patients with venous hypertension: A possible mechanism for trophic changes in the skin. Br Med J 296:1693-1695, 1988.
71. Scott HJ, McMullin GM, Coleridge Smith PD, Scurr JH. Venous ulceration and the role of the white blood cell. J Med Sci Tech 14:184-187, 1990.
72. Bollinger A, Haselbach P, Schnewlin G, Junger M. Microangiopathy due to chronic venous incompetence evaluated by fluorescence videomicroscopy. In Negus D, Jantet G, eds. Phlebology '85. London: John Libbey, 1986.

73. Franzeck UK, Speiser D, Haselbach P, Bollinger A. Morphologic and dynamic microvascular abnormalities in chronic venous incompetence (CVI). In Davy A, Stemmer R, eds. Phlebologie '89. Montrouge, France: John Libbey Eurotext, 1989, pp 104-107.
74. Braide M, Amundson B, Chein S, Bagge U. Quantitative studies of leukocytes on the vascular resistance in a skeletal muscle preparation. Microvasc Res 27:331-352, 1984.
75. Engler RL, Dahlgren MD, Peterson MA, Dobbs A, Schmid-Schönbein GW. Accumulation of polymorphonuclear leukocytes during three-hour myocardial ischemia. Am J Physiol 251:H93-100, 1986.
76. Romson JL, Hook BG, Kunkel SL, et al. Reduction of the extent of ischemic myocardial injury by neutrophil depletion in the dog. Circulation 67:1016-1023, 1983.
77. Wilson JW. Leukocyte sequestration and morphologic augmentation in the pulmonary network following haemorrhagic shock and related forms of stress. Adv Microcirc 4:197-232, 1972.
78. Linas SL, Shanley PF, Whittenburg D, Berger E, Repine JE. Neutrophils accentuate ischemia-reperfusion injury in isolated perfused rat kidneys. Am J Physiol 255:F728-735, 1988.
79. Yamakawa T, Suguyama I, Niimi H. Behaviour of white blood cells in microcirculation of the cat brain cortex during hemorrhagic shock: Intravital microscopic study. Int J Microcirc Clin Exp 3:554, 1984.
80. Braide M, Blixt A, Bagge U. Leukocyte effects on the vascular resistance and glomerular filtration of the isolated rat kidney at normal and low-flow rates. Circ Shock 20:71-80, 1986.
81. Weissman G, Smolen JE, Korchak HM. Release of inflammatory mediators from stimulated neutrophils. N Engl J Med 303:27-34, 1980.
82. Babior BM. Oxidants from phagocytes: Agents of defense and destruction. Blood 64:959-966, 1984.
83. Coleridge Smith PD, Thomas P, Scurr JH, Dormandy JA. Causes of venous ulceration: A new hypothesis. Br Med J 296:1726-1727, 1988.
84. Cheatle TR, Chittenden SJ, Coleridge Smith PD, Scurr JH. The effect on skin blood flow of short-term venous hypertension in normal subjects. Angiology 42:114-122, 1991.
85. Adams DO, Hamilton TA. The cell biology of macrophage activation. Ann Rev Immunol 2:283-318, 1984.
86. Pober JS. Cytokine-mediated activation of vascular endothelium. Am J Pathol 133:426-433, 1988.
87. Schleef RR, Bevilaqua MP, Sawdey M, et al. Cytokine activation of vascular endothelium: Effects on tissue-type plasminogen activator and type 1 plasminogen activator inhibitor. J Biol Soc 263:5797-5803, 1988.
88. Scott HJ, McMullin GM, Coleridge Smith PD, Scurr JH. A histological study into white blood cells and their association with lipodermatosclerosis and ulceration. Br J Surg 78:210-211, 1990.
89. McCollum CN. Personal communication.
90. Chittenden SJ, Shami SK, Scurr JH, Coleridge Smith PD. Vasomotion in the leg skin of patients with chronic venous insufficiency. Vasa 2:138-142, 1992.
91. Bollinger A, Isenring G, Franzeck UK. Lymphatic microangiopathy: A complication of severe chronic venous incompetence. Lymphology 15:60-65, 1982.
92. Layer GT, Stacey MC, Burnand KG. Stanozolol and the treatment of venous ulceration: An interim report. Phlebology 1:197-203, 1986.
93. Sullivan GW, Carper GT, Novick WJ, Mandell GL. Inhibition of the inflammatory action of interleukin-1 and tumor necrosis factor (alpha) on neutrophil function of pentoxifylline. Infect Immun 56:1722-1729, 1988.
94. Colgan M-P, Dormandy JA, Jones PW, Schraibman IG, Shanik DG. Oxpentifylline treatment of venous ulcers of the leg. Br Med J 300:972-975, 1990.
95. Oxpentifylline for venous leg ulcers. Drug Ther Bull 29:59-60, 1991.
96. Rudovsky G. Intravenous prostaglandin E_1 in the treatment of venous ulcers—A double-blind, placebo-controlled trial. Vasa (Suppl) 28:39-43, 1989.

Chapter 4

Common Anatomic Patterns of Varicose Veins

John J. Bergan

A fundamental tenet in the treatment of any condition is that therapy must be directed at the cause. With varicose veins, the cause of the abnormality is multifactorial. Theories of causation of varicosities are many, and no unifying hypothesis has been offered.

The most important hypotheses of the pathogenesis of primary varicose veins are twofold. The first ascribes varicosities to incompetence of valves located above the saphenofemoral junction and exposure of the saphenofemoral valve rings to transient high pressures.[1] Such varicosities cause the valves to stretch and become incompetent. Repetition of the process ultimately results in dilation and elongation of the saphenous vein and its thin-walled tributaries. This gravitational reflux is aggravated by dynamic forces of intra-abdominal pressure. This theory of descending incompetence agrees with observation of long-standing varicosities in which the entire greater saphenous system, from thigh to midcalf, is involved with the varicose process.

The second hypothesis postulates that the initiating factor in varicose disease is a generalized or focal weakness of vein walls. According to this theory, the thin-walled tributaries to the greater saphenous vein become varicose when they are exposed to normal hydrostatic pressure. Support for this theory is demonstrated in patients with rather uniform and prominent reticular veins in the subcutaneous tissue, any of which have become varicose. Opposition to this hypothesis underlies the regular finding of focal saccular lateral wall blowouts in saphenous veins or tributary veins. A variation of the theory of generalized vein wall weakness is the hypothesis that the initial defect is valvular incompetence in communicating veins of the leg. Such valve failure allows the relatively unsupported subcutaneous veins to be subjected to high pressures generated during intercompartmental muscular exercise.

These hypotheses are not mutually exclusive. Therefore it is possible to bring

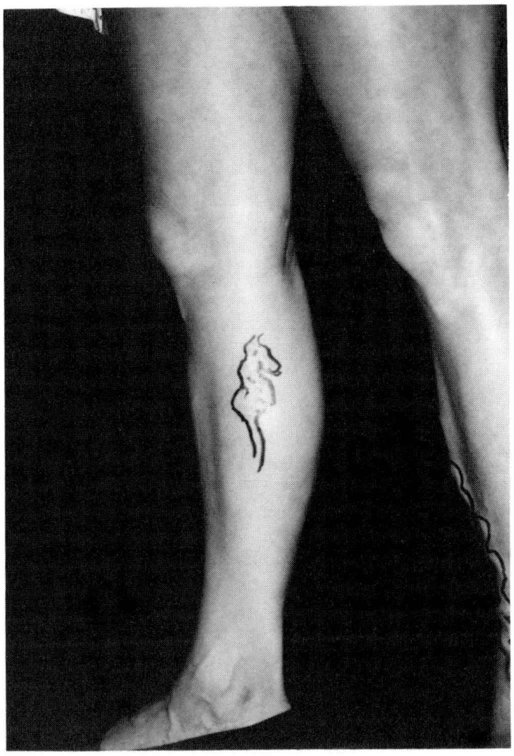

FIGURE 4-1. In some patients with early-developing varicosities, the first cluster appears in the anteromedial calf in association with a Boyd perforating vein, as shown here. Symptoms are aching, heaviness, and localized pain, which can be relieved by local pressure. Ultimate treatment with sclerotherapy or surgical removal of the varicose cluster and perforating vein will relieve the symptoms.

together these theories in order to recognize the patterns of varicosity formation, which is the objective of this chapter.

Observation of patients with varicose veins suggests that in some individuals perforator incompetence becomes the source of varicosities that form a distinctive and recognizable pattern (Figure 4-1). For example, the Boyd perforating vein in the anteromedial calf may become incompetent early in the varicose process. Then the anterior and posterior tributary veins of the greater saphenous system in that location may become varicose as the first finding in varicose disease.[2] Patients with this condition later may develop proximal or distal saphenous venous incompetence. Eventually this condition may lead to reflux in the entire greater saphenous vein (Figure 4-2). Secondary varicosities would appear wherever tributary veins are subjected to resultant high hydrostatic pressure. Furthermore, varicosities could develop from any of the other perforating vein sites and form patterns that are easily recognized or completely aberrant.

Recognition of patterns and relating them to specific perforating veins, many

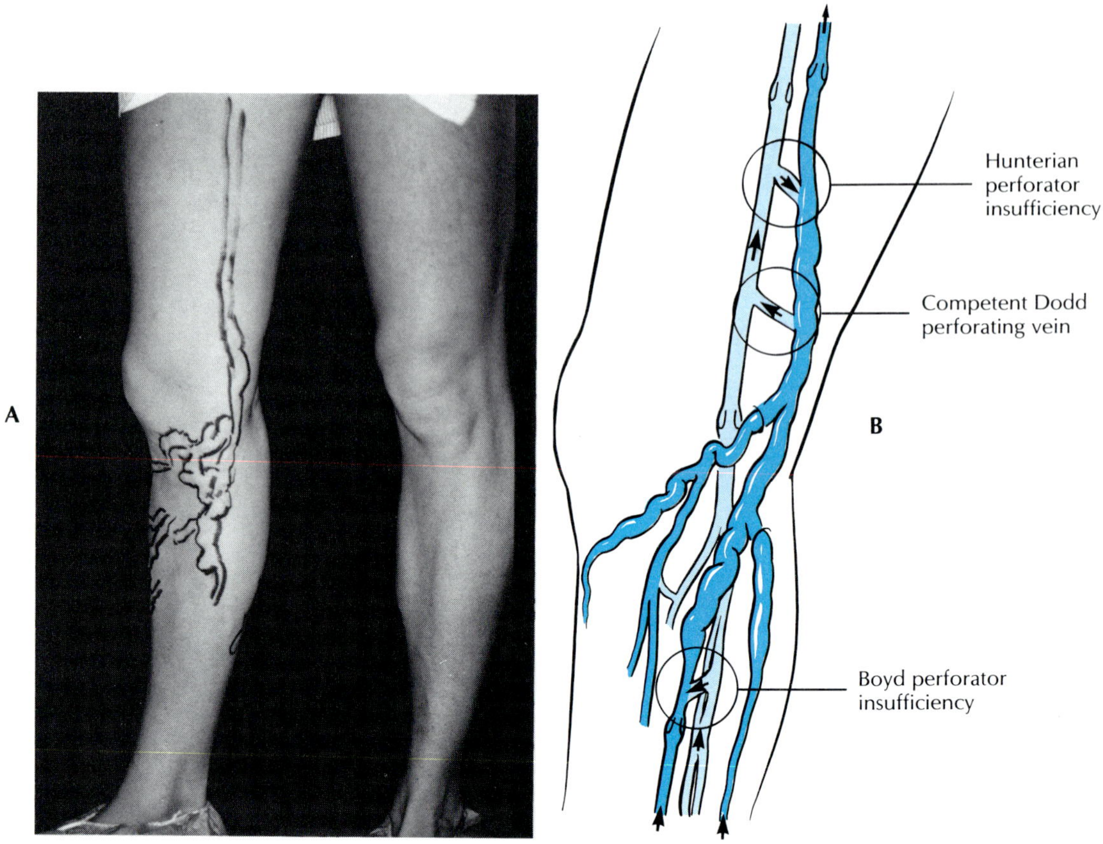

FIGURE 4-2. This photograph (**A**) and accompanying diagram (**B**) show the next stage in progression of varicosities that originate in the anteromedial calf. The refluxing greater saphenous vein in the distal thigh is seen to be dilated, whereas the refluxing greater saphenous vein in the middle third and proximal third of the thigh is less involved but still shows gross reflux.

of which are identified by name, increase our familiarity with various types of primary venous stasis and allow for planning of operations and comparison of patients. Fundamental to recognition of the patterns is a knowledge of superficial venous anatomy and the location of important perforating veins.

NORMAL VENOUS ANATOMY OF LOWER EXTREMITY

Figures 4-3 and 4-4 show the main patterns of normal venous anatomy. Each named vein may be doubled (totally or partially) or absent (entirely or segmentally). This situation accounts for the wide variation in patterns observed in normal veins of the lower extremity.

Of greatest concern to the physician treating venous problems in the lower extremity is the greater saphenous vein (Figure 4-3). The term "saphenous" is derived from the Greek word for "visible."[3] The saphenous vein originates on the dorsum of the foot in the dorsal venous arch, passes anterior to the medial malleolus, progresses through the medial calf across the posteromedial aspect of the

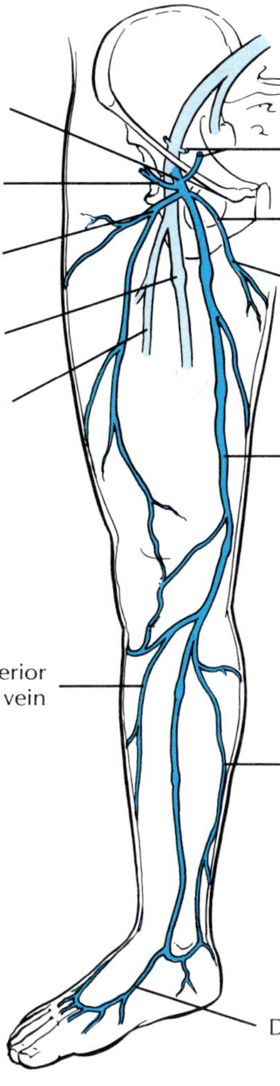

FIGURE 4-3. Normal anteromedial superficial venous anatomy is depicted. The greater saphenous vein ascends from the dorsal venous arch and dominates the anteromedial superficial drainage system. It receives the posterior arch vein (vein of Michelangelo). It also receives variable anterior and posterior tributary veins in the anteromedial calf just below the knee. As the saphenous vein reaches its termination, it receives important tributaries medially and laterally. These tributaries are commonly visualized in duplex ultrasound examinations, which may identify reflux in one or both of these vessels.

popliteal space, ascends in the medial thigh, and terminates in the femoral vein.

The anatomy of the greater saphenous vein is relatively constant. It is well appreciated that this vein lies on the deep fascia of the leg and thigh. However, it is less well recognized that it lies below or deep to the superficial fascia. Even contemporary descriptions of the anatomy of the veins of the lower extremity do not make this distinction.[4] Yet this fact is important to knowledge of the development of varicosities.

In varicose venous anatomy, the important tributaries to the greater saphenous vein extending upward from below are the posterior arch vein, which receives the three Cockett perforating veins; the anterior tributary vein to the saphenous system, which lies below the patella and collects blood from the anterior and lateral surface of the leg; and the posterior tributary vein, which also empties into the greater saphenous vein in the upper anteromedial calf. Other tributaries that may terminate high in the saphenous system near the groin are the posterior medial thigh vein and the anterior lateral thigh vein. Either or both of these veins may become the site of varicose clusters.

Less common in primary varicosities, and more important in recurrent varicose veins after surgery, are other tributaries to the greater saphenous vein as it terminates in the fossa ovalis. These include the superior external pudendal vein, the superior epigastric vein, and the superficial circumflex iliac vein.

Posteriorly, the most important of the axial veins is the lesser saphenous vein (Figure 4-4). This vein originates on the lateral aspect of the foot in the dorsal

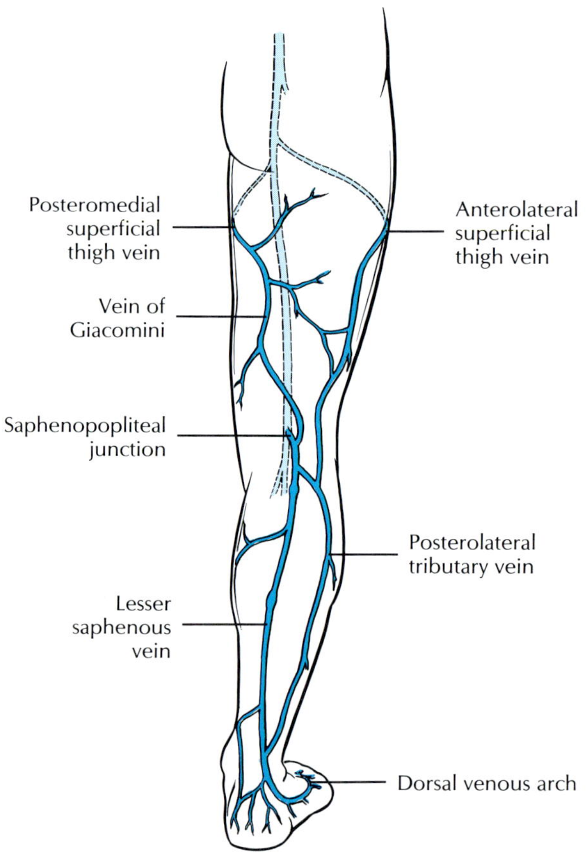

FIGURE 4-4. The lesser saphenous vein dominates the posterolateral superficial venous drainage. It originates in the dorsal venous arch; at the posterolateral ankle, it is intimately associated with the sural nerve. Note the important posterolateral tributary vein and the posterior thigh vein, which ascends and connects the lesser saphenous venous system with the greater saphenous venous system. The anterolateral superficial thigh vein and the posterolateral tributary vein can be very important in congenital venous anomalies such as Klippel-Trenaunay syndrome.

venous arch and ascends virtually in the midline of the calf. Unlike the greater saphenous vein, the lesser saphenous vein may penetrate the deep fascia at any point from the middle third of the calf upward. This fact explains the segmental rather than total nature of reflux that is found in the lesser saphenous vein.

Important tributaries to the saphenous vein are inconstant but may include the posterolateral tributary vein. Superiorly, this tributary may be associated with a lateral thigh vein called the anterior lateral superficial thigh vein. Another important and frequently encountered vein is the ascending superficial vein, which leaves the popliteal space and progresses proximally to join the saphenous vein medially at a point high in the thigh. This vessel is the vein of Giacomini.

The importance of knowing the regular features of the gross anatomy of the superficial veins of the lower extremity is that any one of the systems may be the site of growth of clusters of varicosities. Such clusters can be referred to by the name of the normal vein in that location. All named tributaries to the greater and lesser saphenous system lie superficial to the membranous fascia and are relatively unsupported in comparison to the greater and lesser saphenous vein and the deep veins of the muscular compartments (Figure 4-5).

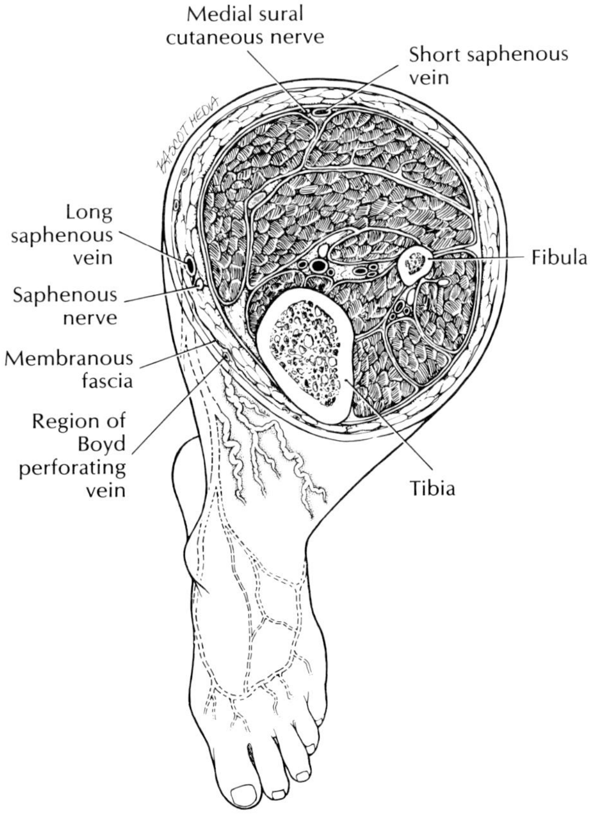

FIGURE 4-5. This diagram illustrates the fact that varicosities lie superficial to the membranous fascia while the saphenous vein lies on the deep fascia and is externally supported by the membranous fascia. Note the proximity of the saphenous nerve to the saphenous vein below the knee. (From Bergan JJ, Kistner RL, eds. Atlas of Venous Surgery. Philadelphia: WB Saunders, 1992, p 36.)

IMPORTANT PERFORATING VEINS

Veins that connect the superficial venous system to the deep venous system and penetrate the fascia are properly called perforating veins. Any one of these veins, or any combination of them, may be the source of the hydrodynamic forces of venous hypertension that produce superficial varicosities. It is the abnormally high pulses of hydrodynamic pressure transmitted through incompetent valves that affect relatively unsupported superficial veins. Such pulses of increased fluid force originate to some extent from increased abdominal pressure and to a greater extent from increased compartmental pressure during muscular contraction.

The best recognized connections between the superficial venous system and the deep venous system are the saphenofemoral and saphenopopliteal junctions. Incompetence of the check valves at their termination has been suggested as the cause of distal varicosities from gravitational reflux. This reverse flow is said to dilate more distal veins in a progressive fashion. As noted earlier, such reflux is neither always present nor is it the cause of highest hydrodynamic pressure.

Because it is frequently the site of the first varicose veins or the first reticular veins that become varicose, the Boyd perforating vein in the anteromedial calf (Figure 4-6) now receives great attention by physicians who treat venous problems.[5] Experience with the duplex scanner reveals that venous incompetence at this level may be isolated and may be the first reflux to appear. Such incompetence may be asymptomatic. However, when the incompetence is symptomatic, it produces aching pain, fatigue, and even a throbbing discomfort. These symptoms can be relieved by firm local pressure. In some patients the next perforator system to become incompetent is the distal thigh perforating vein(s) (Figure 4-7).

The frequency of varicosities in this location is documented in a graph by Cotton[6] that tabulates the number of varices in limbs from the monumental and informative study performed by him in 1957. It was Cotton who pointed out that the "most extreme degree of tortuosity is exhibited by small tributaries which are found close to, and draining into, communicating [perforating] veins." In the figures illustrating Cotton's thesis, one can see the normal deep veins and the abnormal communicating veins *receiving* blood from "intensely tortuous veins which are seen to be varicose tributaries entering the communicating veins."

Reversing this observation, one can visualize pulses of compartmental exercise pressure being delivered to unsupported superficial veins through incompetent perforators (Figure 4-8). Once it is realized that intercompartmental pressure can be transmitted through incompetent check valves of perforating veins to unsupported tributaries of these veins, it can easily be seen how the hydrostatic forces of gravitational reflux are additive to the hydrodynamic forces of muscular contraction. These very high pressures approach 100 mm Hg as they are generated within the muscular compartments. When transmitted outward, they produce localized blowouts or varicosities.

Progressing proximally from the Boyd communicating vein are the perforating veins in the distal third of the thigh. These veins, named for Harold Dodd, may be found in any location along the saphenous pathway in the distal third of the thigh.

The third important series of communicating veins, named for John Hunter, are found in the midthigh. Lea Thomas has surveyed phlebograms to study the

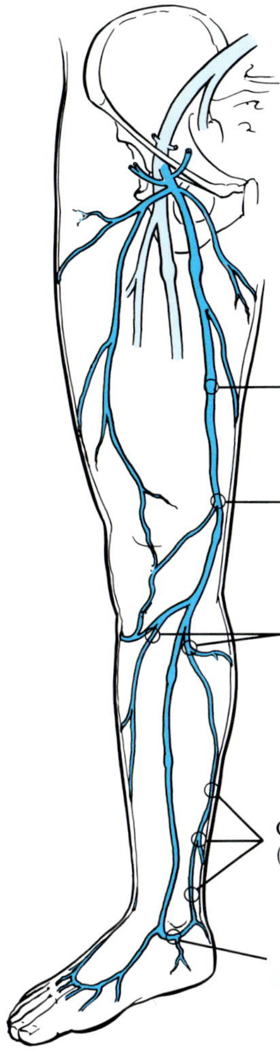

FIGURE 4-6. The location of the most important perforating veins associated with the greater saphenous system are shown. Note that the Cockett and inframalleolar perforating veins are actually separate from the greater saphenous system. The Boyd perforating vein is constantly present, but it may drain the saphenous vein or its tributaries. Perforating veins in the distal third of the thigh are referred to as Dodd perforators, whereas those in the middle third of the thigh are referred to as Hunterian perforators.

anatomy of midthigh perforating veins.[7] He found that 61% of limbs had one or more communicating veins in the middle third of the thigh; in addition, he noted that 27% of the limbs had a perforating vein in the lower third of the thigh. Only 11% of the 100 phlebograms showed no evidence of communicating veins.

A concurrent study from St. Mary's Hospital in London revealed that the incompetent thigh perforating veins were found to occur anywhere in the thigh from the upper edge of the patella to a few centimeters below the saphenofemoral junction. Seventy-one percent were found in the middle third of the thigh, and 20% of the limbs had more than one perforating vein.[8] All the incompetent thigh perforating veins communicated directly with the long saphenous vein. It is interesting to

A

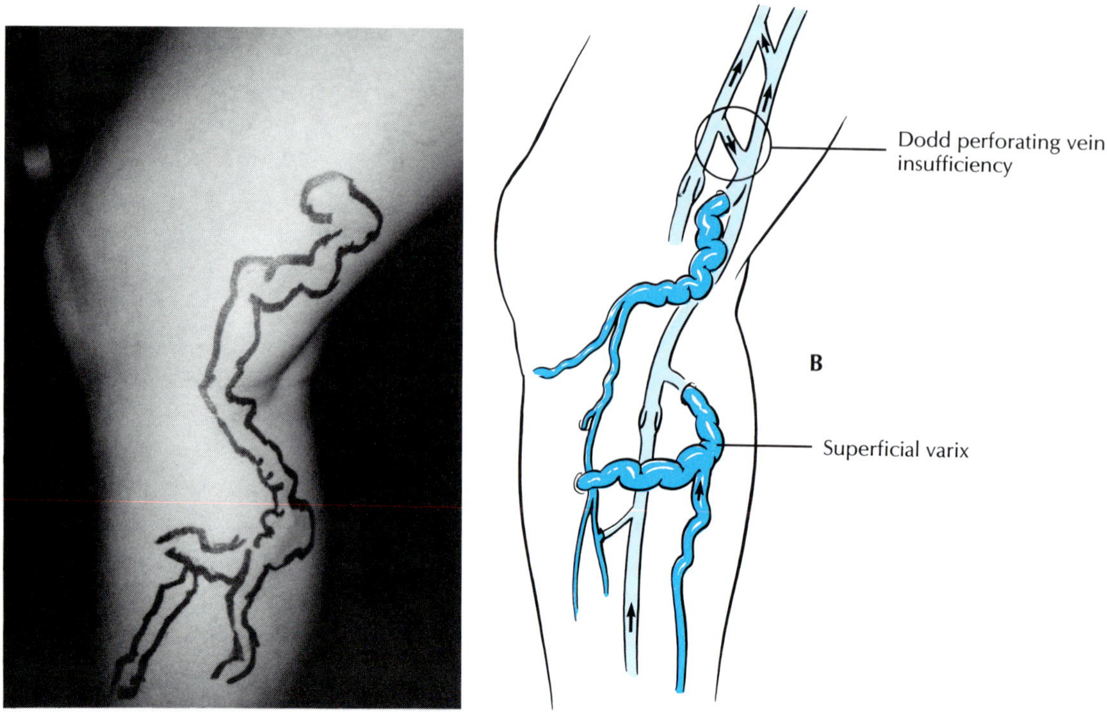

FIGURE 4-7. **A,** This photograph shows varicosities arising from the Boyd perforating vein in the posteromedial calf and the Dodd perforating vein in the distal third of the thigh. Doppler study and duplex confirmation failed to reveal greater saphenous reflux in any other locations. **B,** Depiction of the varicosities and their relationship to localized venous incompetence.

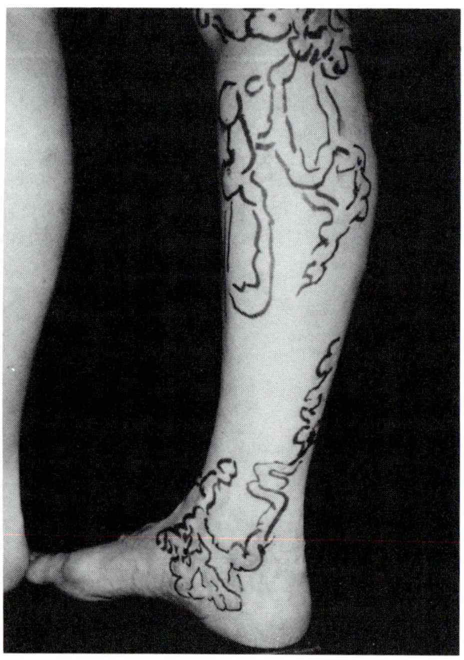

FIGURE 4-8. Combinations of perforating veins producing varying patterns of superficial varicosities present a confusing picture to the untrained eye. Yet a careful look illustrates that the inframalleolar perforating vein (perhaps a Cockett I), a posterior midcalf perforating vein, and the Boyd perforating vein contribute to the pattern seen here.

note that five patients with incomplete saphenous stripping also demonstrated connections of thigh perforating veins to residual saphenous trunks. This observation emphasizes the need for removal of the entire refluxing saphenous vein in the thigh.

Another important perforating vein may be found on the anterior aspect of the thigh, usually in its middle third. This vein connects the deep venous system with superficial clusters of varicosities coursing laterally or medially across the thigh itself. This perforator and its clusters have no relationship to the saphenous veins.

In the leg, the principal communicating veins have been named for Frank Cockett. Many surgeons incorrectly assume that the perforating veins on the medial aspect of the ankle and calf connect the deep system to the greater saphenous vein. That concept is false. These perforating veins actually connect the posterior tibial deep venous system with the posterior arch vein (vein of Michelangelo). Posterior tibial veins are frequently paired, and phlebography may show their connection through perforating veins to the superficial system and the posterior arch vein.[9] Cockett has described the medial communicating veins as if they were relatively constant in location, but they are not. The location is commonly given as the distance from the medial malleolus or the sole of the foot. Figures given above the malleolus are 7, 12, and 18 cm from this point.

Other important perforating veins in the most distal part of the extremity are the inframalleolar perforating vein, frequently the site of a retromalleolar or an inframalleolar painful ulceration. A flare of intradermal telangiectasias below this perforating vein is called the corona phlebectatica (Figure 4-9).

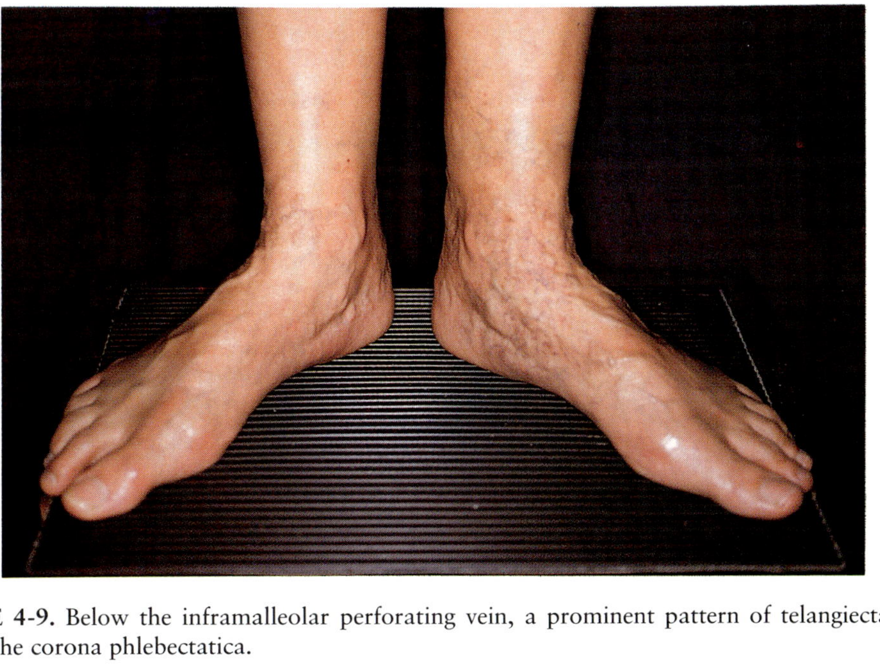

FIGURE 4-9. Below the inframalleolar perforating vein, a prominent pattern of telangiectasias is termed the corona phlebectatica.

Perforating veins on the posterior aspect of the lower extremity are much less well known. However, several are encountered frequently and are found to be the site of origin of varicose clusters. Among these are the lateral thigh perforating vein, which may be located in the middle third of the thigh on its lateral aspect, and the lateral leg perforating vein, also variably located in the middle or proximal third of the calf on its lateral aspect.

PATTERNS OF VARICOSITIES

Recognizing the normal anatomy and the most common perforating vein sources of varicosities makes identification of patterns of varicosities relatively easy. As noted earlier, varicosities arising from the location of the Boyd perforating vein may be the first to appear and may occur in the absence of varicose veins elsewhere in the lower extremity. Such varicosities may consist of the anterior tributary vein varicose cluster or, more commonly, a posterior varicose cluster. Their first manifestations may be pain, aching, and heaviness. Relief may be obtained by applying local pressure and then by performing local excision of the cluster of varicosities and its perforating vein. Whether or not sclerotherapy for this pattern of varicosities will give long-term benefit is undetermined.

Of some importance is the relationship of the saphenous nerve to the Boyd perforating vein and its varicose clusters. In a study of this relationship, the most common vein-nerve pattern was found to be the saphenous vein and saphenous nerve that meet a few centimeters below the knee.[10] Below this point the vein and the nerve were inseparable as far as the medial malleolus. This pattern was noted in 41 of 60 limbs studied. The next most common pattern seen in 10 limbs was the nerve joining the saphenous vein a few centimeters more proximally. Thus, in 50 of 60 limbs, nerve injury could be a problem in limbs in which the saphenous vein was dissected below the Boyd perforating vein. Clusters of varicosities may be isolated or connected with saphenous reflux. They may or may not empty into named perforating veins (Figure 4-10).

Another isolated pattern of varicosities arises from the anterior thigh perforating vein and the anterior lateral tributary vein. These veins may form prominent, ropelike varicosities across the anterior surface of the thigh, coursing laterally and descending on the lateral aspect of the thigh. They may cross the popliteal space and arborize distally on the calf.

Other prominent varicose cluster patterns originate from the perforating veins of Hunter and of Dodd and are sometimes isolated clusters of varicosities. Usually they occur in association with greater saphenous reflux throughout its length. In fact, recognition that these clusters of varicosities are markers of saphenous reflux will alert the interested physician. The probable occurrence of greater saphenous insufficiency, when varicose clusters of the midthigh or the distal thigh are present, then can be confirmed by Doppler study.

In a study intended to classify the clinical appearance of uncomplicated varicose veins, Goren and Yellin[11] found that 71% of the limbs of patients studied demonstrated typical saphenous varicosities. Of the 164 limbs, 147 demonstrated greater saphenous incompetence, whereas only 17 limbs showed lesser saphenous

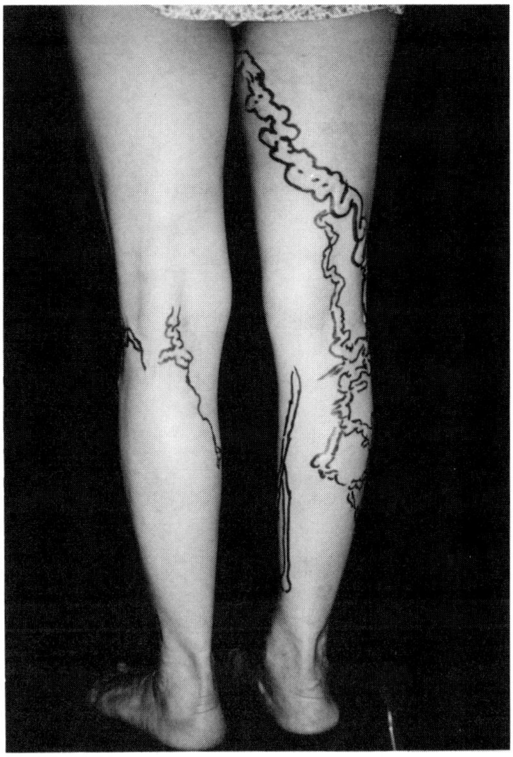

FIGURE 4-10. In this patient, the vein of Giacomini has become varicose in its connection between the lesser saphenous system and the greater saphenous system.

incompetence. Twenty-two percent of the limbs did not show saphenous incompetence; instead they showed isolated perforator vein incompetence. The necessity of reconciling preservation of the saphenous vein for subsequent arterial surgery[12] to the needs of varicose vein surgery is considerably aided by recognizing that greater saphenous incompetence may not be present in some limbs with gross varicosities. In such instances (22% of the limbs in the study by Goren and Yellin), the greater saphenous can be spared, yet the operation can be done properly to remove symptomatic varicosities. The Doppler evaluation and duplex confirmation aid considerably in planning such surgical interventions. However, it also should be understood that in more than 75% of limbs the greater saphenous vein may need to be sacrificed.

Knowledge of the anatomy of the perforating veins, especially those in the medial thigh, has explained why the formerly advocated operation, high ligation of the greater saphenous vein, failed to achieve any of its objectives. Duplex ultrasound scanning has revealed that as many as 80% of these ligated saphenous veins remain patent and that more than half of those showing some thrombosis demonstrated a <10 cm occlusion.[13] Two other duplex ultrasound studies performed in limbs after high saphenous ligation also have confirmed these findings.[14,15]

CONCLUSION

Despite many abnormalities in superficial venous anatomy, patterns of varicose clusters can be recognized. These patterns usually are found in association with named perforating veins. Successful surgical treatment is dependent on removal of the varicosities without the absolute need for identification of the perforating vein itself (see Chapter 10).

REFERENCES

1. Ludbrook J. Primary great saphenous varicose veins revisited. World J Surg 10:954-958, 1986.
2. Thibault P, Bray A, Wlodarczyk J, Lewis W. Cosmetic leg veins: Evaluation using duplex venous imaging. J Dermatol Surg Oncol 16:612-618, 1990.
3. Goldman MP, Fronek A. Anatomy and pathophysiology of varicose veins. J Dermatol Surg Oncol 15:138-145, 1989.
4. Nehler MR, Moneta GL. The lower extremity venous system. I. Anatomy and normal physiology. Perspect Vasc Surg 4(2):104-116, 1991.
5. Boyd AM. Treatment of varicose veins. Proc Roy Soc Med 41:633-639, 1948.
6. Cotton LT. Varicose veins: Gross anatomy and development. Br J Surg 48:589-598, 1961.
7. Tung KT, Chan O, Lea Thomas M. The incidence and sites of medial thigh communicating veins: A phlebologic study. Clin Radiol 41:339-340, 1990.
8. Papadakis K, Christodoulou C, Christopoulos D, et al. Number and anatomical distribution of incompetent thigh perforating veins. Br J Surg 76:581-584, 1988.
9. O'Donnell TF Jr. Surgical treatment of incompetent communicating veins. In Bergan JJ, Kistner RL, eds. Atlas of Venous Surgery. Philadelphia: WB Saunders, 1992.
10. Holme JB, Holme K, Sorensen LS. The anatomic relationship between the long saphenous vein and the saphenous nerve. Acta Chir Scand 154:631-633, 1988.
11. Goren G, Yellin AE. Primary varicose veins: Topographic and hemodynamic correlations. J Cardiovasc Surg 31:672-677, 1990.
12. Mellière D, Cales B, Martin-Jonathan C, Schadeck M. Necessité de concilier les objectifs du traitement des varices et de la chirurgie artérielle: Consequences pratiques. Journal des Maladies Vasculaires 16:171-178, 1991.
13. Friedell ML, Samson RH, Cohen MJ, et al. High ligation of the greater saphenous vein for treatment of lower extremity varicosities: The fate of the vein and therapeutic results. Ann Vasc Surg 6:5-8, 1992.
14. Hammarsten J, Pedersen P, Cederlund C-G, et al. Long saphenous vein–saving surgery for varicose veins: A long-term follow-up. Eur J Vasc Surg 4:361-364, 1990.
15. Rutherford RB, Sawyer JD, Jones DN. The fate of residual saphenous vein after partial removal or ligation. J Vasc Surg 12:422-428, 1990.

PART TWO

Diagnostic Evaluation

Chapter 5

Laboratory Evaluation of Varicose Veins

Paul S. van Bemmelen and David S. Sumner

Noninvasive evaluation of patients with varicose veins is used to detect or rule out valvular incompetence in venous segments that may be difficult to assess through physical examination. Accurate identification of incompetent superficial veins serves the dual purpose of ensuring complete treatment of all involved veins while preserving those that are normal. Such testing also helps to distinguish primary from secondary varicose veins by determining the status of the deep venous system. Ideally, objective methods can be used to replace the more subjective physical examination and offer quantitative information regarding the severity of venous reflux. Application of reliable methods ultimately may improve our understanding of venous pathophysiology and its therapy.

This chapter is concerned with the most useful tests for patients with varicose veins. Emphasis is placed on noninvasive tests that give the clinician information that affects therapeutic decisions. The tests are discussed in historical order, with invasive methods preceding noninvasive methods. In clinical practice, noninvasive tests are done before invasive ones.

DIAGNOSTIC TESTS

Ambulatory Venous Pressure

Although measuring foot vein pressure after exercise may provide important physiologic information, this method is cumbersome and therefore is not routinely used. For two reasons, ambulatory venous pressure (AVP) cannot be considered a preferred method for evaluating varicose veins: (1) venous puncture on the dorsal foot can be painful and technically demanding, and (2) interpretation of results may be difficult.[1]

When varicose veins are accompanied by changes in chronic cutaneous venous stasis, finding an elevated AVP merely confirms the clinical diagnosis of venous hypertension. Early studies of this method compared AVP with ascending venography. Patients were usually stratified on the basis of history and physical examination. Improvement of refilling time with application of a tourniquet was assumed to indicate uncomplicated superficial vein incompetence. These early AVP studies have not been repeated with varicography, saphenography, or descending venography, which would provide a more solid basis for topographic accuracy.

Theoretically, normalization of refilling time would not take place if proximal perforators connect the superficial hydrostatic column to the deep system. In practice, many patients have patterns of combined deep and superficial vein incompetence that are uncontrollable by tourniquet application even if selective occlusion of superficial veins were possible.[2] Based on a study of the highly variable (40 to 300 mm Hg) tourniquet pressures required to occlude incompetent superficial veins, it seems unlikely that tourniquets would provide reliable compression.[3] After it was suggested that similar information could be obtained noninvasively through the use of photoplethysmography, direct pressure measurements virtually disappeared from daily practice.[4]

Photoplethysmography

Photoplethysmography (PPG), like light reflection rheography, measures the reflection of infrared light by red blood cells in cutaneous capillaries. Dorsal or plantar flexion of the foot reduces the amount of blood in the dermal plexus. On cessation of exercise, a curve is obtained that is similar in shape to an AVP recording. Since this method is simple and inexpensive, it is a useful screening tool for initial assessment of venous disease.[5] The original validation of the method in 1979 compared PPG results to those of direct venous pressure measurements.[4] A high correlation coefficient was found when groups of patients with severe venous disease were compared to normal controls. The original patient group studied contained only 14 patients with uncomplicated varicose veins, and the expectation that PPG would be useful to localize incompetence in the great saphenous system was never prospectively verified with an imaging technique. The claim was made that a tourniquet occluding an incompetent superficial vein would normalize an abnormally short refilling time.[5,6] A prospective study in 1990 compared the results of PPG to those of segmental duplex scanning in 151 symptomatic legs.[2] The kappa coefficient of overall agreement was 0.12 ± 0.06, a value approaching zero. When attention was focused on the calf segment of the greater saphenous vein (which was considered to be readily amenable to tourniquet occlusion), the greater saphenous vein was found to be incompetent more often when the PPG refilling time was normal than when the PPG indicated superficial incompetence. Thus the use of tourniquets represents a large source of error in the evaluation of venous insufficiency.[3]

When attention was turned to the results of PPG obtained without the use of a tourniquet, refilling times could not be used to discriminate between normal patients and those with venous incompetence at one, two, or three levels of the leg. Only in the most extensive degree of incompetence, level four, did PPG have a sensitivity greater than 49%; this group of patients is easily recognized clinically by ulceration or obvious skin changes. PPG offered no improvement over clinical inspection of gaiter area skin made prior to laboratory evaluation.

Since PPG recordings in different areas of the same leg have led to different results, it seems that PPG refilling time is more apt to reflect local superficial hemodynamics than the hemodynamics of the entire limb venous system.[7] PPG refilling time may be related to dermal microscopic valvular status.[8] It is likely that PPG and light reflection rheography measurements will continue to provide information regarding microcirculatory changes, but PPG should not play a role in the decision to treat saphenous veins.

Air Plethysmography

In the 1960s, plethysmography was pioneered and applied to the study of varicose veins. Allan[9] described changes in leg vein volume that occur as a result of varicose disease. Recently, a new air plethysmograph has become available commercially. It differs from previous devices in that it has a larger chamber to surround the entire calf. A sensitive recorder makes possible volume readings as small as 2.5 ml. With this device, quantitative measurements of reflux from above-knee to below-knee veins are feasible. The amount of reflux has been related to disease severity and incidence of ulceration.[10,11] The foot is not enclosed in the air cuff, and reflux from ankle to foot would, at least in theory, affect APG measurements paradoxically. Reduction of the volume of venous reflux after removal of varicosities has been documented.[12] Leg volume after exercise correlates to direct venous pressure measurements when legs of normal volunteers are compared to legs with active or healed ulceration reminiscent of those of the first photoplethysmography studies.[13]

To distinguish between superficial and deep reflux, the air plethysmography device relies on proper application of a tourniquet that occludes superficial veins. As noted previously, the tourniquet is a source of error: at times successful occlusion of a long saphenous vein is accomplished easily, but occlusion of the subfascial lesser saphenous vein may be impossible in the legs of obese individuals, leading to a false diagnosis of deep vein incompetence. Although air plethysmography equipment is less expensive than a duplex scanner, topographic information is paramount in the treatment of varicose veins.

Portable Doppler Ultrasound

The portable continuous-wave Doppler device is probably the single most helpful tool for experienced clinicians. It can quickly and noninvasively detect incompetent veins, even when these veins are not visible.[14,15]

The purpose of continuous-wave Doppler examination is to discern the relationship of existing varicose veins to the saphenous system, to assess the competency of the greater and lesser saphenous veins, and to determine if the deep venous system is obstructed. For optimal examination, the patient should be in a standing position. Standing allows for the filling of incompetent venous reservoirs so that when compression of these reservoirs is released, flow can be detected with the

Doppler probe. Examination of the patient in a supine position may yield erroneous results since thin-walled accessory branches are often collapsed or will collapse with external pressure from the Doppler probe. The examination of venous segments distal to the groin is unreliable with regard to retrograde flow elicited by a Valsalva maneuver.[16] Proximal compression of the limb by hand is not a reliable way to promote retrograde flow and valve closure, although a qualitative, subjective impression often can be obtained through this approach.[17] The best method for examining the popliteal fossa and the rest of the leg is with the patient standing,[18] with his/her weight supported by the contralateral leg and the knee of the leg under study slightly flexed.[19,20] A systematic approach from top to bottom includes the venous confluence in the groin and the greater saphenous vein in the thigh, including its anterolateral and posteromedial branches. At the knee level, the medial aspect is examined for both the main greater saphenous vein and the accessory or secondary saphenous vein. Often, the greater saphenous vein runs posterior to the femoral condyle and connects to the deep or lesser saphenous system.

Examination is continued from the anterolateral aspect of the patella to the lateral aspect of the knee. Superficial veins in this area may be anterolateral branches of the greater saphenous vein[21] or may form part of a separate lateral system of dilated subdermal veins.[22] Examination of the popliteal fossa is most demanding. The examiner can best determine the location of the popliteal vein by first locating the popliteal arterial signal. It is possible, however, to mistake sural arteries for the popliteal artery in obese patients and, subsequently, to mistake the gastrocnemius vein or the lesser saphenous vein for the popliteal vein. The distinction between the lesser saphenous vein and more superficially located subcutaneous branches can be difficult. A prudent approach is to consider an all-negative examination of the popliteal fossa as constituting sufficient screening. With reflux at the popliteal fossa, additional study with an instrument that has imaging capabilities usually is necessary for accurate diagnosis.

Examination of the lower leg must be tailored to the individual patient since virtually all areas of the lower leg can be affected with varicosities. The anatomic relationship between superficial branches and the greater and lesser saphenous veins can be assessed by positioning the probe over the saphenous veins and listening during release of compression of the superficial convolutions. Pretibial branches usually are connected to the greater saphenous vein. Posterior tibial veins at the level of the ankle are located alongside the artery and are assessed by release of foot compression. Reflux at this level often occurs because superficial veins are located in the path of the ultrasound beam; it rarely is associated with the deep ankle veins themselves. Therefore the use of a portable Doppler to localize incompetent ankle perforators has limited accuracy.[23]

Failure to detect incompetent veins with the continuous-wave Doppler technique in clinical practice is possible when the patient is obese and superficial varicose veins are located at a depth of several centimeters. In this situation the use of a lower-frequency Doppler probe is indicated. Often only one portable probe is used (8 MHz), an approach that is less versatile than using separate low-frequency (5.4 MHz) and high-frequency (9.3 MHz) probes.

Duplex Scanning and Color Flow Imaging

Some clinicians might question the need for the expensive equipment involved in duplex scanning and color flow imaging to view simple varicosities. Certainly, many patients have adequate diagnosis and treatment of their varicose veins without duplex scanning. This argument depends in large part on the weight of the patient involved. Obesity is very common in the United States, with 25% of the population weighing in excess of 120% of their ideal body weight. In many of these patients the visible varicosities represent the tip of an "iceberg," with the "iceberg" itself not amenable to clinical examination. The consequences of incomplete therapy due to incomplete examination are often more troublesome than performing duplex scanning prior to therapy.

The basic principle of ultrasonic duplex scanning is the combination of B-mode echographic imaging and pulsed-wave Doppler ultrasound beams to allow examination of vessels at a specific depth. This approach is based on the principle that the amount of time between emission and reflection of the ultrasound beam is related to the distance that the ultrasound travels in tissue. The sample volume can be directed at the vein at a specific angle. With the newer color flow machines, the Doppler signals are depicted as colored pixels in the B-mode image. The Doppler principle of maintaining an angle smaller than 90 degrees to the direction of blood flow is paramount in obtaining reliable data with these devices.

The automatic cuff inflator consists of an air compressor that inflates and deflates pneumatic cuffs within 0.3 seconds. This device is used instead of manual compression of the leg and has replaced the Valsalva maneuver, which can generate reflux only in proximal veins and depends on the variable presence of iliac vein valves.[17]

The patient is examined in the standing position as described for continuous-wave Doppler examination.[24] Since the patient needs to place his/her weight on the contralateral leg and keep the knee slightly flexed, a frame or walker is needed for balance. The reflux test maneuver can be standardized with pneumatic cuffs. This technique was originally devised for examination of deep veins[25] and may not be as important in the examination of superficial varicose veins, which often can be emptied by manual compression. Some authors, who subsequently adopted this method, also have used distal cuff deflation at multiple levels of the leg.[26] Since the status of deep veins is often unpredictable from clinical information alone, a complete examination is recommended.[27]

The examination begins at the groin, with the examiner directing the duplex probe at the confluence of the common femoral and greater saphenous veins. A pneumatic cuff (24 cm wide) placed around the thigh is inflated to 80 mm Hg for 3 seconds. Reflux then is measured as the cuff is rapidly deflated. The sample volume is placed in the common femoral vein, the greater saphenous vein, and the proximal superficial femoral vein, in turn. In normal limbs, reflux during closure of competent valves does not exceed 0.45 seconds. When the color flow scanner is used, reflux is evident as persistent flow. In borderline incompetence, the use of spectrum analysis is recommended for more precise timing.

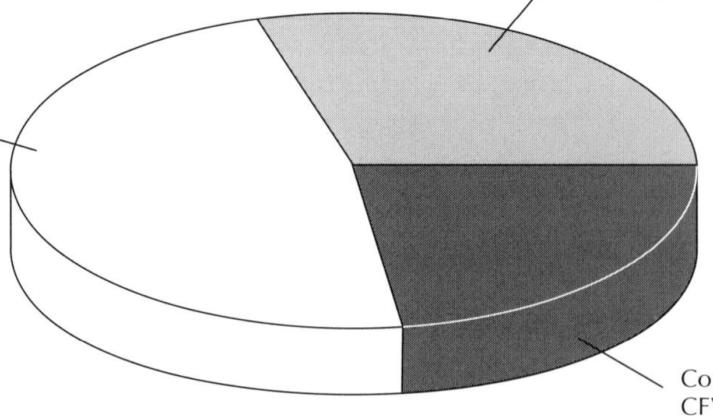

FIGURE 5-1. Association of deep and superficial incompetence near the inguinal ligament. Combined incompetence of the common femoral vein and the greater saphenous vein (true saphenofemoral incompetence) occurs in a minority of patients. N = 55 unoperated legs with reflux. CFV, common femoral vein; GSV, greater saphenous vein.

Even though saphenofemoral incompetence is frequently noted in clinical practice, 78% of 55 unoperated legs with reflux in this area involved isolated incompetence of either the common femoral vein only or isolated incompetence of the proximal great saphenous vein with a normal common femoral vein (Figure 5-1). This finding has important implications for the rationale of simple ligation: if no saphenofemoral incompetence is present initially, the hemodynamics will be unchanged after simple ligation of the proximal great saphenous vein.

A quick screening test to evaluate outflow can be done at this point by rapidly inflating a cuff applied to the calf to a pressure of 100 mm Hg. If the antegrade velocity in the proximal superficial femoral vein reaches 143 ± 29 cm/sec during cuff inflation, significant obstruction in the popliteal–superficial femoral vein segments is unlikely.[28] This test adds only a few minutes to the study and helps to distinguish patients with primary varicose veins from those with secondary varicose veins.

The popliteal fossa is examined with a cuff placed below the knee. After inflation of the cuff for 3 seconds, reflux in the popliteal vein and lesser saphenous vein is measured as the cuff is deflated (Figure 5-2). Although the lesser saphenous vein usually enters the popliteal vein, the termination point is highly variable and must be accurately localized. Both atypical termination of the lesser saphenous vein into the greater saphenous vein and high termination into the superficial femoral vein or profunda vein have been described.[29] Continuation of the lesser saphenous vein as a sciatic vein is more common than the arterial counterpart of this anatomic variation. Multiple connections of the lesser saphenous vein to the gastrocnemial and popliteal veins also occur.

The medial side of the knee is examined to assess flow in the greater saphenous vein and additional accessory veins (Figure 5-3). Incompetent greater saphenous

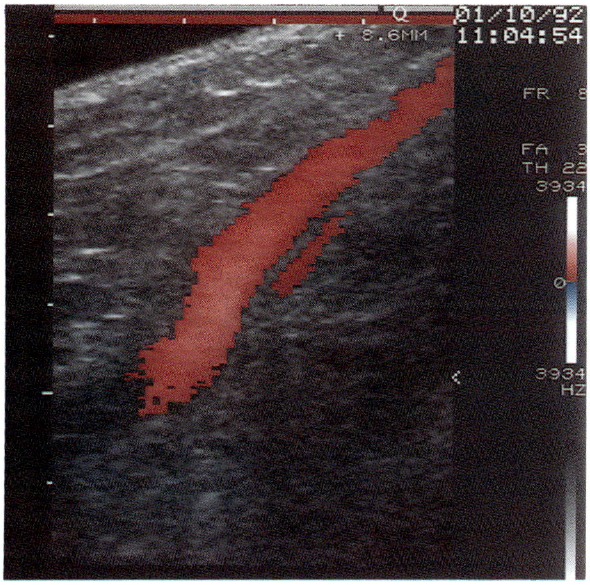

FIGURE 5-2. Incompetent lesser saphenous vein at back of knee. Incompetence of this vein was not evident clinically because of deep location of the vein in the subcutis. Head of patient is toward left. Flow toward the feet is depicted in red.

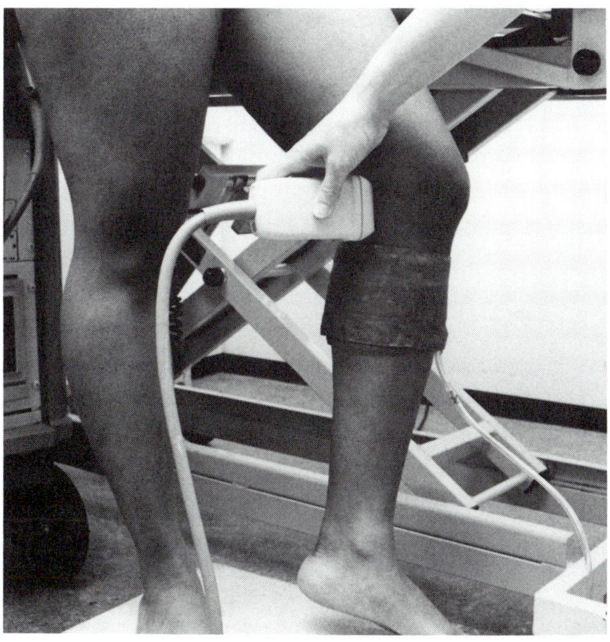

FIGURE 5-3. Examination of medial aspect of the knee. Reflux is measured during deflation of cuff.

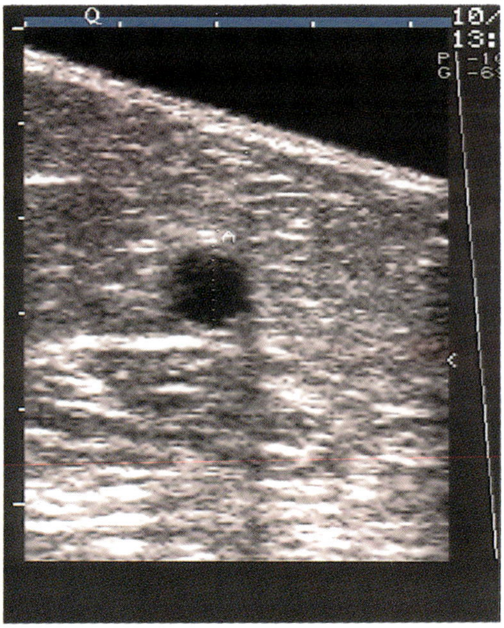

FIGURE 5-4. Cross-sectional view of incompetent greater saphenous vein of male patient presenting with severe weeping stasis dermatitis. Diameter at the knee is 8.3 mm. Depth from the skin is 13.8 mm.

veins can present as straight dilated vessels (Figure 5-4). It is possible to calculate the volume of reflux flow from the diameter of incompetent veins and the velocity of retrograde flow.[30,31] In spite of previous stripping operations or sclerotherapy, incompetent veins are frequently present on the medial side of the knee.[32] After a previous stripping operation, recurrent or accessory saphenous veins can remain as straight vascular structures (Figure 5-5). In other cases the greater saphenous vein is replaced by a conglomerate of convoluted veins (Figure 5-6) in which it is impossible to identify the flow direction. The anterolateral branch of the greater saphenous vein can be identified only if significant dilatation has occurred. In one study, scanning the anterolateral aspect of the thigh near the patella yielded incompetent anterolateral branches in 20% of referred patients.[2]

The calf level is examined with the cuff placed around the ankle. At this level the greater saphenous vein often consists of two branches. Evaluation of the deep calf veins, including the peroneal veins, is facilitated by color imaging.[33] The lesser saphenous vein can be identified at the midcalf level by its straight course and deep position in the posterior midline. Reflux within this segment of the lesser saphenous vein can occur without concomitant incompetence of the proximal part.

Veins at the ankle level are examined with a small (7 cm wide) cuff placed around the foot. An inflation pressure of 120 mm Hg is used. The posterior tibial veins are easily located behind the medial malleolus and alongside the artery. Unless the greater saphenous vein has been previously removed, it can be examined at its premalleolar site. Anterior branches of the greater saphenous vein can be identified

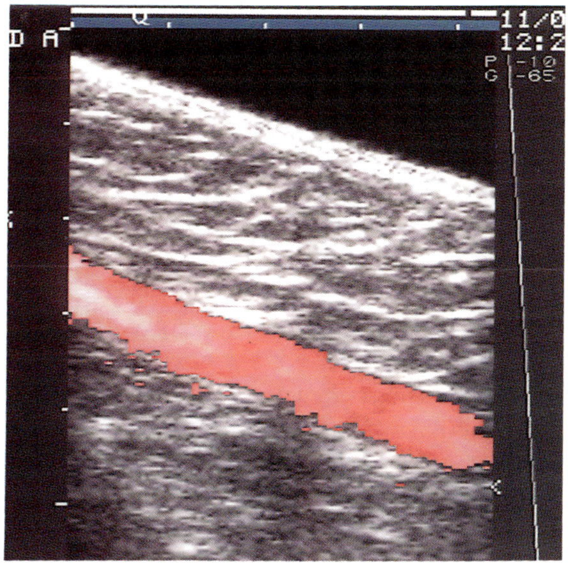

FIGURE 5-5. Recurrent incompetence of the great saphenous vein above the knee, after previous stripping operation. Head of patient is toward left. Reflux is depicted in red.

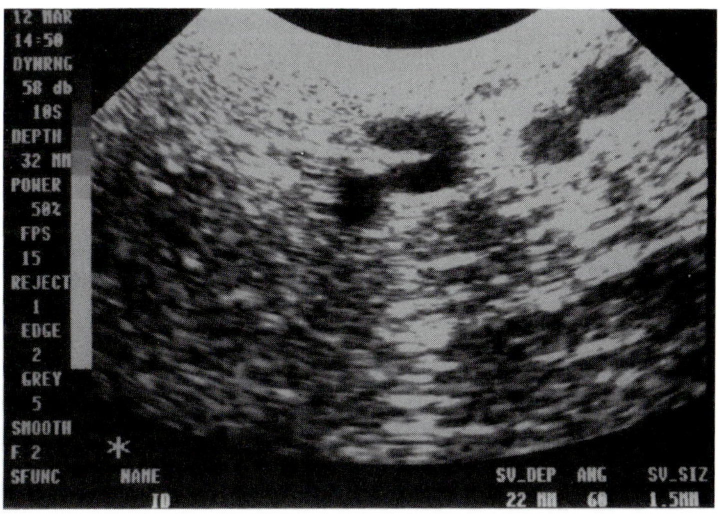

FIGURE 5-6. Typical tortuous varicosities are located in the subcutis at medial aspect of the knee.

in the pretibial area in 13% of subjects. Further imaging of the posterior arch veins and gaiter area can be done if changes in chronic venous stasis complicate the picture. Using duplex scanning, certain authors have confirmed the high incidence of superficial disease in patients with stasis ulceration.[34] A detailed search of the gaiter area for incompetent perforating veins has been described,[35] but the hemodynamic significance of small perforating veins near the ankle is unclear.

DISCUSSION

Laboratory evaluation of patients with varicose veins is useful if it makes a difference with regard to the modality or extent of treatment. For example, accessory veins on the medial side of the leg are easily mistaken for the greater saphenous vein (Figure 5-7), a problem that may account for some controversy regarding the relative efficacy of sclerotherapy and surgery. Comparison of treatment results is possible only if saphenous vein identification is done with a reliable method and if patients are accurately stratified according to the presence of saphenofemoral incompetence with reflux in the common femoral vein vs. isolated reflux limited to the greater saphenous vein in conjunction with a normal common femoral vein. The most reliable method for exact classification is duplex ultrasound. This technique also provides important follow-up data after surgery or sclerotherapy.

With regard to recurrent varicose veins, they may be either actual residual varicose veins caused by incomplete removal during the first operation or they may represent true recurrences. With early recurrence the possibility of secondary varicose veins resulting from deep venous disease must be kept in mind. A complete duplex evaluation of both deep and superficial veins can help identify this situation prior to treatment. Reducing the extent of surgery by limiting treatment to incompetent venous segments ensures the preservation of normal veins and reduces the incidence of inadvertent damage to saphenous and sural nerves.

The distinction between multiple recurrences of primary varicose veins and chronic venous insufficiency is often unclear in practice; evaluation of venous calf pump function with the air plethysmograph can be relevant in complicated situations.

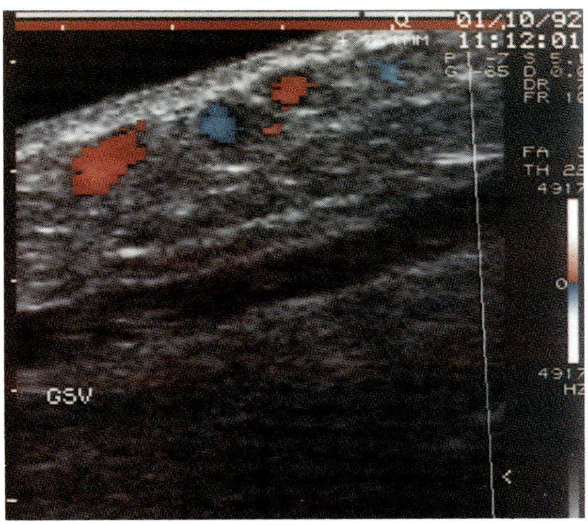

FIGURE 5-7. Longitudinal view at medial side of the knee. Incompetence of superficially located tortuous accessory vein is noted. Reflux is depicted in red and blue because of tortuosity with varying Doppler angles. Absence of reflux in the normal, more deeply located greater saphenous vein is shown in black. This absence was noted during deflation of a cuff placed around the calf.

CONCLUSION

For lean patients with readily visible varicosities, examination of the popliteal fossa and the saphenofemoral area with a portable Doppler device may be all that is needed. If, however, reflux is noted at the back of the knee or if patency of the popliteal vein is in question, duplex examination is recommended. Duplex scanning also is indicated for obese patients with varicose veins, patients with recurrent varicose veins, and those with complaints of severe stasis or ulceration.

REFERENCES

1. Randhawa K, Dhillon S, Kistner RL, Ferris EB. Assessment of chronic venous insufficiency using dynamic venous pressure studies. Am J Surg 148:203-209, 1984.
2. van Bemmelen PS, van Ramshorst B, Eikelboom BC. Photoplethysmography reexamined: The lack of correlation with duplex in venous insufficiency. Surgery 112:544-548, 1992.
3. McMullin GM, Coleridge Smith PD, Scurr JH. A study of tourniquets in the investigation of venous insufficiency. Phlebology 6:133-139, 1991.
4. Abramowitz HB, Queral LA, Flinn WR, Nora PF, Peterson L, Bergan JJ, Yao JST. The use of photoplethysmography in the assessment of venous insufficiency: A comparison to venous pressure measurements. Surgery 86:434-441, 1979.
5. Flinn WR, Queral LA, Abramowitz HB, Yao JST. Photoplethysmography in the assessment of chronic venous insufficiency. In Nicolaides AN, Yao JST, eds. Investigations of Vascular Disorders. New York: Churchill Livingstone, 1981, Chapter 32.
6. Barnes RW. Noninvasive techniques in chronic venous insufficiency. In Bernstein EF, ed. Noninvasive Diagnostic Techniques in Vascular Disease. St. Louis: CV Mosby, 1985, Chapter 84.
7. Rosfors S. Venous photoplethysmography: Relationship between transducer position and regional distribution of venous insufficiency. J Vasc Surg 11:436-440, 1990.
8. Braverman IM, Keh-Yen A. Ultrastructure of the human dermal microcirculation. IV. Valve containing collecting veins at the dermal-subcutaneous junction. J Invest Dermatol 81:438-442, 1983.
9. Allan JC. Volume changes in the lower limb in response to postural alterations and muscular exercise. South African J Surg 2:75-90, 1964.
10. Christopoulos D, Nicolaides AN, Szendro G. Venous reflux: Quantification and correlation with the clinical severity of chronic venous disease. Br J Surg 75:352-356, 1988.
11. Christopoulos D, Nicolaides AN, Cook A, Irvine A, Galloway JMD, Wilkinson A. Pathogenesis of venous ulceration in relation to the calf muscle pump function. Surgery 106:829-835, 1989.
12. Christopoulos D, Nicolaides AN, Galloway JMD, Wilkinson A. Objective noninvasive evaluation of venous surgical results. J Vasc Surg 8:683-687, 1988.
13. Welkie JF, Kerr RP, Katz ML, Comerota AJ. Can noninvasive venous volume determinations accurately predict ambulatory venous pressure? J Vasc Technol 15:186-190, 1991.
14. Sumner DS. Evaluation of the venous circulation using the ultrasonic Doppler velocity detector. In Rutherford RB, ed. Vascular Surgery. Philadelphia: WB Saunders, 1977.
15. Folse R, Alexander RH. Directional flow detection for localizing venous valvular incompetency. Surgery 67:114-121, 1970.
16. van Bemmelen PS, Beach K, Bedford G, Strandness DE. The mechanism of venous valve closure. Arch Surg 125:617-619, 1990.
17. van Bemmelen PS, Bedford G, Beach K, Isaac CA, Strandness DE. Evaluation of tests used to document venous valve incompetence. J Vasc Technol 14:87-90, 1990.
18. Mitchell DC, Darke SG. The assessment of primary varicose veins by Doppler ultrasound—The role of saphenopopliteal incompetence and the short saphenous systems in calf varicosities. Eur J Vasc Surg 1:113-115, 1987.

19. Nicolaides AN, Fernandes é Fernandes J, Zimmerman H. Doppler ultrasound in the investigation of venous insufficiency. In Nicolaides AN, Yao JST, eds. Investigation of Vascular Disorders. New York: Churchill Livingstone, 1981, Chapter 28.
20. Schull KC, Nicolaides AN, Fernandes é Fernandes J, Miles C, Horner J, Needham T, Cooke ED, Eastcott FHG. Significance of popliteal reflux in relation to ambulatory venous pressure and ulceration. Arch Surg 114:1304-1306, 1979.
21. Goren G, Yellin AE. Primary varicose veins: Topographic and hemodynamic correlations. J Cardiovasc Surg 31:672-677, 1990.
22. Albanese AR, Albanese AM, Albanese EF. Lateral subdermic varicose vein system of the legs. Vasc Surg 3:81-89, 1969.
23. O'Donnell TF, Burnand KG, Clemenson G, Lea Thomas M, Browse NL. Doppler examination vs. clinical and phlebographic detection of the location of incompetent perforating veins. Arch Surg 112:31-35, 1977.
24. Szendro G, Nicolaides AN, Zukowski AJ, Christopoulos D, Malouf GM, Christodoulou C, Myers K. Duplex scanning in the assessment of deep venous incompetence. J Vasc Surg 4:237-242, 1986.
25. van Bemmelen PS, Bedford G, Beach K, Strandness DE. Quantitative segmental evaluation of venous valvular reflux with duplex ultrasound scanning. J Vasc Surg 10:425-431, 1989.
26. Czeredarzuk M, Branas CC, Weingarten MS. Duplex imaging and distal cuff deflation to measure venous reflux time. J Vasc Technol 15:196-208, 1991.
27. van Bemmelen PS, Bedford G, Beach K, Strandness DE. Status of the valves in the superficial and deep venous system in chronic venous disease. Surgery 109:730-734, 1991.
28. van Bemmelen PS, Bedford G, Beach K, Strandness DE. Functional status of the deep venous system after an episode of deep venous thrombosis. Ann Vasc Surg 5:455-459, 1990.
29. Franco G, Nguyen Khac G, Nguyen Morere MC. Intérêt de l'écho Doppler de la saphène externe. Confrontation clinique. Phlebologie 43:135-145, 1990.
30. Vasdekis SN, Clarke GH, Nicolaides AN. Quantification of venous reflux by means of duplex scanning. J Vasc Surg 10:670-677, 1989.
31. Bergan JJ, Beeman S, Poppiti R. Quantitative segmental evaluation of venous valve reflux: Impact on clinical practice. Vienna, Vascular European-American Symposium on Venous Diseases. Nov 7-10, 1990.
32. Bishop CRC, Fronek HS, Fronek A, Dilley RB, Bernstein EF. Real-time color duplex scanning after sclerotherapy of the great saphenous vein. J Vasc Surg 14:505-510, 1991.
33. van Bemmelen PS, Bedford G, Strandness DE. Visualization of calf veins by color flow imaging. Ultrasound Med Biol 16:15-17, 1990.
34. Hanrahan LM, Araki CT, Rodriguez AA, Kechejian GJ, LaMorte WW, Menzoian JO. Distribution of valvular incompetence in patients with stasis ulceration. J Vasc Surg 13:805-812, 1991.
35. Hanrahan LM, Araki CT, Fisher JB, Rodriguez AA, Walker TG, Woodson J, LaMorte WW, Menzoian JO. Evaluation of the perforating veins of the lower extremity using high-resolution duplex imaging. J Cardiovasc Surg 32:87-97, 1991.

Chapter 6

Pretreatment Testing of Patients With Varicose Veins and Telangiectatic Blemishes

Ulrich Schultz-Ehrenburg

A physical examination is conducted before sclerotherapy or surgical treatment of varicose veins for many different reasons. These reasons are related to the therapeutic indications and contraindications, anatomic and functional venous findings, treatment plans, and prospects for lasting results.

The contraindications for sclerotherapy include (1) deep vein thrombosis, (2) lymphedema, (3) arterial occlusive disease, (4) immobility, and (5) severe general disease. A deep vein thrombosis is an absolute contraindication. The induced phlebitis triggered by sclerotherapy can impair venous hemodynamics and lead to unpredictable thrombotic reactions. In cases of chronic lymphedema, injections involving the affected leg, as well as surgical measures, are usually inadvisable. The iatrogenic inflammation can further damage the defective lymphatic system, causing further deterioration of lymphatic flow.[1]

Arterial occlusive disease is a relative contraindication to sclerotherapy. Combinations of arterial occlusive disease and varices are encountered particularly after 50 years of age. In these cases the pathophysiologic state is such that negative interactions occur among the various therapeutic measures. At an advanced stage, arterial occlusive disease can interfere with all effective forms of therapy for chronic venous insufficiency (CVI). Patients with this type of mixed vascular disease are unable to elevate their legs, wear compression stockings, or walk with bandaged legs to improve the impaired venous return. For this reason, measuring systolic pressure of the malleolar arteries with the Doppler probe is the first diagnostic measure undertaken before sclerotherapy for patients older than 50 years. This approach also applies to younger patients with corresponding clinical symptoms. If a decrease in systolic blood pressure relative to systemic pressure can be demonstrated, it is advisable to proceed with extreme caution. The hyperemia induced by sclerotherapy can increase the disproportion between blood supply and blood requirements. Poorly healing ulcerations may result.

The following figures serve as a rule of thumb: at pressures <100 mm Hg, varix operations and injections of the lower leg should not be considered; at pressures <80 mm Hg, compression treatment generally is not tolerated since compression may cause the arterial perfusion pressure to decrease to critical values.[2]

Additional contraindications include immobility and severe general diseases. As a general rule, it is stipulated that patients should walk for 30 minutes after sclerotherapy. Otherwise there is a danger that the sclerosing agent will drain poorly and pass into the deep veins, causing a deep vein thrombosis.

CLINICAL EXAMINATION

The medical history provides information about the patient's past and present complaints and his/her motives for seeking consultation. Visual inspection and palpation permit clinical classification with respect to many different factors, especially the type of varix and the clinical stage of CVI.

Varices can be subdivided clinically into two groups comprising the five types of genuine varicose veins:

1. Large varicose veins
   a. Trunk varicosities
   b. Branch varicosities
   c. Incompetent perforators
2. Small varicose veins
   a. Reticular varicosities
   b. Telangiectasias

Refluxes play a decisive role in the pathogenesis of large varices. They are usually detected over the saphenofemoral junction or the saphenopopliteal junction. Identification of these refluxes represents an important area of application for Doppler ultrasonographic techniques. When perforators become incompetent, they may become an additional source of refluxes. Such refluxes are called "blowouts." Usually a protrusion in the area of the blowout is detected by visual examination, and palpation reveals an enlarged fascial gap.

The second important clinical objective is to correctly assess the degree of CVI. Not all varices meet the requirements for CVI. For example, telangiectasias and reticular veins do not represent a disturbance of venous function. Likewise, mild forms of trunk and branch varices (and even incompetent perforators) do not necessarily trigger functional disturbances. Not until these major varices exert a hemodynamic effect do they meet the requirements for venous insufficiency, which is naturally chronic (i.e., a CVI). Approximately 80% of all cases of CVI are caused by a decompensation of varicose veins, whereas the remainder are caused by a post-thrombotic syndrome. Functionally, CVI is characterized by a deterioration of venous function. Another name for CVI is calf pump insufficiency.

Venous function can be evaluated quantitatively by inserting a catheter into a dorsal foot vein to measure venous pressure. Noninvasive examination methods also are available, in particular, photoplethysmography.

CVI can be divided into three clinical stages (see box, p. 87). Edema and corona phlebectatica characterize stage I. Stage II is distinguished by various cutaneous complications occurring below the level of a leg ulcer. I believe that eczema and pigmentation are not linked to any particular clinical stage. They may appear during stage I and may be missing at more advanced stages. Stage III is manifested

CLINICAL STAGES OF CHRONIC VENOUS INSUFFICIENCY

Stage I
- Edema
- Corona phlebectatica

Stage II
- (Eczema, dermatitis)
- (Purpura, pigmentation)
- Fibrosing panniculitis
- Lipodermatosclerosis
- White atrophy (atrophie blanche)
- Stasis papillomatosis

Stage III
- Venous ulcer
- Ulcer scar

by a healed or current venous ulcer. These three clinical stages do not correspond to the division into three degrees of venous insufficiency that can be done on the basis of photoplethysmography.

Highly effective, noninvasive examination methods are available for further evaluation of varicose veins. A distinction must be made between anatomic and functional apparative methods. For routine diagnostic purposes, venous Doppler ultrasonography is the most important anatomic method, and photoplethysmography is the most important functional examination method. I believe that clinical tests such as the Perthes test, the Linton test, and Trendelenburg's test, all of which are frequently recommended in textbooks, can be dispensed with entirely because they are imprecise by modern diagnostic standards.

DIAGNOSTIC METHODS

Photoplethysmography

Photoplethysmography is a method of quantitatively evaluating venous function. The devices used measure changes in the blood volume of the skin brought about by calf pump activity. These devices include an optical sensor that emits infrared light. The infrared light penetrates the skin to a depth of approximately 3 mm; the light is partly absorbed and partly reflected. Blood vessels reflect about 10 times less infrared light than does cutaneous tissue. If the blood volume in the area being measured is decreased, for example, by muscular activity, the average skin reflection rises.

During measurement the patient needs to perform 8 or 10 dorsiflexions while sitting. The probe usually is located 10 cm above the inner ankle. During muscle exercise a curve is produced similar to that obtained by invasive measurement of venous pressure. Muscle movement causes a change in the degree of filling of cutaneous blood vessels and thus in the degree of light reflection, until the maximum amount of blood has been pumped out of the leg. In the subsequent resting phase,

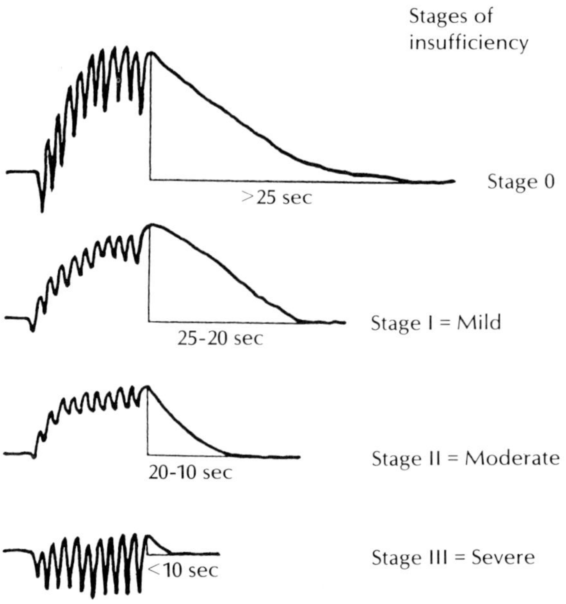

FIGURE 6-1. Assessment of calf pump function by photoplethysmography.

the vessels of a healthy person refill slowly by arterial inflow. In patients with varices, the vessels refill more quickly by means of venous refluxes. This action leads to a shortening of the refilling time.

The refilling time thus provides a quantitative measure of the capability of the calf muscle pump. According to a generally accepted system of classification, there are three degrees of insufficiency.[3] Degree III corresponds to a refilling time of <10 seconds; degree II, to a refilling time of 10 to 20 seconds. Degree I corresponds to a refilling time of 20 to 25 seconds; values >25 seconds are considered normal (Figure 6-1). Although only these refilling time values (T_0) could be evaluated with older devices, modern quantitative photoplethysmographic devices also enable a determination of amplitude of venous pump power (V_0).[4] Further details of photoplethysmography are described in other sources.[5-8]

The muscle pump test measures venous function as a whole. A more detailed picture of the underlying CVI can be obtained with the aid of a tourniquet test. The examination distinguishes between improvable and nonimprovable CVI, which will be explained later in this chapter.

Doppler Ultrasonography

Venous Doppler ultrasonography is the second important diagnostic method for evaluating venous function. This examination provides information about the competence or incompetence of an individual vein. During examination, S sounds must be differentiated from A sounds. S sounds represent spontaneous flow sounds and are important in the diagnosis of a thrombosis. A sounds, or augmented sounds, represent artificial accelerations of flow caused by manual compression. In combination with Valsalva's maneuver, A sounds are used to diagnose reflux in the varicosis.

Doppler ultrasonography is most frequently used for examination of the long saphenous vein, which is verified by Valsalva's maneuver. By means of abdominal pressure, blood is forced in a retrograde direction. Retrograde blood flow is not possible, however, if the venous valves of the long saphenous vein are intact. When valvular incompetence of the saphenofemoral junction exists, reflux occurs and is registered by the Doppler probe as a sharp flow sound. With the Doppler probe, the reflux can be followed along its entire length; therefore this technique can be used to determine the origin and course of a varicose reflux.

Valsalva's maneuver is not suitable for examining the short saphenous vein since this vein does not have a connection of its own to the pelvic region. For this reason manual compression and decompression are performed in the lower part of the vein while the Doppler probe is positioned above the saphenopopliteal junction. The decompression phase is decisive for diagnosis. In the event of valvular incompetence, the pull exerted by the decompression leads to a reflux that can be heard with the Doppler probe. If the valves are intact, no reflux sound is heard.

The Doppler probe is suitable not only for examining the superficial veins but also for diagnosing refluxes of the deep veins.[9] By using five test methods, it is possible to accurately detect refluxes of the deep venous system. These methods are calf compression, calf decompression, thigh compression, thigh decompression, and Valsalva's maneuver. Two examples are provided here to illustrate the use of these methods.

Refluxes in the ankle region play an important role in the pathogenesis of CVI. They can be examined by means of calf compression (Figure 6-2). The Doppler probe is placed in the ankle region above the anterior or posterior tibial veins, and a deep calf compression is performed. In the event of incompetent valves, a loud reflux sound is heard over the malleolar vein; this sound is absent if the valves are intact.

The popliteal vein can be tested by means of calf decompression, thigh compression, and Valsalva's maneuver (Figure 6-3). During the entire examination the Doppler probe is positioned above the popliteal vein. A Doppler sound heard during calf decompression is evidence of reflux extending from the hollow of the knee downward, whereas a Doppler sound noted during thigh compression is evidence of reflux extending from the thigh downward to the hollow of the knee. A Doppler sound heard during Valsalva's maneuver indicates reflux extending from the pelvis to the hollow of the knee.

By systematically applying the diagnostic methods available for detecting superficial and deep venous refluxes, it is possible to obtain a detailed picture of the superficial and deep veins in the leg. This approach plays an important role in formulating an accurate treatment plan.

The efficiency of the Doppler probe can be seen, in particular, in cases of atypical saphenous varices. These are trunk varices of the long saphenous vein with a negative Valsalva segment proximally and a positive Valsalva segment distally. This condition also is called a paradoxical reflux. In reality, the reflux is not para-

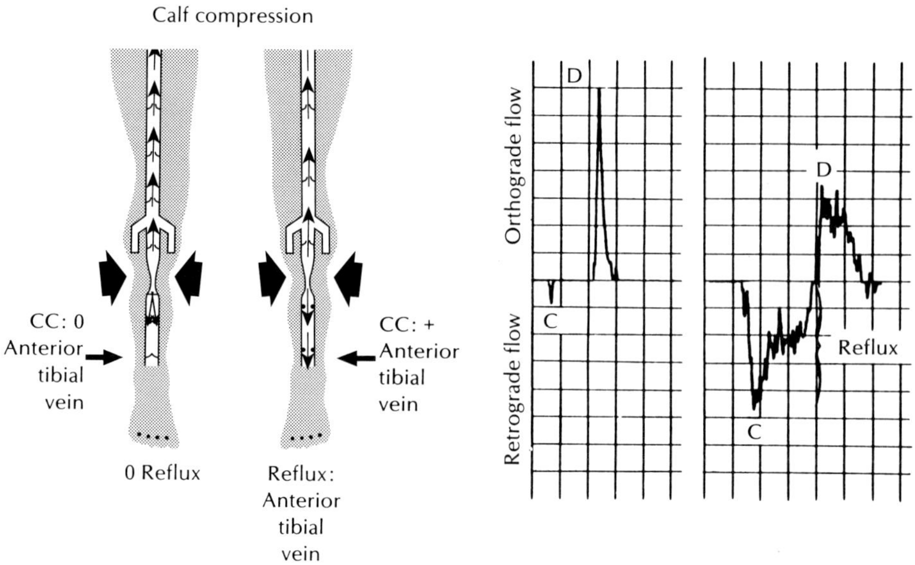

FIGURE 6-2. Diagnosis and documentation of deep refluxes in ankle region. CC, compression of calf; C, compression; D, decompression.

doxical; the intact proximal venous segment is circumvented via collateral veins. In this context two types of atypical refluxes can be differentiated: (1) simple atypical refluxes with a superficial collateral circulation, and (2) hidden atypical refluxes with a deep collateral circulation (see box, p. 95). Additional methodological details and exact instructions regarding examination techniques have been described.[9]

The benefits of noninvasive diagnostic methods make them an indispensable part of the routine diagnostic workup. The examination methods provide a great deal of information without placing a burden on the patient; consequently they can be repeated as often as desired. Today photoplethysmography and Doppler ultrasonography are part of the basic phlebologic diagnostic arsenal. They represent the examination methods of choice and in most cases obviate the necessity for resorting to invasive methods. There is no reason to deny photoplethysmographic or Doppler ultrasonographic examination to a patient with a genuine varicosis or more severe phlebological findings. In the event of contradictory results, however, the diagnosis should be confirmed with invasive methods (e.g., direct venous pressure measurement or phlebography).

CHRONIC VENOUS INSUFFICIENCY

The results of the photoplethysmographic examination do not provide information as to whether the underlying vein incompetence is superficial or deep. For this reason the examination is repeated with the tourniquet test, in which a cuff placed below the knee occludes varicose refluxes in the long and short saphenous

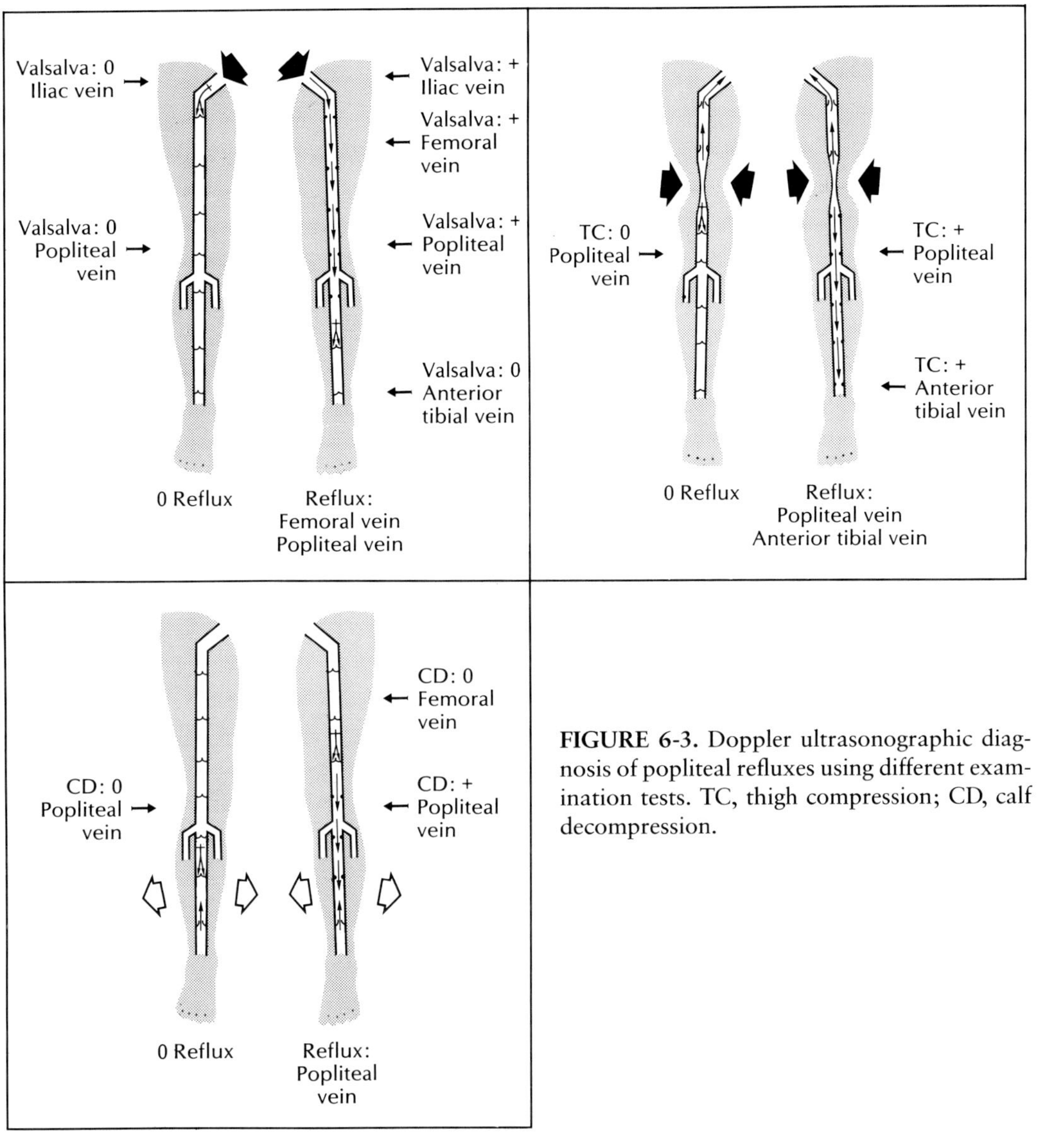

FIGURE 6-3. Doppler ultrasonographic diagnosis of popliteal refluxes using different examination tests. TC, thigh compression; CD, calf decompression.

veins. Two different results can be obtained: improvement or nonimprovement of venous function, referred to as improvable or nonimprovable CVI (Figure 6-4).

Improvable CVI generally indicates superficial vein incompetence, whereas nonimprovable CVI most often indicates deep vein incompetence, usually in connection with a postthrombotic syndrome. Incompetent perforators also can simulate nonimprovable CVI within the scope of a genuine varicosis; this condition is called falsely nonimprovable CVI (see Figure 6-4). Finally, deep vein thrombosis also can result in nonimprovable CVI. Therefore several explanations are possible for a tourniquet test result of nonimprovable CVI.

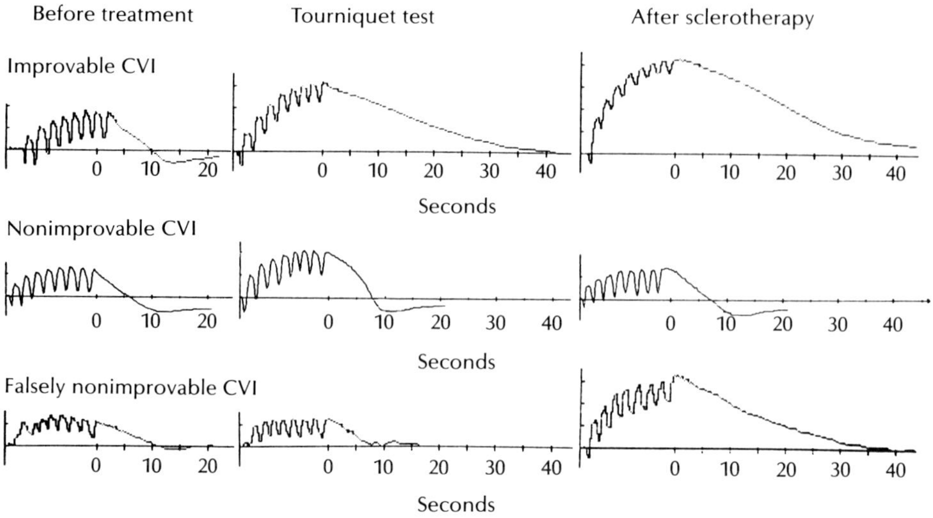

FIGURE 6-4. Photoplethysmographic findings in improvable, nonimprovable, and falsely nonimprovable chronic venous insufficiency (pretherapeutic tourniquet test and findings after complete varix elimination).

Improvable Chronic Venous Insufficiency

Improvable CVI constitutes a clear indication for invasive varix treatment (i.e., surgery and/or sclerotherapy). In these cases the tourniquet test has clearly demonstrated that calf pump insufficiency can be improved by eliminating the varices. The foremost value of photoplethysmographic examination thus lies in this objective identification of an indication. Consequently this technique also should be used after the treatment has been completed and to detect recurrences at follow-up examinations.

Nonimprovable Chronic Venous Insufficiency

The management of nonimprovable CVI is quite different. Since the majority of cases are caused by deep vein incompetence, eliminating the varices makes little sense. In this situation the dominant pathologic condition is the deep venous disturbance, which cannot be corrected by treating the superficial varicose veins. Patients must wear medical compression stockings their entire lives, especially when they exhibit cutaneous complications or edema or have subjective complaints. This kind of treatment cannot cure CVI; however, it can compensate for the condition. Complete varix elimination is no longer necessary and, in fact, is not advisable. Such therapy would not eliminate the need for compression therapy, which the patient may be tempted to discontinue because of the improved cosmetic results.

The Doppler probe should be used in every case to confirm whether a nonimprovable venous function is actually caused by a deep venous incompetence. In many cases Doppler ultrasonography reveals a completely normal deep venous system. In the clinical setting these patients regularly show multiple incompetent perforators of the lower leg, so that the missing improvement during the tourniquet test can be explained by the blowout refluxes. In these cases the result of the Doppler examination of the deep veins is of prime importance for deciding on therapy.

Falsely Nonimprovable Chronic Venous Insufficiency

If Doppler ultrasonographic examination shows competent deep veins, I do not base a treatment plan on the tourniquet test result. Instead, I perform a complete varix treatment for these patients, with preference given to sclerotherapy. After completion of therapy, the functional result is checked with photoplethysmography. In most cases a normalization of venous function is observed, which confirms the diagnosis of falsely nonimprovable CVI retrospectively.

In such situations the incompetent perforators are probably the reason for the negative result of the tourniquet test. This theory presupposes that the incompetent perforators are located below the tourniquet and that they have a hemodynamic effect, which appears to be the case in only a minority of patients with clinically incompetent-appearing perforating veins. The question arises whether the effect of these perforating veins can be excluded by lowering the tourniquet. Since the photoplethysmographic sensor normally should be placed 10 cm above the inner ankle, the advantages gained by lowering the tourniquet are limited. Even when the tourniquet is lowered, perforating veins often remain more distally.

Combined Photoplethysmography and Doppler Ultrasonography

The diagnostic possibilities of photoplethysmography increase when this method is used in conjunction with Doppler ultrasonography. With the Doppler method, the competence of the deep veins can be checked directly rather than indirectly. In this way contradictions can be discovered quickly and the conclusions can be used to determine the most effective treatment for the patient. It is necessary only to correlate the findings from photoplethysmography with those from Doppler ultrasonography to differentiate among improvable CVI, nonimprovable CVI, and falsely nonimprovable CVI (Figure 6-5).

Determination of Need for Doppler Ultrasonography

The question may arise about whether it is necessary to use Doppler ultrasonography in every case of CVI. Figure 6-5 provides guidelines for making such a determination. If photoplethysmography reveals improvable venous function, the results are clear-cut. In such situations Doppler ultrasonography can be dispensed with since the indication for an invasive treatment (i.e., stripping and/or sclero-

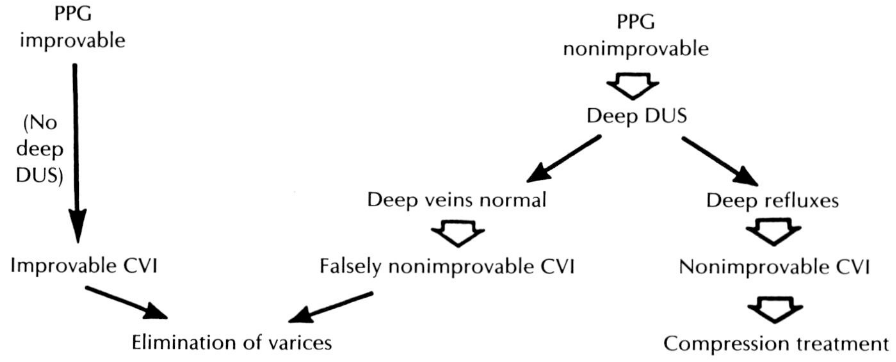

FIGURE 6-5. Flow chart of noninvasive checkup before invasive varix treatment for chronic venous insufficiency. PPG, photoplethysmography; DUS, Doppler ultrasonography.

therapy) is unquestionable. If photoplethysmographic examination shows nonimprovable venous function, Doppler ultrasonographic examination of the deep veins of the leg is required to distinguish between truly and falsely nonimprovable venous function. Patients with falsely nonimprovable CVI also should receive complete treatment of varicose veins. Since venous function can be completely normalized in many cases, the phlebologist should not “shy away” from this indication. I prefer successive sclerotherapy to one-time surgical treatment because injection treatments can be followed up step by step both clinically and photoplethysmographically.

SAPHENOUS VARICES

One of the greatest mistakes made by physicians who are performing sclerotherapy is that they limit injections to those venous segments that can be recognized by the naked eye as varicose veins. A comparable mistake made by surgeons performing vein surgery is that they often prefer standard operations, even when the actual findings call for a modified procedure. The pitfalls accompanying both of these frequently observed modes of behavior are seen, in particular, in connection with atypical saphenous varices.

Atypical Saphenous Varices

Atypical saphenous varices are characterized by atypical reflux paths, whereas typical saphenous varices are distinguished by typical reflux paths. Typical saphenous refluxes exhibit junctional valvular incompetence, with reflux passing through the proximal trunk. Visible varices may affect the trunk and branches. Atypical refluxes are refluxes that circumvent proximal venous segments via collateral circu-

ATYPICAL SAPHENOUS VARICOSE VEINS

Simple Atypical Refluxes

Reflux in long saphenous vein transmitted by a lateral branch
Reflux in double long saphenous vein
Reflux in long saphenous vein transmitted by external pudendal veins
High-ending, incompetent long saphenous vein
Reflux in short saphenous vein transmitted by long saphenous vein

Hidden Atypical Refluxes

Reflux in long saphenous vein transmitted by perforating veins
Reflux in lateral veins transmitted by perforating veins
Reflux in short saphenous vein transmitted by femoropopliteal vein
Reflux in short saphenous vein transmitted by a high-ending femoropopliteal vein

lation. A distinction can be made between simple and hidden atypical refluxes (see box), as illustrated by the two examples presented here.

One well-known example is incomplete trunk varicosis of the perforator type. Doppler examination reveals a negative Valsalva segment in the junctional region and the proximal long saphenous vein; a clear reflux sound is noted in the distal truncal segment. For purposes of classification, a deep reflux examination of the external iliac vein and the femoral vein is necessary. The reflux runs from the external iliac vein and the femoral vein across one or more perforating veins into the long saphenous vein (Figure 6-6).

This type of reflux belongs to a group of hidden atypical refluxes that consist of a combination of superficial and deep venous segments. The proximal trunk of the long saphenous vein is sufficient and is circumvented by deep venous reflux. A complete ankle-to-groin stripping should not be done because it would sacrifice an intact venous segment. The most proximal location for surgery or sclerotherapy is the uppermost incompetent perforator, which must be ligated or injected before treatment is directed toward the dependent insufficient segments.

In contrast to hidden atypical refluxes, simple atypical refluxes consist of superficial venous segments along their entire length. The most well known example is a branch type of incomplete trunk varicosis in which the proximal trunk of the long saphenous vein is circumvented by an insufficient tributary and a connecting vein (Figure 6-7). The entire length of the reflux can be followed by the Doppler probe, even if there is no visible varicose dilatation.

Atypical saphenous varices occur in 20% of all genuine varices.[10] In addition to the two reflux paths described, seven types of atypical refluxes can be differentiated. Because of the diversity exhibited by these refluxes, clinical examination alone

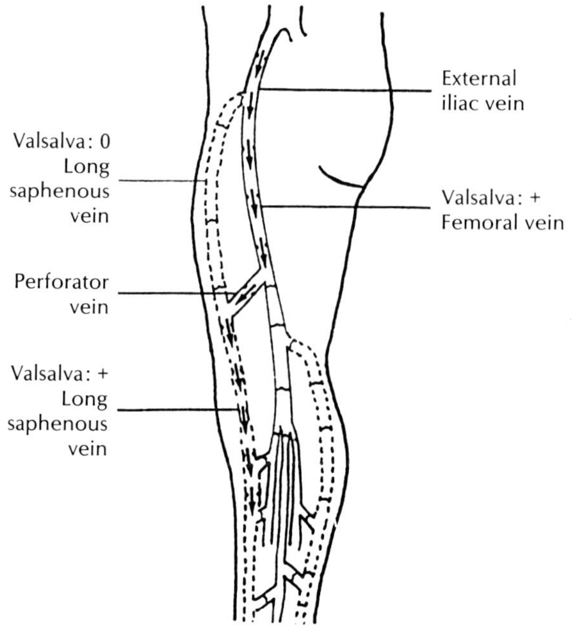

FIGURE 6-6. Doppler findings with hidden atypical reflux of long saphenous vein transmitted by perforating veins.

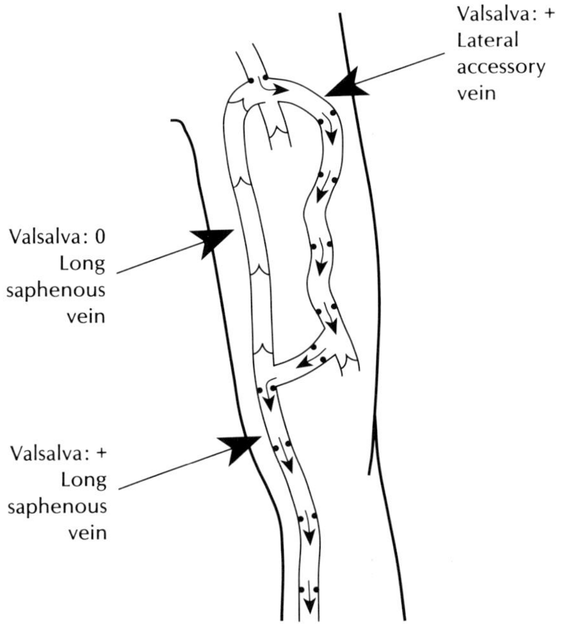

FIGURE 6-7. Doppler findings with simple atypical reflux of long saphenous vein transmitted by a lateral branch.

is not sufficient for establishing an optimal treatment plan. Frequently it is not possible to determine the origin of reflux during clinical examination. For this reason Doppler examination of the superficial venous system is essential in every case of genuine varicosis. This type of examination is the best way to determine the origin, length, and course of venous reflux.

The trend in modern phlebology is clearly away from sacrificing competent venous segments. The long saphenous vein is a valuable "spare part" used in arterial bypass surgery. For this reason routine stripping of the long saphenous vein cannot be accepted as a treatment for atypical saphenous varices. It is necessary to exclude the most proximal escape point and the pathologic reflux path and to occlude or remove the varicose segments via surgery and/or sclerotherapy. In cases of hidden atypical refluxes, the uppermost incompetent perforating vein of the long saphenous vein is the uppermost therapeutic location. In cases involving simple atypical refluxes, the superficial collateral reflux path located "upstream" also must be eliminated.

Atypical saphenous varices constitute an excellent indication for sclerotherapy. The disappearance of collateral refluxes can be demonstrated by normalization of Valsalva reflux from positive to negative.

Typical Saphenous Varices

For typical saphenous varices, high ligature and stripping of the long saphenous vein are now considered the treatment of choice. The remaining branches lend themselves to sclerotherapy. Thus the patient is spared unnecessary (and often disfiguring) scars. Nevertheless, there are patients, probably more in Europe than in America, who would prefer no treatment rather than undergo surgery. In these cases sclerotherapy with injection of the saphenous junction is an alternative treatment that is particularly recommended for the short saphenous vein. Although all trunk varices can be treated surgically, patients eligible for sclerotherapy must be selected carefully.

The risk associated with sclerotherapy that is not associated with varix surgery is recanalization. However, the recanalization rate is not the same for all patients. A decisive factor is whether the patient has reflux of the popliteal or femoral vein in addition to saphenous reflux. Five years after successful primary junction obliteration of the short saphenous vein, my associates and I observed recanalization in 73% of patients with reflux of the popliteal and femoral veins. In those patients with only saphenous reflux, the recanalization rate was only 27%.[9] A similar situation exists with respect to the long saphenous vein. These Doppler-controlled long-term observations show that lasting saphenous junction obliteration can be achieved in a high percentage of patients who have trunk and branch varicosis but no deep refluxes. Thus a precise Doppler diagnosis offers at least some patients the possibility of receiving conservative treatment.

In order to select suitable patients, Doppler examination of the superficial and deep venous system is necessary. Investigation of the deep venous system can be limited to examining the femoral and popliteal veins by means of Valsalva's maneuver. Those patients in whom a deep reflux is demonstrated at these locations should be advised of the high risk of recanalization and referred for surgery.

INJECTION SCLEROTHERAPY FOR TELANGIECTATIC BLEMISHES

In contrast to large varices, small varices represent a condition in which refluxes and hemodynamic factors do not play an important role. If no contraindications are known, in principle no impediment to injection treatment of telangiectatic blemishes and reticular varices exists. Sclerotherapy is the treatment of choice, one for which there is no surgical alternative. The injections are performed according to cosmetic visual criteria, with sclerotherapy always being started with the vessel in front of the branching. Apart from this requirement, no hierarchic treatment plan is required.

In their pure form, small varices do not require any apparative diagnostic measures. However, they may occur in combination with large varicose veins. Therefore I recommend that, even for these two types of varices, photoplethysmography and Doppler ultrasonography be performed to measure venous function and to detect refluxes of the saphenous veins. This approach ensures that medically relevant findings are not overlooked.

SUMMARY

Examinations performed before an invasive varix treatment have different objectives. These objectives are related to indications and contraindications, anatomic and functional findings, and the treatment plan. A schematic stripping of the entire saphenous trunk in all cases should be rejected. Likewise, uncritical sclerotherapy that involves injection of only the visible varices should not be done. The operative diagnostic measures should consist of an anatomic and a functional test. Two noninvasive examination methods are now available for this purpose: Doppler ultrasonography (diagnosis of superficial and deep venous refluxes) and photoplethysmography (venous function test with tourniquet test).

An improvable CVI can be distinguished from a nonimprovable CVI by means of photoplethysmography. Truly nonimprovable CVI can be distinguished from falsely nonimprovable CVI by means of an additional deep Doppler examination. Improvable and falsely nonimprovable CVI constitute indications for invasive varix therapy (i.e., surgery and/or sclerotherapy).

Before formulating a treatment plan, the physician should perform an exact Doppler examination of the saphenous system and the deep venous system. Surgery is the treatment of choice for typical saphenous varices. Atypical saphenous varices are highly suitable for sclerotherapy. Reticular varices and telangiectatic blemishes can be injected, regardless of location, according to visual and cosmetic criteria. Complete elimination of large varices is not advisable in patients with nonimprovable CVI. In such cases treatment with medical compression stockings is indicated as soon as cutaneous complications, edema, or subjective complaints develop.

REFERENCES

1. Földi M, Casley-Smith JA, eds. Lymphangiology. Stuttgart: Schattauer, 1983.
2. Schultz-Ehrenburg U, Weindorf N. Problemsituation Ulcus mixtum. Swiss Med 6(9 a):41-44, 1984.
3. Blazek V, May R, Stemmer R, Wienert V. Die Standardisierung der LRR-Untersuchung. In May R, Stemmer R, eds. Die Licht-Reflexions-Rheographie (LRR). Erlangen: Perimed, 1984, pp 151-155.
4. Blazek V, Schmitt HJ, Schultz-Ehrenburg U, Kerner J. Digitale Photoplethysmographie (D-PPG) für die Beinvenendiagnostik. Medizinisch-technische Grundlagen. Phlebol Proktol 18:91-97, 1989.
5. Blazek V, Wienert V. Licht-Reflexions-Rheographie: Eine nichtinvasive Technik zur Beurteilung chronisch-venöser Insuffizienz. Wiss. Berichte d. Österr. Ges. f. Biomed Tech 261-277, 1981.
6. Blazek V, Schmitt HJ, Schultz-Ehrenburg U. Digitale Photoplethysmographie: Ein neues mikroprozessorgesteuertes Meßsystem für die Beinvenendiagnostik. Biomed Tech 33 (Suppl 2):307-308, 1988.
7. Fronek A. Noninvasive Diagnostics in Vascular Disease. New York: McGraw-Hill, 1989.
8. Weindorf N, Schultz-Ehrenburg U. Der Wert der Photoplethysmographie (Lichtreflexionsrheographie) in der Phlebologie. Vasa 15:397-406, 1986.
9. Schultz-Ehrenburg U, Hübner HJ. Reflux Diagnosis With Doppler Ultrasound. Significance for Diagnosis, Indication and Objective Followup in Phlebology. Stuttgart: Schattauer, 1989.
10. Goren G, Yellin AE. Primary varicose veins: Topographic and hemodynamic correlations. J Cardiovasc Surg 31:672-677, 1990.

PART THREE

Treatment Options

Chapter 7

Compression Therapy

H.A. Martino Neumann and Dig. J. Tazelaar

Compression therapy is one of the most powerful instruments of the phlebologist, and it is the one most commonly used. In the treatment of venous diseases, this therapy plays an important role both when used alone and as an adjunct to other forms of therapy.

Compression techniques are used to improve venous and lymphatic circulation. Different techniques of compression include the following types[1]: (1) bandages: elastic, half elastic, and nonelastic; (2) stockings: elastic; (3) mechanical: pneumatic (intermittent).

Although compression therapy is usually used for leg disorders, it also can be used with great success for arm problems. In daily practice, compression therapy is often called "ambulant compression therapy" because the interaction between the bandage and the muscular contraction associated with walking is important in accomplishing the aims of treatment. Mechanical techniques, like intermittent pneumatic compression, however, are not performed in association with ambulation.

Compression therapy is divided into two phases: initial therapy and maintenance. The first phase usually involves the use of nonelastic bandages until total reduction of edema or healing of ulceration has been achieved. Since compression is not a permanent solution, it is necessary to assess and correct the pathologic alterations of venous flow (if possible). To be effective, compression must be maintained during the daytime. The maintenance phase involves use of elastic therapeutic hosiery. This type of hosiery is indicated when pathologic hemodynamics cannot be permanently corrected by interventional treatment, surgery, or the use of drugs.

Chronic venous insufficiency (CVI) refers to all late results of nonoptimal venous system function. CVI can develop from superficial, deep, and perforator venous insufficiency (Figure 7-1). The clinical picture is well known and consists of pitting edema, cutaneous pigmentation, abnormal keratosis, atrophie blanche, and corona phlebectatica. CVI may develop into leg ulceration.

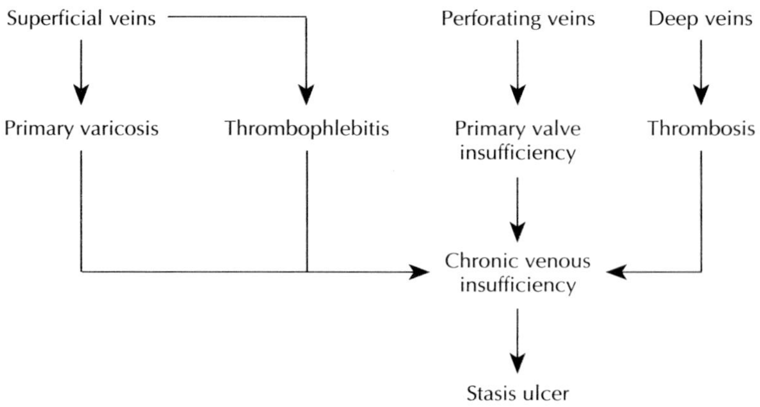

FIGURE 7-1. Development of chronic venous insufficiency.

Human circulation is a closed system characterized by high pressure in the arteries and low pressure in the veins. Capillaries separate one type of pressure from the other. Pressure, especially in the veins, also is influenced by gravity. In the standing position, hydrostatic pressure is added to resting pressure (as measured in the supine position). This explains why pressure in the posterior tibial vein is only 20 mm Hg when an individual is in the supine position but it is approximately 90 mm Hg in the standing position. Since venous valves are open in the standing position, they cannot close the blood column. Thus they do not reduce the foot venous pressure. In other words, the valves will not influence hydrostatic pressure when the patient is standing. (Properly, this hydrostatic pressure is often called standing venous pressure.) The implication is that patients suffering from CVI, those with only varicose veins, and nonpatients will have the same standing venous pressure, which is influenced only by the length of the blood column (right atrium–to-foot distance).

Since the pumping action of the heart is much more like that of a pressure pump than a suction pump, other mechanisms are needed to obtain an adequate venous return and thus a reduction of venous pressure. The mechanisms for venous return are (1) vis a tergo (force from behind), (2) vis a fronte (force from in front, (3) venous tonus, and (4) muscle pump. The muscle pump, which is the most important mechanism for venous return to the heart, reduces standing venous pressure to ±20 mm Hg during walking (walking venous pressure). With insufficient valve function or reduced muscle activity (dependency), this degree of pressure reduction will not occur. The leg blood volume is increased and the Starling equilibrium is disturbed because of rising transmural pressure (intracapillary pressure reduced by tissue pressure). Decompensation of the venous and lymphatic systems occurs, which, in turn, adversely affects the microcirculation[2] (Figure 7-2). Most clinical signs of CVI directly reflect this failure of the microcirculation.

In 1956, Charpy and Audier[3] stated that "all problems start when the patient leaves the hospital after a deep venous thrombosis in a so-called healed condition." Good compression therapy is an inexpensive and effective method preventing serious sequelae, including leg ulcers, in this group of patients.

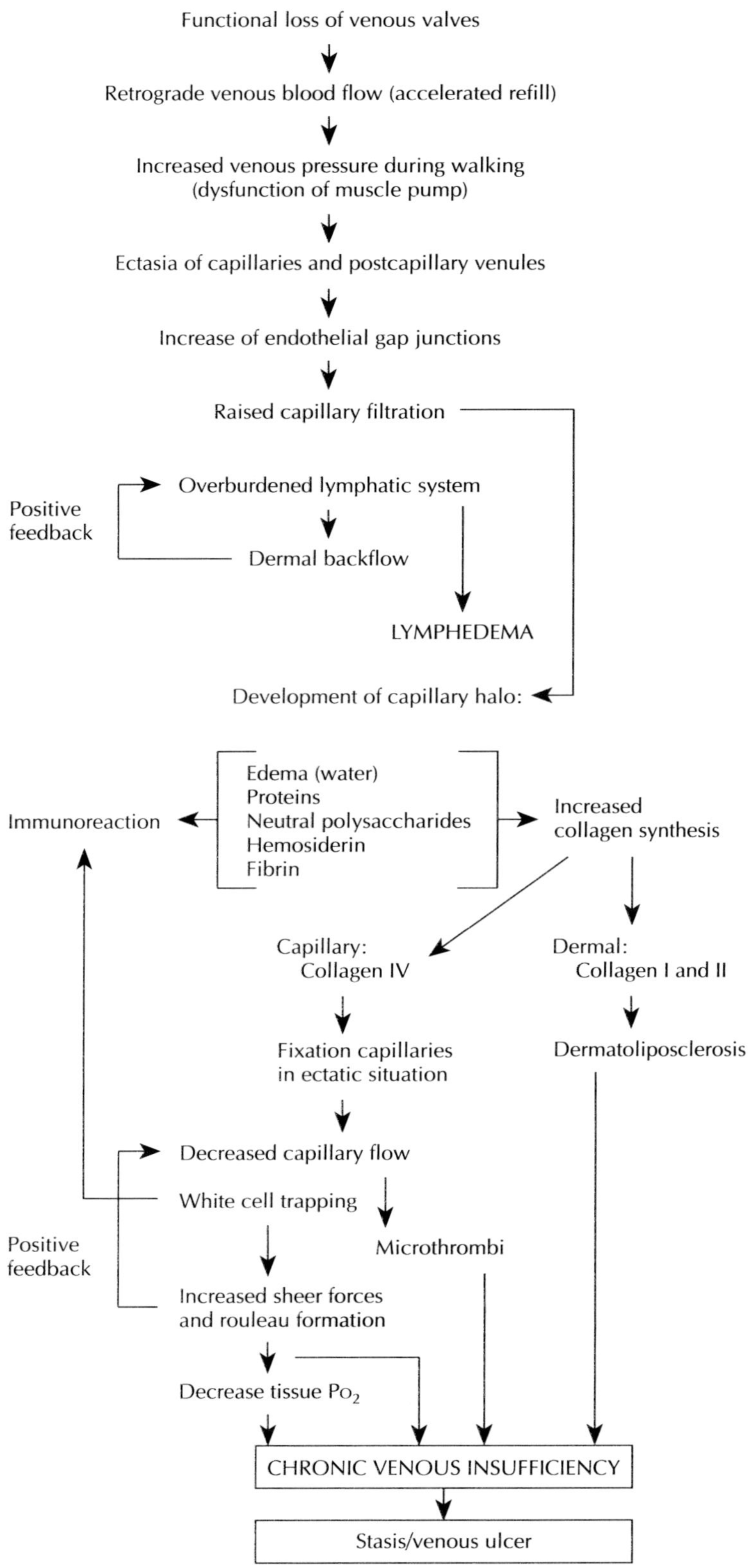

FIGURE 7-2. Microcirculation in relation to chronic venous insufficiency. (From Neumann HAM. Het ulcuc cruris. Medifo 2:22-30, 1991.)

CONTRAINDICATIONS FOR COMPRESSION THERAPY

Diminished arterial inflow (arterial pressure <70 mm Hg)
Acute deep vein thrombosis without sufficient collaterals
Severe congestive heart disease
Undefined ulcers (e.g., carcinoma cutis, leishmaniasis)

There is no doubt about the effectiveness of compression therapy. However, much attention to detail is necessary to obtain good results. Poor compression and inadequate support can lead to serious side effects and disappointing results (see box). In a 5-year follow-up, Callam et al.[4] reported 147 cases of ulcers and necroses caused by inadequate compression therapy.

Compression as therapy has a long history. In the Old World, the Egyptians used compression bandages for treatment of leg ulcers. The Bible (Isaiah) also indicates that compression therapy was used for venous disease. Hippocrates used linen bandages for compression. The first modern report of compression therapy dates from 1768, when Wieseman used dog-skin "hosiery" around the leg. William Brown introduced rubber-inlaid threads for hosiery in 1848. Jonathan Sparks made these rubber threads more comfortable by surrounding them with cotton.[5]

Today, synthetic elastomers are used for making therapeutic compression stockings. The European Economic Community plans to introduce a European standard for medical compression hosiery. This standard will include different compression classes and requirements for such factors as compression gradation and maintenance.

Compression therapy influences deranged venous flow in CVI at different levels. With phlebography, Fischer[6] proved that the diameter of both epifascial and subfascial veins diminishes under compression. More recently, phlebography and Doppler ultrasound have been used to confirm that reflux in deep veins is decreased by external compression.[6-8] Extra pressure from special padding as a compression aid may make incompetent valves become competent[9] and insufficient perforating veins will resume function.[10]

Compressing veins of the legs reduces the blood volume. Bandages decrease this volume by 72% in the standing position.[10] Furthermore, the mild compression (6 to 10 mm Hg) produced by antithrombosis stockings reduces blood volume in the sitting position in comparison to the volume in the supine position.[11] A reduction in blood volume combined with more competent valves enables the muscle pump to increase venous return.[12]

INDICATIONS FOR TREATMENT

It is essential to emphasize that compression therapy plays an important role in the treatment of CVI. Since CVI is already a substantial socioeconomic problem,

INDICATIONS FOR COMPRESSION THERAPY

Chronic venous insufficiency
Therapy phase of varicose vein treatment with sclerotherapy or surgery
Superficial phlebitis
Deep vein thrombosis
Angiodysplasia
Lymphedema
- Primary
- Secondary

Other edemas
- Posttraumatic
- Postinflammatory
- Postsurgery
- Dependent
- Diabetic angiopathy
- Erysipelas/cellulitis
- Cardiac or renal

Some dermatologic diseases
- Vasculitis
- Erythema nodosum
- Schamberg's disease

increased mean life expectancy of an aging population will only increase its impact in the future. Compression therapy is an inexpensive and effective treatment for a very large number of patients. In addition, this therapy is used not only for CVI but also for a variety of other conditions (see box).

CHRONIC VENOUS INSUFFICIENCY

All the stages and clinical manifestations of CVI benefit from compression therapy. Therefore this therapy is the basic treatment for all patients with CVI, (including those with postthrombotic syndrome). Edema, induration, stasis dermatitis, lipodermatosclerosis, and venous leg ulcer all should be treated with compression therapy. Today, with the more frequently encountered mixed ulcer (a combination of CVI and diminished arterial influx), special care must be given to the technique of compression.

In cases of primary varicosis without hemodynamic disturbances (normal venous refill time), treatment is not needed from a medical point of view. However, in patients with this condition it is wise to prescribe the use of compression hosiery during pregnancy or for extended periods of sitting or standing. Treatment by sclerotherapy is another possibility. The effectiveness of compression in CVI is mainly the result of improving venous drainage through a more competent muscle pump and by increasing lymphatic drainage.

A substantial correlation exists between CVI and microcirculation (see Figure 7-2). Most clinical signs (e.g., pigmentation and edema) are the visible results of decompensated microcirculation. Although the effect of compression therapy on microcirculation is not yet fully understood, compression does increase venous refill time and expelled blood volume.[13] However, it is unclear whether or not venous hypertension is influenced by compression. A decreased pressure can be observed by direct venous pressure measurements.[14,15] Unfortunately, most investigations have not proved an influence on ambulatory venous pressure.[16,17] Therefore, on the venous side of the microcirculation, pressure remains high. As a result, physiologic recovery of microcirculation is not possible. The Starling equilibrium shifts toward a decrease in capillary filtration and an increase in reabsorption. Thus the capillary filtration rate diminishes. This reduction is mainly caused by a loss of water rather than protein.[18] When compression is discontinued, edema will quickly recur. Therefore compression therapy must be a continuous therapy modality.

One technique for evaluation of microcirculation is transcutaneous oxygen measurement ($tcPO_2$). This measurement is performed with a modified Clark electrode.[19] In patients with CVI, $tcPO_2$ is diminished[20,21] and there seems to be a direct correlation between morphologic factors and the severity of CVI.[20] Partsch[22] found very low $tcPO_2$ values (12.9 ± 12.5 mm Hg) in the borders of venous leg ulcers. Through positron emission tomography, Gowland Hopkins et al.[23] studied the borders of venous leg ulcers in areas with lipodermatosclerosis. Blood flow was increased, and diminished fractional oxygen extraction was noted.

With reduction of edema during compression therapy, capillary density increases.[24] Blood flow increases[23,25] and $tcPO_2$ rises.[26-28] It is interesting to note, however, that pneumatic compression does not increase $tcPO_2$.[29]

Fibrin plays a special role in CVI. Burnand et al.[30] found that perivascular fibrin cuffs were present in lipodermatosclerosis. This finding was confirmed by others.[31,32] Fibrin cuffs may lead to an increase in the collagen layer of the capillaries.[33] The initial presumption that fibrin cuffs are a barrier for oxygen is not true.[34] Compression therapy has no influence on fibrin cuffs,[31] although fibrinolytic activity increases during compression.[35,36] For example, intermittent compression of an arm leads to increased fibrinolytic activity.[37] This observation is of interest for the prevention of venous thrombosis.

ADJUNCTIVE COMPRESSION THERAPY

Immediately after varicose vein surgery, harvesting of vein grafts, or sclerotherapy for varicosity, the use of a compression bandage is effective in reducing and minimizing side effects and complications. The compression bandage prevents edema formation and enhances wound healing. For sclerotherapy, it is essential to apply compression immediately after injection.[38] Compressing superficially injected veins is helpful, especially when pads are placed over the veins to achieve extra local compression. This method may prevent intravascular thrombus formation. Thrombi that occur after sclerotherapy may cause early recannalization, pigmentation, and inflammation.

Although there is no consensus about the duration of compression after sclerotherapy, a period of 3 to 6 weeks is usually sufficient, depending on vein size and extent of reflux. Compression done immediately after the treatment of telangiectasias also is recommended.[39] The duration of compression in this particular situation can be limited to 3 to 7 days.

Superficial Phlebitis After Sclerotherapy

Treatment of superficial phlebitis comprises incision and expression of the thrombus. This approach will relieve pain and discomfort for the patient. After the thrombus has been removed, a compression bandage is applied, and an extra pressure pad is placed over the treated vein to avoid refilling.

Compression and Deep Vein Thrombosis

Although limited to patients with sufficient arterial circulation, deep vein thrombosis is a very good indication for compression therapy. Such therapy is the treatment of choice for thrombosis that is limited to calf veins.[40] Compression therapy can be performed without bedrest when it is combined with the administration of oral anticoagulants. Even deep vein thrombosis that extends into the pelvis does not have a higher risk of pulmonary embolism when treatment involves ambulation.[41] However, confirmatory reports will be required before such treatment is fully accepted.

Since deep veins can be compressed to narrow cords,[6] blood velocity increases in these veins after compression therapy.[10,42] In addition, with compression, thrombi are thought to be fixed to the vein wall, and various enzymes and mediators are released from endothelial cells, which results in an immediate relief of pain and a reduction of edema. The actual influence of enhancing fibrinolysis with compression and its effect on the growing thrombus are not fully understood.[35-37]

Angiodysplasia

Conditions such as Klippel-Trenaunay syndrome, Servelle-Martorell syndrome, and Parkes-Weber syndrome can be complicated by varicose veins. Apart from possible arteriovenous anastomoses, it is wise to take a conservative attitude regarding intervention in treatment of these varicose veins. Therefore maintenance of compression therapy with elastic compression hosiery is of great value.

Lymphedema

Compression therapy is the most important type of treatment for all types of lymphedema. For best results, a high degree of compression is needed. Initially, long mechanical pneumatic compression should be used, and it should be followed by maintenance compression with a high-compression stocking (Table 7-1). Such treatment requires experience in fitting hosiery since the condition requires precision in

TABLE 7-1. Indications for elastic stockings correlated with compression class

Indication	Class
Prevention of thrombosis in hospitalized patient	I
Minor complaints with normal venous refill time	I
Prevention of thrombosis during pregnancy	II-III
Prevention of thrombosis in postthrombotic syndrome	(II)-III-(IV)
Sclerotherapy	II-(III)
Edema	II-III
Varicose veins	II-III
Angiodysplasia	III-IV
Lymphedema, grade II	III-IV
Lymphedema, grade III	IV
Lymphedema, grade IV	Maximum in class IV

measurements. Custom-made, flat-woven, gradient, high-compression hosiery with closed toes is best for treatment of lymphedema.

Other Edemas

In principle, all forms of edema can be treated with compression: posttraumatic, postinflammatory, and postrevascularization. In addition, compression therapy can be used for posttraumatic and postsurgical hematomas. Furthermore, dependency edema caused by a deficient muscle pump resulting from paralysis or joint deviations responds to compression; in this situation, the therapy is helpful even though pump function is not influenced. Treatment of cardiac and renal edemas also can be diminished by compression therapy as long as overfilling of the circulation does not occur. Prevention of congestive heart failure remains a prime consideration in patients with these conditions.

Diabetic neuropathy, when associated with microangiopathy, can lead to edema. In such cases compression therapy is effective.[43] Only light compression should be applied since the patient will not experience pain because of the neuropathy. Severely diminished arterial inflow must be ruled out through appropriate noninvasive examinations.

Other Dermatologic Diseases

It is well known that some vascular-mediated cutaneous disorders, such as vasculitis and erythema nodosum, are likely to occur on the lower legs. This occur-

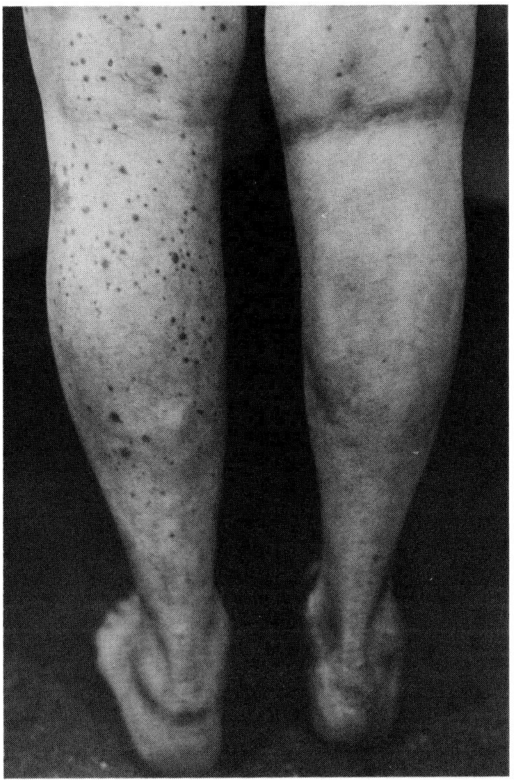

FIGURE 7-3. Leukocytoclastic vasculitis. Right leg has been treated with a compression bandage. Note total absence of eruptions due to compression on the lower right leg.

rence can be explained by induction of flow in capillaries so that immune complexes, antigens, antibodies, and other agents adhere more easily to the vessel wall. Also, CVI will exacerbate some skin diseases, such as progressive pigmental purpura and Schamberg's disease. Vasculitis, especially leukocytoclastic vasculitis and erythema nodosum, are typical examples of conditions that resolve quickly with good compression bandaging (Figure 7-3). The underlying cause of the disease, of course, also must be treated.

PHYSICAL AND PATHOLOGIC ASPECTS OF COMPRESSION

The extent to which the intended effects of compression are achieved depends largely on the pressure with which the bandage is applied.[44] This pressure (P) is directly correlated with bandage tension (S) and indirectly correlated with the radius (R) of the surface ($P = S/R$). This relationship is known as Laplace's law. Pressure on the leg can vary according to the surface curvature. On areas of decreased radius, for example, the malleolus, over the distal Achilles tendon, and at the sharp edge of the tibia, there is a danger of producing excessive pressure. The curvature must be flattened with padding to avoid pressure necrosis.[45] On the other hand, pressure may be insufficient over areas in which the convex curvature is naturally low, such as the retromalleolar sulci, or convex areas, such as the dorsum of the foot. Therefore the radius needs to be altered artificially in these areas by means of prominent pads. From Laplace's law, it can be concluded that less pressure is needed to achieve the same amount of pressure on a thin leg as on a leg of larger circumference.

Bandage pressure changes during walking. Working pressure develops during muscle contraction, and a resting pressure is obtained during muscle relaxation. The extent of the variation in pressure is determined to a considerable extent by the bandage material.[45,46] Nonelastic fibers have a large working pressure because they do not stretch during muscle contraction. Also, the resting pressure they produce is low because the material does not shrink during muscle relaxation. For these reasons, nonelastic bandages can be worn at night. The large pressure differences induced by walking augment the muscle pump, providing a strong antiedema effect.[47-49] Nonelastic and short-stretch bandages are preferable for use in cases of lymphedema and deep venous insufficiency.

Long-stretch elastic material is used in patients without edema but with superficial reflux. The pressure differences with such material are less than those of nonelastic materials. The working pressure is less because of the stretching bandage. The resting pressure is high because the bandage must be applied with a certain amount of tension. In the supine position, when the influence of gravity on the circulation is absent, high resting pressure can cause ischemia, especially if arterial circulation is impaired. Similarly, an elastic bandage or elastic hosiery with pressure of ±25 mm Hg around the ankle must be removed at night.[50,51] The question arises about whether the high rate of ulceration and necrosis in patients with compression bandages and elastic hosiery, as reported by certain Scottish surgeons,[4] correlates with this bandaging technique.

COMPRESSION BANDAGES

Application of a compression bandage is not easy. Experience is necessary to develop good technique. Although it is not possible to learn this application from a book, the main problems of bandaging are illustrated in Figures 7-4 through 7-10 and will be helpful in training.

Requirements for Compression Bandages

1. Pressure needs to be modified for the type of underlying disease. We believe that in primary varicoses or mild CVI a pressure of 25 to 35 mm Hg is sufficient. In severe CVI or in the postthrombotic state, we recommend at least 40 mm Hg. Lymphedema and indurated edema can be treated successfully only with bandages that produce a working pressure of 60 to 80 mm Hg in the ankle region.[52-56] However, some authorities do use less pressure.[57,58]

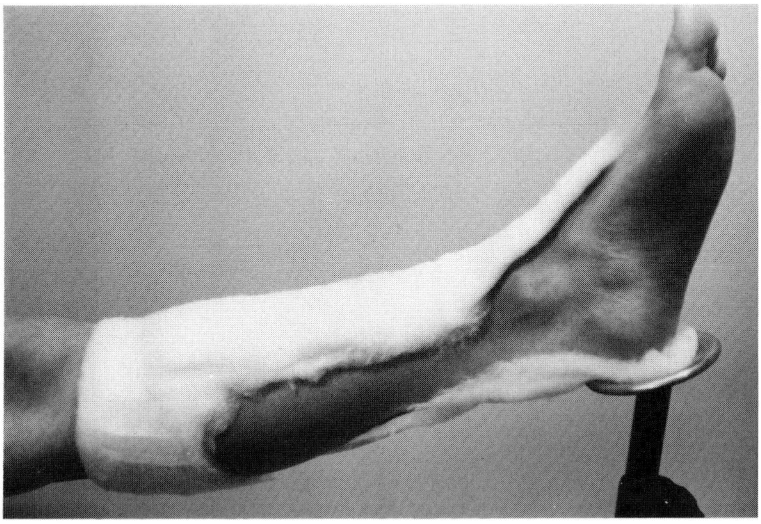

FIGURE 7-4. Leveling of all areas with a strong curvature, such as ankles, Achilles tendon, instep, and sharp edges of the tibia.

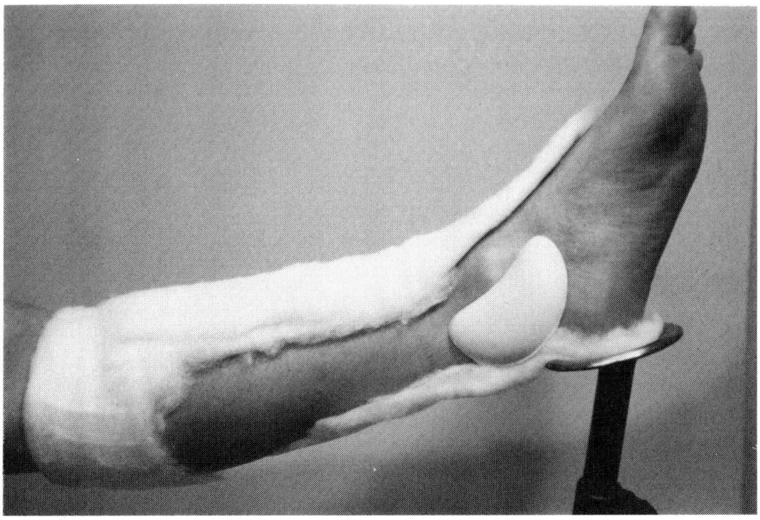

FIGURE 7-5. Raising the retromalleolar space with pads to achieve a good bend with the Achilles tendon.

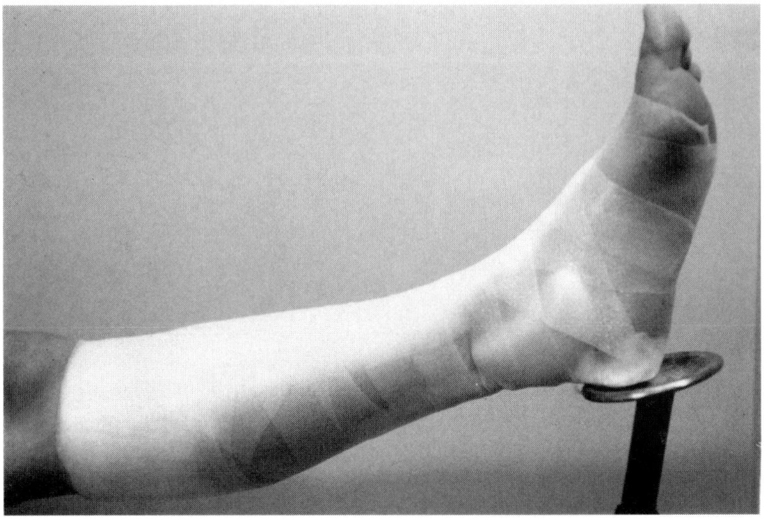

FIGURE 7-6. Fixing cotton wool and pads.

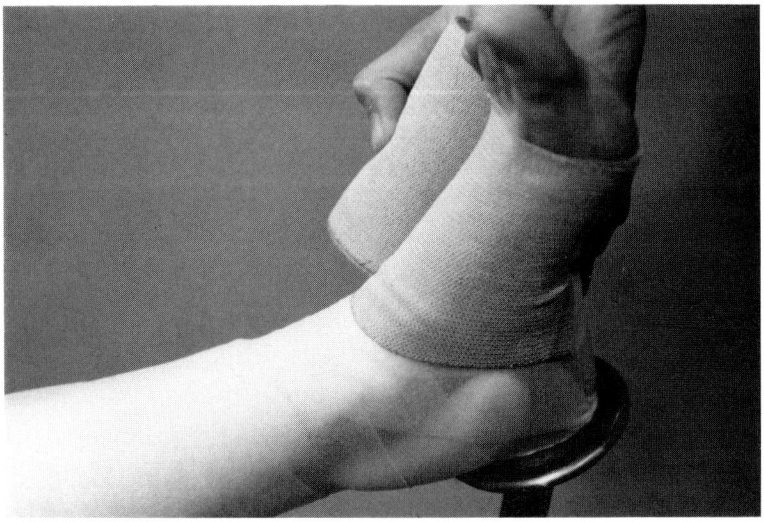

FIGURE 7-7. Bandaging is begun at median dorsal area with foot in dorsiflexion.

A

B

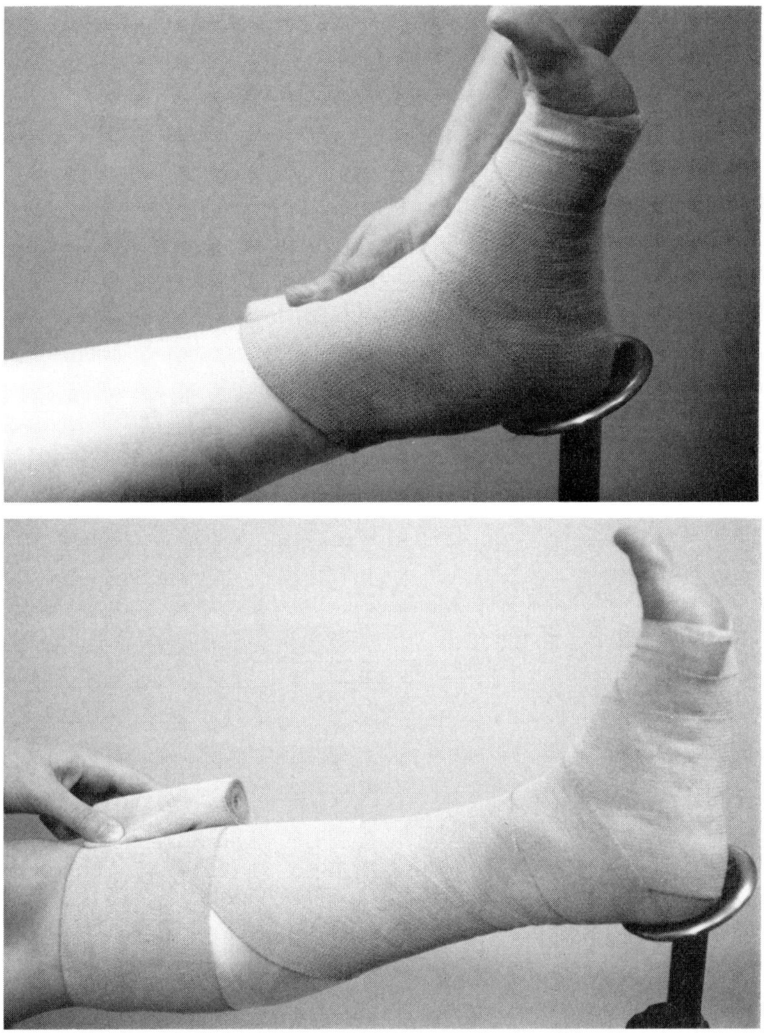

FIGURE 7-8. A, With each turn, two thirds of the bandage is covered, except for a turn under the knee, B, where there is no circular bandaging but the bandage turns across the leg and the contour of the leg is followed naturally. Such a bandage produces no constriction and eliminates slippage.

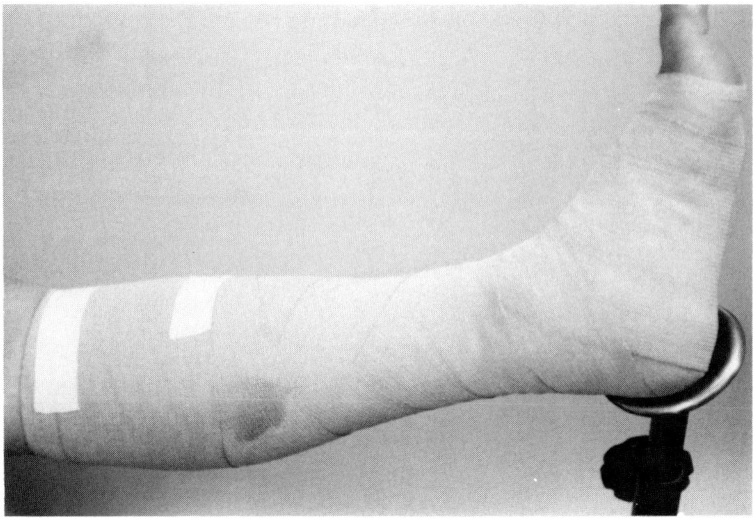

FIGURE 7-9. First bandage is applied.

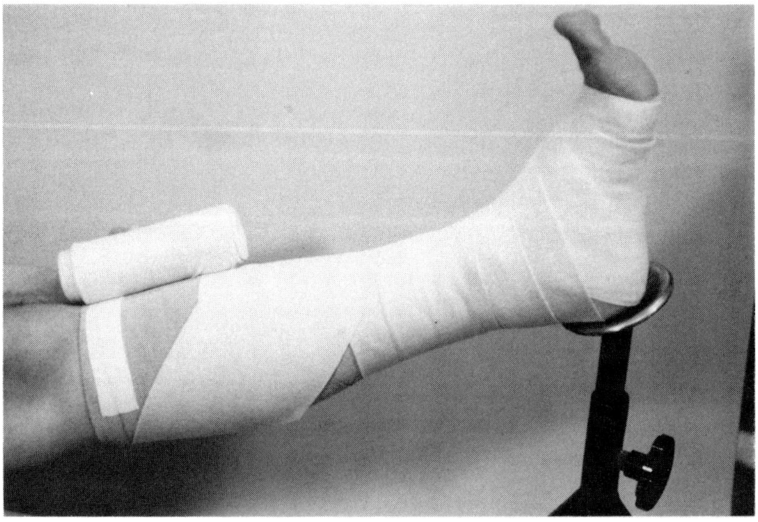

FIGURE 7-10. Second bandage is applied, from the opposite direction, starting from the lateral dorsal area.

We must recognize the importance of arterial circulation in every patient. In patients with nonpalpable arteries, a determination of the ankle systolic pressure through Doppler ultrasound is necessary before any compression bandage is applied. When a bandage is applied, the amount of pressure is dependent on the person who applies the bandage. The individual will usually bandage within the same pressure range each time. However, the amount of pressure applied can be increased or decreased. It should be noted that the pressure does decrease quickly after application of the bandage.[59] As long as there are no practice objective methods for measuring the pressure applied, physician experience is the most important factor for successful treatment.

2. For optimal support of muscle pump function, a gradient of pressure reduction from distal to proximal is needed.[60,61] Laplace's law states that in cases of bandage stretch pressure located distally will be higher than that found proximally on the leg.
3. The retromalleolar sulci must be filled with cottonwool, and the tibial area must be protected with the same material. Above indurated tissue, for identifiable insufficient perforators or ulcers, increased pressure is necessary.[45]
4. The bandage must not constrict the skin. When the bandage is applied, circular turns must be avoided. The use of oblique turns avoids constriction and leads to a bandage that crosses over to a firm but flexible tube, thereby fitting the leg as an external fascia.[9,62]
5. Muscle pump function is possible only when the patient is able to walk. For this reason the bandage must not be too thick since the patient will need to wear shoes.
6. Bandage materials must be nonallergic to avoid the development of dermatitis.

COMPRESSION STOCKINGS

Compression hosiery is very effective in maintaining compression. When no cure is possible (e.g., in postthrombotic syndrome or angiodysplasia), compression hosiery is the treatment of choice.[14,63]

Patient education is the key to good maintenance of compression. In the Netherlands, half of the prescribed medical hosiery is not worn by the patient.[63] In such cases the stockings often are poorly fitted, inconvenient, or ugly.

Compression hosiery also can be used in the therapeutic phase of compression, such as when varicose veins are being treated with sclerotherapy. In such instances the hosiery is not intended to reduce edema, only to keep the leg edema-free.

The classification of elastic hosiery compression is summarized in Table 7-2. Since the effect of compression on deep veins occurs above 30 mg Hg of pressure, and since in postthrombotic syndrome the mean pressure in the calf veins will be approximately 60 mm Hg, elastic hosiery of class III or IV is recommended. A patient with a relatively large leg circumference and long-standing high pressure also will need a high level of pressure for compression.

TABLE 7-2. Classification of elastic hosiery by pressure

Class	Pressure (mm Hg)	Effect
I	<25	Small effect on superficial veins
II	25-35	Clear effect on superficial veins; small effect on deep venous system
III	35-45	Effect on superficial and deep superficial venous system
IV	>45	Clear effect on deep venous system

Requirements for Elastic Hosiery

Methods for obtaining exact pressure, independent of hosiery size, are possible.[64,65] The hosiery must remain durable for at least 6 months without demonstrating a significant decrease in pressure.[66] After 6 to 12 months, pressures usually decrease.[46,67] Therefore it is best to replace hosiery every 6 months. For proper hygiene, it is advisable to prescribe two stockings at a time for each leg requiring therapy so that compression can be continued while one stocking is being washed.

Taking accurate measurements for elastic hosiery is key to a proper fit. Such measurement is possible only when the patient's legs are edema-free. Therefore if edema is present, a compression bandage is used until the edema has disappeared totally. Leg circumference is measured at defined locations (Figure 7-11).

Two types of elastic hosiery are available: flat-knit and circular-knit. Both kinds can be ready-made or custom-made, but the most exact elastic hosiery can be made only by using the flat-knit technique. With this technique, the exact number of stitches can be decreased and/or added at each turn. In circular-knit hosiery, the circumference can be influenced only by increasing or decreasing the tension of the inlaid thread. For this reason the pressure produced by circular-knit stockings will never be as precise as that of flat-knit ones. Because of the constant tension of the inlaid thread, circular-knit hosiery also is more difficult to apply.

Hosiery pressure is not the only factor that keeps the leg edema-free. The so-called slope value of elastic compression is also important. "Slope" means that with increasing circumference the pressure also will increase because of the elasticity of the material. A high slope value indicates a hosiery with a high edema-protection factor. However, a high slope value also has some disadvantages. Hosiery with a high slope value is difficult to apply and requires a more exact fit.

If a prescriber must choose between ready-made and custom-made hosiery, he/she realizes that all patients with significant CVI and all patients with lymphedema do much better with custom-made hosiery. In contrast, when sclerotherapy is done, ready-made hosiery nearly always suffices.

Ready-made hosiery never will fit (1) when there is a difference between the A and B value or (2) when the D value is equal or higher than the C value (see Figure 7-11).[68]

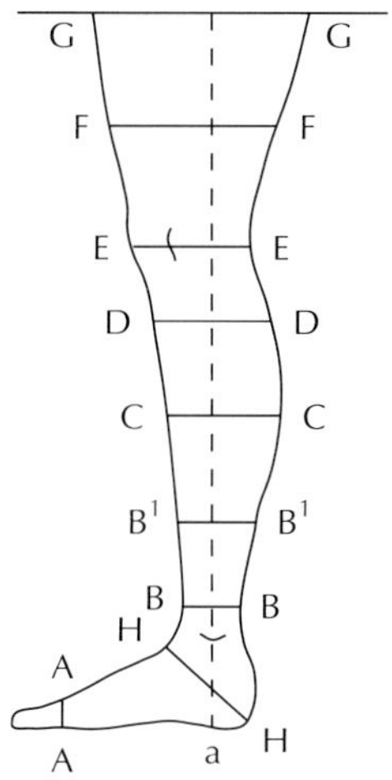

FIGURE 7-11. Standardized measuring points on the leg for elastic hosiery.

CONTRAINDICATIONS FOR COMPRESSION THERAPY WITH MEDICAL HOSIERY

All contraindications noted in the box on p. 106
Skin diseases that need topical treatment; ointments will quickly damage rubber and synthetic threads
Inflammatory process
Inability to put on and take off hosiery (as in rheumatoid arthritis)

In many patients, there is a difference in the relation between length and girth. Ready-made hosiery is knitted for the average leg. Prescription is possible only when the leg circumference corresponds to the manufacturer's size table. If the leg circumference does not agree with the size table, good compression will not be possible. In such cases prescription of custom-made hosiery is the best solution.[69]

Compression with hosiery has the same contraindications as compression therapy in general (see box, p. 106), but there are also some special contraindications related specifically to the use of hosiery (see box above). For most maintenance therapy in patients with below-knee symptoms, AD hosiery will meet therapeutic demands. These short stockings will be more comfortable for the patient than long, above-knee AF or AG ones (see Figure 7-11).

To determine the effectiveness of compression stockings, the major indicator is the absence of edema. An experienced physician and a well-motivated patient are necessary to ensure successful ongoing therapy. If either of these two factors are inadequate, treatment with elastic hosiery will lead to disappointing results.[70]

If pressure must be increased, such as when edema formation occurs during treatment with medical compression hosiery, either of the following steps should be taken:

1. Hosiery from a higher compression class should be chosen (see Table 7-2).
2. Two stockings should be worn, one over the other on the same leg. Pressure is then complementary. For example, two stockings that produce an ankle pressure of 25 mm Hg will have the same effect as one with a pressure of 50 mm Hg. The use of two types of stockings will enable many elderly patients to obtain the correct compression because one strong stocking is too difficult for them to apply. In practice, the so-called antithrombosis stocking (13 to 17 mm Hg) is often used as a primary hosiery.

To maintain the desired effect of compression and to ensure patient compliance with therapy, it is essential for the patient to visit the physician at least twice a year. During these visits, the best objective parameter for checking the effectiveness of compression is edema formation. Measuring the circumference at point B (see Figure 7-11) generally will give sufficient information about compression. However, from time to time, the circumference of the leg at all levels needs to be measured.

REFERENCES

1. Molen van der HR. Physikalische Therapie im Rahmen der Lymphodembehandlung mit Extubatio. Aktuel Probl Angiol 35:58-64, 1977.
2. Neumann HAM. Het ulcus cruris. Medifo 2:22-30, 1991.
3. Charpy J, Audier M. Les troubles trophiques des membres inférieurs d'origine veneuse. Paris: Masson, 1956.
4. Callam MJ, Buckley CV, Dale JJ, Harper DR. Hazards of compression treatment of the leg: An estimate from Scottish surgeons. Br Med J 295:1382, 1987.
5. Hohlbaum GG. Zur Geschichte der Kompressionstherapie, Part I. Phlebol Proktol 16:241-255, 1987.
6. Fischer H. Action de la compression sur les veins. Phlebologie 32:171-178, 1979.
7. Christopoulous D, Nicolaides AN, Szendro G. Venous reflux: Quantification and correlation with the clinical severity of chronic venous disease. Br J Surg 75:352-356, 1988.
8. Partsch H. Reduktion der venosen ambulatorischen Hypertonie durch Veneneinengung. Z Arztl Fortbild (Jena) 80:123-126, 1986.
9. Tazelaar DJ. Het compressieverband, keuze en techniek van aanleggen. The practitioner, Ned Uitg 973-978, 1987.
10. Lofferer O. Kompressionstherapie—Wirkungsweise und Andwendungsgebiet. Z Hautkr 57:633-642, 1982.
11. Partsch H, Rigal K. Reduktion des venosen Pooling in der Wade durch Antithrombosestrumpf und Beinhochlagerung. Phlebol Proktol 12:58-62, 1983.
12. Christopoulous D, Nicolaides AN, Belcaro G, Duffy P. The effect of elastic compression on calf muscle pump function. Phlebology 5:13-19, 1990.
13. Kuiper JP. Venous pressure determination (direct method). Dermatologica 132:206-217, 1966.
14. Somerville JJF, Brow GO, Byrne PJ, Quill RD, Fegan WG. The effect of elastic stockings on superficial venous pressures in patients with venous insufficiency. Br J Surg 61:979-981, 1974.
15. Kuiper JP, Brakkee AJM. Uber die haemodynamischen Auswirkungen von Kompressionsstrumpfen. Phlebol Proktol 17:202-207, 1988.
16. O'Donnell TF, Rosenthal DA, Callow AD, et al. Effect of elastic compression on venous haemodynamics in postphlebitic limbs. JAMA 242:2766-2768, 1979.
17. Mayberry JC, Moneta GL, DeFrang RD, Porter JM. The influence of elastic compression stockings on deep venous hemodynamics. J Vasc Surg 13:91-100, 1991.

18. Partsch H, Mostbeck A, Leitner G. Experimentelle Untersuchungen zur Wirkung einer Druckwellenmassage (Lymphapress) beim Lymphodem. Phlebol Proktol 9:124-128, 1980.
19. Huch R, Huch A, Albani M, et al. Transcutaneous Po_2 monitoring in routine management of infants and children with cardiorespiratory problems. Pediatrics 57:681-690, 1976.
20. Franzeck UK, Bollinger A, Huch R, Huch A. Transcutaneous oxygen tension, capillary morphology, and the density in patients with chronic venous incompetence (CVI). Circulation 70:806-811, 1984.
21. Neumann HAM, Leeuwen van M, Broek van den MJThB, Berretty PJM. Transcutaneous oxygen tension in chronic venous insufficiency syndrome. Vasa 13:213, 1984.
22. Partsch H. Hyperaemic hypoxia in venous ulceration. Br J Dermatol 110:249-250, 1984.
23. Gowland Hopkins NF, Spimks TJ, Rhodes GC, et al. Position emission tomography in venous ulceration and liposclerosis: Study of regional tissue function. Br Med J 286:333-336, 1983.
24. Mahler F, Cher D. Intracavital microscopy for evaluation of chronic venous incompetence. Int J Microcirc Clin Exp (Suppl) 106:1, 1990.
25. Partsch H, Lofferer O, Mostbeck A. Zur Beurteilung der Lymph- und Venenzirkulation am Bein mit und ohne Kompression. In Zeitter E, ed. Diagnostik mit Isotopen bei arteriellen und venosen Durchblutungsstorungen der Extremitaten. Akt Probl Angiol 19. Wien: Huber, 1973.
26. Neumann HAM. Transcutaneous Po_2 measurements in chronic venous insufficiency syndrome. In Merlin NJ, ed. Phlebologie 1983. Brussels: Medical Media International, 1984, pp 199-200.
27. Neumann HAM. Possibilities and limitations of transcutaneous oxygen tension measurements in chronic venous insufficiency. Int J Microcirc Clin Exp (Suppl) 105:1, 1990.
28. Kolani PJ, Pekan Muki K. Effects of intermittent compression treatment on skin perfusion and oxygenation in lower legs with venous ulcers. Vasa 16:312-317, 1986.
29. Nemeth AJ, Falanga V, Alstadt SA, Eaglestein WH. Ulcerated edematous limbs: Effect of edema removal on transcutaneous oxygen measurements. J Am Acad Dermatol 120:191-197, 1989.
30. Burnand GK, Whimster I, Naidoo A, Browse NL. Pericapillary fibrin in the ulcer-bearing skin of the leg: The cause of lipodermatosclerosis and venous ulceration. Br Med J 285:1071-1072, 1982.
31. Neumann HAM, Broek van den MJThB. Stanozolol and the treatment of severe chronic venous insufficiency. Phlebology 3:237-246, 1988.
32. Falanga V, Moosa HH, Nemeth AJ, Alstadt SP, Eaglestein WH. Dermal pericapillary fibrin in venous disease and venous ulceration. Arch Dermatol 123:620, 1987.
33. Neumann HAM, Broek van den MJThB. Increased collagen IV layer in the basal membrane area of the capillaries in severe chronic venous insufficiency. Vasa 1:26-29, 1991.
34. Neumann HAM. Skin oxygen tension values in patients with and without pericapillary cuffs in chronic venous insufficiency and porphyria cutanea tarda. In Leaper DJ. International Symposium of Wound Management. Bussum, The Netherlands: Medicom, 1991, pp 47-49.
35. Clarke RL, Orandi A, Cliffton EE. Tourniquet induction of fibrinolysis. Angiology 11:367-370, 1960.
36. Haas S, Altenkämper H, Lill G, et al. Einfluss der intermittierenden pneumatischen Kompression auf die fibrinolytische Activitate der Venewand. Phlebol Proktol 16:107-111, 1987.
37. Knight MTN, Dwason R. Effect of intermittent compression of the arms on deep thrombosis in the legs. Lancet 1:1265-1267, 1976.
38. Fegan WC, Fitzgerald DE, Milliken JC. The results of simultaneous pressure recordings from the superficial and deep veins of the leg. Ir J Med Sci 6:363, 1964.
39. Goldman MP. Compression in the treatment of leg telangiectasias: Theoretical considerations. J Dermatol Surg Oncol 15:184-188, 1989.
40. Voorhoeve J, Bruyninckx CMA. Het thrombosebeen, een bedriegelijk ziektebeeld. Ned Tijdschr Geneeskd 128:2289-2292, 1989.
41. Oburger K, Mostbeck A, Partsch H. Mobilitat bei patienten mit Beckenvenenthrombose. Vasa (Suppl) 30:161-163, 1990.
42. Mostbeck A, Partsch H, Hahn P, Tham B. Nuklearmedizinische Untersuchungen zur Beurteilung von regionalem Blutvolumen und venosen Stromungsgeschwindigkeit. Z Phlebol Proktol 13: 111-115, 1984.

43. Belcaro G, Laurora G, Cesarone MR, Pomante P. Elastic stockings in diabetic microangiopathy. Vasa 21:193-197, 1992.
44. Molen van de H, Kuiper J. Mesure de la compression en therapeutique phleboloque et notament de la pression permanente efficace après reduction de l'oedema. Phlebologie 13:21, 1960.
45. Stemmer R. Konzentrische und exzentrische Kompression. Phlebol Proktol 13:53-57, 1984.
46. Gregory von R. Eigenschaften elastischer Binden. Phlebol Proktol 7:171-182, 1978.
47. Hargens AR, Millard RW, Petterson K, Johansen K. Gravitation haemodynamics and oedema prevention in the giraffe. Nature 329:59-60, 1987.
48. Wupperman TH, Pretschner DP, Holm I, Emter M. Nuklearmedizinische Messung des Intravasal- und Extravasalraumes an Wade und Fuss beim Gehen und Sitzen zum Vergleich zweier Arten der Kompressionstherapie. Phlebol Proktol 16:175-183, 1987.
49. Ohlert P, Weinert V. Zum Wirkungsnachweis von Kompressionsverbanden. Vasa 17:262-266, 1988.
50. Berg van den F, Wupperman TH. Plethysmographische Ermittlung des Andruckes elastischer Kompressionsstrumpfe—"Anti-Thrombose-Strumpfe." Swiss Med 2:4a, 1980.
51. Callam MJ, Haiart D, Farouk M, et al. Effect of time and posture on pressure profiles obtained by three different types of compression. Phlebology 6:79-84, 1991.
52. Orbach EJ. Compression therapy and lymph vessel disease of the lower extremities. Angiology 30:95-103, 1979.
53. Jones NAG, Webb PJ, Rees RI, Kakkar VV. A physiological study of elastic compression stockings in venous disorders of the leg. Br J Surg 67:569-572, 1980.
54. Stemmer R, Marescaux J, Furderer CH. Die Kompressionsbehandlung der unteren Extremitaten speziell durch Kompressionsstrumpfe. Hautartz 31:355-365, 1980.
55. Blair SD, Wright DDI, Backhouse ChM, Riddle E, McCollum CN. Sustained compression and healing of chronic venous ulcers. Br Med J 297:1159-1161, 1988.
56. Stoberl CH, Gabler S, Partsch H. Indikationsgerechte Bestrumpfung—Messung der venosen Pumpfunktion. Vasa 18:35-39, 1989.
57. Fentem PH. Claims about compression treatment for venous disease. Br Med J 285:16, 1982.
58. Struckmann J. Low-compression, high-gradient stockings in patients with venous insufficiency: Effect on the musculovenous pump evaluated by strain gauge plethysmography. Phlebology 1: 189-196, 1986.
59. Raj TB, Goddard M, Makin GS. How long do compression bandages maintain their pressure during ambulatory treatment of varicose veins? Br J Surg 67:122-124, 1980.
60. Sigel B, Edelstein AL, Savitch L, et al. Type of compression for reducing venous stasis. Arch Surg 110:171-175, 1975.
61. Horner J, Fernandes e Fernandes J, Nicolaides AN. Value of graduated compression stockings in deep venous insufficiency. Br Med J 297:820-821, 1980.
62. Schneider W, Fischer H. Die chronisch-venose Insuffizienz. Stuttgart: Enke, 1969.
63. Korstanje MJ, Neumann HAM. Compressietherapie door middel van elastische kousen. Ned Tijdschr Geneesk 134:799-802, 1990.
64. Stolk R. Ein pneumatisches Druckmessgerat für direktes Messen von Druckwerten bei Kompressionsstrumpfen. Phlebol Proktol 9:176-182, 1980.
65. Weber G, Gohr O. Eine neuartige Methode zur Ermittlung der Druckeigenschaften von Kompressionsstrumpfen. Phlebol Proktol 11:34, 1982.
66. Bernink BP. Elastische Strumpfe und ihre Qualitats Beurteilung. Medita 8:152-157, 1978.
67. Stemmer R. Vorschlage zur Verbesserung der Kompressionsstrumpfe. Phlebol Proktol 9:129-137, 1980.
68. Olsen G. Zur Praxis der Versorgung von Beinkranken mit Gummistrumpfen. Fortschr Med 83:697-699, 1965.
69. Hohlbaum GG. Mass- oder Konfektionsstrumpf. Phlebol Proktol 11:42-49, 1982.
70. Ellerbroek U. Arzt und Kompressionsstrumpfverordnung. Therapiewoche 26:2376, 1976.

Chapter 8

Historical Development of Varicose Vein Surgery

Sidney S. Rose

The treatment of varicose veins has developed over a period of more than 2000 years (Figure 8-1) and includes a wide variety of methods. Most surgical treatments for varicose veins that were used in the past failed to give satisfactory results. Even when the results seemed reasonable in the short term, they did not prove to be successful in long-term follow-up. Many of the operations failed from both a functional and a cosmetic point of view. Some surgeons, in an attempt at radical vein removal, produced disfiguring scars. One example is the horrifying result of the Rindfleisch-Friedel operation of 1908. After ligation of the internal saphenous vein in the thigh, a spiral gutter was cut into the leg, encircling the leg four to seven times, down to deep fascia, with superficial veins being tied as they came into view. The wound was left open to granulate in an attempt to prevent infection!

The disregard for cosmetic result that typified early attempts at surgical treatment was unfortunate since leg appearance has been in the past, and remains today, the most common patient complaint and reason for referral. Throughout the years many family practitioners probably have dismissed women who were genuinely distressed by their ugly but asymptomatic varicose veins because the surgical results would be unsatisfactory and would not produce a good cosmetic appearance. In general, varicose vein surgery has been relegated to the junior members of a surgical team, and this practice has been reflected in the results.

In the past, the approach to treatment of varicose veins focused on the mechanical effect of back pressure on the varicosity. Such pressure was perceived to be its underlying cause. A modern trend toward the additional removal of varicosities has developed because of better results with this modification. This trend is more in accord with the weak vein wall theory, which explains the basic cause of venous dilatation. In light of that theory, back pressure is viewed as a secondary effect. Only recently has the cause of varicosities begun to become clear.

In the following discussion, we will look backward throughout history to follow the evolution of medical and surgical techniques used in the treatment of

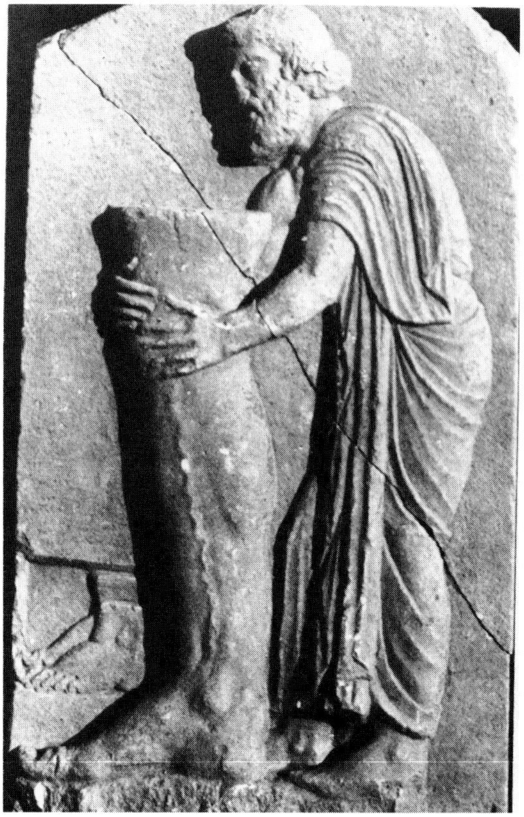

FIGURE 8-1. Votive tablet found on the site of the sanctuary of Dr. Amynos near the Acropolis dates from the fourth century. It is the earliest known depiction of varicose veins. (From Browse NL, Burnand K, Lea Thomas M, eds. Diseases of the Veins. London: Edward Arnold, 1988.)

varicose veins. After a summary of three important periods of progress, the discussion turns to the nineteenth century and goes back through the preceding centuries, ending with the Greco-Roman era.

PERIODS OF PROGRESS

The War Years and Postwar Trends: 1941-1953

The opinions expressed in this chapter are the result of experience gained throughout almost 50 years of my practice of varicose vein surgery. This experience included the personal treatment and follow-up of approximately 15,000 patients. It began in 1941, just 50 years after Trendelenburg's classic paper on varicose vein surgery, when this type of surgery was beginning to escape the domination of his teaching. The operation that my associates and I practiced then was called the Trendelenburg procedure, but our approach involved two important differences

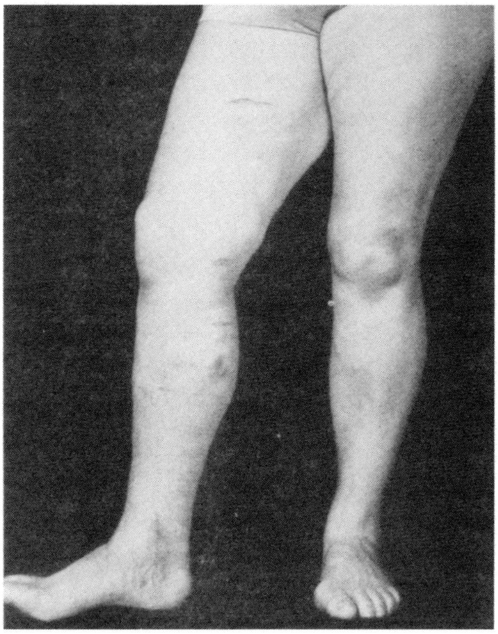

FIGURE 8-2. At the turn of the century the dominant varicose vein operation was the Trendelenburg procedure, in which the upper incision was placed in the midthigh, as shown here. After World War I the modified Trendelenburg procedure, which involved the groin incision and a high saphenous ligature, became increasingly popular. (From Foote RR. Varicose Veins. London: Butterworth, 1952.)

from Trendelenburg's classic description. First, the uppermost incision and ligation was done in the groin, not in the middle third of the thigh (Figure 8-2). Second, the operation included adjunctive sclerotherapy done simultaneously.

In 1941 there was no shortage of patients with varicose veins in either civilian or military practice in Great Britain. The notable frequent occurrence of varicose veins among members of the armed forces demonstrated that this complaint was by no means limited to women. However, varicosities in men were largely asymptomatic and usually were discovered on routine medical examination. The worst cases had been identified earlier, at the original military medical examination. Nevertheless, the complaint of varicose veins was exceedingly common. Perhaps the appeal of a few days in hospital, light duty, excused drill, and sick leave made the complaint of an aching leg seem an attractive alternative to many. Whatever the reason, the highest surgical admission rate to the Emergency Medical Service hospitals during World War II was for treatment of varicose veins. In fact, this type of high admission rate is a common experience in wartime. In 1811 Sir Everard Home, brother-in-law of John Hunter, wrote, "No surgical complaint, incident to the soldier, has deprived His Majesty's Service of so many men as that of ulcers of the leg due to varicose veins."

The operation I performed in 1941 was high ligation at the saphenofemoral junction, ligation of tributaries, and retrograde passage of a ureteric catheter down the cut end of the vein until it would go no further. About 6 to 8 ml of 5% to 10% sodium morrhuate was injected down the catheter as it was slowly withdrawn. The entire procedure was carried out with the patient under local anesthesia and done on an outpatient basis. The result was an immediate massive reaction along the line of the saphenous vein from ankle to groin. A chemical thrombophlebitis was produced that required heavy bandaging and caused considerable disability. The patients were painfully incapacitated during the 2 to 4 weeks it took for the condition to resolve. The ultimate fate of the thrombosed vein was recanalization, which took place sooner than expected.

The differences from the classic Trendelenburg operation did not seem to make much difference in regard to the results. A follow-up of cases operated on in the war years was impractical. However, the inadequacies of that surgery become apparent because large numbers of patients returned for further treatment. Recurrences were largely the result of the recanalized saphenous vein.

Use of the ureteric catheter was discontinued in 1945, and the practice of simultaneous sclerotherapy was ended in 1946. The operation performed with the patient under general anesthesia was simplified in 1947. The simplified version involved high ligation of the internal saphenous vein in the groin and low ligation in the distal third of the thigh and just below the knee. The main benefit of this approach was early ambulation, but the patient was kept in hospital for a week. The results of the operation were not noticeably different from those of the more complicated method.

TURN-OF-THE-CENTURY CONTRIBUTIONS

In 1896 William Moore, a Melbourne surgeon, advocated groin ligation performed with the patient under local anesthesia and done on an outpatient basis. In those days communications from Australia took a long time to reach the West, which may account for the fact that Moore's work did not arouse much attention in the surgical world at the time. There was no such excuse for the work of Thelwall Thomas of Liverpool, also published in 1896, which passed almost unnoticed. Thomas also described ligation of the internal saphenous vein at the saphenous opening. Despite this publication, 20 years later, in 1916, credit for suggesting the flush ligation of the internal saphenous vein in the groin was given to John Homans of San Francisco. In 1930 credit for carrying out the operation as an outpatient procedure with the patient being administered a local anesthetic went to Geza de Takats of Chicago.

To discover the origin of simultaneous use of a sclerosant at operation, one must go back to 1908, when this method was practiced by Beniamino Schiassi in Bologna (Figure 8-3). Schiassi used an iodide solution of unpredictable action. Fifteen years later E. Unger introduced the modification of injecting a sclerosant down a ureteric catheter. He used sodium salicylate, the first of the "safe" sclerosant agents.

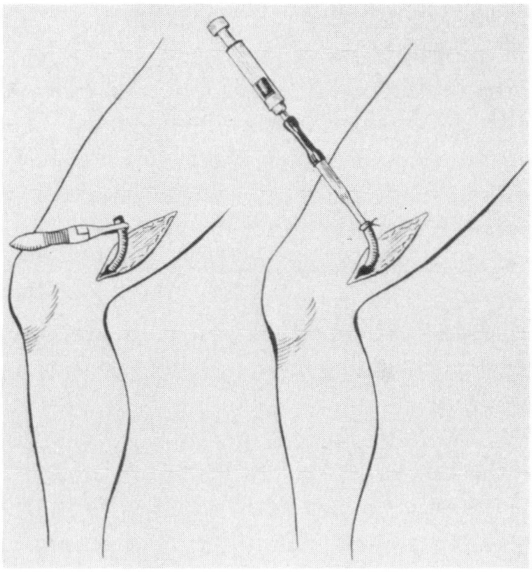

FIGURE 8-3. Simultaneous use of sclerosants and surgery was introduced by Schiassi in 1908 with the technique demonstrated here. Fifteen years later Unger developed a technique that consisted of injection of a sclerosant down a ureteral catheter from the groin. (From Foote RR. Varicose Veins. London: Butterworth, 1952.)

Sclerotherapy

Sclerotherapy as a treatment for varicose veins once was practiced by nonsurgeons as an alternative to surgery. However, more recently sclerotherapy has assumed the role of an adjunct to surgery.

For accuracy, sclerosants should be divided into two categories, thrombosants and true sclerosants. This categorization should be done in accordance with the agent's method of action, whether it causes (1) clotting of blood or (2) an inflammatory action in the vein wall. In the latter situation, if the vein is compressed, its walls will adhere to each other and produce luminal occlusion. Salicylates, quinine urethan, hypertonic saline, and sodium morrhuate all are thrombosant agents. Ethamoline (monoethanolamine oleate) is closer to being a true sclerosant. Ideally, a true sclerosant is required since intraluminal thrombosis usually leads to recanalization. Such thrombotic recanalization was the reason for introduction of the empty vein injection technique and pressure sclerotherapy.

The sclerosants in general use in 1941 were ethamoline and sodium morrhuate. Ethamoline, introduced into the United States in 1937 by H. Biegeleisen, was not widely used because of a long-standing antipathy to injection therapy. This agent was not in general use in England until the later years of World War II. Sodium morrhuate was widely used both in England and in the United States in 1941. In Europe, where centers of sclerotherapy arose and became increasingly popular after the war, the perceived need for a true sclerosant led to the decline of sodium morrhuate. Reports of unpleasant side reactions, such as allergy and skin necrosis, also contributed to the unpopularity of this agent.

A cycle of popularity follows the introduction of every sclerosant and thrombosant. In the nineteenth century perivenous injection was practiced by the influential Viennese school, sometimes with disastrous effects. The Surgical Congress of Lyons of 1894 condemned this technique as unsafe, and this censure was probably the cause of this method's traditional unpopularity in the United States. Later, Paul Ehrlich, whose world stature as a chemist commanded attention, was able to show that when properly injected, some agents could produce a thrombosis safely. This demonstration by Ehrlich led to Professor L. Sicard's successful introduction of the first "safe thrombosant," sodium salicylate, in 1911. For the next 30 years arguments for and against sclerotherapy raged. However, in 1947 N. Garber of Johannesburg wrote a very convincing paper arguing against the use of sclerosants. Garber advocated high resection of the saphenous vein followed by multiple resection of varices. This approach is basically what is practiced today, although techniques differ and sclerotherapy is used as an adjunct to surgery. Sclerosants in general use today include polidecanol, sodium tetradecyl sulfate, and chromated glycerin.

Introduction of the Stripper

The introduction of the stripper has been attributed to William Keller in 1905, Charles Mayo in 1906, and Stephen Babcock in 1907. The Keller instrument was a flexible intraluminal wire that turned the vein inside out. The Mayo instrument was an external ring that was passed along the vein, cutting the tributaries as it went. Babcock used an intraluminal stripper with an acorn-shaped head that pleated the vein along its length, as do strippers in use today. The Keller operation was given up because it was ill conceived; the Mayo, because of severe hemorrhage; and the Babcock, probably because the instrument was too short, too straight, and inflexible.

The Trendelenburg Years: 1841-1891

Friedrich Trendelenburg (Figure 8-4) described a transverse incision at the junction of the upper and middle third of the thigh. He could not have attempted to carry out a groin dissection through this incision, and he believed that step was not necessary. Since Trendelenburg simply ligated the vein in the midthigh, it seems strange that his operation won worldwide acclaim. Probably this acclaim was the result of his reputation for manual dexterity and the general tenor of his presentation. In his paper describing the operation, Trendelenburg paid tribute to those who had gone before him. He singled out Sir Benjamin Brodie for recommending midthigh ligation of the saphenous vein. Trendelenburg felt that such ligation was a logical procedure to relieve the effects of proximal valvular incompetence. It was, however, practiced before the discovery of blood circulation, when it was believed that the blood drained down the leg under its own weight. In fact, it would have

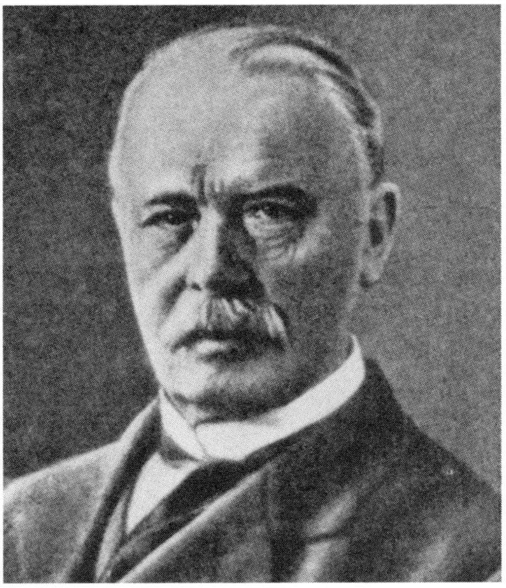

FIGURE 8-4. Friedrich Trendelenburg dominated vascular surgery at the end of the nineteenth century. His technique of ligation of the greater saphenous vein in the upper third of the thigh was a logical development from his observations of greater saphenous vein reflux as a powerful influence on varicosities and venous ulceration. (From Foote RR. Varicose Veins. London: Butterworth, 1952.)

been illogical to those who followed the teaching of Harvey to tie the saphenous vein if the blood were flowing in the opposite direction. Trendelenburg pointed out that after his operation the blood during exercise would flow through competent perforators and thus alleviate back pressure. He also created a stir by claiming that he could do the operation so quickly that no anesthetic was required. The operation required only a 3 cm incision, an aneurysm needle, and division between ligatures. Therefore one wonders why the patient was kept in hospital for 5 weeks after so minor a procedure.

When Trendelenburg published the results of patients he operated on and personally followed 4 years later, he admitted a 22% recurrence rate. This rate was probably an optimistic assessment. In those halcyon days no one would have the temerity to suggest an independent audit to a distinguished professor of surgery. In fact, Trendelenburg's work was followed up 4 years later by his disciple Georg Perthes, who advocated a much higher level of saphenous vein ligation and gave a glowing account of success with varicose ulcers with a recurrence rate of 18% in 41 cases. In his paper Perthes introduced his extension of what would later be known as the Trendelenburg test, first described by Sir Benjamin Brodie in 1846. The "Trendelenburg" operation was practiced in the Bonn Surgical Clinic in Germany for the next 35 years.

HISTORICAL APPROACHES TO TREATMENT
Nineteenth Century

If one goes back to the nineteenth century, one would expect that lack of anesthesia in the first half of that century would have severely inhibited surgical practice. However, such was not the situation. Instead, the battle against the varix was unabated, and in some instances the action was remarkably modern. For example, a little-known Italian surgeon, Giovanni Rima (1777-1843), not only advocated but practiced midthigh ligation of the saphenous vein without inducing anesthesia. In Rima's operation, done almost 100 years before the time of Trendelenburg, speed was of the essence.

Sir Benjamin Brodie (1783-1862) (Figure 8-5), of St. George's Hospital in London, was the first to demonstrate reflux in the saphenous vein; in 1846 he described in great detail what later was to be known as the Trendelenburg test. Actually Trendelenburg was inspired by work done in the previous century and admired Brodie. Brodie was a distinguished surgeon and clinician who made valuable contributions to the literature on venous disease. Toward the end of his life, disillusioned by his operative results, Brodie disagreed with his colleague Sir Everard Home about varicose vein surgery. This disagreement was based largely on the matter of sepsis. Brodie eventually advocated conservative treatment for all but the most severe cases. Therefore he developed a system of double bandaging with flannel for treatment of varicose ulcers and instructed patients on how to apply the

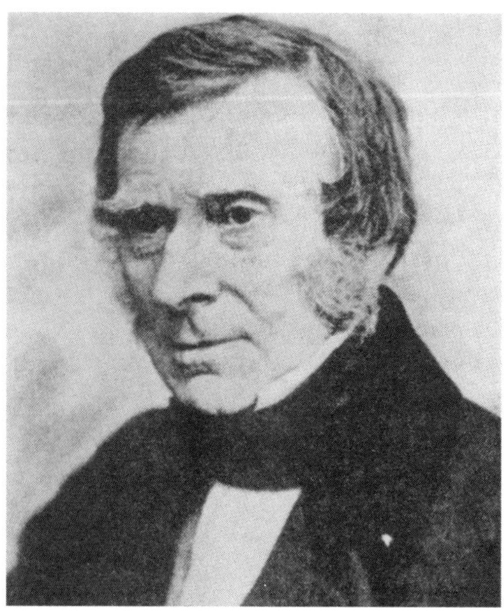

FIGURE 8-5. Sir Benjamin Brodie is shown at the height of his career at St. George's Hospital in the early nineteenth century. (From Foote RR. Varicose Veins. London: Butterworth, 1952.)

bandages. The patients were taught to include the foot in the bandage to prevent swelling and to apply the pressure from below in an upward direction. Although Brodie's treatment was ambulatory, he recommended elevation of the limb whenever possible and especially in bed at night. Brodie knew the value of calf muscle exercises, was aware of skin allergies to various medicaments, and was especially averse to sticky bandages.

Brodie was at the height of his fame when Queen Victoria came to the throne of England in 1837. She promptly knighted him for his services to medicine. At that time Brodie was reputed to be earning £10,000 a year, and, on hearing of his honor, he was quoted as saying to his entourage, "Gentlemen, there is more in veins than just blue blood."

Eighteenth Century

In the early eighteenth century the leading phlebologists were in France. Jean Louis Petit (1674-1750) (Figure 8-6), first director of the Academy of Surgery of Paris, taught that the cause of varicose veins was "anything that obstructed the

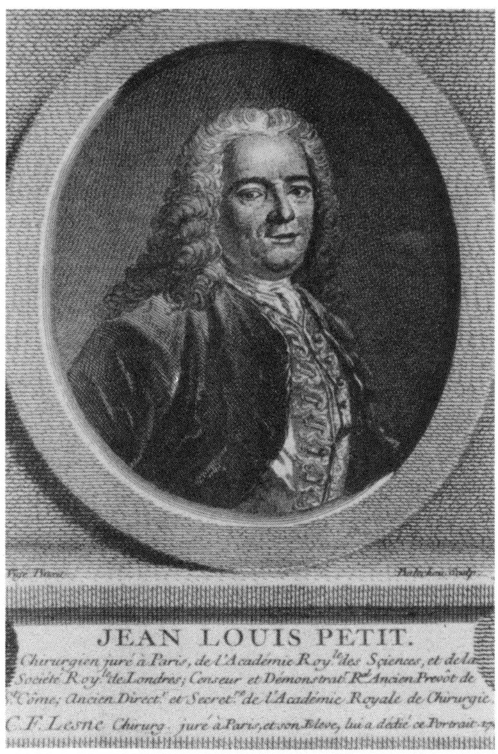

FIGURE 8-6. Jean Louis Petit performed radical excision of varices without inducing anesthesia. (From Haeger K, ed. The Illustrated History of Surgery. Gothenburg, Sweden: AB Nordbok, 1988.)

rising of blood in the veins." Petit practiced radical excision of varices. We know nothing of his use of anesthesia, if he used it at all. Petit's distinguished predecessor, Pierre Dionis (1668-1718), Surgeon-in-Ordinary to the Queen of France and the Empress Maria Theresa, believed that the cause of varicosity was "gross blood that caused the vein to make a small purse to allow blood both space and liberty." Dionis's poetic description of a varicose blow-out was equaled by his allegorical reference to venous valves. "These [valves]," he said "form steps to help the ascension of the blood and so facilitate its return to its source." Dionis strongly advocated the use of compression bandages on the leg and the use of support hose fashioned of linen or dog skin. In surgical treatment he made multiple longitudinal incisions over the veins and used cautery to destroy the veins (Figure 8-7). Like Sir Benjamin Brodie, Dionis became disillusioned with varicose vein surgery. Several of his works, which influenced many generations of surgeons to come, were even translated into Chinese as footnotes to the *Nei Ching* (*Canon of Medicine*), which had been handed down verbally for many centuries until it was first recorded in the third century and updated thereafter. The other writings of Dionis received the accolade of highest quality when they were burned during the French Revolution as a symbol of aristocratic decadence.

The French Revolution and the rise to prominence of John Hunter moved the centers of excellence from Paris to London. John Hunter (1728-1793) offered his most important contribution to vein surgery in his work on thrombophlebitis and pulmonary embolus. He emphasized differentiation between septic phlebitis, which was a frequent occurrence requiring drainage, and spontaneous (traumatic) thrombophlebitis, which did not require surgical treatment.

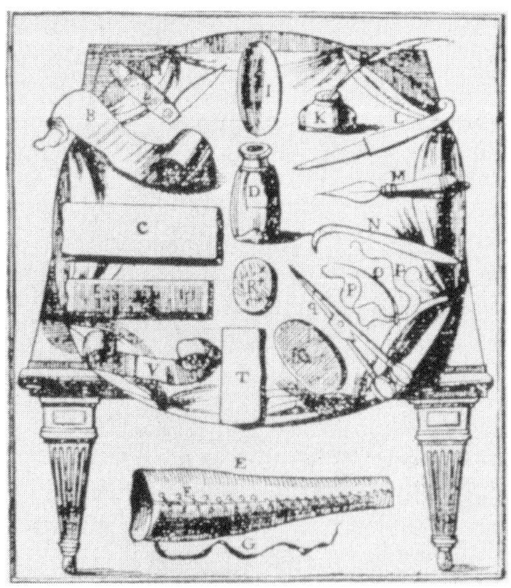

FIGURE 8-7. Instruments used by Pierre Dionis for treatment of venous stasis in the eighteenth century. Note the tapered legging fashioned of linen or canine skin to effect compression therapy. (From Foote RR. Varicose Veins. London: Butterworth, 1952.)

Seventeenth Century

The seventeenth century was one of the most turbulent periods in history. It was the century of the pilgrim fathers, the civil war in England, Cromwell's protectorate, the Great Plague, the Great Fire, the restoration of the monarchy, and, most dramatically, the execution of King Charles I. In attendance was the man who had made one of the greatest medical discoveries of all time, the royal physician, William Harvey (1578-1657) (Figure 8-8). After publication of his *De Motu Cordis* in 1628, Harvey endured a 20-year struggle for acceptance against the prevalent humeral theory of Galen, which had held sway for almost 1400 years. Harvey was attacked by members of the medical profession and by such distinguished philosophers as Descartes and Bacon. Harvey's theory of circulation was formulated through his study of venous valves and heart valves. Through this approach, Harvey came to two conclusions that had escaped all other investigators: (1) that blood could flow only one way in blood vessels, and (2) that blood was pumped throughout the body by the heart. Strangely enough, Harvey still subscribed to Galen's teaching that the vital spirit dwelt in the heart. Descartes accused Harvey of being obsessed with the Aristotelian principle that true perfection lay in the completion of the circle.

As Trendelenburg pointed out, discovery of the function of valves in assisting return of blood to the heart meant a complete reversal of attitude toward surgery of varicose veins. It could no longer be maintained that blood moved downward under its own weight. Although treatment remained much the same, the rationale changed.

Venous stagnation must have been in the mind of Richard Wiseman, sergeant

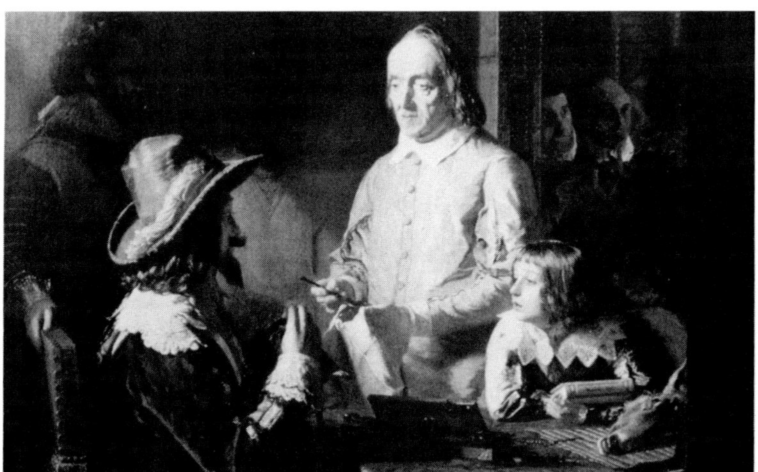

FIGURE 8-8. William Harvey formulated his theory of circulation of the blood through a study of venous valves and valves in the heart. He is seen demonstrating a point of anatomy to his royal patron and patient, the ill-fated Charles I of England (left). The future Charles II (right) is an interested onlooker. (From Haeger K, ed. The Illustrated History of Surgery. Gothenburg, Sweden: AB Nordbok, 1988.)

surgeon to King Charles II, in 1666, the year of the Great Fire, when he treated leg ulcers by a "rowled up compress and bandage from foot to gartering." When healed, the leg was supported by a "laced up stocking." Thus Wiseman demonstrated that he was a man ahead of his time.

Sixteenth Century

The subject of varicose veins was exercising the great surgical minds of the sixteenth century, as evidenced by the writings of Ambroise Paré (1510-1590) (Figure 8-9). It must be remembered, however, that at this time medical thinkers did not understand how blood circulated. Galenical theory prevailed, and it was believed that blood in the heart oscillated back and forth through fine pores in the interventricular septum to produce a pulse. It was Harvey's denial of this idea that provoked so much opposition.

Paré wrote concerning varicose veins: "The matter of them is usually melancholy blood, for varices often grow in men of a melancholy temper, who usually feed on gross meats, or such as breed and grow melancholy humors. Also women with

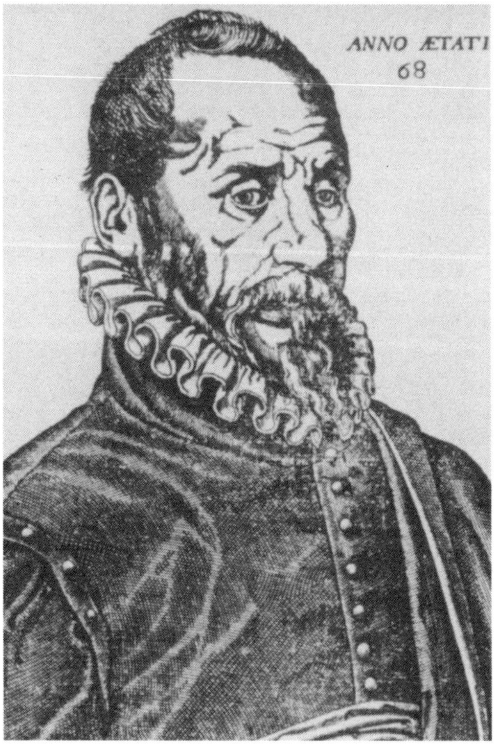

FIGURE 8-9. Ambroise Paré is credited with several milestones in surgery, including reintroduction of the ligature, which he used in midthigh ligation for treatment of varicose disease. (Courtesy New York Academy of Medicine.)

child are commonly troubled with them by reason of the heaping together of their suppressed menstrual evacuation. It is best not to meddle with them."

The breadth of Paré's surgical experience was demonstrated by the sophistication of his operative treatment of varicose veins. His approach should not surprise us. Once again, it was midthigh ligation.

To appreciate the level of Paré's surgical skill in the context of his time, one must recall that it was during his period of preeminence in Europe that King Henry VIII granted the charter to the barber-surgeons in England to found the Royal College of Surgeons.

Middle Ages

In the centuries from the Renaissance back to the fall of the Roman Empire, there are few accounts of advances in surgery. This period comprised the Dark Ages, when most records were destroyed from time to time by the barbaric hordes that swept across Europe in waves. Nevertheless, some illustrious names survive. In fourteenth-century France, Guy de Chauliac, the physician to three popes, produced his great book on surgery, *La Grande Chirurgie*. In this work he wrote extensively about varicose veins and influenced teaching on many surgical subjects for the next 300 years. De Chauliac treated varicose veins by opening the vein and cauterizing the bleeding ends. If this method was not successful, he advised avulsion. We do not know about de Chauliac's success rate, but since he practiced long before the advent of blood transfusion, it might be just as pertinent to ask about his patient survival.

When the Moors conquered Spain toward the end of the seventh century, they brought with them the cultures of the eastern Mediterranean. From Greece, Persia, Cyprus, Egypt, the Holy Land, and Byzantium came the culture that, when wedded to Spanish subculture, flowered to create great centers of learning in the cities of the Iberian peninsula. Among these centers was Cordova, where a mixture of Arabic, Hebraic, and European knowledge formed the basis for establishing an eminent center of medical excellence in the eleventh century. The famous Maimonides (1135-1204) was born here. However, the most illustrious surgeon of this academy was Albucasis of Cordova (936-1013), who bore the medical tradition of his Arabic forebears with great distinction. In raising the standards of surgery, he deplored the fact that it "had passed into the hands of vulgar and uncultivated minds and had fallen into contempt." By this statement, Albucasis showed his disapproval of those colleagues whose ignorance and malpractice had given support to the ancient fallacy of the intellectual supremacy of the physician, an attitude that has stayed with us throughout the ages. Albucasis was an extremely cautious surgeon. However, he described the operation of multiple vein ligation and stripping with an external vein stripper 900 years before it was advocated by Charles Mayo.

In the tenth century, another Arabic surgeon, Haly Abbas (d. 994), who also subscribed to the humoral theory of varicosity, described the clinical picture of varicose veins most vividly. He said that the dilated veins were caused by "overloading with viscous blood that sinks into the legs under its own weight. It therefore happens mostly in peasants, porters and sailors, and women with child . . . and these veins become tortuous and thick and inclined to become green or black in colour." Abbas advised multiple puncture, bleeding, and cautery, which constituted standard practice at the time.

Approximately 300 years earlier in Byzantium, Paul of Aegina (607-690), who trained in Alexandria, seems to have been not only a competent surgeon but also one who adopted a very modern approach. He described in great detail his sophisticated operation for varicose veins. He made novel use of tourniquets, applied above and below the knee, and then made the patient walk until the appropriate vein was filled with blood. The veins were marked with a special ink. The patient was then positioned on a table with legs extended, and an incision was made over the vein. The vein was quickly mobilized, and double sutures were passed around the upper and lower ends. The sutures were tied and cut, with a length of vein left between them that was removed. The wound was left open and was packed with an "oblong compress soaked in wine and oil." The vein removed was the internal saphenous vein in the midthigh.

After a search of fourteen centuries, we have found the originator of the midthigh ligation in Paul of Aegina. He demonstrated not only impeccable technique but also removal of a length of vein; moreover, he was aware that the way to avoid sepsis was to pack the wound open and leave it to granulate.

Greco-Roman Era

The great men of surgery who were regarded by Paul of Aegina and his distinguished Byzantine colleague Aetius of Amida as their source of inspiration were two Greeks and a Roman. The Greeks were Galen and Hippocrates, and the Roman was Celsus.

Galen (c. 130–c. 200), born in Pergamon in Asia Minor, was groomed in medicine and surgery from a very early age. It was his father who recognized his aptitude. Galen started his surgical career as physician to the gladiators. He was the first to realize that if a gladiator could be saved to fight again, it would be a great advantage to all concerned, especially the gladiator. Too many gladiators had been left to die of their wounds. Galen soon gained great renown and was invited to Rome, where he set up what now would be called a casualty and intensive care center at the Colosseum. There his skill came to the attention of Emperor Marcus Aurelius, who appointed Galen as his personal surgeon. Galen became a great expert in trauma and is credited with inventing the ligature, without which most surgery would be impossible. He removed varicose veins through three to six incisions with a hook that has been reinvented several times since its introduction. In addition, Galen developed a method of bandaging that held the wound edges together, and occasionally he was known to use a needle to transfix the wound edges to keep them in apposition. As noted earlier, Galen's theory of circulation was to remain standard theory for the next 1400 years. His voluminous works became a medical bible that dominated the Western World for the next 1500 years, even though only a third of them escaped destruction after the fall of Rome.

Cornelius Celsus (53 BC–AD 7), born a year after Julius Caesar invaded Britain for the second time, had no formal medical training. Being a physician in early Roman times was an arbitrary status. There is no record of Celsus's surgical apprenticeship, but there is no doubt that he became a very skillful operator. He questioned everything he saw and soon developed his own opinions, which he recorded most assiduously. Celsus was an inveterate chronicler of events who established himself as an authority in a vast number of medical fields. He became a legend in his own lifetime, and his opinions were sought on a great variety of matters both within and outside the field of medicine. Celsus developed a method of operating on varicose veins in which he made multiple incisions along the varicosity four fingerbreadths apart and touched the vein with a cautery through each incision. He then grasped the ends of the vein and extracted as much vein as he could. Those who practice multiple avulsion today will derive great comfort from the fact that this method was highly recommended by so great an authority as Celsus.

Greek civilization reached its height in the fourth century BC. The island of Cos was the center of medical learning, and there Hippocrates reigned supreme. His advice on the subject of varicose veins consisted of making multiple punctures in the varicosities and then bandaging the limb firmly. This practice was intended to let out blood along with whatever "evil" it contained. Hippocrates was opposed to excision because of the possibility of ulceration and infection. A great believer in cautery, he was quoted as saying, "What cannot be cured by medicaments is cured by the knife, what cannot be cured by the knife is cured by the searing iron, whatever this cannot cure must be considered incurable."

Long before the Hippocratic era, Greeks were treated by the priests of the god Asclepios, who were known as Asclepiads. To be treated, the patient brought a votive offering to the altar. Figure 8-1 shows such an offering, a tablet that dates from 350 BC. The slab was found near the Acropolis in Athens at the shrine of a physician named Amynos. The tablet, showing a sculptured leg with a large varicose vein, was placed on the altar presumably as an offering for a cure. It shows that the ancient Greeks had knowledge of varicose veins and that they considered there to be a need for treatment of varicosities. Since the Greeks of this time believed that evil humors were present in the thickened blood, they were adverse to bandaging. They thought that bandaging would drive the humors back into the body and produce dire results. Faith healing for varicose veins, which was popular 2000 years ago, is currently exemplified by the miracle cures offered in the popular press.

History therefore teaches that the common denominator of treatment throughout the years has been midthigh ligation and venous excision, often with the addition of venous sclerosis by one means or another. Thus we are reminded that there is nothing new under the sun.

MODERN SURGICAL TECHNIQUES—A PERSONAL VIEW: 1941-1991

The Trendelenburg operation described at the beginning of this chapter technically should have been called the Moore-Unger modification, a somewhat different procedure. In the Moore-Unger modification, sclerotherapy, considered a fundamental part of the operation, was done postoperatively. However, from approximately 1945 to 1948, sclerotherapy was deliberately avoided because of concern about sodium morrhuate. Radiologic evidence had helped to establish the fact that material injected into the thigh could find its way into the deep veins with all the consequences implied. The recommended method of treatment was changed to include an even more meticulous groin ligation and a midthigh and below-knee ligation plus, if necessary, short saphenous exploration and ligation. No veins were removed, and simultaneous sclerotherapy was not performed. The number of residual veins that accumulated postoperatively, however, required another look at sclerotherapy. Since ethamoline had become increasingly acceptable, being viewed as a safer and more appropriate sclerosant, this agent began to be used for residual veins and as definitive treatment for veins not considered large enough to warrant surgery. This method became standard practice from 1949 to 1952. In regard to development, these were somewhat unproductive years because the method in common use was a mere modification of the prewar practice.

In order to trace the modern development of surgery of veins, a personal history can be used for demonstration.

The Stripping Technique

In the course of a visit to the Mayo Clinic in 1952, I learned the stripping technique. The use of a modified Babcock technique of vein stripping by Thomas T. Myers at the clinic in the late 1940s had led to a revival of the stripping operation, which had been abandoned in 1907. A newly designed, long, flexible stripper that pleated up the vein along its length proved to be immensely popular. The worldwide prestige of the Mayo Clinic coupled with Tom Myers's personal charm and hospitality contributed much to the widespread and immediate acceptance of the procedure.

The essence of the operation was a careful groin dissection followed by high ligation of the internal saphenous vein just distal to the saphenofemoral junction. Tributaries of the saphenous vein at the junction were ligated and divided. Stripping was carried out in the following way. An incision large enough to accommodate the sizable stripper head was made over the medial malleolus. The saphenous vein was isolated at the ankle, with care taken not to damage the saphenous nerve. The vein was supported by two untied ligatures. An incision was made into the lumen of the vein, and the guide end of the stripper was inserted into the vein. The distal ligature was tied, and the stripper was passed from below upward so that it would not catch in a valve. The stripper was extracted from the saphenous vein at the upper incision. The lower end of the vein was then tied firmly with a ligature around the neck of the stripper, and the vein was divided in front of the ligatures. The stripper head was eased into the malleolar incision with continuing firm traction that moved the stripper up the leg until it emerged from the groin incision with the vein pleated upward behind the head of the stripper.

I was surprised to find that the stripping technique sometimes demanded a blood transfusion because of bleeding along the stripper track. Such bleeding was the result of an attempt to avoid a hematoma by dragging a roll of gauze along the track by a length of ligature previously attached to the stripper. As would be expected, this method only caused further bleeding. Subsequently this practice was abandoned and substituted by the use of aspiration combined with manual pressure along the stripper track and firm bandaging from toe to groin as the vein was stripped.

Experience With Instrumentation

On returning to England in 1953, I began performing the operation with guarded optimism. Groin dissection and high ligation at the saphenofemoral junction were carried out as before. All tributaries of the saphenous vein at the junction were divided and ligated.

I began by using the stripper presented to me by Dr. Tom Myers. This instrument had a fixed head and guide. It soon became apparent that it would be advantageous to have detachable heads of various sizes and a detachable guide and handle. Thus the Rose stripper (Down Brothers, London) was developed. As I gained experience through the use of this stripper, I modified my technique. First, this stripper allowed me to gauge which head seemed to be least traumatic at the ankle and yet large enough to perform efficient stripping. Further, the stripper could be used in reverse if necessary. The ankle incision, in this situation somewhat smaller, was made in the submalleolar hollow and not over the malleolus so that it was safely away from the pressure point over the bone. The ankle dissection of the saphenous vein was done as before. The use of a smaller ankle acorn exposed the saphenous nerve to less trauma. The limb was compressed along the stripper track and firmly bandaged as the stripper was taken slowly up the leg in a series of short lengths.

At first, lengths of sponge rubber were laid along the track of the stripper to enhance the local pressure, but this practice was discontinued when careful bandaging proved to be equally effective. Peripheral varices were ignored since most were expected to disappear after they had been cut off from the main saphenous veins. One of the obvious attractions of the operation was the speed with which it could be performed.

Those who advocated stripping believed that the technique would achieve three main objectives. First, it would remove the main saphenous vein, which was always thought to be incompetent, in most (if not all) of its length. Second, it would isolate the varicose tributaries that would then thrombose. Third, it would interrupt any incompetent deep perforators that might feed the varicose clusters. It soon became obvious that only the first objective was being achieved. The most important observation that emerged was that all the tributaries of the saphenous vein that were interrupted by the stripper could be prevented from bleeding by the use of firm pressure. This was a well-known surgical fact concerning blood vessels that had not been applied before in this situation. Ligation was still necessary at the main saphenofemoral and saphenopopliteal junction, but the fact that broken ends of the smaller tributaries would seal off spontaneously made it apparent that varicosities could be removed without the need to tie the ruptured ends, especially if the varicosities were removed by traction rather than after clean division.

As experience with this procedure grew, three very interesting facts emerged. First, the stripper often passed unhindered under a scar at the site of a supposed previous ligation, and second, the peripheral varicosities had survived unchanged. The latter was the usual source of concern to the patient and constituted the indication for repeat surgery. Third, and most important, it became apparent from examination of the stripped vein that whole lengths of the vein were normal. This observation did not arouse much comment at that time since there was no stimulus to preserve the vein; arterial bypass surgery was not yet a common part of practice.

Coincidentally, from approximately 1956 to 1957, a revival of interest in sclerotherapy was spearheaded by Fegan's compression injection technique, which was soon rigorously practiced in the follow-up clinics. The immediate results of Fegan's procedure were satisfactory, but in the long term they proved to be disappointing. Such, however, was the volume of cases in postoperative clinics that, when limited to 50 cases per session twice a week, the caseload soon became unmanageable. By 1957 it was decided that stripping, as practiced at that time, was only a partial answer. It was thought that the only way to avoid overcrowded postoperative outpatient clinics was to excise the larger peripheral varicosities at the time of the original stripping.

Development and Experimentation: 1957-1964

The years from 1957 to 1964 were a period of further experimentation. The operations that my associates and I performed were based on stripping, with other procedures added as appropriate. In late 1957 we adopted a policy of making incisions over larger peripheral varicosities and excising them. At first it was thought prudent to ligate larger veins with fine catgut sutures. We were still not confident that blind avulsion would not give rise to difficult bleeding. This approach considerably lengthened the operation but gave a much more acceptable result to the patient. Coincidentally, the number of postoperative injections declined. Later we became bold enough to rely on pressure applied to smaller veins as a means of stopping bleeding. This practice was extended to larger veins provided that they were at a safe distance from a main junction. From 1963 onward, the trend in surgery turned further away from routine stripping and increasingly toward multiple avulsion. This trend marked the development of the currently accepted operative technique, limited axial stripping with the addition of extensive multiple avulsion.

Incompetent Perforating Veins

At this point we began to reconsider the role of perforating veins in relation to varicose clusters. Supposedly these clusters were caused by underlying incompetent deep perforators. When it was possible to demonstrate such perforators through phlebography, it was thought that cause and effect had been established. Some surgeons went further and considered these perforators to be the main cause of many mainline varicosities as well as the outlying varicose clusters. They thought these perforators were the explanation for all varicosities that occurred below a competent valve. Therefore it seemed logical to identify and ligate incompetent perforators. So strong was belief in this doctrine that eventually ligation of these veins alone was advocated and practiced by many. Even eminent surgeons followed this practice. Prior to operation, incompetent perforators were identified by Doppler ultrasonography, thermography, and/or phlebography. Though the phlebogram was the gold standard, even with a practiced eye there was difficulty in interpretation. Although some perforators were found and ligated in relation to the varicosities, many explorations were tedious and carried out in vain. Even when these perforators were identified, simple ligation alone failed to produce the desired effect, and many varicosities remained. Worse still, the operation could be a cosmetic disaster because of the length of the incisions required. Such a result was particularly unfortunate when the complaint was cosmetic in the first place. Therefore the majority of surgeons preferred to both strip and ligate perforators, but results of this treatment were marginally better, although they did not justify widespread acceptance of the procedure.

We decided to investigate the role of incompetent deep perforators, and we started a lengthy but unrewarding period of searching for and ligating them. When the technical difficulties of locating the perforator in relation to the varicosity became apparent, and when these perforators could not be found through cosmetically acceptable incisions, we restricted this approach to limbs where such a result was a secondary consideration. One could justify this procedure only for operations for varicose ulcer.

The stripping operation demonstrated that many peripheral varicosities were independent of the main saphenous system. Also, in many cases the main systems themselves were either not involved or only partially involved. This fact has been confirmed recently by several centers using duplex ultrasonography. This technique has shown that the relationship between saphenofemoral incompetence and peripheral varicosities can be inconsistent. In fact, some varicose clusters were completely isolated without demonstrable deep connection.

If incompetence of perforating veins is not exclusively caused by back pressure, loss of valvular competence can be explained if the perforator itself becomes dilated as the result of the varicose process (Figure 8-10). In such a case it might be argued that ligation is still necessary. However, ligation by itself would not cause the overlying varicosity to regress. On the other hand, if the overlying varicosity were removed, this action would not only solve that problem but also would divide any connecting perforator by traction. Pressure hemostasis then would occlude it. Even if it were theoretically possible for such perforators to remain patent, there would be no superficial varicosity into which to feed (Figure 8-11). These observations caused us to abandon the search for incompetent perforators. In addition, general enthusiasm for the procedure by others has diminished.

The evolution of this theory of incompetent perforating veins has made us concentrate on removing the outlying varicosities ever more thoroughly. Also, it has caused us to refocus on the vein wall and in particular to review the weak vein wall

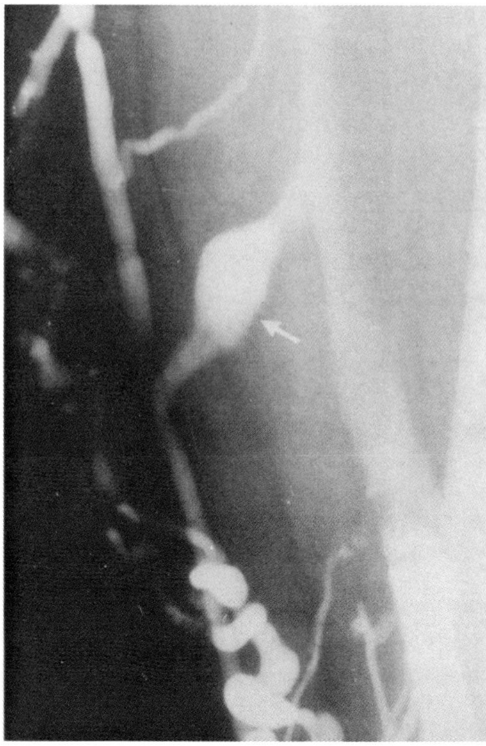

FIGURE 8-10. This phlebogram dramatically shows involvement of a perforating vein in the varicose process. Note the grossly varicose greater saphenous vein (arrow). (From Browse NL, Burnand K, Lea Thomas M, eds. Diseases of the Veins. London: Edward Arnold, 1988.)

theory more seriously. This line of thought started an investigation, the development and conclusions of which are fully described in Chapter 2.

Currently we avulse all irregular varicosities through much smaller incisions because we are confident of hemostasis achieved by firm pressure. The immediate results of this approach are far superior to those obtained earlier. It is obvious that the improvement is the result of removal of the varicose veins themselves.

Careful clinical examination and Doppler insonation have revealed that saphenous dilatation may begin in the lower third of the thigh approximately at the site of the Hunter perforator or further down below the knee at the site of the Boyd perforator. It was through this vein that Boyd was concerned that sclerosants injected around the knee could gain access to the deep venous system, an effect that he demonstrated by phlebography. In the early 1960s we began to do less stripping and more avulsion. This approach has meant that we are able to perform more outpatient and day-case procedures with the patient under a local anesthetic when a full groin exploration is not considered necessary. This practice has helped to lessen the demand for hospital beds and shorten waiting lists. It was this approach, in fact, that had made compression sclerotherapy so popular in the early 1960s in a time of

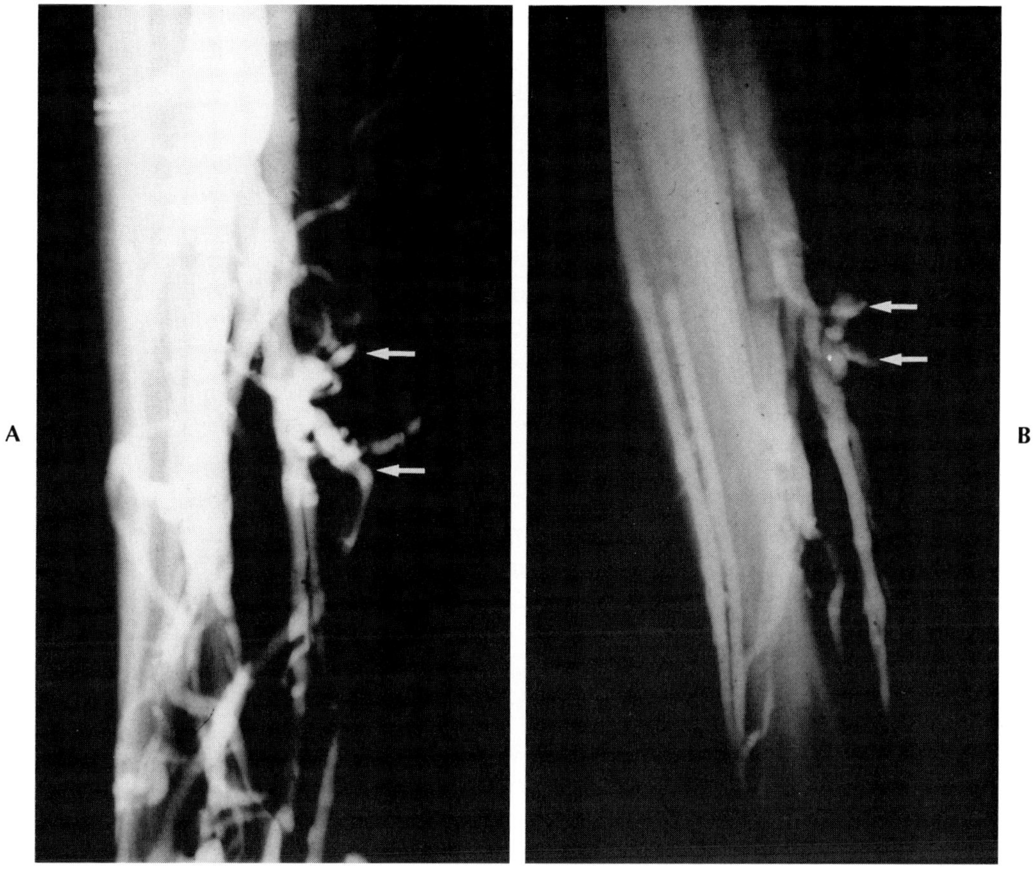

FIGURE 8-11. A, Preoperative phlebogram shows below-knee varicosities (arrows) in a clearly demonstrated perforating vein. A large communication exists between the greater and the lesser saphenous systems. **B,** After multiple avulsion of the superficial varicosities without any stripping, the perforating vein is still patent but there is no superficial varicosity into which the vein can feed (arrows). Considerable improvement in the varicose condition is noted.

financial stringency. As we began to strip the internal saphenous vein less often, the question arose whether we should strip the internal saphenous vein at all.

ISSUES IN SURGERY

Stripping the Internal Saphenous Vein

The relevance of saphenofemoral incompetence to the occurrence and development of peripheral varicosities needs to be examined. In particular, the pros and cons of stripping the internal saphenous vein must be elucidated.

Let us consider some technical objections. First, it is recognized that reflux in the groin is not present in all cases of varicose veins. Second, there is always the possibility of sural or saphenous nerve damage during stripping. Third, increased postoperative morbidity is associated with stripping. Although stripping is a comparatively painless procedure, it often involves postoperative bruising, tenderness, and induration along the line of the stripped vein. Certainly there is more discomfort after stripping than after simple local avulsion. Fourth, and perhaps the most potent argument for not removing the main saphenous vein, is the possibility of future arterial bypass requirements. However, an obviously dilated varicose vein is not likely to be suitable for such a purpose. Nor is it certain that a normal section of a saphenous vein that is only moderately dilated should be used as an arterial bypass. It could be argued that this section might become varicose at some future time. Yet cases have been described in which no extension of the varicosity develops. Some arterial surgeons have reported success in using borderline veins for arterial repair. However, this method must be considered as a calculated gamble.

The main argument in favor of stripping the saphenous vein is that it will further the aims of treatment. Therefore one must ask whether this approach will contribute to the eradication of varicose veins and the prevention of recurrence. With regard to the first objective, the answer must be that stripping alone does not seem to be sufficient. As already described, many of the offending varicosities remain after stripping.

In order to assess the part played by removal of the internal saphenous vein, it is necessary to consider the incidence of recurrence with and without stripping of this vein. These investigations are now taking place at numerous surgical centers, but a significant period of time must elapse before meaningful results can be obtained.

Indications for Surgery

Not all patients with varicose veins require treatment. Many are asymptomatic and remain so for most of their lives. On the other hand, some patients complain of aching pain that varies from mild to severe. Pain in the leg and varicose veins are both common conditions. However, the important point is to establish whether the symptom and the cause are related. Pain of skeletal and arterial origin always must be eliminated. Male patients often present with severe varicose veins with well-developed skin pigmentation, eczema, and ulceration. They may have surprisingly little pain from the varicose veins themselves, but the ulcers become painful if infected. Often these patients have evidence of tinea pedis, which may predispose them to superficial phlebitis. Varicose veins are not confined to those individuals in an occupation that involves long periods of standing, but naturally the symptoms are more likely to be noted under these conditions. A history of a sudden hemorrhage or a dilated vein in a site vulnerable to trauma, such as the shin, the ankle, or the dorsum of the foot, is often an urgent indication for surgery. Athletes often have large asymptomatic veins, and many of those involved in track and team sports must undergo surgery because of the risk of large traumatic hematomas or superficial phlebitis. Superficial phlebitis also can arise spontaneously or after a local or general infection. This condition usually foretells morbidity, especially if it is repeated.

A history of previous deep phlebitis is not a contraindication to surgery if no evidence of persisting deep vein obstruction exists. Since such obstruction occurs in only 10% of cases, most patients will have some degree of deep venous reflux. Venous return from the leg will be hampered if superficial reflux also is present. With exercise, venous pressures show that if the superficial veins are dealt with, the fall in pressure associated with exercise is improved and in some instances will return to normal. If deep venous occlusion is present and persists, the patient will complain that firm bandaging makes the condition worse, even to the point of venous claudication. In such patients superficial veins are part of the collateral venous return.

Last, but by no means least, is the cosmetic problem. Many women complain of varicose veins for purely cosmetic reasons. Such complaints are often not considered seriously by physicians. Women who make these complaints constitute a wide age group. They may be multiparous and are drawn from all social classes and occupations. Despite such disparity, these patients all have one thing in common. They regard their veins as unacceptable disfigurements. Their complaint is as distressing to them as any painful affliction would be, and it is often less well tolerated. When fashion decrees that skirts are to be worn shorter, these women seek treatment at once. I think that they are entitled to our attention and that no surgeon should turn them away if he or she can assure them of a good cosmetic result.

Finally, some patients have no symptoms but are driven to seek advice because of some drastic happening to other members of their family who had varicose veins. Each such case needs to be treated on its own merits.

Contraindications to Surgery

Varicose veins should not be operated on during pregnancy; nor should such surgery be done in the presence of peripheral arterial disease, any contraindication to general anesthesia, any bleeding diathesis, or active skin infection in the lower limb. In addition, surgery for varicose veins should not be performed in association with lymphedema or in the presence of venous claudication. In any case of unusual presentation, a congenital malformation should be considered. The contraceptive pill should be discontinued 1 month before and 1 month after this type of surgery.

Preparation for Surgery

As stated in our goals, the only practical way of eradicating varicose veins is by a meticulous and radical removal of all the varicosities, with the addition of ligation, if necessary, at the saphenofemoral and saphenopopliteal junction and/or localized stripping of the main saphenous veins.

Veins are carefully charted after the patient has been standing for 10 minutes. The extent of varicosity is estimated by palpation, propagation of the cough impulse, and Doppler ultrasound. This approach establishes connections with the long saphenous vein. The short saphenous vein should be examined in the same way, but palpation is easier to do with the patient's knee slightly flexed to relax the deep fascia. A full abdominal examination is performed, and the peripheral pulses are palpated. Sciatic pain is eliminated by using the straight leg–raising test. The conditions of the ankle, knee, and hip are estimated. It is important to note any existing blemishes on the limb. The patient must be told that the veins can be removed but the tendency to varicosity is inborn and cannot be eliminated. Therefore maintenance treatment, consisting of injections or surgical removal done on an outpatient basis, may be necessary from time to time. An instruction sheet outlining the preoperative and postoperative routine is helpful. Great emphasis is placed on postoperative walking exercise of six 10-minute brisk bursts rather than a 60-minute walk since the latter tends to be more time-consuming and not as efficient in stimulating venous return.

SUMMARY

The history of the development of varicose vein surgery throughout the ages has been described, and the evolution of the modern operation has been followed over the last 50 years. The time-honored attitude to surgery that has been directed toward the doctrine of primary valvular incompetence has been questioned because it has been shown that varicose veins can develop in the absence of incompetence in the feeding veins. It has been postulated that the answer must lie in weakness of the vein wall and that, on examination, this theory will readily explain the anomalies described. Evidence for this theory is presented in Chapter 2.

As the modern trend in varicose vein surgery turns away from routine stripping and toward multiple avulsion, results have improved. There are, however, a number of circumstances in which limited stripping of the internal saphenous vein is indicated. Our approach to this problem is to combine limited stripping with multiple avulsion.

We suggest an operative technique that places great emphasis on elimination of varicosities wherever they occur while also achieving a good cosmetic result. Although we believe that a specialist clinic could achieve the best results from the patient's point of view, one of the most important functions of medicine is the training of young people in appropriate varicose vein surgery. This training must include an indoctrination that sees the high attainment of good results as a challenge. This challenge is to be met in a much neglected but most important branch of surgical art.

BIBLIOGRAPHY

Babcock WW. A Textbook of Surgery, 2nd ed. Philadelphia: WB Saunders, 1935.

Barros D'Sa Aires AB, Bell PRF, Darke SG, Harris PL. Vascular Surgery—Current Questions. Oxford: Butterworth Heinemann, 1991.

Bernsten A. Des varices du membre inférieur, spécialement au point de vue de l'étiologie et du traitement chirurgical. Acta Chir Scand 62:61, 1927.

Browse NL, Burnand K, Lea Thomas M, eds. Diseases of the Veins. London: Edward Arnold, 1988.

Buck AH. The Growth of Medicine. New Haven, Conn.: Yale University Press, 1917.

Edwards EA. The treatment of varicose veins: Anatomical features of ligation of the great saphenous vein. Surg Gynecol Obstet 59:916, 1934.

Foote RR. Varicose Veins, ed 2. London: Butterworth, 1954.
Garrison FH. Introduction to the History of Medicine, 4th ed. Philadelphia: WB Saunders, 1929.
Genevrier M. Soc de Med Mil Franc 15:169, 1921.
Greenhalgh RM. Vascular Surgical Techniques. An Atlas, 2nd ed. Philadelphia: WB Saunders, 1989.
Haeger K. The Illustrated History of Surgery. Gothenburg, Sweden: AB Nordbok, 1988.
Higgins TT, Kittel AB. The use of sodium morrhuate in treatment of varicose veins by injection. Lancet 1:68, 1930.
Homans J. The operative treatment of varicose veins and ulcers based upon a classification of these lesions. Surg Gynecol Obstet 22:143, 1916.
Homans J. Varicose veins and ulcer: Methods of diagnosis and treatment. Boston Med Surg J 187:258, 1922.
Keller WL. A new method of extirpating the internal saphenous and similar veins in varicose conditions; A preliminary report. NY Med J 82:385, 1905.
Keller WL. Combined extirpation and obliteration in the treatment of varicose veins. Ann Surg 79:907, 1924.
Lyons AS, Petrucelli RJ. Medicine: An Illustrated History. New York: Harry N. Abrams, 1978.
Maingot RH, Carlton CH. The injection treatment of varicose veins. An estimate of its place in practice. Lancet 1:806, 1928.
Mayo CH. Treatment of varicose veins. Surg Gynecol Obstet 2:385, 1906.
McPheeters HO, Anderson JK. The Injection Treatment of Varicose Veins, 2nd ed. Philadelphia: Davis, 1939.
Nicolaides AN, Sumner DS. Investigation of Patients With Deep Vein Thrombosis and Chronic Venous Insufficiency. London: Med Orion, 1991.
Ochsner A, Mahorner H. Varicose Veins. St. Louis: CV Mosby, 1939.
Paré A. Journeys in Diverse Places. Translated by S. Paget. New York: Collier, 1910.
Perthes G. Über die Operation der Unterschenkelvaricen nach Trendelenburg. Dtsch Med Wochenschr 21:253, 1895.
Schiassi B. Sem Med Paris 28:601, 1908.
Sicard JA, Gaugier L. Les Traitements des Varices par les Injections Locale Sclérosantes. Paris: Masson, 1927.
de Takats G. Ambulatory ligation of the saphenous vein. JAMA 94:1194, 1930.
de Takats G, Quillin L. Ligation of the saphenous vein. A report on two hundred ambulatory operations. Arch Surg 26:72-88, 1933.
de Takats G, Quint H. The injection treatment of varicose veins. Surg Gynecol Obstet 50:545, 1930.
Trendelenburg F. Beitr Klin Chir 7:195, 1891.
Warwick WT. The Rational Treatment of Varicose Veins and Varicocoele. London: Faber & Faber, 1931.

Chapter 9

Treatment of Varicosities of Saphenous Origin: Comparison of Ligation, Selective Excision, and Sclerotherapy

Peter Neglén

Patients suffering from varicose veins have many complaints. Some may be concerned about minute localized varicosities for cosmetic reasons, whereas others do not seek medical advice until they have major varicose veins with swelling, aching, and eczema. Naturally, the treatment expectations of the two groups differ. This chapter focuses on the treatment of varicose veins with main-stem insufficiency.

Several different treatments have been recommended for patients with long (greater) saphenous vein or short (lesser) saphenous vein reflux. Flush ligation combined with stripping, avulsion of local varicosities, and perforator interruption is still the most common operation. An alternative is to spare the long saphenous vein by performing proximal ligation with excision of local visible varices and ligation of incompetent perforators. Sclerotherapy, accomplished by injecting the visible vein perforators and/or the main stem, performed alone or in combination with flush ligation of the long saphenous vein at the saphenofemoral junction, has been advocated.

Since venous varicosity is a progressive, incurable disease, the treatment is only palliative without guarantee of a cure. Therefore the objectives should be the same for all modes of treatment, that is, to provide a satisfactory cosmetic result, relieve symptoms, avoid complications, and prevent recurrences.

GENERAL ASPECTS OF SURGICAL TREATMENT

Treatment of insufficiency of the long saphenous stem by ligation of the vein's termination was described in the late 1800s. The importance of performing flush ligation of the main stem and its tributaries close to the femoral vein to prevent recurrences was pointed out by Homans[1] in 1916. In the early 1900s, Mayo[2] introduced stripping of the long saphenous vein with the technique refined by Babcock[3] and later by Myers and Cooley.[4] In addition, proper excision of local varicosities with meticulous disconnection of all incompetent perforators is the "classic" surgery of varicose veins. Very low recurrence rates have been claimed for this type of radical surgery.[5,6]

Several arguments have been made for restricting the removal of saphenous veins, either to avoid any stripping of the vein or to limit it to the thigh portion. With a limited operation the patient may not require hospitalization and will have a shorter convalescence. Increased morbidity, pain, bleeding, and wound infection, although minimal, are associated with complete stripping. A well-recognized complication of ankle-to-groin stripping of the long saphenous vein is damage to the distal portion of the saphenous nerve, resulting in skin anesthesia of the medial ankle and foot.[7] Stripping the vein in a distal direction (groin-to-ankle) decreases the incidence of nerve injury.[8] Thus it appears to be advisable to strip the long saphenous vein below the knee in a distal direction. If stripping the main stem is limited from the groin to just below the knee, nerve injury is markedly reduced from 39% to 4% to 7%.[9,10] In addition, the remaining distal portion may be used later for arterial reconstructive surgery.

The greater demand for arterial reconstructive surgery has accentuated the fact that unnecessary stripping of the long saphenous vein removes the most favorable graft conduit. On the other hand, a grossly dilated, tortuous, incompetent main stem is a poor arterial substitute. Nevertheless, the main reason for limited saphenous vein surgery is that the long saphenous vein is spared for future arterial surgery. The important issues are whether saphenous vein–saving surgery compromises the objectives of varicose vein treatment and whether the remaining veins can be used as grafts.

FLUSH LIGATION OF LONG SAPHENOUS VEIN

Flush ligation done without stripping of the long saphenous vein was the first operation recommended for saphenous vein incompetence. It has definite advantages because it is a simple operation that can be performed with the patient under local anesthesia; it involves little or no postoperative sick leave. Although the patient is initially relieved of symptoms, the recurrence rate is significantly reduced if removal of the long saphenous vein also is performed.[11]

Inappropriate flush ligation without interruption of all tributaries invites recurrence of varicose veins. If proper ligation of the saphenofemoral junction has been done, another explanation for recurrence is incompetence of the superficial and deep communicating veins of the leg and thigh, often called perforators. Although numerous perforators are present in the calf, three or four medial calf perforators are fairly constant in position. It is important to note that they do not communicate directly with the distal long saphenous vein but with the posterior arch vein. Therefore stripping the long saphenous vein below the knee does not correct all perforator incompetence. This is a valid argument for abandoning stripping of the distal long saphenous vein unless the vein is tortuous, dilated, and incompetent.

In contrast to calf perforator veins, thigh perforators drain the long saphenous

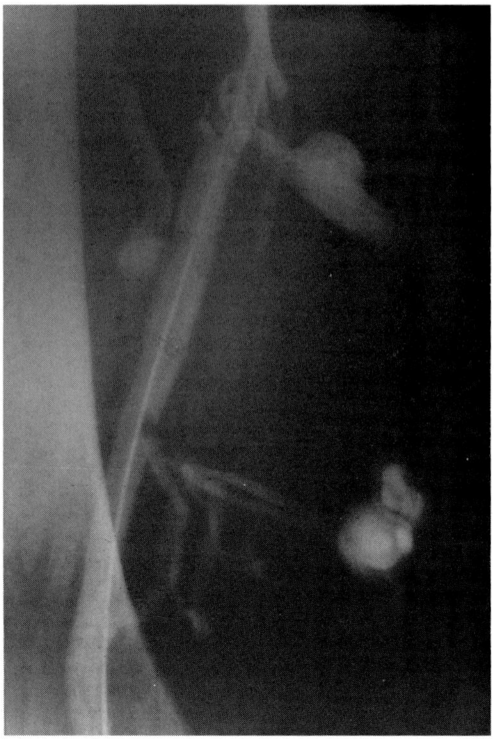

FIGURE 9-1. Popliteal venogram showing two midthigh perforators filling a distally incompetent long saphenous vein. (Courtesy Professor Bo Eklöf.)

vein directly to the superficial femoral vein (Figure 9-1). Retrograde saphenography has demonstrated at least one thigh perforator in 87% of patients.[12] Incompetent thigh perforating veins may be multiple and have been shown to occur anywhere in the thigh. However, in the majority of patients (80%) only one perforator is identified, with two thirds of them found in the middle third of the thigh.[13] Stripping the long saphenous vein at the thigh usually, but not invariably, disrupts these communications. Thus recurrence caused by dilatation of Hunter's thigh perforators and reflux into a preserved, patent long saphenous vein is prevented.[14]

What happens to the vein after simple ligation? It does not seem to be occluded completely by thrombosis. The long saphenous vein of the thigh remains patent in more than 85% of operated legs.[15] Presumably, the vein stays open to the point of the most proximal perforating vein, with thrombosis likely above this level. If this perforating vein becomes insufficient, the entire saphenous system again may undergo reflux and varicosities are likely to recur.

Another explanation for recurrence after a properly performed flush ligation of the saphenofemoral confluence has been suggested by Sheppard.[16] He found that connections between the long saphenous stump and the remaining saphenous vein

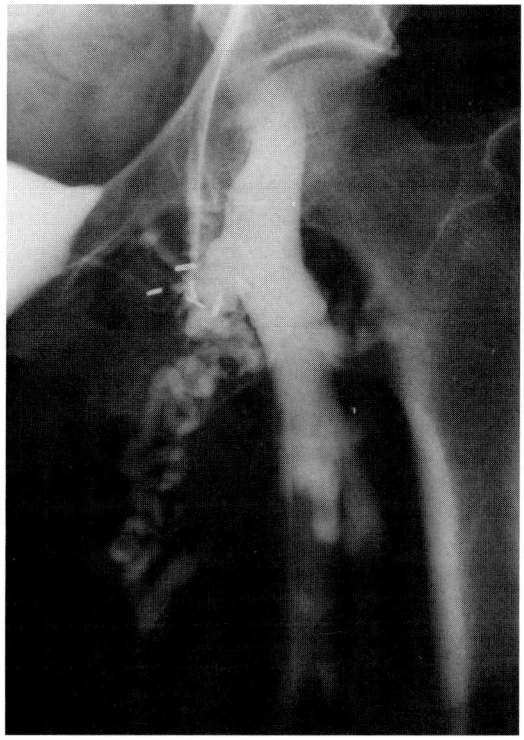

FIGURE 9-2. Popliteal venogram showing neovascularization in the groin after previous high ligation of the long saphenous vein. (Courtesy Professor Bo Eklöf.)

or its tributaries may be reestablished by neovascularization of granulation tissue at the site of the flush ligation. Recurrence develops from reflux into the remaining incompetent saphenous vein (Figure 9-2).

Varicography of recurrent varicose veins was performed in 41 lower limbs 2 to 33 years after proximal ligation of the saphenous vein without stripping.[17] On examination, continuous-wave ultrasound indicated a source of reflux from above the knee. The varicogram revealed midthigh perforator incompetence in 34% of the lower limbs and a patent portion of the saphenous vein in the thigh in 54%. The most common cause of recurrence (80%), however, was a residual or recurrent communication between the femoral vein and the remaining long saphenous vein.

In one prospective study, 54 patients had long saphenous vein incompetence verified by duplex ultrasound prior to flush ligation of the long saphenous vein.[18] At follow-up 6 to 12 months later, scanning of the saphenofemoral junction was repeated. The surprising finding was that two patients still had a patent and incompetent saphenofemoral junction. In addition, 46% of the remaining long saphenous veins were present and incompetent. In two patients reflux stemmed from a demonstrable midthigh perforator, with the remaining saphenous veins fed by small veins branching from the femoral vein. This observation supports the concept of collateral formation by neovascularization.

Regardless of whether recurrence is most commonly caused by remaining perforating thigh veins or by reestablishment of communication at the saphenofemoral confluence, stripping of the long saphenous vein of the thigh appears to be crucial in minimizing recurrence. A prospective trial in which limbs with saphenofemoral incompetence were randomly selected for saphenofemoral flush ligation alone or ligation combined with stripping of the long saphenous vein has been performed by Munn et al.[11] At follow-up 2.5 to 3.5 years later, an independent objective assessment revealed that stripping the vein conferred significantly greater protection against recurrence. Based on these observations, I strongly believe that it is inadequate to restrict surgery to proximal flush ligation of the incompetent long saphenous vein, and I firmly advocate stripping of the thigh portion of the long saphenous vein.

SELECTIVE EXCISION: LONG SAPHENOUS VEIN–SAVING SURGERY

Removal of the long saphenous vein from the groin to the knee leaves the distal portion of the vein for potential use as an arterial graft and avoids injury to the saphenous nerve. If the distal long saphenous vein is normal and since the calf perforating veins do not join the main stem, this limited stripping does not endanger the objectives of the operation. Negus[10] has reported a low recurrence rate (12.5%) in 96 limbs, with an average follow-up of 3.7 years.

Attempts have been made to limit surgery to flush ligation of the saphenofemoral/popliteal veins with avulsions of obvious varicosities through multiple stab incisions and the incompetent saphenous vein left in situ. Large[19] has reported excellent results in a retrospective follow-up done 3 years after this procedure in a randomly selected group of 171 from a total of 1000 patients with 295 affected limbs. A satisfactory result was observed in 90% of patients. Whether or not the remaining saphenous vein was useful for arterial grafting was not indicated.

Hammarsten et al.[20] have reported the results following random allocation of 42 patients to either "classic" operation, including ankle-groin stripping of the saphenous vein, or flush ligation of the saphenous vein at the saphenofemoral junction. Both procedures were combined with local excision of varicosities and ligation of incompetent perforators. Perforators were visualized by phlebography or were noted clinically. It is not clear whether thigh perforators were interrupted. At follow-up done more than 4 years later, the recurrence rate was low in both groups (12%). This finding was supported by a significant increase in venous return time as measured by strain-gauge plethysmography. Ultrasound scanning of the remaining long saphenous veins showed that 78% of these veins could be used for arterial grafting. This observation contradicts the findings of Sutton and Drake.[12] On retrograde saphenography performed during varicose vein surgery, 65% of long saphenous veins were found to be varicose with an average length of normal-appearing vein $<$16 cm, which made them unsuitable for arterial grafts.

Koyano and Sakaguchi[21] chose to remove only those segments of the long saphenous vein that involved reflux detected by Doppler ultrasound in 337 lower limbs with primary varicose veins. These authors found incompetence of the saphenofemoral junction and long saphenous vein from groin to at least knee level in 91% of limbs. An additional 7% of limbs had reflux of the saphenofemoral junction with limited or no incompetence of the long saphenous vein, whereas only 2% had segmental incompetence with no reflux at the junction. Almost 50% of the patients with varicosities of short saphenous vein origin had no reverse flow in the distal saphenous vein. The distribution of incompetence is probably different in another catchment area, but there is no doubt that most patients who complain of varicose veins have saphenofemoral or saphenopopliteal insufficiency with varying degrees of trunk involvement.

Selective stripping of incompetent veins was performed in 80 patients. The results were compared to those of 189 limbs in which standard stripping was done during the same time period, after an average follow-up of 3.2 years. Plethysmographic measurement of venous reflux volume in a limited number of the limbs and clinical examination of 80% of them at follow-up revealed no difference between the two groups. Whether the remaining veins were adequate for use as vascular grafts is not clear. As expected, a reduction in the rate of saphenous and sural nerve injury was observed.

Use of noninvasive modalities such as duplex scanning will undoubtedly facilitate the investigation of each segment of superficial and deep veins with detection of incompetent perforators. The ability to map superficial incompetence will make it possible to perform selective, directed surgery of incompetent segments. However, preservation of a diseased segment is of no proven value and may jeopardize the objectives of varicose vein surgery. The intention still must be to remove diseased incompetent superficial veins and to control reflux.

SURGERY VS. SCLEROTHERAPY

Sclerotherapy has been used in central Europe for decades. However, the method had its true revival when Fegan[22] published his basic studies on the effects of the sclerosant and stressed the necessity of effective elastic compression after injection. Having become firmly established in Great Britain and Scandinavia, sclerotherapy is now being enthusiastically accepted in North America. The advantages of compression sclerotherapy are obvious: no anesthesia, no hospitalization, and no loss of work are required. These factors substantially decrease the cost to the patient and the community.[23] Advocates of sclerotherapy treatment also maintain that the cosmetic results are better. The advantages are real, however, only if sclerotherapy done alone or in combination with saphenofemoral flush ligation produces results equivalent to those of surgery. The initial economic advantage is greatly eroded if regular follow-up examinations and repeated treatments are necessary.

The results of "adequate" initial surgery, including stripping of the saphenous vein with flush ligation of the proximal vein, meticulous avulsion of all tributaries, and interruption of all perforating veins, have been reported to be extremely good in some reviews, with very low 10-year recurrence rates (<15%) noted.[6,24] Enthusiastic sclerotherapists have reported similar excellent results, 80% to 90% success following sclerotherapy performed alone.[22,25,26]

These studies probably exaggerate the results of both surgery and sclerotherapy. It is well known that varicose vein disease is a chronic condition and that intervention is palliative. With a long observation time, new varicosities invariably develop. Objective assessment of any treatment for varicose veins is extremely difficult because of the varying definition of what a recurrence is and how to measure it. This lack of uniformity also makes comparisons of studies difficult. In studies it is vital that the follow-up be long enough (at least 5 years) and that results be assessed as objectively as possible, preferably by someone who is not involved in treatment. In most studies treatment outcome is described by patients as a subjective opinion, with the objective findings reported by a surgeon. It is well known that agreement is oftentimes poor between what the surgeon and the patient consider a good result. Physiologic tests of calf pump function following the two forms of treatment are most valuable. From a socioeconomic viewpoint, the need for additional treatment is of greatest importance.

Despite the fact that modern compression sclerotherapy was introduced 25 years ago, controversy still exists as to whether sclerotherapy or surgery is the most effective treatment for varicose veins involving long saphenous vein or short saphenous vein insufficiency. Several studies have attempted to compare the two treatments in prospective controlled random trials.[27-32]

In 1972, Chant et al.[27] reported no significant difference in results between injection compression sclerotherapy in which Fegan's technique was used and radical surgery for varicose veins 3 years after initial treatment. However, by 5 years, 40% of patients who initially received sclerotherapy had further treatment compared with 24% of those treated surgically[28] (Figure 9-3). This difference was statistically significant. Patients more than 35 years of age and those with signs of chronic venous insufficiency, such as edema and ankle flare, fared better with surgery than with sclerotherapy.

In 1975, Doran and White[29] described the results of another controlled study in favor of compression sclerotherapy over surgery after 1 year (24% vs. 45% failures). After 2 years the difference was not significant (21% vs. 16.4% failures).

These two trials found no contraindications to sclerosis of primary saphenofemoral incompetence, but neither study identified the type of superficial insufficiency. Both studies can be criticized for being short-term or for having an unclear endpoint, which was set as the need for further treatment (e.g., prescription of stockings). In addition, patients who underwent retreatment were included in 2- and 5-year follow-up, which rendered judgment of the initial treatment impossible.

In 1979, Jakobsen[30] studied 483 patients with incompetence of the long saphenous vein or the short saphenous vein or a combination of the two types. Patients were randomized into three comparable groups. Radical surgery was performed in 161 patients, and 167 patients received compression sclerotherapy. The third group of 165 patients had a combination of these treatment approaches. Objective success after 3 years was 90% for surgery and 37% for sclerotherapy alone (Figure 9-4). Injection sclerotherapy was performed according to Sigg.[31]

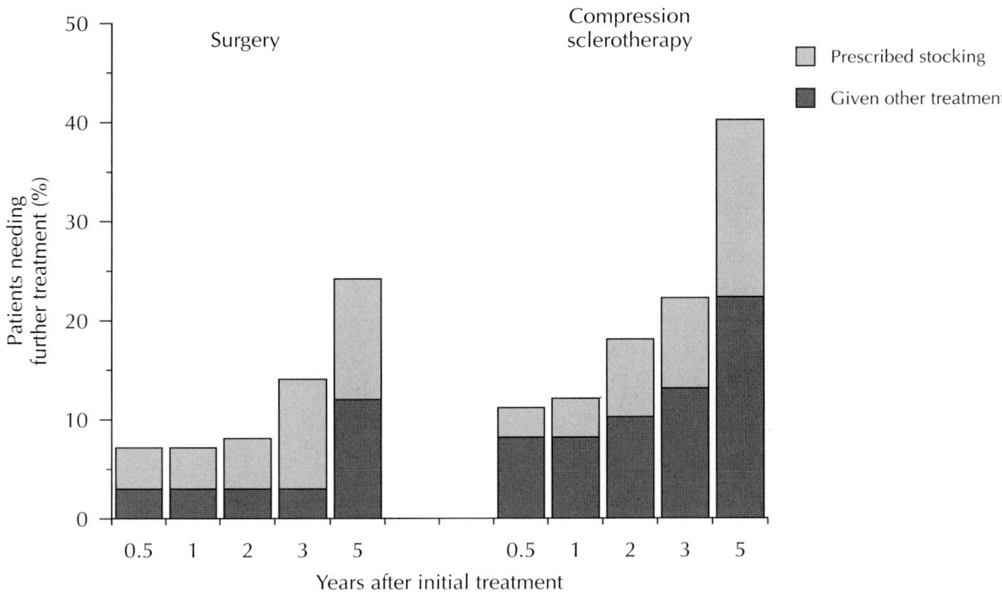

FIGURE 9-3. Chant's comparison of surgery and compression sclerotherapy. Although no statistical difference was noted after 3 years, at 5-year follow-up significantly more patients who had initial treatment with sclerotherapy needed further treatment. (Data from Chant ADB, Jones HO, Weddell JM. Varicose veins: A comparison of surgery and injection/compression sclerotherapy. Lancet 2:1188-1191, 1972; Beresford SAA, Chant ADB, Jones HO, Piachaud D, Weddell JM. Varicose veins: A comparison of surgery and injection/sclerotherapy. Five-year follow-up. Lancet 1:921-924, 1978.)

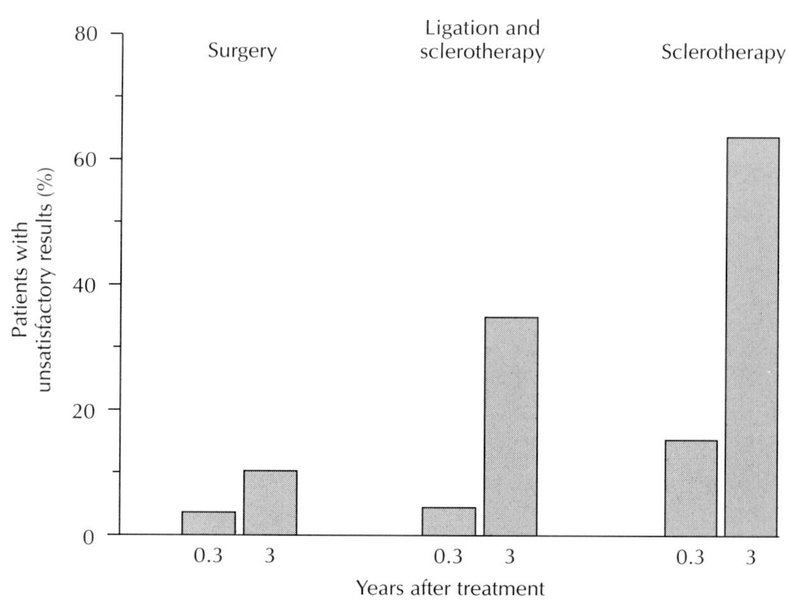

FIGURE 9-4. Recurrence rate was significantly lower for surgery compared to ligation combined with sclerotherapy. At 3 years after treatment, recurrence rate was significantly lower for combined treatment than for sclerotherapy alone. (Data from Jakobsen B. The value of different forms of treatment for varicose veins. Br J Surg 66:182-184, 1979.)

In 1974 and 1984, Hobbs[32,33] reported the results of the most comprehensive randomized long-term study done to date, comparing sclerotherapy and surgery for varicose veins in 500 patients. The large number of patients permitted stratification into defined groups according to short saphenous vein or long saphenous vein insufficiency, isolated perforator incompetence, or dilated local varicose veins. Although compression sclerotherapy initially seemed effective even when proximal incompetence was present, later objective results were substantially better with surgery (surgery vs. compression sclerotherapy at 5 years 79% vs. 30% [excellent] and at 10 years 71% vs. 6% [good], respectively) (Figure 9-5). Patients with mainstem insufficiency had a higher recurrence rate than the others. Hobbs[32,33] concluded that saphenous vein insufficiency is best managed by radical operation but that compression sclerotherapy is superior for treatment of local varicosities, isolated leg perforator incompetence, and residual or recurrent veins after appropriate surgery.

In a prospective study done by our group, 152 lower limbs with primary varicose veins and long saphenous vein incompetence were studied closely.[34] Of these, 78 limbs had been randomized for compression sclerotherapy and 74 limbs for radical stripping. Injection therapy was performed according to Hobbs's modification of the Fegan technique,[32] and surgery was performed as previously described. These patients were followed up not only for rate of recurrence after 5 years but also for assessment by foot volumetry. Expelled volume, which expresses calf muscle pump function, and refilling flow ratio, which is directly related to the amount of venous reflux, were estimated before and after treatment.

At follow-up, three groups were defined through inspection and palpation by the surgeon: (1) cured, in which no true varicose veins were seen or palpated (except for minor reticular veins); (2) improved, in which limited residual or recurrent varicosities or a long saphenous vein was palpable as recanalized at the injection site (even if no varicosities were seen); and (3) failed, in which large varicosities with incompetent perforators or retrograde flow in the long saphenous vein were noted. When treatment failed according to objective assessment, these limbs were considered failures throughout the study and were not reevaluated by foot volumetry.

As early as 6 months after treatment, the surgeon's findings showed a smaller cure rate with compression sclerotherapy compared to surgery, although the failure rate was minimal in both groups. After 5 years, a striking difference was found between the surgically treated patients (60% "cured" and 35% improved) and the sclerotherapy group (51% failure rate) (Figure 9-6).

Foot volumetric results are shown in Table 9-1 and Figure 9-7. Throughout the study period of 5 years, the radical surgery group showed significantly greater functional improvement than did the sclerotherapy group (i.e., higher expelled volume and lower refilling flow). At 5 years, foot volumetric results had returned to pretreatment levels in the injected limbs, despite the fact that failures, which involved additional treatment, were not included. This study firmly supports previous reports in concluding that compression sclerotherapy cannot replace radical surgery for varicose vein disease that involves saphenous vein incompetence.

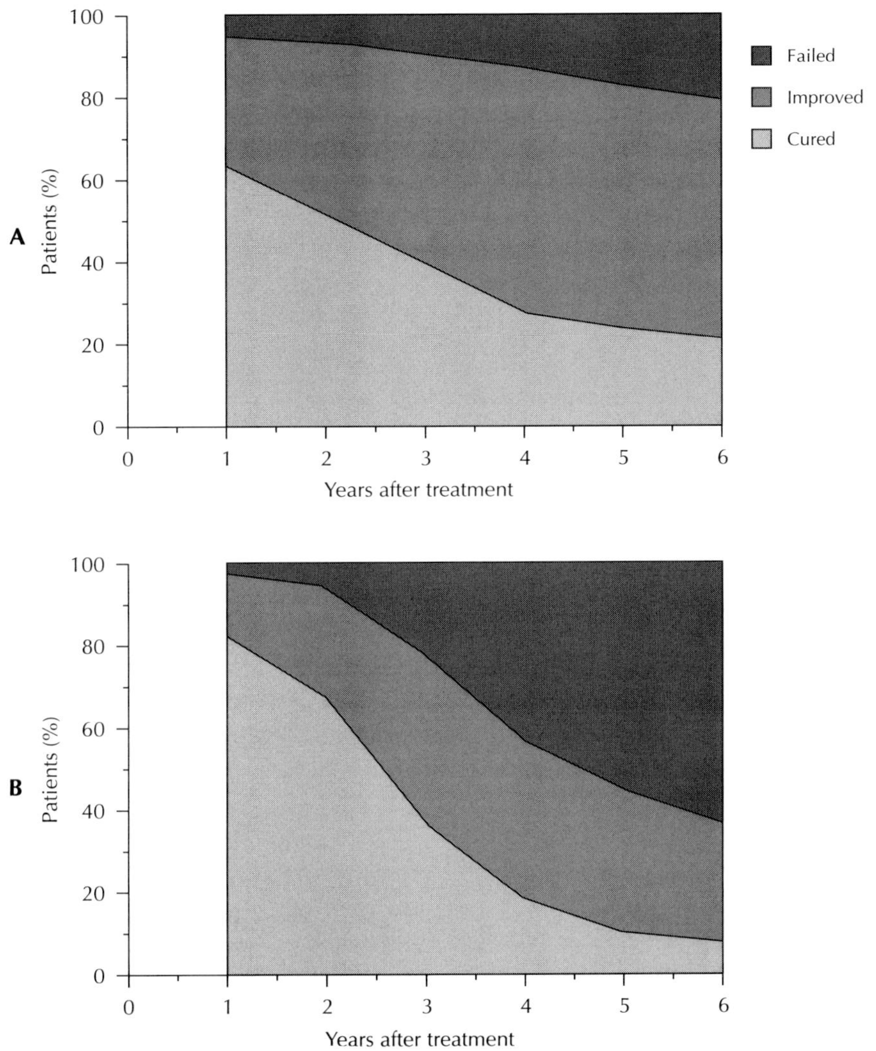

FIGURE 9-5. Comparison of results with surgery (**A**) and sclerotherapy (**B**). Early failure rates are similar, but after 6 years more patients were cured or improved with surgery. (Redrawn from Hobbs JT. Surgery and sclerotherapy in the treatment of varicose veins. Arch Surg 109:793-796, 1974. Copyright 1974, American Medical Association.)

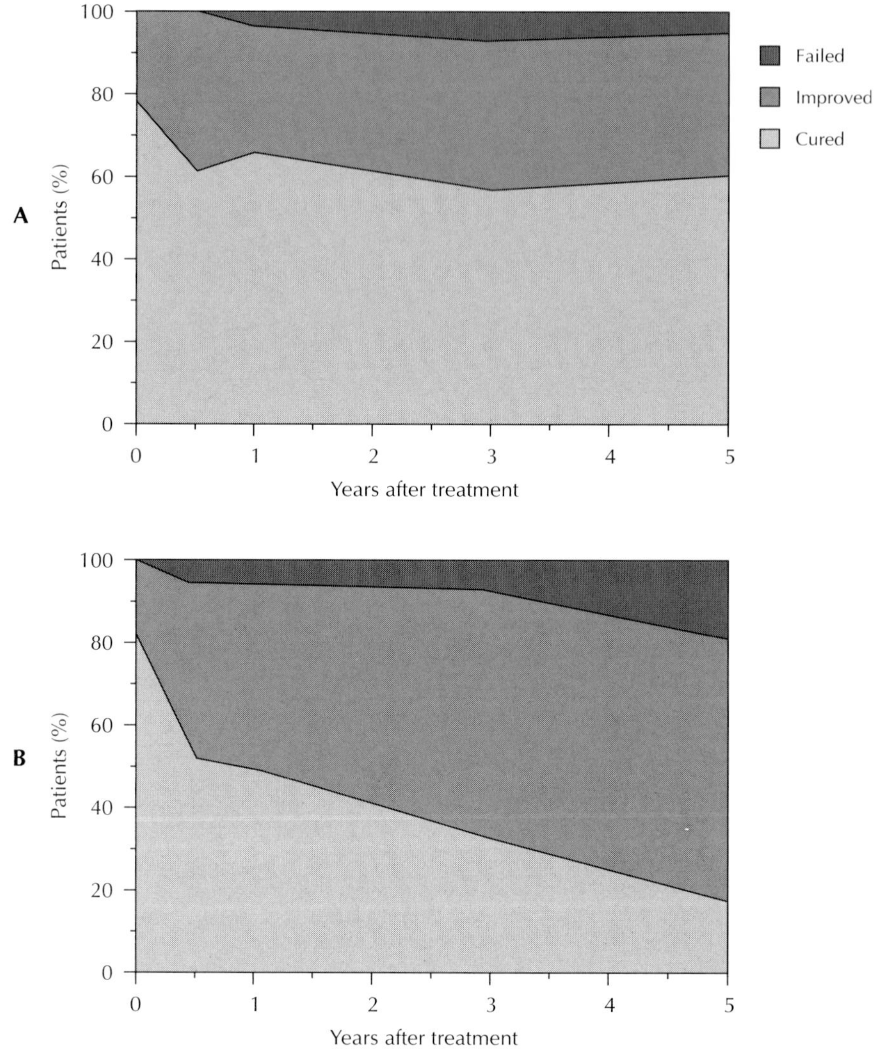

FIGURE 9-6. Results with surgery (**A**), ligation combined with sclerotherapy (**B**), and sclerotherapy alone (**C**) in patients with incompetent long saphenous vein. After 5 years more cured and improved patients were found among the groups that had surgery or combined treatment than in the group that had sclerotherapy alone. (Data from Einarsson E. Compression sclerotherapy of varicose veins. In Eklöf B, Gjöres JE, Thulesius O, Bergqvist D, eds. Controversies in the Management of Venous Disorders. London: Butterworth, 1989, pp 203-211; Neglén P, Einarsson E, Eklöf B. High tie with sclerotherapy for saphenous vein insufficiency. Phlebologie 1:105-111, 1986.)

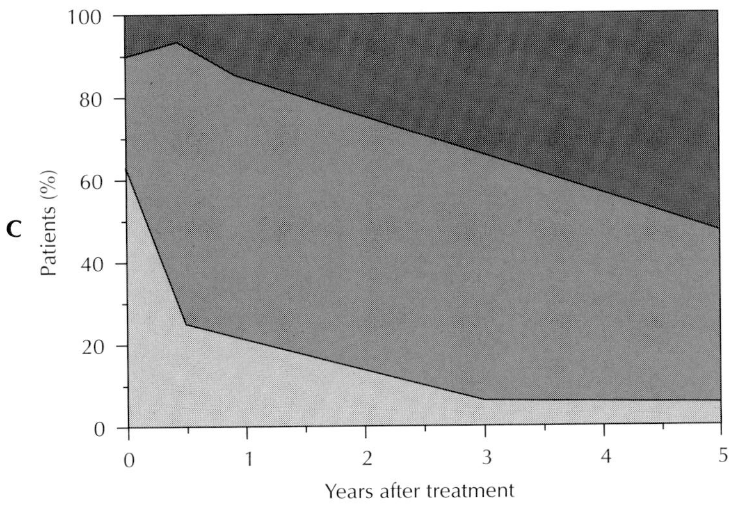

FIGURE 9-6, cont'd. For legend see opposite page.

TABLE 9-1. Results of foot volumetric measurements compared to baseline values in patients having three different modes of varicose vein treatment

Treatment	Foot Volumetric Measurement	Baseline Value	Best Result	5-Year Result
Compression sclerotherapy	EV	10.0 ± 0.5	13.2 ± 0.9*	10.0 ± 0.7^{ns}
	Q/EV_{rel}	5.1 ± 0.4	4.2 ± 0.3†	5.3 ± 0.7^{ns}
		(n = 78)	(n = 58)	(n = 39)
Combined ligation and compression sclerotherapy	EV	9.5 ± 0.7	13.3 ± 0.9*	10.7 ± 0.7^{ns}
	Q/EV_{rel}	4.8 ± 0.4	3.5 ± 0.2*	4.6 ± 0.4^{ns}
		(n = 63)	(n = 60)	(n = 47)
Radical surgery	EV	10.4 ± 0.6	14.9 ± 0.8*	14.0 ± 0.8*
	Q/EV_{rel}	4.4 ± 0.3	2.3 ± 0.2*	3.2 ± 0.3‡
		(n = 74)	(n = 57)	(n = 57)

EV, ejection volume (ml); Q/EV_{rel}, refilling flow ration (1/min).
*$p = < 0.05$
†$p = < 0.01$
‡$p = < 0.001$
Note: Mean ± SEM; ns, not significant.

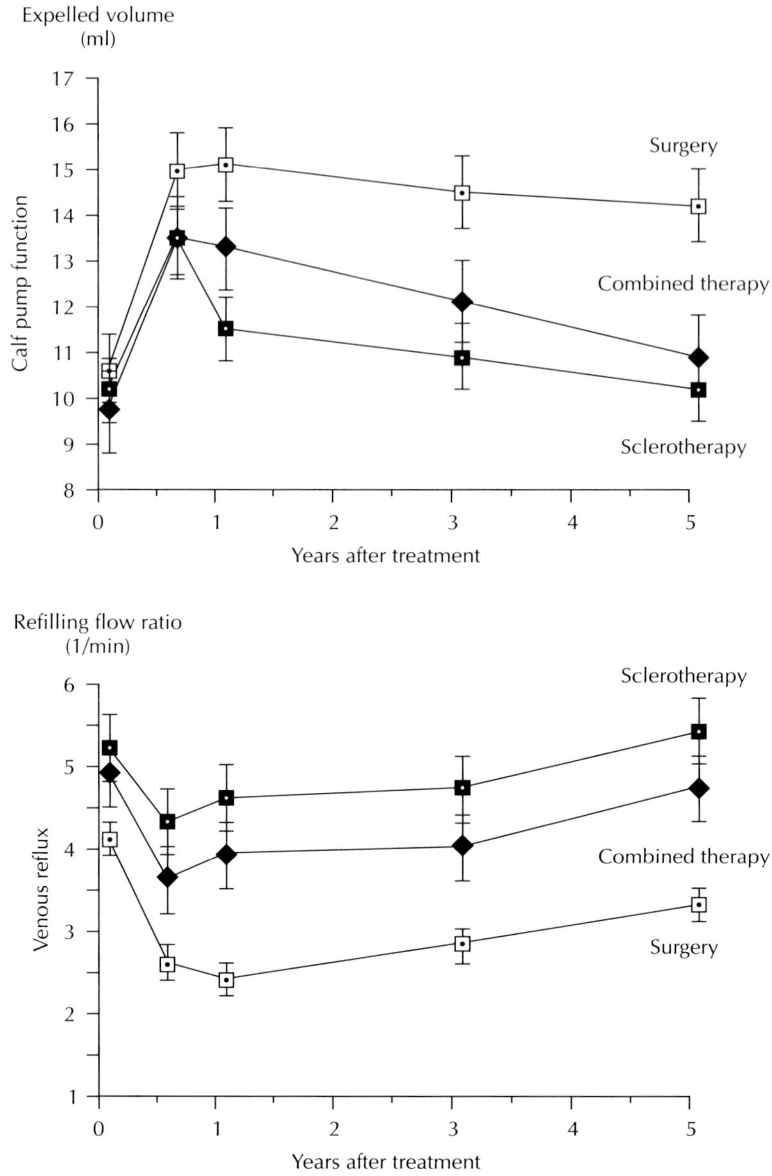

FIGURE 9-7. Foot volumetric results in patients from two separate studies. With the exception at 6 months, expelled volume was significantly higher following surgery compared to combined treatment or sclerotherapy alone. Refilling flow ratio was significantly lower for surgically treated patients throughout the observation period. (Data from Einarsson E. Compression sclerotherapy of varicose veins. In Eklöf B, Gjöres JE, Thulesius O, Bergqvist D, eds. Controversies in the Management of Venous Disorders. London: Butterworth, 1989, pp 203-211; Neglén P, Einarsson E, Eklöf B. High tie with sclerotherapy for saphenous vein insufficiency. Phlebologie 1:105-111, 1986.)

COMBINED SCLEROTHERAPY AND LIGATION OF LONG SAPHENOUS VEIN

The concept of combining ligation of the long saphenous vein with distal sclerotherapy had been discussed by the turn of the century, but it was popularized in the 1930s by de Takats and Quillin.[35] However, the early sclerotherapy technique differed from present methods. At the time of high ligation, sclerosant was injected distally in the vein without compression. Lofgren[36] reported poor results in 60% of patients assessed objectively after 5 years. Sladen[37] found that patients with main-stem insufficiency prior to treatment with injection sclerotherapy alone invariably developed saphenous vein incompetence 2 to 3 years later. If sclerotherapy was combined with ligation of the main stem, there were few recurrences.

Jakobsen[30] not only randomized patients with main-stem vein insufficiency for surgery or compression sclerotherapy alone but also had a third group of 165 patients who received combined treatment. With the patient under local anesthesia, he performed flush ligation of the long saphenous vein or the short saphenous vein and ligation of incompetent perforators. This procedure was followed by injection sclerotherapy done with Sigg's technique. Jakobsen found that after 3 years 65% of patients had a satisfactory result. Although this finding was significantly better than the results following sclerotherapy alone (37%), it did not attain the level of that following surgery (90%) (see Figure 9-4).

Our group studied 63 lower limbs in 60 patients with long saphenous varicose vein incompetence.[38] Half of these patients had varicosities in the thigh. Injection treatment was performed as described by Hobbs, and the whole lower limb was firmly bandaged. After all tributaries were divided, flush ligation was performed at the saphenofemoral junction with the patient under local anesthesia. As in the previously described randomized study, patients were followed up for 5 years and assessed clinically and functionally by foot volumetry at regular intervals.

Although the initial results were good, a steady deterioration occurred throughout the study period, with only 16% of patients cured after 5 years. All limbs with treatment failure had recurrent insufficiency of the saphenous vein despite a properly performed high tie. Among the improved patients, almost half had a patent palpable (although not obviously insufficient) long saphenous vein. When the results for limbs with only minor local recurrent varicosities were combined with those of the cured legs, 67% were noted as satisfactory after 3 years and 40% after 5 years (Figure 9-8). Although combined therapy produced better results than sclerotherapy alone, the results were not comparable to those of radical surgery and appeared to deteriorate rapidly with time (see Figure 9-6).

Through foot volumetry measurements, the function of calf muscle was demonstrated to be improved with a decrease in venous reflux (see Figure 9-7). After 3 years venous reflux decreased considerably, and after 5 years the values had returned to pretreatment levels (see Table 9-1). Although the average best physiologic value in each group is similar, the deterioration in patients having sclerotherapy and those

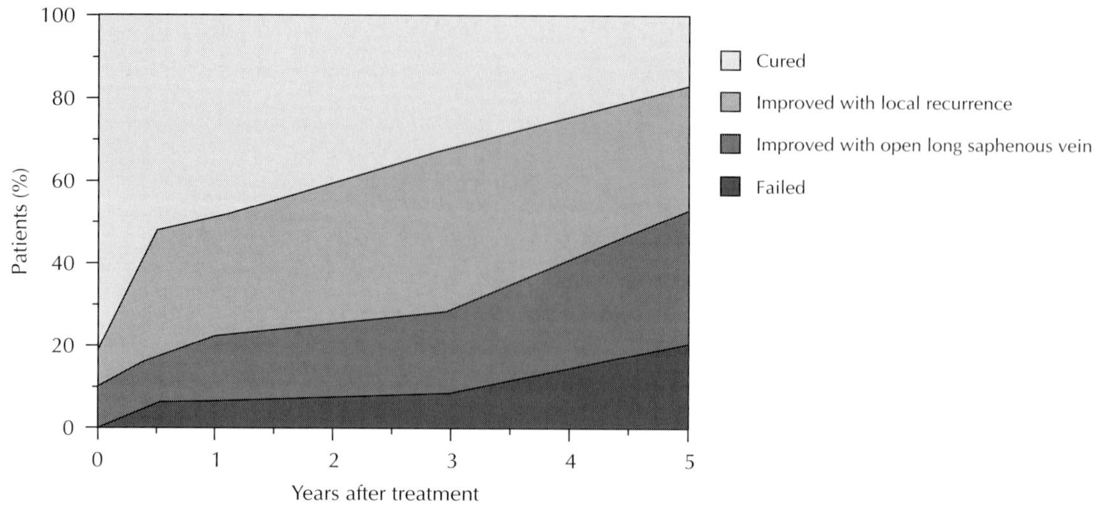

FIGURE 9-8. Results of combined high ligation and sclerotherapy in patients with varicose veins and long saphenous vein incompetence. After 3 years the number of recanalized long saphenous veins increased significantly and appeared to precede complete failure. (Modified from Neglén P, Einarsson E, Eklöf B. High tie with sclerotherapy for saphenous vein insufficiency. Phlebologie 1:105-111, 1986.)

having the combined treatment is striking after 5 years. Recanalization of the main stem seems to precede complete treatment failure.

The aim of sclerotherapy is to produce an inflammation of the vein wall, which obliterates the lumen and eventually results in a fibrosed cord. Pressing the vein walls together is thought to facilitate this development. Swelling of the vein caused by induced inflammation may create the same situation. However, the thigh portion of the long saphenous vein may be more difficult to sclerose because it has a large diameter with a higher flow rate; it is more difficult to compress effectively during and after injection. If the injection of sclerosant results in intraluminal red thrombus alone, recanalization will commonly occur later and the vein will become incompetent. With reopening of the saphenous vein, a situation similar to that described for flush ligation of the saphenofemoral confluence alone may occur. Reflux may recur through thigh perforators or newly formed collaterals between the saphenous stump and the remaining vein, and varicosities may return.

Both clinical and functional results after combined treatment indicate that it is a better method for patients with varicose veins and long saphenous vein incompetence compared to compression sclerotherapy alone. However, combined therapy does not appear to be as efficient as radical surgery, and results indicate that with longer follow-up further deterioration may occur with combined therapy. Combined therapy should be the treatment of choice for patients who are unwilling to undergo complete surgery and for those who are old, unfit, or in whom general or epidural anesthesia is contraindicated.

SELECTIVE TREATMENT FOR MAIN-STEM INSUFFICIENCY

Despite the availability of sclerotherapy and surgery for decades, the controversy regarding which patient to treat with a particular method still exists. The results of long-term prospective randomized studies strongly suggest that compression sclerotherapy as practiced during the 1970s and the early 1980s is a poor treatment for varicose veins involving short saphenous vein or long saphenous vein incompetence. On the other hand, sclerotherapy is the ideal treatment for patients with isolated primary varicosities and residual or recurrent varicosities following adequate main-stem surgery. Its role in the treatment of perforator insufficiency has not been clarified.

In recent years new methods for injecting the long saphenous vein and its junction with the femoral vein have been described.[39] Directed injection done under the guidance of ultrasound, modified compression bandaging, and new sclerosants may have greater efficacy in closing saphenous veins permanently. However, long-term randomized studies that include these recent developments have not been published. Until such studies appear, surgery remains the treatment of choice for main-stem insufficiency.

New diagnostic techniques also will influence surgical technique. Not every patient with varicose veins of saphenous origin needs a complete ankle-groin stripping of the saphenous vein. Segmental incompetence can be identified by Doppler ultrasound or duplex scanning, and insufficiency of the superficial venous system can be mapped. Therefore surgery can be directed toward ligation of main-stem confluences involving reflux, thereby limiting the stripping of the trunk to incompetent segments. With more emphasis on atraumatic technique and minimal incisions, cosmetic results are excellent even after radical surgery.

CONCLUSION

It appears that stripping to the knee can be performed with few late recurrences in the majority of patients and without involvement of distal portions of the saphenous vein. The chronicity of varicose vein disease and the frequent presence of direct deep-to-superficial perforating veins in the thigh have been thoroughly discussed here. Leaving the thigh portion of a long saphenous vein, even though it is competent, may invite long-term recurrences. However, it is desirable to save the long saphenous vein for future use as a vascular graft. Therefore competent portions of saphenous trunks may be saved. There is no proven value in preservation of incompetent dilated saphenous trunks. The aim of varicose vein surgery still should be the removal of diseased incompetent vein segments and the control of reflux.

REFERENCES

1. Homans J. Operative treatment of varicose veins and ulcers. Surg Gynecol Obstet 22:143-158, 1916.
2. Mayo CH. Treatment of varicose veins. Surg Gynecol Obstet 2:385-388, 1906.
3. Babcock WW. A new operation for the extirpation of varicose veins of the leg. N Y Med J 86:153, 1907.

4. Myers TT, Cooley JC. Varicose vein surgery in the management of the post-phlebitic limb. Surg Gynecol Obstet 99:733-744, 1954.
5. Lofgren KA. Management of varicose veins: Mayo Clinic experience. In Bergan JJ, Yao JST, eds. Venous Problems. Chicago: Year Book, 1978.
6. Rivlin S. The surgical cure of primary varicose veins. Br J Surg 62:913-917, 1975.
7. Cox SJ, Wellwood JM, Martin A. Saphenous nerve injury caused by stripping of the long saphenous vein. Br Med J 1:415-417, 1974.
8. Jakobsen BH, Wallin L. Proximal or distal extraction of the internal saphenous vein? Vasa 4:240-242, 1975.
9. Holme JB, Skajaa K, Holme K. Incidence of lesions of the saphenous nerve after partial or complete stripping of the long saphenous vein. Acta Chir Scand 156:145-148, 1990.
10. Negus D. Should the incompetent saphenous vein be stripped to the ankle? Phlebologie 1:33-36, 1986.
11. Munn SR, Morton JB, Macbeth WA, McLeish AR. To strip or not to strip the long saphenous vein? A varicose vein trial. Br J Surg 68:426-428, 1981.
12. Sutton R, Drake SG. Stripping the long saphenous vein: Preoperative retrograde saphenography in patients with and without venous ulceration. Br J Surg 73:305-307, 1986.
13. Papadakis K, Christodoulou C, Christopoulos D, Hobbs J, Malouf GM, Grigg M, Irvine A, Nicolaides A. Number and anatomical distribution of incompetent thigh perforating veins. Br J Surg 76:581-584, 1989.
14. Lofgren EP, Lofgren KA. Recurrence of varicose veins after the stripping operation. Arch Surg 102:111-114, 1971.
15. Rutherford RB, Sawyer JD, Jones DN. The fate of residual saphenous vein after partial removal or ligation. J Vasc Surg 12:422-428, 1990.
16. Sheppard M. A procedure for the prevention of recurrent saphenofemoral incompetence. Aust N Z J Surg 48:322-326, 1978.
17. Corbett CR, Runcie IJ, Thomas ML, Jamieson CW. Reasons to strip the long saphenous vein. Phlebologie 41:766-769, 1988.
18. McMullin GM, Coleridge Smith PD, Scurr JH. Objective assessment of high ligation without stripping of the long saphenous vein. Br J Surg 78:1139-1142, 1991.
19. Large J. Surgical treatment of saphenous varices, with preservation of the main great saphenous trunk. J Vasc Surg 2:886-891, 1985.
20. Hammarsten J, Pedersen P, Cederlund CG, Campanello M. Long saphenous vein–saving surgery for varicose veins. A long-term follow-up. Eur J Vasc Surg 4:361-364, 1990.
21. Koyano K, Sakaguchi S. Selective stripping operation based on Doppler ultrasonic findings for primary varicose veins of the lower extremities. Surgery 103:615-619, 1988.
22. Fegan G. Varicose veins. Compression sclerotherapy. London: Heineman Medical, 1967.
23. Neglén P, Jönsson B, Einarsson E, Eklöf B. Socio-economic benefits of ambulatory surgery and compression sclerotherapy for varicose veins. Phlebologie 1:225-230, 1986.
24. Larsson RH, Lofgren E, Myers TT, Lofgren KA. Long-term results after vein surgery: Study of 1000 cases after 10 years. Mayo Clin Proc 49:114-117, 1974.
25. Reid RG, Rothnie NG. Treatment of varicose veins by compression sclerotherapy. Br J Surg 55:889-895, 1968.
26. Dejode LR. Injection compression treatment for varicose veins. Br J Surg 57:285-286, 1970.
27. Chant ADB, Jones HO, Weddell JM. Varicose veins: A comparison of surgery and injection/compression sclerotherapy. Lancet 2:1188-1191, 1972.
28. Beresford SAA, Chant ADB, Jones HO, Piachaud D, Weddell JM. Varicose veins: A comparison of surgery and injection/sclerotherapy. Five-year follow-up. Lancet 1:921-924, 1978.
29. Doran FSA, White M. A clinical trial designed to discover if the primary treatment of varicose veins should be Fegan's method or by an operation. Br J Surg 62:72-76, 1975.
30. Jakobsen B. The value of different forms of treatment for varicose veins. Br J Surg 66:182-184, 1979.

31. Sigg K. Treatment of varicosities and accompanying complications (ambulatory treatment of phlebitis with compression bandage). Angiology 3:355-379, 1952.
32. Hobbs JT. Surgery and sclerotherapy in the treatment of varicose veins. Arch Surg 109:793-796, 1974.
33. Hobbs JT. Surgery or sclerotherapy for varicose veins; 10-year results of a random study. In Tesi M, Dormandy J, eds. Superficial and Deep Venous Diseases of the Lower Limbs. Turin: Edizione Minerva Medica, 1984, pp 243-246.
34. Einarsson E. Compression sclerotherapy of varicose veins. In Eklöf B, Gjöres JE, Thulesius O, Bergqvist D, eds. Controversies in the Management of Venous Disorders. London: Butterworth, 1989, pp 203-211.
35. de Takats G, Quillin L. Ligation of the saphenous vein. A report on two hundred ambulatory operations. Arch Surg 26:72-88, 1933.
36. Lofgren KA. Management of varicose veins: Mayo Clinic experience. In Bergan JJ, Yao JS, eds. Venous Problems. Chicago: Year Book, 1978, pp 71-83.
37. Sladen JG. Flush ligation and compression sclerotherapy for the control of venous disease. Am J Surg 152:535-538, 1986.
38. Neglén P, Einarsson E, Eklöf B. High tie with sclerotherapy for saphenous vein insufficiency. Phlebologie 1:105-111, 1986.
39. Raymond-Martimbeau P. Two different techniques for sclerosing the incompetent sapheno-femoral junction: A comparative study. J Dermatol Surg Oncol 16:626-631, 1990.

Chapter 10

Treatment of Varicosities of Saphenous Origin: A Dialogue

Ralph G. DePalma, Sidney S. Rose, and John J. Bergan

Whenever a surgical condition is common, a plethora of operations is applied. Contrary opinions abound, and no single method becomes standard. Yet our constant objective is to improve surgery so that results are optimized, complications are minimized, and patient satisfaction is maximized. To achieve these goals, we have established the following dialogue among experienced vascular surgeons who bring a variety of background experiences and observations to one focal point, surgery of varicose veins.

Dr. Bergan: In practice, four goals must be kept in mind when planning the treatment of varicose veins.[1] Although the treatment needs to be individualized, the following objectives remain: (1) permanent removal of the varicosities, (2) determination and ablation of the source of venous hypertension, (3) achievement of the best cosmetic result possible, and (4) minimization of complications. Mr. Rose, what is your opinion about the indications for surgery?

Mr. Rose: First, not all patients with varicose veins require treatment. Many are asymptomatic and remain so for most of their lives.[2] On the other hand, it must be noted that aching pain from varicose veins can vary from mild to severe, any pain of skeletal or arterial origin must be eliminated in the differential diagnosis, and many patients, especially women, complain of varicosities for purely cosmetic reasons. Male patients may have surprisingly little pain from the veins and may encounter severe discomfort only when superficial ulceration occurs. In regard to female patients, in Chapter 2 of this book, I have described the hormonal relationship of varicose vein pain during pregnancy and menstrual cycles.

Dr. DePalma: I would agree. In my practice, about five times as many women as men present with primary varicose veins in the saphenous system distribution. Characteristically, symptoms of aching and fullness worsen during the day, particularly after periods of standing and activity. Recumbency and leg elevation relieve these symptoms and help to differentiate them from musculoskeletal and arterial causes. The severity of complaints of aching, fullness, pain, easy fatigability, and tiredness do not necessarily relate to the gross appearance of the varicosities. This situation is especially relevant to men who have gross, protuberant saccular varicosities but no symptoms. In women, the symptoms are clearly related to the progesterone phase of the menstrual cycle and appear maximally during the first or second day of a menstrual period, paradoxically when the predominant progesterone hormone level decreases and the estrogen level increases.

Prominence or protuberance of the varicosities appears to depend more on subcutaneous tissue thickness and venectasia rather than on the hemodynamic or physiologic effect from the varices.

Although women often seek consultation for the cosmetic appearance of tortuous varicosities related to the saphenous system or for microvarices or telangiectasias, in fact, these abnormalities also may be the source of symptoms. The telangiectasias especially can cause a burning or bursting discomfort and frequently, but not always, are associated with truncal or saphenous vein branch varicosities. The authors of Chapter 20 have described the symptom complex associated with telangiectasias, and they have pointed out the similarities of their pathophysiologic origin to gross varicosities and truncal or perforating venous reflux.

Dr. Bergan: It is clear that we agree that symptoms of aching pain, easy fatigability, tiredness, and even the appearance of gross, protuberant saccular varicosities are indications for surgical intervention. Are there other indications for surgery?

Dr. DePalma: Superficial thrombophlebitis of varices or of the saphenous trunk is another indication for surgery. Surgery may be required in the acute situation in which thrombophlebitis of the saphenous vein may propagate upward and encroach on the saphenofemoral junction. Furthermore, a cluster of varicosities may remain acutely inflamed for a long time, even with good, conservative care. In such a situation, I recommend surgical intervention. When surgery is necessary, I use perioperative anticoagulant therapy with heparin and always examine the patient with the color flow duplex scanner to investigate the deep venous system. When deep venous thrombosis is not present, I would proceed with saphenous vein ligation and retrograde stripping to remove the foci of inflamed varicose clusters.

Mr. Rose: To this I must add that a history of external bleeding or sudden hemorrhage from a dilated vein in a site vulnerable to trauma, such as the shin, ankle, or dorsum of the foot, is often an urgent indication for intervention.

I must emphasize that women who complain of varicosities for purely cosmetic reasons should be considered seriously. They regard their varicose veins as unacceptable disfigurements, and their complaint is as distressing to them as any painful affliction and it is often less well tolerated. When fashion decrees that skirts be shorter, such patients rush to the physician's door. I think that these patients are equally entitled to our attention and that no surgeon should turn them away, providing that he or she can assure them of a good cosmetic result.

Dr. Bergan: Dr. DePalma, tell us about your preoperative evaluation of the patient.

Dr. DePalma: We have discussed the patient's history, which will elucidate the indications for surgical intervention for varicose veins or sclerotherapy for telangiectasias. In addition, the comprehensive consultation must include inquiry about possible risk factors for arterial disease, which might later require the saphenous vein to be used in peripheral or coronary artery revascularization. The intensity and duration of each of the risk factors that predispose the patient to atherosclerosis should be recorded. These factors include a history of cigarette smoking with an estimate of pack-years. Inquiry should be made into familial predispositions, such as hypercholesterolemia, diabetes, and hypertension. It is also important to record any familial pattern of varicose veins and to note whether deep venous thrombosis has occurred in the patient or his or her siblings. In addition, investigations into coagulapathy, including evaluation of protein C, protein S, antithrombin III, anticardiolipin antibodies, and lupus anticoagulant, should be done. Examination of the arterial system should be performed, with ankle-to-arm pressure indices recorded and peripheral pulses palpated. The saphenous vein should not be routinely removed in patients who have major risk factors for arterial occlusive disease (except when severely varicose), such as a male with an excess of 20 pack-years of smoking history in conjunction with another risk factor.

Mr. Rose: What Dr. DePalma has described is a complete evaluation of the patient. Such an evaluation is certainly necessary in every case involving a history of phlebitis, especially the recurrent type, and any situation in which arteriosclerotic disease is a risk factor. Of course, this type of evaluation is essential if basic research is being undertaken. Many clinics, however, are not equipped for such evaluations and are not research oriented. In addition, it must be recognized that many cases do not require this type of full investigation. It is a matter of clinical experience to separate those that do deserve such attention from those that do not. Initially, we rely heavily on the physical examination in evaluating patients for surgical intervention. After the patient has been standing for 10 minutes, the varicose vein pattern is carefully charted. The extent of varicosities is estimated by palpation, propagation of the cough impulse, and examination with the continuous-wave, hand-held Doppler instrument. The Doppler device establishes connection with the greater saphenous vein, and the short saphenous system should be examined similarly with the knee slightly flexed to relax the deep fascia. The patient undergoes a full abdominal examination, after which the peripheral pulses are palpated. The presence of sciatic pain is eliminated through the straight leg–raising test, and the condition of the ankle, knee, and hip are estimated—through flexion, abduction, and external rotation. All these findings are duly recorded.

Dr. Bergan: Dr. DePalma, would you tell us about your preoperative testing routine?

Dr. DePalma: Rational treatment of saphenous varicosities requires delineation of points of reflux from the deep venous system as well as delineation of specific areas of truncal incompetence.[3] The patient is examined while standing, and the examiner is seated.

Palpation should include inspection; use of the tap, cough, and thrill tests; and insonation of the saphenofemoral and popliteal regions and the major trunks with use of a hand-held continuous-wave Doppler pencil probe (Figure 10-1). While the patient is standing, careful inspection is done to detect major perforating vein

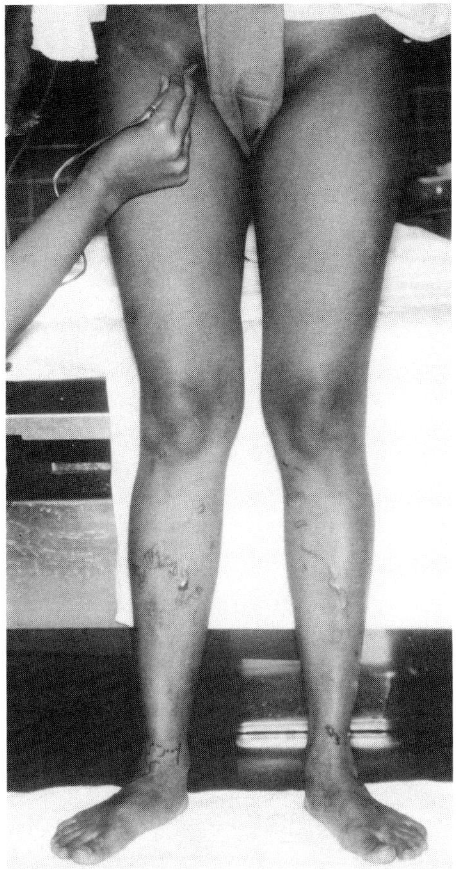

FIGURE 10-1. This photograph shows Doppler venous examination as part of preoperative evaluation of this 28-year-old woman with symptomatic, below-knee varicosities, which are easily seen. The patient demonstrated severe truncal reflux on Doppler evaluation, and it was later confirmed through duplex scanning. Note absence of visible thigh varices despite greater saphenous reflux found bilaterally.

reflux. The most common area of deep to superficial connection is the anteromedial aspect of the upper calf in the region of the Boyd perforating vein. The next most common important perforating vein connection is located in the midthigh in the region of Hunter's canal.[4,5] The third most common and important perforating vein is the one named for Dodd, which is located in the distal third of the thigh.[5] It should be noted that the Boyd perforating vein may be the first to give rise to primary varicosities in the anterior tributary group or the posterior tributary group or in both. Furthermore, this vein may be connected to the greater saphenous system, the lesser saphenous system, or even the popliteal vein. Appropriate superficial to deep disconnection will be required.

Dr. Bergan: What about the classical tourniquet tests that are taught in surgical services and medical schools?

Dr. DePalma: The classical tourniquet tests have been taught and are currently receiving attention. However, in my experience, I have found the tourniquet tests to be disappointing. Figure 10-2 illustrates some of the problems encountered with tourniquet application.

Dr. Bergan: What about use of the color flow duplex scanner?

Dr. DePalma: After the results of physical examination and Doppler study have been recorded on the patient's chart, duplex scans are routinely obtained in our surgical service. We have completed a study in which we prospectively evaluated 80 limbs in 40 symptomatic patients prior to treatment of primary saphenous varicosities. We compared sensitivity, specificity, positive and negative predictive values of physical examination, and Doppler insonation with color flow duplex scanning. When color flow duplex scanning was used as a standard, physical examination had a sensitivity of only 48%. Its specificity was 73%, and there was a positive predictive value of 75% and a negative predictive value of 46%. The addition of Doppler insonation improved specificity and positive predictive values. Its sensitivity was 48%; specificity, 83%; and positive predictive value, 83%. The negative predictive value remained 49%.

As a result of this study, and with further experience, I recommend that a color flow duplex scan be done prior to surgical intervention for varicose veins involving the saphenous system.[6] The color flow scanning is particularly effective at the saphenofemoral junction. I have not yet recommended or practiced selective ligation at the saphenofemoral junction.[7,8] With major or gross saphenous reflux, I

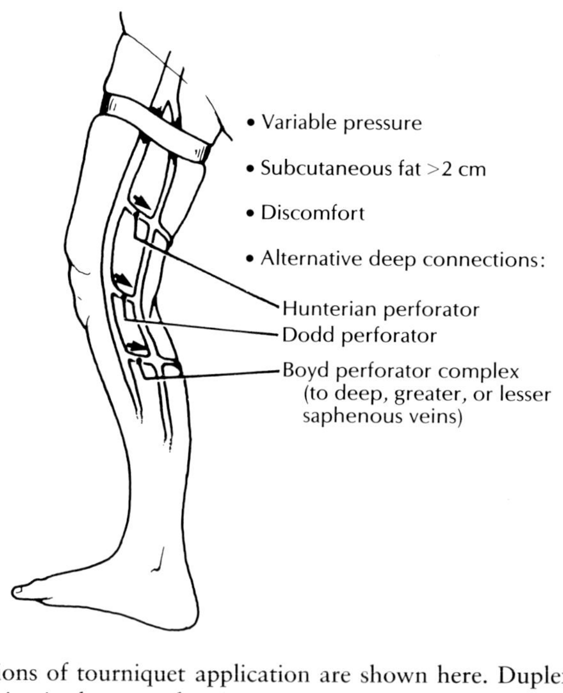

FIGURE 10-2. Limitations of tourniquet application are shown here. Duplex reflux evaluation has replaced tourniquet testing in the care of varicose veins at most institutions.

think that surgical intervention and removal of the saphenous trunk are needed. Others have practiced proximal ligation and distal sclerotherapy with success, but that approach is not our practice.[9,10]

Duplex scanning is particularly useful in patients with prior operations; in fact, it is invaluable. We have discovered retained lateral or medial saphenous trunks and missed groin communicating veins in 14 of 18 limbs in which groin scars existed and symptoms of primary varicosities continued.[11] Of equal importance is the fact that when saphenofemoral incompetence is not present the main saphenous trunk can be spared.[12] Surgery then will consist of selective ligation and removal of specific branches and deep disconnections.[13]

Mr. Rose: I would support what Dr. DePalma says about duplex scanning. It is the most valuable noninvasive technique for venous and arterial investigation thus far developed. However, although most major clinics have this equipment, it is not yet universally available, and many clinics will need to rely on the older methods of assessment. However, as Dr. DePalma has said, when our experience with duplex scanning offers us more information about the pros and cons of selective groin ligation, surgery then may consist of selective ligation and removal of specific branches and deep disconnections.

Dr. Bergan: When should operations for lower extremity varicosities not be done?

Mr. Rose: Patients with varicose veins should not be operated on during pregnancy, in very old age, or when peripheral arterial occlusive disease is present. Furthermore, if a patient has any contraindication to general anesthesia, a history of bleeding diathesis, or active skin infection in the limb, the operation should not be done until the condition is investigated or rectified. When varices are present in a limb with lymphedema, surgery should not be performed. Also, surgery should not be done when venous claudication is present; instead, extensive investigation should be undertaken.

Dr. DePalma: Actually, effective symptomatic treatment can be achieved through the use of prescription lightweight support pantyhose or below-knee support hosiery. It is important that these aids be obtained from a supplier who can be relied on for accuracy in specific fitting and will make adjustments to correct a poor "fit." Prescription of elastic support hosiery with less than 20 mm Hg pressure usually will suffice. Higher pressures must be prescribed if lipodermatosclerosis or dermatitis complicates primary saphenous varicosities. In patients who are not surgical candidates because of their age or medical condition, or for those who wish to delay therapy for any reason, the consistent use of elastic support hosiery can be quite satisfactory.

Sclerotherapy is an alternative to surgery or compression therapy. I use sclerotherapy for treatment of veins that do not communicate directly with the main trunks and for those that are less than 3 to 4 mm in diameter. In fact, I use sclerotherapy during surgery to identify small varices and telangiectasias. At the time of surgery, I introduce 11.7% or 23.4% saline solution while the patient is anesthetized.

Mr. Rose: We use the same criteria that Dr. DePalma does for sclerotherapy, but we tend not to use it perioperatively. The small varicosities and telangiectasias

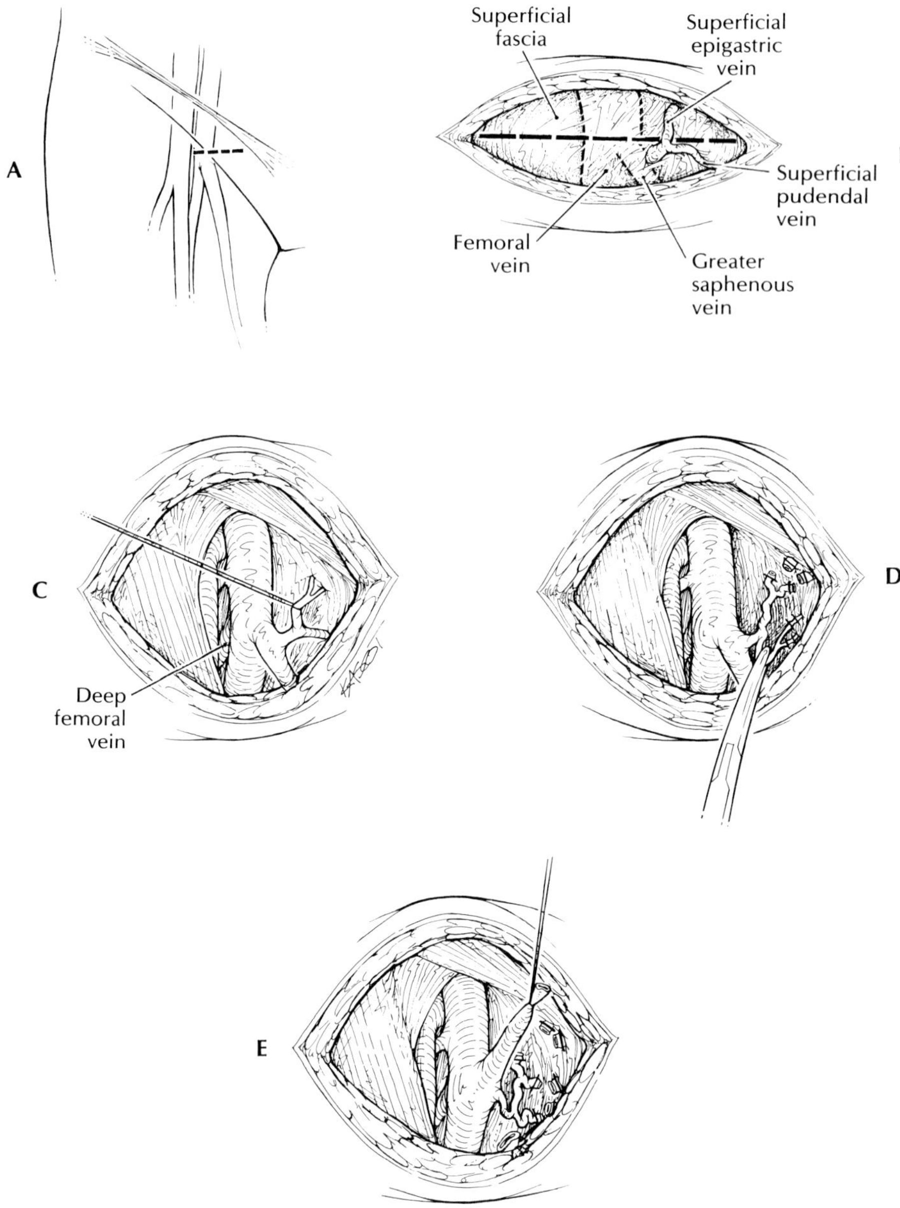

FIGURE 10-3. A, Placement of groin incision for interruption and ligation of greater saphenous vein is shown. Incision is placed proximal to inguinal crease in appropriate skin lines, depending on the physiognomy of the particular patient. **B,** With skin and subcutaneous tissues divided, the superficial fascia comes into view. Frequently, medial and superior tributaries to the saphenous vein are seen lying on this fascia. Fascia is incised transversely. **C,** Division of fascia will expose saphenous vein at its termination with a variable number of tributaries entering saphenous vein or femoral vein. Complete exposure of 2 cm of femoral vein is necessary to ensure division of all tributaries in this location. **D,** Each tributary to saphenous vein and femoral vein is pulled into the incision and ligated or clipped; the tributary is divided beyond its bifurcation, as shown here. **E,** Saphenous vein is divided and lifted into view so that suture ligature can be placed carefully, obliterating any cul-de-sac that might form. Suture ligature should not impinge on femoral vein. (From Bergan JJ, Kistner RL. Atlas of Venous Surgery. Philadelphia: WB Saunders, 1992, p 66.)

are not as easy to identify during surgery, and I worry that the sclerosant will leak into the tiny incised areas and cause an intradermal inflammatory response. It is probably true, however, that the use of hypertonic saline is less likely to cause any harm under these circumstances than is the detergent class of sclerosing agents. With regard to surgical technique, it is important to recognize that the only practical way of eradicating varicose veins is by meticulous and radical removal of all the varicosities with, if necessary, the addition of ligation at the saphenofemoral and saphenopopliteal junction and/or localized stripping of the main saphenous veins.[14] The operation can be performed as an outpatient procedure, a day-stay case, or an inpatient procedure with an overnight stay. A two-night stay is rarely necessary. Prior to surgery, the patient is examined while standing and the veins are marked very carefully. Particular attention must be paid to any localized painful areas or varicosities that cause special discomfort since these are the focal points of the patient's complaint and must not be missed.

Dr. Bergan: I think that there are two principles that should be used as a guide to successful varicose vein surgery. The first is ablation of reflux from the deep to the superficial venous system. The second is removal or destruction of all varicosities existing at the time of surgical intervention.[15] Ablation of reflux from the deep system should be done at the points indicated by Dr. DePalma. Detection of such reflux is obtained by physical examination and inspection and by use of the Doppler instrument; its presence is verified with the duplex scanner.[16] When gross saphenous reflux is present, the saphenous vein should be removed to encompass the perforating veins of Hunter, Dodd, and Boyd. Simple proximal ligation without segmental stripping has proven to be unsatisfactory.[17-19] Adherence to the second principle of varicose vein surgery allows correction of any errors made in preoperative detection of deep to superficial reflux; that is, if all varicose veins and varicose clusters are excised, the end organs of perforator reflux are removed. Thus missed identification of perforating veins is corrected by thorough removal of all varicosities.

Mr. Rose: To follow what Dr. Bergan was saying, if the principle of meticulous removal of isolated clusters is adhered to, the time-consuming search for elusive perforators is eliminated and a satisfactory operation can be carried out, even when a duplex scanner is not available.

The important points to observe in the groin dissection are as follows. The femoral pulse is palpated so that the position of the saphenous vein opening medial to that pulse is identified. The incision should be long enough to gain good access to the saphenous vein opening; the length will vary somewhat, depending on the obesity of the patient and the experience of the surgeon.

Dr. Bergan: All incisions must be carefully placed in the exact skin lines of the individual patient.[20,21] The most common error in saphenous vein surgery is placement of the upper incision too far distally. In the past, it was taught that the incision should be placed distal to the groin crease, but that method is distinctly erroneous. At present, advocacy of placement of the incision in the groin crease also seems to be erroneous. In general, the transverse incision should be placed 1 to 2 cm proximal to the oblique groin crease (Figure 10-3). The incision should extend medially from the palpable femoral pulse, and every tributary to the saphenous vein should be sought and divided. Stanley Rivlin[15] has said:

> Attempts have been made to list the variations in so-called normal venous anatomy at the saphenofemoral junction. In fact, there is no normal. The arrangements of the venous tributaries are seemingly infinite and the ways in which they join the long saphenous or femoral vein seem to be decided only by the laws of chance.

Mr. Rose: At first sight it may appear that the anatomic abnormalities occur by chance, but in fact they are merely variations on a basic theme that is described as the normal anatomy. Either a high or a low insertion of the internal saphenous vein in the groin is possible, and accordingly variations occur in the path followed by the main tributaries, which generally enter the main saphenous vein. The anterolateral and posteromedial saphenous veins are similarly displaced according to their site of entry; when either one is enlarged alone, it constitutes an accessory saphenous vein that is sometimes referred to as a twin saphenous vein. Therefore the main patterns actually can be drawn without reference to an anatomy textbook and with a basic knowledge of what to expect. To obtain an adequate exposure of the operative field, I believe that it is best to use the oblique incision parallel to the groin crease. This incision is easy to enlarge to give better access, if necessary, without leaving an ugly scar. At operation, once the saphenofemoral junction has been dissected, with the understanding that it may be located above or below the normal position, the disposition of the tributaries then can be determined easily. The only troublesome variation is when an accessory saphenous vein opens posteromedially. I think that the mystique of the saphenofemoral junction has been overemphasized. It must be understood that, no matter how variable, the tributaries must not be allowed to escape ligation. Nevertheless, young surgeons should be closely supervised throughout their training course.

Dr. Bergan: In regard to surgical technique, the wound edges undergo atraumatic retraction, and the layers of superficial fascia are divided. The saphenous vein itself lies beneath the superficial fascia, which must be divided. As each of the tributaries comes into view, it should be doubly clamped and ligated, and the saphenofemoral junction itself should be visualized clearly before any clamps are applied. Usually, a small branch of the external pudendal artery runs transversely deep to the saphenous vein. Occasionally, however, this branch lies superficial to the saphenous vein.

Although variations in anatomy are common, all incompetent tributaries should be identified. In particular, the anterior lateral saphenous vein should be identified and removed. This vein is frequently the source of anterior and lateral thigh varicosities. Depending on its size, the anterior lateral saphenous vein is either ligated or avulsed in a distal direction. It should be remembered that an accessory saphenous vein may be an extra tributary of the saphenous system from a medial and posterior position. This vein may enter the saphenous vein as far as 3 to 4 inches below the saphenofemoral junction. An accessory saphenous vein should be identified by finger dissection, ligated, divided, and removed segmentally.

Dr. DePalma: In the groin, the main trunk at the saphenofemoral junction is carefully dissected. All collateral branches and the lateral tributary are divided, with care taken to spare lymphatic trunks. A stripper usually can be passed from the groin distally, easily traversing the incompetent valves that have been detected by color flow Doppler imaging (Figure 10-4). The stripper is recovered through a

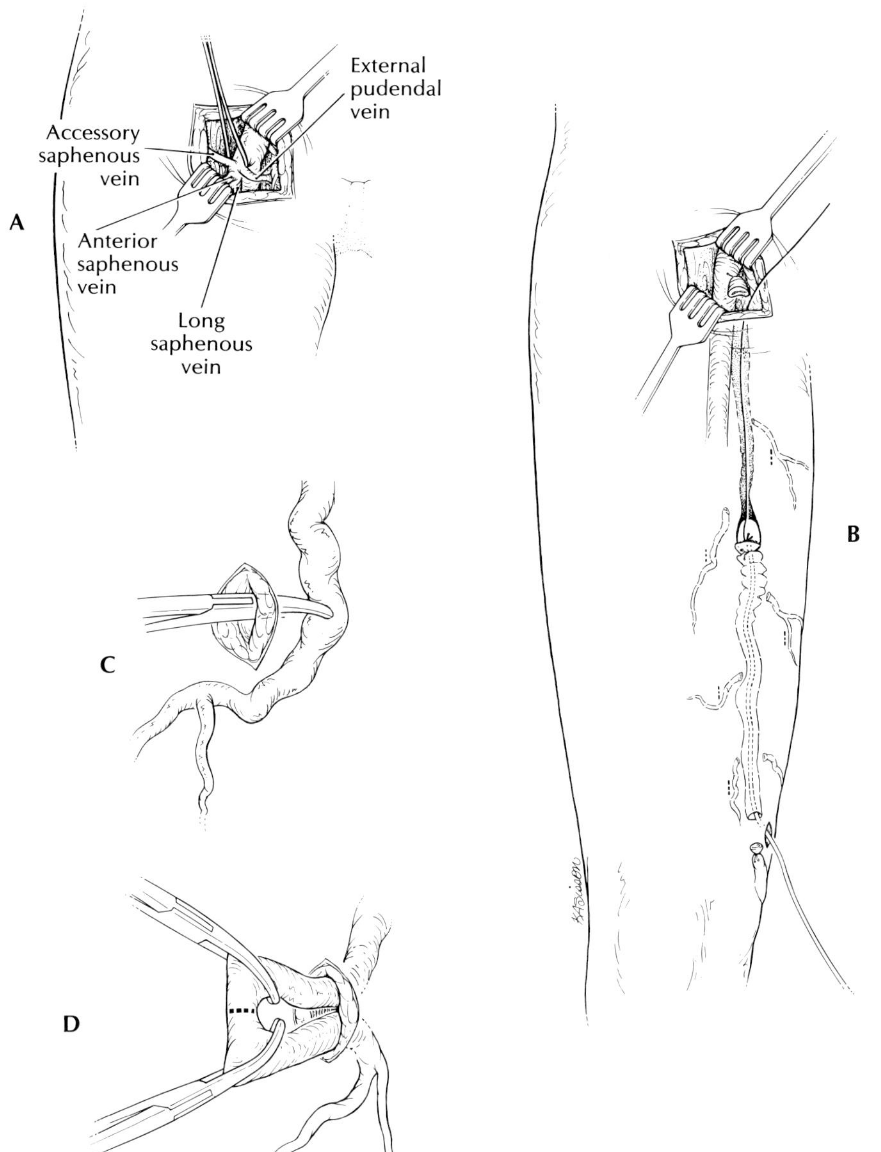

FIGURE 10-4. Gross axial reflux in greater saphenous vein will dictate removal of that vein at least to distal thigh or proximal calf. **A,** Exposure of saphenous vein in groin is done as illustrated in Figure 10-3. Stripper is introduced from above in a downward direction. **B,** Stripper and retrieving thread or umbilical tape is pulled distally after stripper has been identified in distal thigh or anteromedial calf. Objective of stripping greater saphenous vein is to interrupt variably placed perforating veins that enter saphenous vein in middle third and distal third of thigh. **C,** While stripper and pack are in place, stab avulsion of previously marked varicose vein clusters can be accomplished by the technique illustrated. **D,** Division of each varicosity allows proximal and distal removal of lengths of varicose vein. (From Bergan JJ. The role of surgery in treatment of varicose veins and venous telangiectasias. In Goldman MP. Sclerotherapy: Treatment of Varicose and Telangiectatic Leg Veins. St. Louis: Mosby–Year Book, 1991, pp 295-297.)

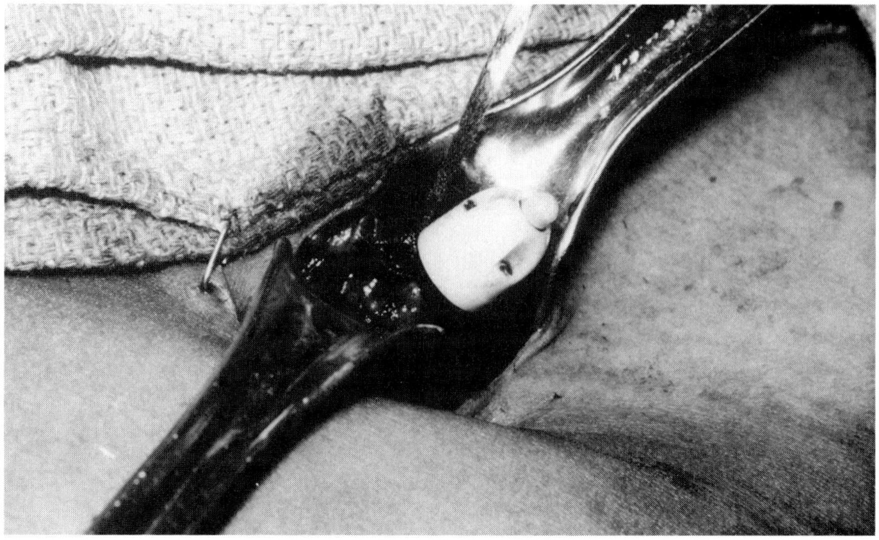

FIGURE 10-5. This photograph illustrates proximal groin incision with stripper in place within saphenous vein and umbilical tape tied to stripper so that stripper can be retrieved. Umbilical tape may be placed into groove of stripper head, where friction will hold it in contact with plastic stripper.

microincision at a point near the knee. Stripping then is carried out over a period of 5 to 10 minutes. The procedure is done from the groin to the distal microincision with the operating table placed in 15 degrees of foot elevation prior to vein removal. Ultimately, the stripper is recovered through the groin incision by means of an attached umbilical tape (Figure 10-5). This adds considerably to the cosmetic efficacy of the procedure.

Mr. Rose: We also strip the vein in a retrograde manner, but we do not pull the head of the stripper through the lower skin opening. Instead, the stripper is removed by upward traction on a long thread attached to the stripper head. Using a stripper with a drilled head facilitates attachment of the thread. Pressure is applied along the path of the stripper as it is pulled proximally, and the stripped vein is removed through the groin incision. This method avoids enlarging the lower incision by pulling the head of the stripper through it. We have used this technique for the past 25 years without a single complication.

Dr. Bergan: We also introduce the stripper from above, attach a narrow umbilical tape to the stripper head, and then tie in a length of roller gauze that is 5 to 10 cm in width and use two to four layers of such gauze as a pack (Figure 10-6). The pack follows the stripper head distally and is left in place during the stab avulsion portion of the operation. We remove the saphenous vein through the distal incision to ensure that the distal tributaries are divided. This approach is especially necessary when the stripper exits below the knee in the region of the Boyd perforating vein tributaries.

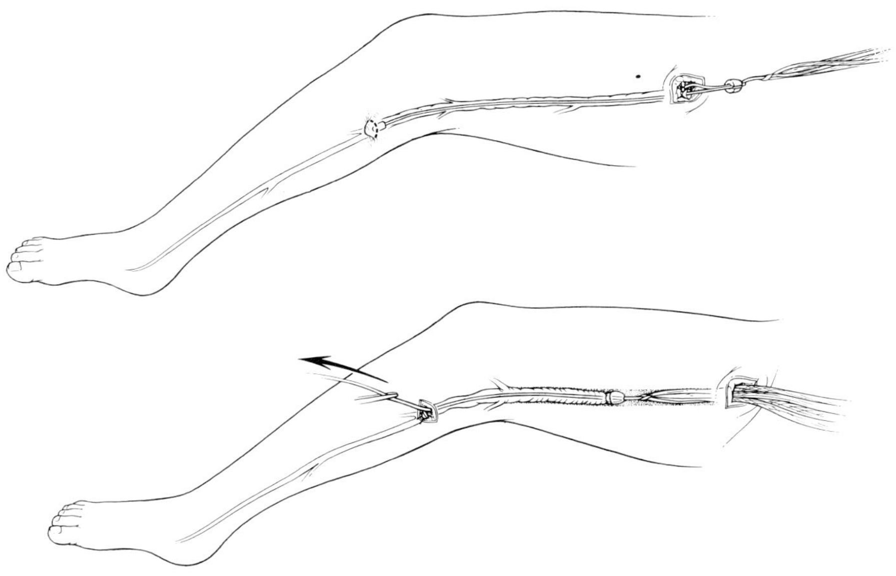

FIGURE 10-6. Stripper introduced from above can be identified by palpation and distal placement of incision. Usually, incision is in a vertical direction, although transverse incision illustrated may be appropriate in skin lines around the knee. Stripper is pulled distally, and saphenous vein is removed from distal incision. In lower illustration, progress can be seen in four-layered gauze pack, which is tied as close as possible to stripper head. This pack is left in place when stab avulsion treatment of varicose clusters is done. After adequate time has been allowed for hemostasis, entire stripper, stripper head, and gauze pack are retrieved through proximal incision. (From Bergan JJ, Kistner RL. Atlas of Venous Surgery. Philadelphia: WB Saunders, 1992, p 67.)

In order to reduce hematoma formation, we do the entire operation with the patient's feet elevated on a picket fence or rack so that the entire limb is extended in a 30-degree elevated position while the table is kept flat. After all other steps of the procedure have been completed, the entire gauze pack, stripper head, and stripper are removed through the proximal incision.

Dr. DePalma: The groin incision is closed with fine subcuticular chromic catgut, and the extremity incisions used for stab avulsion also are closed with subcuticular absorbable sutures. Steri-Strips are applied to all these incisions.

Mr. Rose: Prior to closure of the groin incision, any hematoma that may have developed is squeezed out of the track of the stripper. We prefer not to use the sucker or gauze pack for this step because it can cause rebleeding. It is important to use manual pressure along the line of the strip, as described earlier. The groin incision is closed with subcuticular continuous 3-0 catgut sutures, and the skin edges are opposed with Steri-Strips. We leave this step to the end of the operation so that all oozing has stopped.

Dr. Bergan: Our own choice is for 3-0 Vicryl absorbable sutures for the superficial fascia and 5-0 Vicryl sutures for the subcuticular closure, but we also apply Steri-Strips.

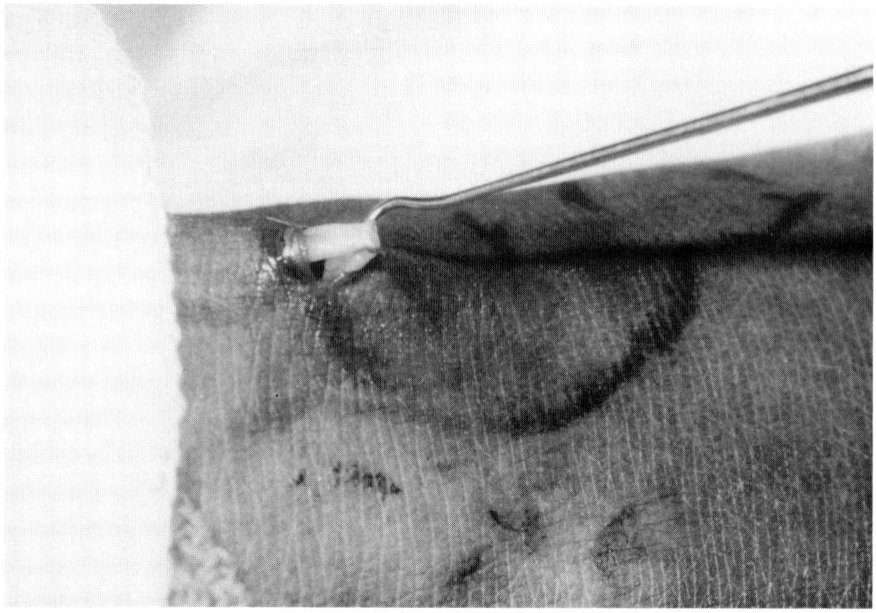

FIGURE 10-7. Use of a skin hook in grasping anterior surface of incompetent greater saphenous vein through an oblique microincision at the ankle. Note complete skeletonization of saphenous vein so that terminal filaments of saphenous nerve can be eliminated from trauma of venous stripping.

Dr. DePalma: For stab avulsion, we use small distal skin-line incisions not greater than 2 to 3 mm in length. The underlying varicosities are best elevated by capturing the vein with a skin hook (Figure 10-7). This method permits smaller access than does a crochet hook, which must be inserted beneath the skin. Alternatively, veins can be grasped with hemostats, and a flexible vein grasper can be inserted through microincisions for removal of the remaining varices by avulsion.

Mr. Rose: We believe that the instruments used for multiple avulsion should be kept as simple as possible (Figure 10-8). We agree with Dr. DePalma about the crochet hook. We do not find it necessary to use a skin hook or a flexible vein grasper. We use a miniknife (Beaver 1600-B), mosquito forceps, heavier curved forceps, and toothed dissecting forceps. The multiple tiny incisions are made with the Beaver blade at intervals over the veins so that the maximal length of vein can be removed with the minimum number of incisions. The incisions are 2 to 3 mm but are not always of the stab incision type. They are made with much more care than a stab incision would imply. Stretching the skin in the line of the vein allows the incision to be made more easily and naturally. The incisions are stab type only when sufficient subcutaneous adipose tissue is present to prevent perforation of the vein. Otherwise the dissection is hampered by bleeding. The incisions are made precisely in the skin lines, and they disappear almost completely in time.[22] It is convenient to make the incisions where the veins are most easily palpable and can be grasped more easily. Incisions should not be made over indurated areas because it will be impossible to avulse the vein where indurated and inflamed subcutaneous tissue is present.

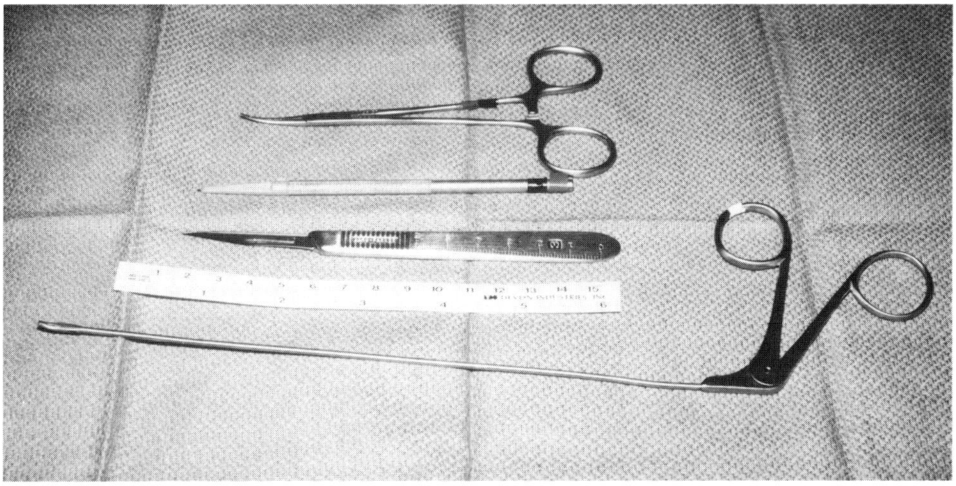

FIGURE 10-8. Instruments used for microincision as well as stab avulsion of varicose clusters. From above to downward, one sees fine-pointed hemostat used for grasping varices and Beaver blade used for creating microincisions. Below is No. 11 Bard-Parker blade used for slightly larger incisions. Below ruler is flexible vein grasper made to specifications by the Pilling Corporation (Philadelphia).

The skin incision should penetrate the dermis. The skin edges are separated, the vein is identified, and the vein is picked up by grasping its adventitia (Figure 10-9). The hold on the vein is consolidated, and the vein is drawn through the surface. When the loop of vein emerges from the incision, a forceps can be passed under it so that the loop can be divided. Each end of the vein is now gradually drawn out by means of an alternate traction and twisting motion. A forceps is reapplied closer to the skin as the vein is avulsed. Care is taken not to pull the vein back across the incision because if the skin has lost its elasticity, the incision will become stretched. This caution applies especially to the posterior aspect of the leg. Ultimately, the vein breaks and hemostasis is secured by application of firm pressure, which is continued until the next incision is explored.

The process is repeated down the leg until all offending and previously marked veins have been removed. It has been postulated that any perforating veins will be automatically interrupted. Care must be taken to distinguish between fine cutaneous nerves and small veins. Avulsion of nerve filaments may produce significant hyperesthesia and sudden stabs of pain.

The leg is cleansed after avulsion of all the marked veins has been accomplished, and the wounds are sealed with Steri-Strips. The Steri-Strips must be simply laid in the line of the wound, and the skin edges must not be opposed under tension since this method may produce blistering of the skin. Careful bandaging is done firmly to complete the procedure.

A number of specialized instruments have been advocated by others, but they are not necessary if the technique described here is followed.[23-25]

Dr. DePalma: Although we have been discussing the usual removal of grossly refluxing saphenous vein and clusters of varicosities, there are situations in which

A

B

C

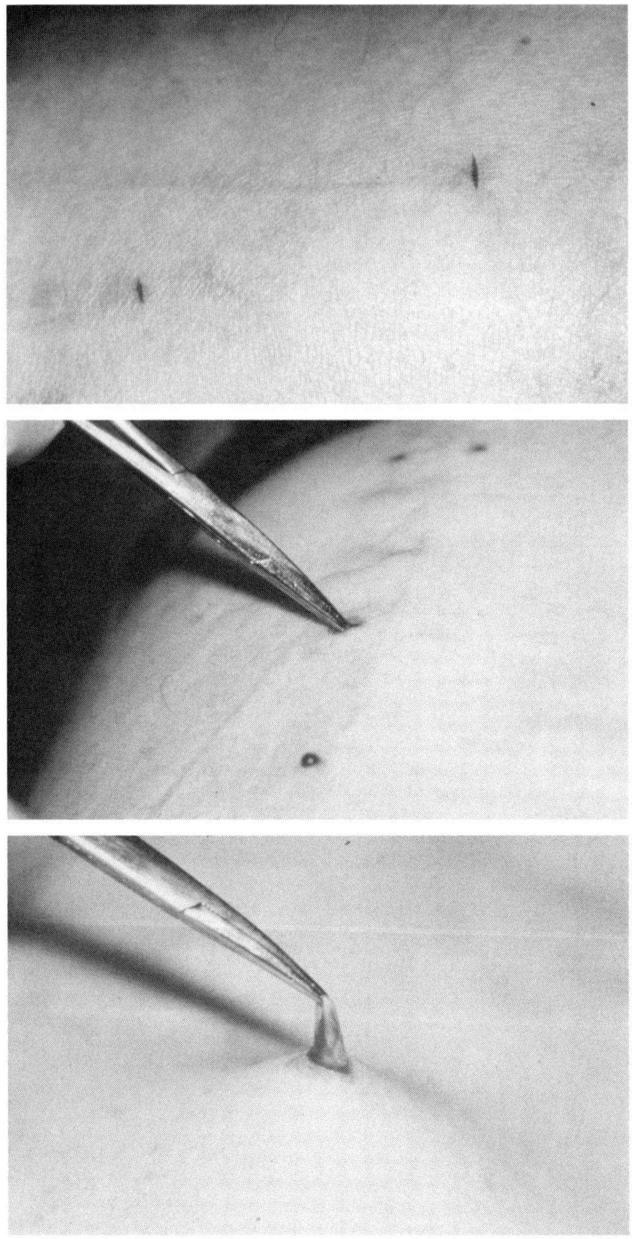

FIGURE 10-9. This operative series shows technique of stab avulsion. **A,** Microincisions are made with Beaver blade, with careful attention given to skin lines. **B,** Underlying varicosity can be grasped with a fine-pointed hemostat. **C,** Varix is raised above skin level.

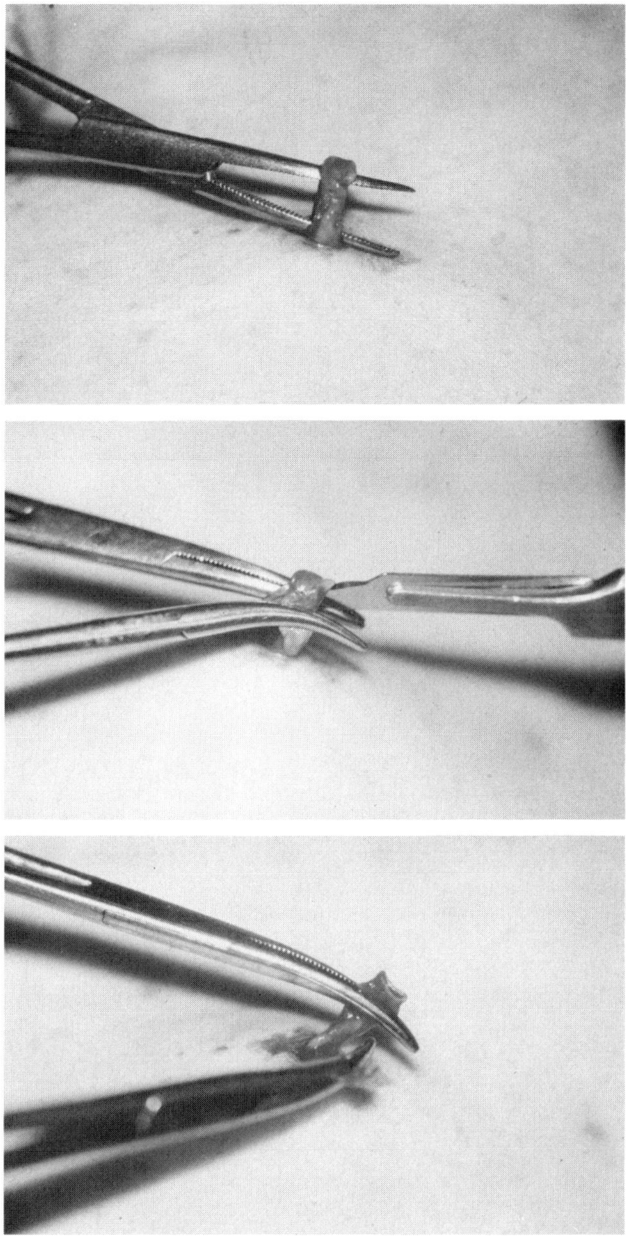

D

E

F

FIGURE 10-9, cont'd. D, A loop of vein, when identified completely, shows a proximal and distal portion of varix. **E,** After varix has been doubly clamped, it is divided sharply, as shown. **F,** Each end of divided vein is winkled out of its subcutaneous position.

Continued.

G

H

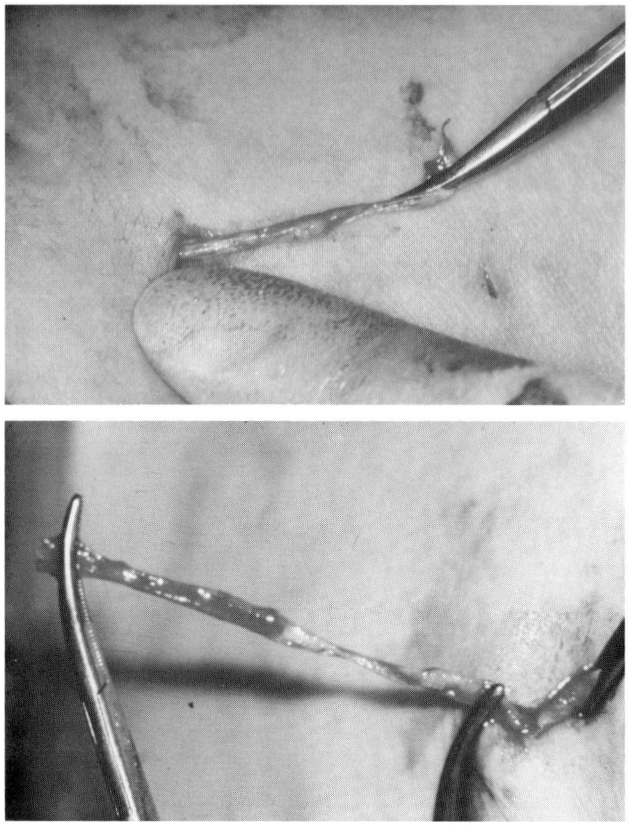

FIGURE 10-9, cont'd. G, Firm traction with hemostat and countertraction with finger allows maximum removal of varicosity in a proximal and distal direction. H, Frequently, great lengths of varicosity can be removed, thus minimizing number of microincisions made in the skin.

specific and unnamed perforating veins must be treated. We have not been satisfied in defining posterior arch tributaries or delineating the detailed anatomy of the infracrural zone with color flow duplex scanning. Therefore our approach is to expose the perforating vein near the knee and to perform intraoperative varicography with 60% Renografin, which is inserted into the varix through a blunt cannula. Control of infracrural incompetence can involve ligation of a deep direct perforating vein from the popliteal vein, excision and ligation of a contribution from the lesser saphenous vein, or division of a main contribution from an otherwise competent greater saphenous vein. Selective intraoperative venography makes possible the precise application of microincisions and rational ligation and excision for disconnection from the deep venous system in the popliteal area.

Mr. Rose: The short saphenous vein is dealt with according to the same principles as the long saphenous vein, but the dissection of the popliteal fossa is a much more complicated procedure. First, there is great variability in the location of the saphenopopliteal junction. Second, the short saphenous vein is deep to the deep

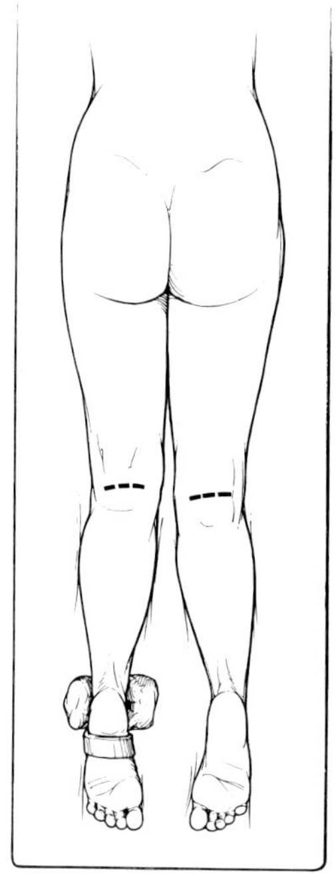

FIGURE 10-10. Surgery to interrupt lesser saphenous vein in popliteal space must allow adequate exposure. Such exposure can be achieved as shown here when operation is done bilaterally. When bilateral operations are planned, the patient should be placed in a prone position on the operating table, and exposure should not be compromised.

fascia. Third, the gastrocnemius veins may be involved. The proximity of the medial popliteal nerve provides an additional hazard. Therefore the patient is operated on in the prone position so that vascular access is unhindered and the anatomy can be easily visualized (Figure 10-10). The incision is placed where the saphenopopliteal junction has been identified preoperatively or through varicography, and the incision is not compromised by cosmetic considerations.

A natural skin line is identified for placement of the incision, and the incision is deepened through the subcutaneous fascia until the deep fascia is reached. The fascia is then incised (Figure 10-11). When the saphenous vein has been identified, the sural nerve should be sought and carefully protected. Proximal dissection allows identification of the saphenopopliteal junction. Frequently, a tributary that runs upward and medially can be identified. This tributary, which joins the internal saphenous system, is the so-called vein of Giacomini. This vessel is an important conduit for superficial blood flow if the deep connection of the saphenous vein to the popliteal vein is abnormally small. All other tributaries that may be varicose and that arise from the gastrocnemium muscle must be divided. Such tributaries may cause troublesome bleeding if they are not carefully ligated. They should never be avulsed. In surgery of the short saphenous vein, we often find varicography to be most useful for identifying anatomic abnormalities and determining the extent of involvement of the gastrocnemius and soleal veins.

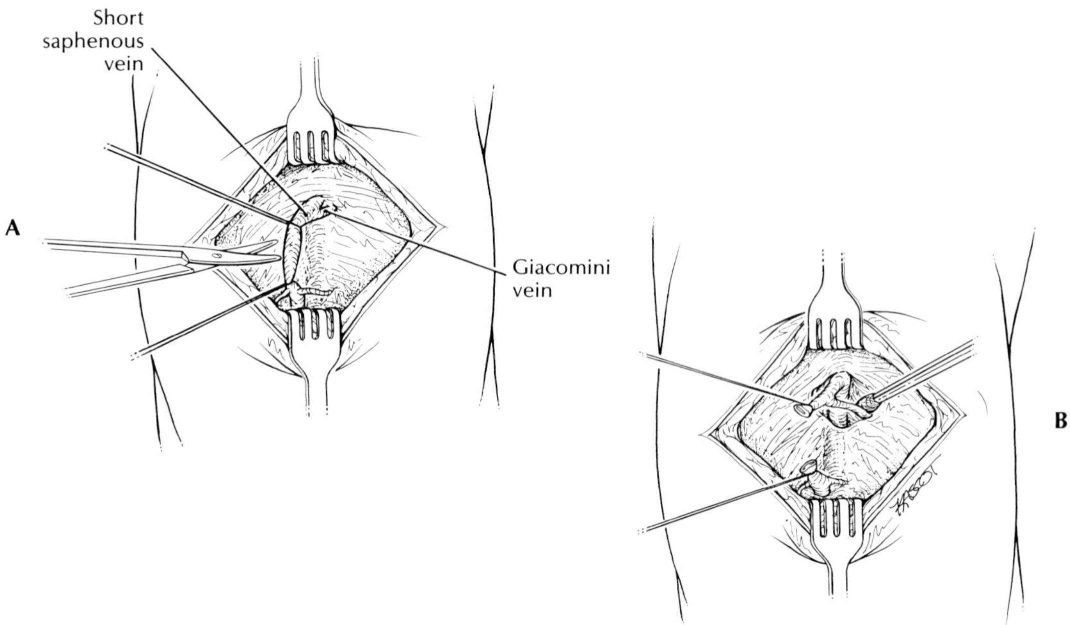

FIGURE 10-11. Short saphenous vein and its termination should be identified by duplex ultrasound or intraoperative varicography. Skin incision placement depends on the location of termination of short saphenous vein. Note exposure of tributaries to short saphenous vein, including vein of Giacomini (**A**). All these tributaries should be drawn into wound and divided so that short saphenous vein can be exposed at its termination in popliteal vein (**B**). All tributaries should be removed, and a segment of short saphenous vein should be excised.

Proximal ligation is performed as close to the popliteal vein as is feasible with safety. The deep fascia is closed with absorbable sutures. We prefer not to strip the short saphenous vein for two reasons. First, the short saphenous vein is usually not varicose throughout most of its length. Second, damage to the sural nerve is possible. Damage to the sural nerve may occur with incisions lateral to the Achilles tendon and behind the lateral malleolus. Such damage can produce a very persistent sensory change on the outer side of the foot that is occasionally accompanied by distressing paresthesia. In general, operations on the upper end of the short saphenous vein are not recommended for the inexperienced surgeon because of the anatomic variability.

Dr. DePalma: The ideal goals of varicose vein surgery include minimum scarring, precise ablation of all varices, and interruption of points of deep venous connection. These goals are accomplished by using well-planned, minimally invasive incisions. Carefully considered, meticulously accomplished, and anatomically sound surgery will produce physiologically and cosmetically acceptable results in almost all patients. Effective treatment relieves aching discomfort and manifestations of dermatitis. Even after these goals have been accomplished, an intrinsic individual recurrence rate can be noted, even though precise and comprehensive treatment has been done. We recommend annual follow-up for interval treatment of recurrent varices. Such treatment may include sclerotherapy or even minor surgical intervention.

Mr. Rose: Although sclerotherapy has always been popular on the European continent for the treatment of truncal and tributary varicosities, it has fallen into almost total disuse elsewhere. Truncal and tributary varicosities can be treated so simply by the surgical means described here that such sclerotherapy is justifiably reserved for patients who cannot be operated on because of age, general physical condition, or local skin complications such as refractory lipodermatosclerosis. Sclerotherapy can be used for postoperative recurrences of varicosities or new varicosities developing because of genetic or hormonal considerations. Furthermore, sclerotherapy is very effective for ablation of venous telangiectasias.

When Dr. DePalma spoke of minor surgical intervention, he made a very important point. Of course, we all aim for perfection in our results, but if saving the saphenous vein as a possible conduit results in having a few minor outpatient surgical interventions, it is a small price to pay. In any event, a patient with an inherent tendency to varicose veins is always a candidate for further procedures, even with the best of surgical treatment, and should be told at the outset that he or she may require therapeutic maintenance from time to time.

Dr. Bergan: No discussion of a surgical procedure would be complete without a description of complications. Who would like to address that subject?

Mr. Rose: Remarkably few complications occur with the procedure we have described. I can recall only one groin hemorrhage in our entire series. This complication resulted from an anterolateral saphenous tributary. It was memorable not only because of its uniqueness but also because it occurred on the day of President John F. Kennedy's assassination. As in other surgery, sepsis may occur, but it is extremely rare. We have seen no more than a case of minor wound infection once in 5 years. Curiously, such infections are found in small incisions and not in the groin. Other complications specific to the procedure include superficial phlebitis, which is often due to a residual hematoma in the path of the stripped vein. Theoretically, deep venous thrombosis should occur, but it is our practice to give one unit of low-molecular-weight Dextran to obese patients or patients older than 50 during anesthesia and to firmly advise the patient to take brisk walking spells postoperatively. The last recorded case in our experience occurred 8 years ago and involved a somewhat overweight 55-year-old woman.

Dr. Bergan: We have paid careful attention to deep venous thrombosis following superficial venous surgery and can only record two instances of this complication. The first occurred in a physician's wife, a 35-year-old woman who experienced dyspnea, tachycardia, and pleuritic pain of a transient nature 3 weeks after varicose vein surgery. Investigations were not performed, and the patient had no other manifestations. The second case involved an extremely tall male patient who experienced idiopathic atrial arrhythmia 48 hours following saphenous vein stripping. The patient was hospitalized, digitalis therapy was begun, and a normal sinus rhythm was restored. The ventilation/perfusion pulmonary scan was negative, but it was presumed that a small embolus had triggered the atrial arrhythmia.

Mr. Rose: In our surgical service, we have had five minor pulmonary emboli cases after surgery in the last 40 years. Two of these situations were similar to your case and even involved a physician's wife. We have had no instance of pulmonary embolus in the past 16 years. I attribute these low figures to the comparatively atraumatic procedure, early ambulation, and the use of low-molecular-weight dextran in patients at risk. I think antiembolus stockings are at their most effective where there is no risk of embolus!

Dr. Bergan: We have noted two instances of lymphocele in which a fluid collection did transilluminate easily. Both lymphoceles were in the pathway of saphenous vein stripping.

Mr. Rose: Occasionally a collection of lymph develops under the groin scar because of damage to the lymphatics during the course of dissection in that area. Such a fluid collection usually resolves spontaneously and rarely requires aspiration. Antibiotics should be given if aspiration is necessary.

Dr. Bergan: Mr. Rose, with your long experience, what would you say are the most important changes that have occurred in varicose vein surgery in recent years?

Mr. Rose: The modern trend in varicose vein surgery has been away from routine stripping of truncal veins and toward multiple avulsion and removal of varicose clusters. As this change has occurred, the results have improved considerably. This improvement is what one would expect if the basic cause of varicosities was weakness in the vein wall.[26] Admittedly, there are still a number of circumstances in which limited stripping of the greater saphenous vein is indicated. Our approach to the problem has been outlined here, and we think that such stripping should be combined with multiple avulsions. Such an operation places great emphasis on elimination of all varicosities, wherever they occur, while also achieving the most cosmetic result.

We think that one of the most important functions of surgical teaching is the training of young surgeons in varicose vein surgery. This training must include indoctrination that focuses on the high attainment of good results as a challenge to be met in a much neglected but most important branch of the surgical art.

Dr. Bergan: Mr. Rose, that statement reminds us that all venous surgery is cyclic. Those techniques that were used and abandoned in the past later return repetitively and are used until better treatments are found to replace them. Your advice recalls the admonitions of Benjamin Brodie. Would you conclude this dialogue by repeating that story for us?

Mr. Rose: In 1846, while lecturing at the bedside of a patient suffering from a varicose ulceration, Benjamin Brodie said:

> . . . this is a case in which there is no question about the patient's life or death. I think it very probable that many among you may pass by the bedside of such a patient without thinking it worthy of attention. But I am not disposed to regard it in this manner. Although the patient will probably not die of this disease, without great care it will render her miserable. The disease may be very much relieved by art, and it is of very common occurrence. Such a case, as may meet you at every turn of practice, and your reputation in early life will depend more upon your understanding a case of this kind than upon your knowledge of one of more rare occurrence.

That story, which was quoted in the monograph by Rowden Foote[27] in 1949, is an appropriate conclusion for this dialogue.

REFERENCES

1. Bergan JJ. The veins. In Nora PF, ed. Operative Surgery. Philadelphia: Lea & Febiger, 1990, pp 991-997.
2. Samuels PB. Technique of varicose vein surgery. Am J Surg 142:239-244, 1981.
3. Goren G, Yellin AE. Primary varicose veins: Topographic and hemodynamic correlations. J Cardiovasc Surg 31:672-677, 1990.
4. Papadakis K, Christodoulou C, Christopoulos D, et al. Number and anatomical distribution of incompetent thigh perforating veins. Br J Surg 76:581-584, 1989.
5. Tung KT, Chan O, Lea Thomas M. The incidence and sites of medial thigh communicating veins: A phlebologic study. Clin Radiol 41:339-340, 1990.
6. Koyano K, Sagaguchi S. Selective stripping operation based on Doppler ultrasonic findings for varicose veins of the lower extremities. Surgery 103:615-619, 1988.
7. de Takats G. Ambulatory ligation of the saphenous vein. JAMA 94:1194, 1930.
8. de Takats G, Quillin L. Ligation of the saphenous vein. A report on two hundred ambulatory operations. Arch Surg 26:72-88, 1933.
9. Kistner RL, Ferris EB III, Randhawa G, et al. The evolving management of varicose veins: Straub Clinic experience. Postgrad Med J 80:51-59, 1986.
10. Sladen JC. Flush ligation and compression sclerotherapy for the control of venous disease. Am J Surg 152:535-538, 1986.
11. Lofgren EP, Lofgren KA. Recurrence of varicose veins after the stripping operation. Arch Surg 102:111-114, 1971.
12. Large J. Surgical treatment of saphenous varices with preservation of the main greater saphenous trunk. J Vasc Surg 2:886-891, 1985.
13. Mellière D, Cales B, Martin-Jonathan C, Schadeck M. Nécessité de concilier les objectifs du traitement des varices et de la chirurgie artérielle: Conséquences pratiques. J des Maladies Vasc 16:171-178, 1991.
14. Rose SS. Surgical techniques in the treatment of varicose veins. In Greenhalgh RM, ed. Vascular Surgical Techniques: An Atlas. Philadelphia: WB Saunders, 1989, pp 374-382.
15. Rivlin S. The surgical cure of primary varicose veins. Br J Surg 62:913-917, 1975.
16. Semroe CM, Laborde A, Buchbinder D, et al. Preoperative mapping of varicosities and perforating veins. J Vasc Tech 14:72-74, 1990.
17. Friedell ML, Samson RH, Cohen MJ, et al. High ligation of the greater saphenous vein for treatment of lower extremity varicosities: The fate of the vein and therapeutic results. Ann Vasc Surg 6:5-8, 1992.
18. Jakobsen BH. The value of different forms of treatment for varicose veins. Br J Surg 66:182-184, 1979.
19. McMullen GM, Scott HJ, Coleridge-Smith PD, et al. An investigation of the effect of ligation without stripping of the long saphenous vein. Surg Res Soc, Jan 1990.
20. Cox HT. The cleavage lines of the skin. Br J Surg 29:234-240, 1941.
21. Flint MH. Langer's lines: A commentary. Surg Ann 8:25-46, 1976.
22. Chester JF, Taylor RS. Hookers and French strippers: A technique for varicose vein surgery. Br J Surg 77:560-561, 1990.
23. Ramelet AA. Muller phlebectomy: A new phlebotomy hook. J Dermatol Surg Oncol 17:814-816, 1991.
24. Ramelet AA. La phlébectomie ambulatoire selon Müller: Technique, avantages, désavantages. J des Maladies Vasc 16:119-122, 1991.
25. Ricci S, Georgiev M. Office varicose vein surgery under local anesthesia. J Dermatol Surg Oncol 18:55-58, 1992.
26. Rose SS, Ahmed A. Some thoughts on the aetiology of varicose veins. J Cardiovasc Surg 27:534-543, 1986.
27. Foote RR. Varicose Veins. London: Butterworth, 1949.

SUGGESTED READINGS

Bjordal RI. Circulation patterns in incompetent perforating veins in the calf and in the saphenous system in primary varicose veins. Acta Chir Scand 138:251-261, 1972.

Cotton TL. Varicose veins: Gross anatomy and development. Br J Surg 589-598, 1957.

Goren G, Yellin AE. Ambulatory stab avulsion phlebotomy for truncal varicose veins. Am J Surg 162:165-174, 1991.

Hammarstein J, Pedersen P, Cederlund CG, et al. Long saphenous vein saving for varicose veins: A long-term follow-up. Eur J Vasc Surg 4:361-364, 1990.

Holme JB, Holme K, Sorensen LS. The anatomic relationship between the long saphenous vein and the saphenous nerve. Arch Chir Scand 154:631-633, 1988.

Larson RH, Lofgren DF, Meyers TT, et al. Long-term results after vein surgery: Study of 1,000 cases after 10 years. Mayo Clin Proc 49:114-117, 1974.

Lefebvre-Vilardebo M. Le carrefour sapheno-fémoral: Etude anatomique et concepts de prévention des récidives variqueuses. J des Maladies Vasc 16:355-358, 1991.

Ludbrook J. Primary great saphenous varicose veins revisited. World J Surg 10:954-958, 1986.

Meyers TT. Results and technique of stripping operation for varicose veins. JAMA 163:87-92, 1957.

Rollins DL, Semrow CM, Friedell ML, et al. Use of ultrasonic venography in the evaluation of venous valve function. Am J Surg 154:189-191, 1987.

Chapter 11

Treatment of Varicose Veins by Sclerotherapy: An Overview

André Cornu-Thenard and Pierre Boivin

Treatment of varicose veins by injection of a sclerosing agent is a very old method.[1-3] Its long history reflects the efficacy of this technique. However, sclerotherapy has evolved over the years, and this method is currently undergoing rapid progress. Clinical experience and controlled studies have defined indications for the technique. Development of new sclerosing agents has made this method more effective, and studies concerning the relationships between the diameter of varicose veins and the concentration of the sclerosant suggest the possibility of standardization of care. Use of Doppler and duplex ultrasound techniques provides better hemodynamic and anatomic precision, which also improves treatment efficacy.

The primary objective of sclerotherapy is to destroy the varicose vein with at least the same degree of efficacy achieved with surgical stripping. To maintain lasting aesthetic and functional results, it is essential to be guided by certain basic principles, comply with indications and contraindications, perform a complete pretreatment assessment, use optimal sclerosing solutions, and adopt a rigorous technique.

Sclerotherapy can be used for treatment of all pathologic superficial venous dilatations. However, this chapter focuses on the treatment of varicose veins >3 mm in diameter.

MECHANISM OF ACTION

When all the necessary conditions are combined—adequate sclerosant, effective dose, and sufficient compression—the intravaricose injection of a sclerosing agent results in sclerosis of the injected segment, followed by its resorption. The process that occurs between the time of injection and resorption can be divided into several stages.

First, injection of a sclerosing agent induces an endothelial and a mural lesion, followed by three phenomena that evolve simultaneously: spasm, inflammatory reaction in the vessel wall, and formation of an adherent thrombus. Spasm is induced by both needle trauma and sclerosing solution. It occurs immediately and may interfere with injections in adjacent sites.

The inflammatory reaction causes thickening of the vessel wall, which then is transformed into indurated scar tissue. The more effective the sclerosing agent, the greater the thickness of the vessel wall caused by this reaction. Ideally, the density of the scar tissue is sufficient to completely occlude the lumen, ensuring complete fibrous transformation of the varicose vein. The fibrous cord is subsequently transformed into a fine network that is totally resorbed. Occasionally venous obstruction is incomplete, and a channel within the fibrosis will persist. In such situations repeated injections must be performed to induce total obstruction. Otherwise recurrence is inevitable after a variable interval.

The formation of a thrombus is related to the endothelial lesion. The lesion induces adhesion and platelet aggregation, with activation of intrinsic pathways of coagulation. No risk of thrombotic embolization is present because the thrombus is firmly adherent to the vessel wall. However, if an excessively large thrombus forms and involves an exaggerated intravascular and extravascular inflammatory reaction, it may interfere with fibrosis, causing a high risk of recanalization. This mechanism is responsible for in situ recurrences associated with apparently perfect sclerotherapy. Effective compression after injections can prevent, or at least reduce, this phenomenon. Compression plays an essential role by limiting formation and extension of thrombosis and by facilitating endothelial fibrosis. Therefore the endothelial lesion induced by intravenous injection of a sclerosing agent must be as complete as possible. The resulting vascular necrosis must be sufficiently extensive to destroy the entire vessel wall without leaving significant thrombus.[3]

INDICATIONS AND CONTRAINDICATIONS

The indications for sclerotherapy of varicose veins may include any varicose veins not demonstrating reflux derived from the deep venous system. The principal indications recognized by major authors are as follows[3-8]:

1. Nonsaphenous varicose veins
   a. Varicose veins in which a normal saphenous trunk is demonstrated
   b. Isolated incompetent perforating veins and their tributaries
   c. Varicose veins derived from the vulvoperineal network
   d. Residual varicose veins after surgical treatment of refluxing saphenous veins
2. Long or short saphenous varicose veins after isolated ligation/division of the saphenofemoral or saphenopopliteal junction.

A more controversial indication for sclerotherapy involves incompetent long or short saphenous trunks for which surgery cannot be performed for reasons such as patient refusal, surgical contraindication, or excessive separation from home.

Contraindications to sclerotherapy are related to either the patient or the sclerosing agent. Patient-related contraindications include concomitant deep venous thrombosis or superficial thrombophlebitis, postthrombotic syndrome when the venous dilatation acts as a collateral vessel, hypercoagulability, confinement to bed, pregnancy, and breast-feeding. Contraindications related to the sclerosing agent include (1) allergy to the agent itself, and (2) the sclerosant polidocanol in patients receiving disulfiram (Antabuse), since it contains 5% ethyl alcohol.

STRATEGY

Sclerotherapy of varicose veins must comply with certain basic principles for a satisfactory result for both patient and physician to be achieved.[2] These principles are easy to understand and are based on logical assumptions. Treatment must be performed from above in a downward direction and proceed from the largest to the smallest vein; it must be complete (all-or-nothing rule) and must include short- and long-term follow-up.

Above-to-Downward Approach

The origin of varicose vein reflux is derived from the proximal part of the varicose vein, that is, at its upper extremity when the patient is standing. When the reflux is interrupted at this level, distal pressure is decreased, leading to a marked reduction in the caliber of distal varicose veins and thus facilitating sclerosis. This is the principle behind the therapeutic combination of ligation/division of the saphenofemoral junction and sclerotherapy of the distal long saphenous vein. When this approach is used, the sclerosing injections also must be started as proximally as possible, with the distal portion being finished over the course of subsequent sessions. If this principle is not followed, in situ recurrence is inevitable. Reflux will penetrate through the fibrotic wall of the varicose vein, leading to recanalization and recurrence.

Therefore before treatment is begun, it is essential to make sure that the obvious varicose vein is not actually supplied by a more proximal unseen varicose vein. Verification can be obtained by means of either a manual compression test or Doppler study (Figure 11-1). If this above-to-downward direction principle is not followed, a large patch of telangiectatic matting, venulectasias, or a new varicose vein parallel to the original one may develop at the injection site (worse yet, a combination of all three may occur).

Largest-to-Smallest-Vein Approach

In general, sclerotherapy of varicose veins is done by starting with largest-diameter veins and finishing with the smallest ones. Schematically, the incompetent perforating vessels must be sclerosed first, followed by large varicose veins, then smaller varicose veins, and finally venulectasias and telangiectasias.[3,9] Treatment of telangiectasias or small varicose veins before sclerosis of the varicose veins supplying these small vessels is associated with risk of treatment failure, early recurrence, or excessive inflammation.

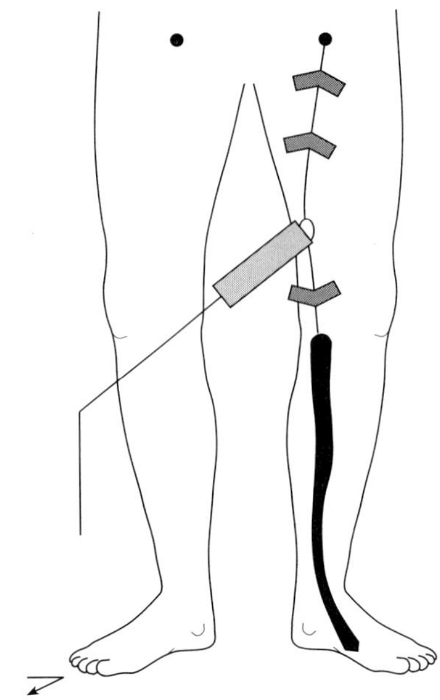

FIGURE 11-1. Palpation-percussion demonstrates varicose veins in leg but not in thigh. Doppler studies identify the origin of reflux: a perforator in adductor (Hunter's) canal.

Complete Approach

To obtain a good long-term result, the entire varicose vein must be sclerosed. Like surgical excision, such sclerosis ensures total disappearance of the varicose cluster without any portions of the varicose vein left intact for possible recurrence.

Follow-up

Regular follow-up, at least once a year, is essential. Such follow-up allows for treatment of new varicosities or those in evolution.

MATERIALS

Syringes

Disposable 2 to 5 ml plastic syringes graduated in 0.1 ml or 0.2 ml increments are the most widely used type. The tip of the syringe may be either central or eccentric, depending on the physician's preference. Glass syringes may be used, but they are less practical and require fastidious cleaning.

Needles

Long beveled needles are used: *usually* 0.4 to 20 mm (or 27-gauge 3/4 inch), 0.45 to 16 mm (or 26-gauge 5/8 inch), 0.5 to 16 mm (or 25-gauge 5/8 inch); *occasionally* 0.6 to 25 mm (or 23-gauge 1 inch); *more rarely* 0.7 to 40 mm (or 22-

TABLE 11-1. Most widely used sclerosing agents

Active Ingredient	Trade Names	Supply	Maximum Dose per Session	Drug Companies
Chromated glycerin	Scleremo (France)	5 ml ampules	France: 10 ml	Laboratoire Bouteille 7 Rue des Belges 87100 Limoges, France Omega 11177 Rue Hamon Montreal, Canada H3M3A2
Polidocanol	Aetoxisclerol (France) Aethoxysklerol (Germany) Sclerovein (Switzerland) Etoxisclerol (Spain)	2 ml ampules (0.5%, 2%, and 3%)	France: 4 ml (0.5%), 2 ml (2% and 3%)	Dexo S.A. 31 Rue d'Arras 92000 Nanterre, France Globopharm AQ P.O. Box 1187 8700 Kusnacht, Switzerland Kreussler & Co. D 6200 Wiesbaden-Biebrich, Germany
Sodium tetradecyl sulfate	Thrombovar (France) Sotradecol (U.S.A.) Thromboject (Canada)	2 ml ampules (1% and 3%)	France, U.S.A., and Canada: 10 ml (3%) Great Britain: 4 ml (3%)	Promedica 41 Rue C. Pelletan 92305 Levallois-Perret, France Elkins-Sinn, Inc. 2 Esterbrook Lane P.O. Box 5483 Cherry Hill, NJ 08034, U.S.A.
Dextrose/ sodium chloride	Sclerodex (Canada)	10 ml ampules	10 ml	Omega 11177 Rue Hamon Montreal, Canada H3M3A2

gauge 1½ inch), 0.8 to 40 mm (or 21-gauge 1½ inch). Certain specialists use butterfly needles. With small varicose veins or veins that are difficult to puncture in the supine position, the varicose vein is punctured while the patient is standing and the sclerosing agent is injected while the patient is lying down.

Sclerosing Agent

Numerous sclerosing agents are available on the market, although the choices vary from one country to another (Table 11-1). Each product has certain advantages and disadvantages, and the choice is based on personal experience. The best sclerosing agent is the one that the practitioner knows best.[10,11] Sclerosing agents can be classified according to the mechanism of action by which they induce the endothelial lesion.

Compression Material

Compression is an integral part of the technique required for sclerosing injection. Stockings and/or bandages may be used.[12] Elastic stockings must exert a pressure of approximately 30 mm Hg at the ankle (e.g., Sigvaris 503). If edema is present, the patient should systematically wear the stockings for 8 days before each injection session. This practice makes the varicose veins more accessible to palpation and therefore easier to inject.

Bandages should be nonelastic rather than elastic.[13] Nonelastic bandages are used to obtain maximum impact on the varicose dilatation. The bandage should not be applied too tightly.[14] In this way the varicose veins, emptied at the time of injection while the patient was in a supine position, are maintained flat by this semirigid bandage. When an adhesive bandage (e.g., Elastoplast or Micropore 8 cm wide) is used, it remains firmly in place. If an elastic bandage is used, segmental compression is obtained by means of four or five turns without tightening. The main problem with this type of bandage is keeping it in place. An elastic stocking is worn by the patient after application of this segmental compression.

TECHNIQUE

Sclerotherapy should be a harmless therapeutic modality. Varicose veins are not a sufficiently serious condition to justify taking the slightest risk. At each session the practitioner must be well prepared, act effectively, and inform the patient wisely.

The pretreatment visit must include clinical examination; ideally, the examination is combined with a Doppler ultrasound study, which offers greater sensitivity.[15,16] Based on the examination findings, a precise map of the varicose lesions is drawn. The origin of the various refluxes, vein morphology, presence of branches or perforating vessels, and varicose vein diameter should be indicated in the patient's medical record.[17]

In preparation for a sclerotherapy session, a clinical history must be recorded and a search for allergic reactions must be done. The latter may require suspension of injections or use of another agent. Injection sites, carefully identified by palpation and percussion, are marked by two parallel lines on either side of the varicose vein. The clinical measurement of diameter is recorded beside these two parallel lines so that the dose of the sclerosing agent can be calculated in relation to the size of the varicose vein.

The patient remains supine because this is the most comfortable position that helps to reduce excessive venous pressure so that the sclerosing agent can be injected into an empty varicose vein.[18] Complete emptying ensures optimal contact between the sclerosing agent and the wall of the varicose vein. The practitioner must assume a stable and comfortable position and needs good illumination of the operating field. Varicose veins are located again because the patient's new position may have modified previous markings by several millimeters.

Puncture, aspiration, and injection are theoretically simple procedures. Puncture must never be performed blindly. It always must be performed on a clearly identified and, better still, palpable varicose vein. The axis of the vessel is indicated by the two parallel lines, with the angle of entry between 30 and 45 degrees. The skin puncture should be swift. Perforation of the vein wall sometimes can be detected easily.

Occasionally, when the varicose vein is small or when it is situated in a dangerous zone such as the popliteal fossa, the puncture is performed with a butterfly needle while the patient is standing.[19] The injection is administered several seconds later with the patient lying down. An inclining table can be very useful in this situation.

Negative pressure within the plastic syringe can be produced by withdrawing the piston so that as the bevel of the needle crosses the wall of the vessel, blood is aspirated into the syringe by suction, immediately indicating the correct position of the needle. Users of glass syringes think that the piston slides sufficiently easily in the chamber of the syringe that it will rise on its own when in contact with arterial blood. One recommendation has been to insert the needle, not attached to the syringe, into the injection site.[20] The color and pressure of the blood coming from the needle are used to confirm correct intravenous position.

The injection must be performed precipitously. It must be painless, and the patient must be asked to describe what he/she feels.[21] The injection should be slowed or even stopped in the event of pain.

Selective compression of the puncture site during injection with the index finger of the free hand keeps the varicose vein flat (distention of the wall can be painful), ensures good contact between the sclerosing agent and the endothelium, and confirms nonextravasation of the sclerosing agent injected.

Treatment Session Report

All the information concerning the injection session is recorded in the patient's medical record, including the side and sites of injection, the diameter of the varicose vein at these sites, the sclerosing agent used (with concentration and volume injected specified), and the results obtained. This information must be clearly presented and understandable to all members of the health care team. The following format for a treatment session report serves as a guide for the practitioner in subsequent treatment sessions:

Right	1	2	3	etc.
Diameter				mm
1% STS				ml
Results				

Compression

Compression is an integral part of treatment, just as it is after surgery.[3,22,23] Injection without compression is generally followed by intravaricose thrombosis associated with an inflammatory reaction and hematoma. Digital compression over the puncture site during or after injection, reinforced by segmental compression, constitutes the best way of preventing thrombosis and generally obviates the need for thrombectomy.

Pigmentation and matting are the principal aesthetic complications. They usually appear alone, but occasionally they are present together. Pigmentation and matting are generally secondary to an intense inflammatory reaction, usually related to lack of control of the sclerosing process by means of a compressive bandage. Therefore a compressive bandage always must be applied, and the patient must be convinced to keep the bandage on for several days to avoid subsequent aesthetic complaints.

Sclerosing Agent and Starting Dose

Sclerotherapy of varicose veins usually gives excellent results, particularly in the hands of an experienced practitioner. Nevertheless, the choice of sclerosing agent and the dose to be injected remain a delicate problem. The most appropriate sclerosing agent should be selected after its advantages and disadvantages have been considered in relation to the patient's clinical context and the lesions to be treated.

The choice of dose is more difficult since it is impossible to predict the effects of a given dose on a particular type of varicose vein. A number of factors are probably involved: age, sex, body weight, elasticity of the cutaneous tissue, skin fragility, skin color, and type of varicose vein (its age, tortuosity or straight appearance, and diameter). For these reasons a standard dose does not exist. However, there is a close relationship between the diameter of the varicose vein and the dose.[24] It is referred to as the "minus one" technique. It can be used to calculate the ideal starting dose for all nonsaphenous varicose veins, with 1% sodium tetradecyl sulfate (STS) used as the sclerosing agent.

The ideal starting dose is the quantity of sclerosing agent sufficient to obtain a good result by the first injection without inducing any harmful effects. It is calculated as follows:

$$\text{Ideal starting dose (ml 1\% STS)} = \frac{\text{Diameter of varicose vein (mm)} - 1}{10}$$

where ideal dose is one that ensures maximum efficacy (resolution or painless cord) with a minimum of side effects (little or no painful induration, pigmentation, or additional telangiectasias) (Table 11-2). The starting dose is the dose injected for the first time into one point of a varicose vein. The dose of sclerosing agent corresponds to the volume (ml) injected multiplied by its concentration. If the initial concentration used is 1%, the dose corresponds to the volume injected. The diameter (mm) of the varicose vein is determined at the injection site by palpation (caliber rule) or by ultrasonography with the patient standing.

TABLE 11-2. Relationship between clinical diameter of nonsaphenous varicose veins and ideal starting dose

Diameter of Varicose Veins* (mm)	Ideal Starting Dose (ml 1% STS)
3	0.2
4	0.3
5	0.4
6	0.5
7	0.6
8	0.7

*Diameter as measured at injection site with patient standing.

TABLE 11-3. Scoring of results of sclerotherapy at injection site

Score	Effect Obtained
0	No result
1	Reduction in diameter by one half
2	Total resolution
3	Cord
4	Cord and inflammatory reaction >8 days
5	Cord and pigmentation
6	Cord and development of telangiectasias

In practice when this "minus one" technique is used with injections every 5 cm, and when principles of dual, segmental, and global compression of the limb are used, the results are excellent in approximately 70% of cases, ineffective in about 20%, and excessive in slightly less than 10%. This technique is easy to use because the diameter is often relatively constant along the varicose vein and rarely exceeds 8 mm. This diameter-dose relationship has been used by other authors with other sclerosing agents.[25]

The therapeutic approach at subsequent sessions is guided by evaluation of the results obtained with the first injections. The system of scoring the results (Table 11-3) has been used in the various statistical studies mentioned here. It is easy to use, can be adapted for computer processing, and effectively completes the treatment session report. This score can be used to complete the fourth line of the treatment session report (see sample report, p. 195). Thus, at a single glance, this report describes the initial session, tells what was done, and notes the results obtained.

When no reaction is observed at the injection site (result scored as 0), the volume injected is increased by 0.1 ml. When the diameter is reduced by one half (result scored as 1) and the entire length of the vein remains patent, the same volume of sclerosing agent is reinjected. When sclerosis of part of the vein occurs, the "minus one" technique is pursued. In the case of total resolution or a cord (scores 2 and 3, respectively), the "minus one" technique is applied to the other varicose veins.

In the case of an excessive reaction, such as a cord with inflammatory reaction lasting more than 1 week, a cord with pigmentation, or a cord with telangiectasias (scores 4, 5, and 6, respectively), the initial dose was excessive and should be decreased by one half for other varicose veins. Rigorous application of compression is essential in such a situation. With intense inflammatory reactions, local anti-inflammatory treatment should be applied. If the thrombus is not reabsorbed after 30 days, thrombectomy must be performed by incising the indurated zone with a large-caliber needle (21 gauge) or a No. 11 scalpel blade and pressing on the edges of the varicose vein. In most cases evacuation of the thrombus will prevent pigmentation of the zone.

Timing of Treatment Sessions

Treatment sessions must not occur too frequently because complete response to treatment can occur as late as 2 to 3 weeks after injections. Therefore an interval of at least 1 month should be allowed between each session for each varicose vein. If other varicose veins need treatment, particularly on the opposite leg, treatment sessions can be scheduled more frequently.

Patient preference concerning frequency of sessions and number of injections also should be considered. It is important to listen and clearly define the patient's reasons for consulting the physician so that the technique can be adapted to achieve the defined objectives.

Injection of Saphenous Veins After Ligation

When the long (greater) saphenous vein (LSV) and short (lesser) saphenous vein (SSV) do not require stripping, simple ligation of the saphenofemoral and saphenopopliteal junctions can be performed. This ligation is generally followed by a reduction in the diameter of the tributary veins. Sclerotherapy should be performed according to the rules defined in the following discussion. Initial doses injected into a palpable saphenous vein correspond to twice the "minus one" technique (e.g., 6 mm dilatation requires a dose of 1 ml of 1% sodium tetradecyl sulfate). The "minus one" technique then is applied to the remaining tributaries.

Treatment of Saphenous Veins With Sclerotherapy Alone

Treatment of long and short saphenous veins by sclerotherapy alone is controversial and does not appear to be indicated as first-line treatment.[8] Sclerosis of the junction regions, where blood flow and reflux are maximal, is difficult to achieve. Even when sclerosis is obtained, recanalization is usually inevitable because of underlying reflux. Therefore surgical treatment with ligation/division of the junctions, with or without stripping of distal varicose veins, appears to be the treatment of choice.

However, sclerotherapy of the LSV and SSV sometimes can be performed with a satisfactory success rate, particularly in the case of long-standing varicose veins. These veins are generally sufficiently large to be palpable over their entire length and therefore are easy to inject, which allows complete treatment to be done from above in a downward direction. Sclerotherapy of the LSV has a greater chance of success when the vein is sinusoid with dilatations at different levels and in male patients. In such cases compression is applied with stockings or superimposed nonadhesive bandages.

Additional indications for sclerotherapy of the SSV include improvement in functional testing after application of a 20 mm Hg elastic stocking and only minor reflux into the deep venous system. Because of the large number of anatomic variants in the popliteal fossa, a complete venous Doppler ultrasound study must be performed systematically. The sclerosing agent of choice is STS at a concentration of 3% for the LSV and 2% for the SSV. The modalities of compression are identical to those used for nonsaphenous varicose veins.

LONG-TERM RESULTS

Patients should be seen at least once a year after treatment. Follow-up should consist of a clinical examination and Doppler studies (whenever possible, combined with duplex to avoid missing a residual patent lumen within the sclerosis). This approach is designed to evaluate the efficacy of previous treatments and to demonstrate the appearance of varicose veins in previously untreated territories. Complementary treatment then can be instituted as a means of limiting disease progression.

Most authors agree that correctly performed sclerotherapy gives very satisfactory results in the majority of cases.[4-7] This view is supported by certain statistical studies.[8] Other authors monitor the intensity of sclerosis obtained and its subsequent course by ultrasound.[26] However, there is no easy way of differentiating among residual varicose veins, recurrent varicose veins, and natural progression of the disease. No method of quantification of varicose disease has been established. These points remain limiting factors for demonstrating the efficacy of any treatments.

A topographic and quantitative assessment of the lesions should be performed before any treatment is repeated, and this assessment should be performed at regular intervals.[27] Topographic differences between subsequent examinations allow for in situ recurrent varicose veins to be distinguished from new varicose veins. Quantitative differences allow for a quantitative assessment of the rate of disease progression.

ULTRASOUND-GUIDED INJECTION

When sclerotherapy is difficult or even dangerous to perform under clinical guidance by palpation or direct vision, ultrasound can be used to visualize the vein and guide the injection.[28,29]

Indications

General indications for ultrasound-guided sclerotherapy are the same as those described previously. Specifically, ultrasound guidance is used for deep varicose veins (in obese patients), nonpalpable incompetent perforators, residual channels resulting from incomplete efficacy of previous sclerotherapy, LSV or SSV when sclerotherapy is indicated, and tributaries of the upper third of the LSV.

Technique

We use real-time ultrasonography with a 7.5 MHz transducer. The sclerosing agent and dose are selected as already described. The needle must be of sufficient caliber to be echogenic, and its length should be adapted to the depth of the varicose veins. We generally use a 0.7 to 40 mm (22-gauge 1½ inch) or 0.8 to 40 mm (21-gauge 1½ inch) needle.

Initially, the varicose vein to be injected is located with the patient in a standing position. Then the location is again checked with the patient lying down. The needle is introduced into the vein until the bevel of the needle is visualized in the form of an isolated white echo in the lumen of the vein between the anterior and posterior walls (Figure 11-2). With standard sclerotherapy, traction on the piston of the syringe confirms the intravenous position of the needle by the presence of dark-red blood. The injection then can be performed. Passage of the solution into the superficial vein sometimes is associated with zones of turbulence, which can be seen on the monitor.

Limitations

Ultrasound-guided sclerotherapy does not eliminate all risks. However, it allows dual visual control through the use of the syringe and the ultrasound monitor. Although not essential, this type of sclerotherapy constitutes a valuable aid for guiding the injection in particular situations. It should be considered as only a complement to clinical examination and standard sclerotherapy.

OTHER METHODS

Doppler-Guided Injection

The injection site is located with a Doppler probe by percussion of the portion of the vein just above or below the varicose vein to be injected. The needle is inserted anterior to and into the axis of the problem area, almost perpendicular to the skin surface. Reflux into the syringe and the flow of the injection are rendered audible by the Doppler effect.

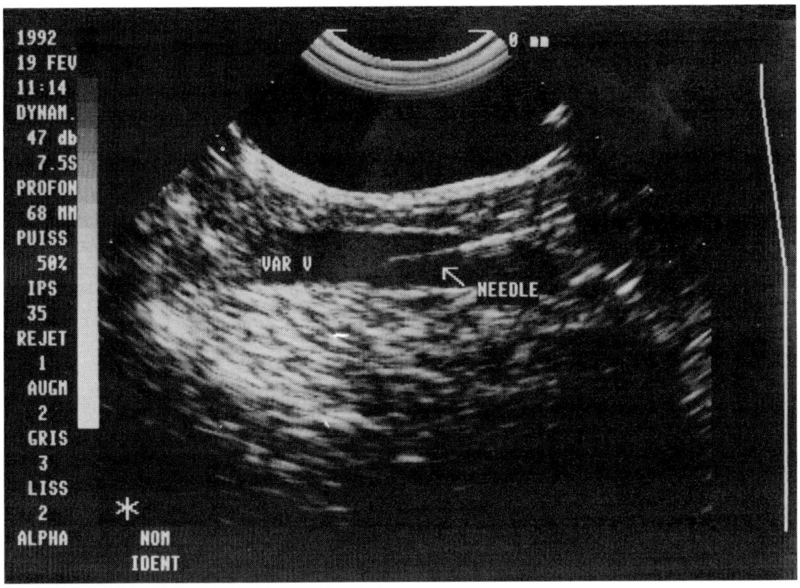

FIGURE 11-2. Ultrasound visualization of needle correctly located in varicose vein to be injected.

Endoscopic Injection

Venous endoscopy allows visualization of the venous endothelium, the valves, and the tributaries. However, this technique is still under investigation, and endoscopic sclerotherapy is only a research technique at present.[30]

SPECIAL CASES

Pregnancy

In general, sclerotherapy is not indicated during pregnancy. The combination of diurnal compression with leg elevation at night halts disease progression during gestation.[31] During pregnancy, compression should exert 30 to 40 mm Hg, and the foot of the patient's bed should be raised 10 to 12 cm. This dual approach should be continued at least until delivery. An assessment should be performed after pregnancy to determine the indications for curative treatment. Depending on the patient's desires, treatment can proceed, but plans for a future pregnancy should not alter the therapeutic approach.

Postthrombotic Syndrome

Sclerotherapy cannot be considered until the thrombosed deep vein has become recanalized and if the superficial dilatation is the site of constant blood flow, indicating a collateral vessel. This problem area can be detected by repeated noninvasive investigations. In fact, noninvasive venous investigation is imperative in such a situation to assess the respective importance of the superficial and deep veins. A clotting survey should be done to eliminate possible hypercoagulability.

■ ■ ■

A 56-year-old woman presented with a painful varicose vein of the right thigh. She had no history of deep venous thrombosis and had not undergone treatment. The diagnosis of nonsaphenous varicose veins was based on clinical examination and Doppler studies. The patient had a large varicose vein (9 mm in greatest diameter) on the anterolateral surface of the right lower extremity (Figure 11-3, *A*) with a clinically normal LSV; no reflux was present on the cough test. Manual compression of the saphenofemoral junction had no effect (the varicose vein filled at the same rate when the patient stood up). Doppler examination confirmed the integrity of the LSV; no reflux was present (Figure 11-3, *B*). However, marked reflux into the varicose vein was noted (Figure 11-3, *C*), and on ultrasound examination the dilatation measured 9 mm at its most proximal point (Figure 11-3, *D*). The remainder of the examination produced normal findings, with no other varicose veins, good patency and competence of the deep veins, and no arterial disease noted.

This patient's nonsaphenous varicose vein constituted a perfect indication for sclerotherapy. Treatment was commenced after the procedure was explained to the patient and

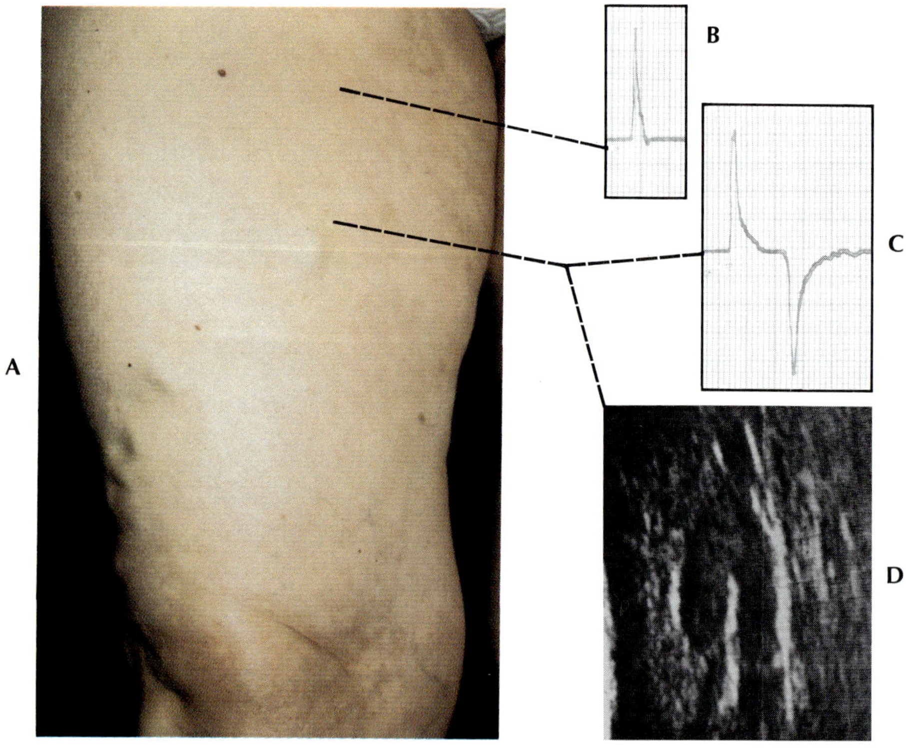

FIGURE 11-3. A, Nonsaphenous varicose vein. **B,** Doppler recording of competent long saphenous vein. **C,** Doppler recording of nonsaphenous varicose vein. **D,** Ultrasound examination.

after informed consent had been obtained (Figure 11-4). Injection sites were marked, and the corresponding diameter was measured with the patient in a standing position (Figure 11-5, *A*).

In this first session, the doses for injection were established according to the "minus one" technique. For the first three injection sites, which measured 9 mm, 6 mm, and 7 mm, the volumes of 1% STS were 0.8 ml, 0.5 ml, and 0.6 ml, respectively. A total of nine injections at intervals of 5 cm were done along this varicose vein (Figure 11-5, *B*). A nurse specialist applied the segmental compression (Figure 11-6, *A*); the bandage was worn for 8 days. The elastic stocking was put on with an extensor (Figure 11-6, *B*). The treatment session report includes all pertinent data (Figure 11-6, *C*).

PATIENT INFORMATION

Sclerotherapy of varicose veins is not devoid of risks. The technique consists of the injection of a sclerosing agent into your varicose veins. This agent acts by inducing irritation of the wall of the varicose vein. When a sufficient dose is injected, it causes complete obstruction of the varicose vein, leaving a more or less sensitive cord for several days. Your body will gradually resorb this cord, which finally disappears completely.

The objective of these injections is to eliminate your varicose veins, exactly as if they were removed surgically. In the same way as after surgery, compressive bandages are extremely important after the procedure. The aesthetic results obtained when these bandages are used are much more satisfactory and longer lasting.

You must comply with the following rules:

1. Lead a normal life during the hours following the injection. Specifically, do not rest but walk and go about your usual activities. Avoid prolonged sitting, such as in a car (stop every 20 minutes for a walk) or in a train (walk up and down the aisle).
2. Over the following 3 to 8 days, avoid excessive heat, shower rather than bathe, and do not cover your legs with heavy blankets. Avoid excessively violent sports.
3. Keep the bandages on for 8 days. If for any reason you must remove them, replace them within hours. If you need to wear an elastic stocking, continue to do so by putting it on over the bandage (without removing the bandage). When showering, protect your leg with a plastic bag.
4. Several minor events may occur in the treated regions, such as a sensitive cord or a hematoma. These are usual phenomena that are no cause for concern.

Do not hesitate to contact me by phone (or leave a message) if you have any questions or concerns.

Doctor ____________________

Patient ____________________

Telephone # ____________________

FAX # ____________________

Date ____________________

FIGURE 11-4. Patient information form for sclerotherapy.

A

B

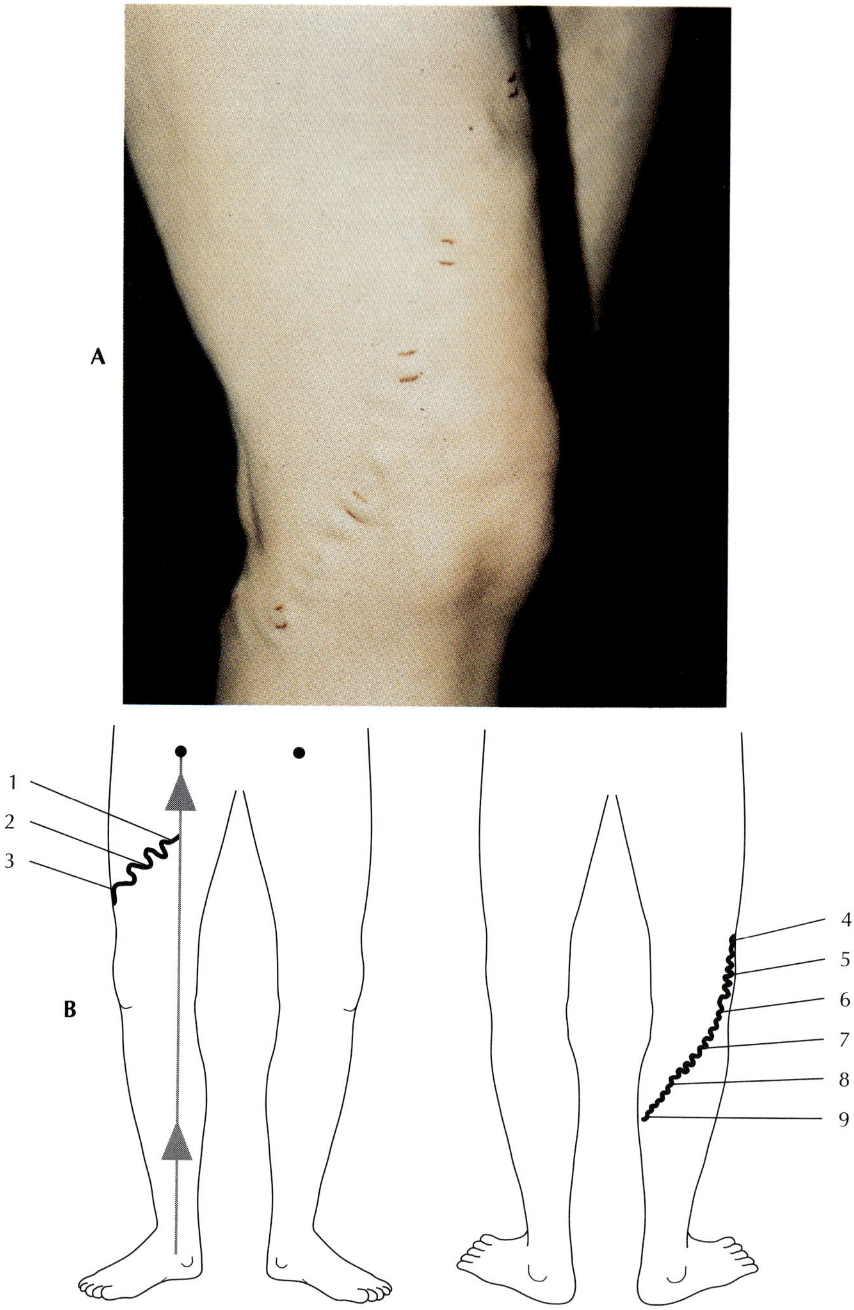

FIGURE 11-5. A, Marking of injection sites and diameters. B, Corresponding case file.

A

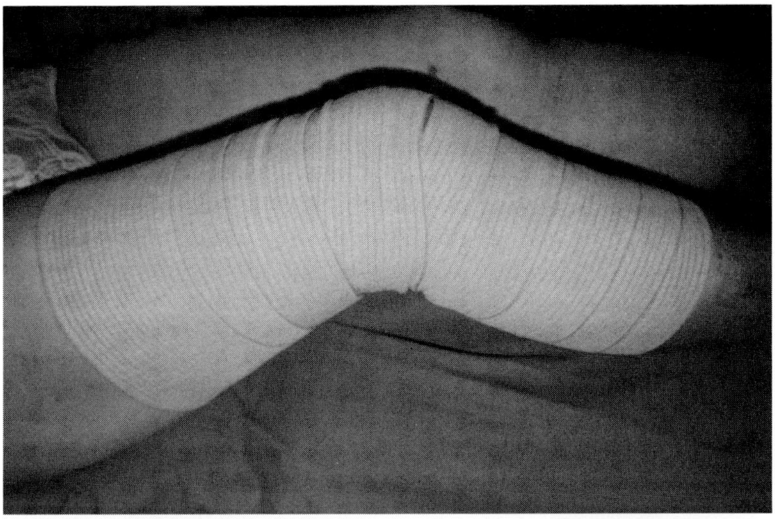

B

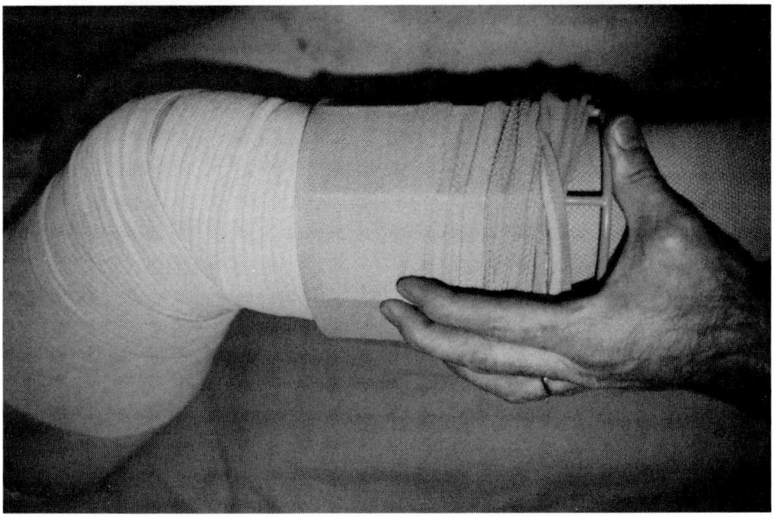

C

Right	1	2	3	4	
Diameter	9	6	7		mm
1% STS	0.8	0.5	0.6		ml
Results					

FIGURE 11-6. A, Application of segmental compression. **B,** Elastic stocking is put on with Sigvaris extensor. **C,** Establishment of treatment session report.

A

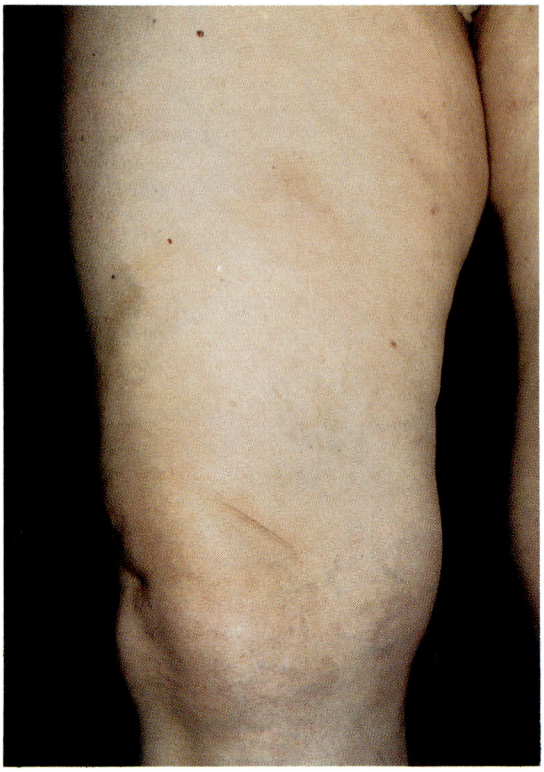

B

Right	1	2	3	4	
Diameter	9	6	7		mm
1% STS	0.8	0.5	0.6		ml
Results	3	3	3		

FIGURE 11-7. Clinical result (**A**) and transcription to treatment session report (**B**).

One month after treatment, the results were assessed (Figure 11-7, *A*) and scored to complete the treatment session report (Figure 11-7, *B*). In this case each injection site was scored as 3, corresponding to a cord. This single session was considered to be satisfactory, and the patient was scheduled for follow-up every 6 months for 2 years and annually thereafter.

CONCLUSION

Sclerotherapy remains a cornerstone in the treatment of superficial venous insufficiency. It occupies an important place among other available treatments. Sclerotherapy always must comply with two essential imperatives: safety and efficacy. A rigorous approach must be taken in defining the indications and administering the treatment.

REFERENCES

1. MacLatchie JD. The Treatment of Varicose Veins by Intravenous Injection. New York: Macmillan, 1929.
2. Tournay R. La Sclérose des Varices, 4th ed. Paris: L'Expansion Scientifique Française, 1985.
3. Goldman MP. Sclerotherapy: Treatment of Varicose and Telangiectatic Leg Veins. St. Louis: Mosby–Year Book, 1991.
4. Eklof B. Modern treatment of varicose veins. Br J Surg 75:297-298, 1988.
5. deGroot WP. Practical phlebology. Sclerotherapy of large veins. J Dermatol Surg Oncol 17:589-595, 1991.
6. Bishop C, Fronek H, Fronek A, Dilley R, Bernstein E. Real-time color duplex scanning after sclerotherapy of the greater saphenous vein. J Vasc Surg 14:505-510, 1991.
7. Perrin M. L'insuffisance Veineuse Chronique des Membres Inférieurs. Paris: Medsi/McGraw-Hill, 1990.
8. Hobbs JT. Surgery and sclerotherapy in the treatment of varicose veins: A random trial. Arch Surg 109:793-796, 1974.
9. Boivin P. Traitement des telangiectasies. Phlebologie 39:233-239, 1986.
10. Hutinel B. Phlebologie Esthetique. Paris: Arnette, 1990.
11. Sapin G, Parpex P. Choix du sclérosant. Phlebologie 38:183-185, 1985.
12. Stemmer R. The choice of compression stocking. Phlebologie 35:107-116, 1982.
13. Stemmer R. Sclérose des varices et compression. Phlebologie 44:49-67, 1991.
14. Ducros R. Intérêt de la compression dans le traitement sclérosant. Phlebologie 27:205-207, 1974.
15. Fronek HS. Noninvasive examination of the venous system in the leg: Presclerotherapy evaluation. J Dermatol Surg Oncol 15:170-173, 1989.
16. Large J. Doppler testing as an important conservation measure in the treatment of varicose veins. Aust N Z J Surg 54:357-359, 1984.
17. Cornu-Thenard A, Boivin P, Parpex P. Essai d'une quantification clinique des varices pour l'épidémiologie, la therapeutique et l'informatique. Phlebologie 39:661-676, 1986.
18. Wallois P. The condition necessary to achieve an effective sclerosant treatment. Phlebologie 35:337-344, 1982.
19. Raymond-Martimbeau P. Sclérotherapie de la saphene interne en position debout et en position assise. Etude comparative. Phlebologie 44:97-110, 1991.
20. Bernbach HR. Le traitement sclérosant selon SIGG. Phlebologie 44:31-36, 1991.
21. Fronek A. Injection compression sclerotherapy of varicose veins. In Ernst CB, Stanley JC, eds. Current Therapy in Vascular Surgery, 2nd ed. Philadelphia: BC Decker, 1991.
22. Fegan WG. Varicose Veins: Compression Sclerotherapy. London: Heinemann Medical, 1967.
23. Sladen JC. Compression sclerotherapy: Preparation, technique, complications, and results. Am J Surg 146:228-232, 1983.
24. Cornu-Thenard A, de Vincenzi I, Valty J. Sclérotherapie des varices—Intérêt de la mesure clinique de leur diamètre avant les premières injections. In Davy A, Stemmer R, eds. Phlebologie '89. Montrouge: John Libbey Eurotext, 1989.
25. Sadick NS. Minimal sclerosant concentration of hypertonic saline and its relationship to vessel diameter. J Dermatol Surg Oncol 17:65-70, 1991.
26. Schadeck M. Doppler and echotomography in sclerosis of the saphenous veins. Phlebology 2:221-240, 1987.
27. Cornu-Thenard A, de Vincenzi I, Maraval M. Evaluation of different systems for clinical quantification of varicose veins. J Dermatol Surg Oncol 17:345-348, 1991.
28. Knight RM, Vin F, Zygmunt JA. Ultrasonic guidance of injections into the superficial venous system. In Davy A, Stemmer R, eds. Phlebologie '89. Montrouge: John Libbey Eurotext, 1989.
29. Miserey G, Reinharez D, Ecalard P. Sclérose sous echographie dans certaines zones à risques. Phlebologie 44:84-96, 1991.
30. Van Cleef JF, Desvaux P, Griton P, Cloarec M. Sclérose de la saphene externe sous contrôle endoscopique. Phlebologie 44:131-136, 1991.
31. Boivin P, Hutinel B. Varices et grossesse. J Mal Vasc 12:218-221, 1987.

Chapter 12

Compression Sclerotherapy for Large Varicose Veins and Perforator Veins: A Personal Technique

Joseph G. Sladen and John D.S. Reid

In North America, the traditional approach to treating large varicose veins and complicated venous disease has been surgical.[1-3] In the last decade sclerotherapy, with or without a few days of compression, has gained popularity for treating small superficial veins and telangiectasias. Cosmetic appearance is usually the primary indication for this procedure, although some of these veins are symptomatic. Compression sclerotherapy for large veins was initially described by Sigg[4] in 1952 and reported in the English literature by Fegan[5] in the 1960s. A random trial comparing surgery with compression sclerotherapy that was published by Hobbs[6] in 1974 demonstrated that compression sclerotherapy controlled perforators effectively. We have practiced compression sclerotherapy with a few modifications during the last 15 years, concentrating on patients with symptoms. For 10 years, flush ligation of the saphenofemoral junction has been used as an adjunct to compression sclerotherapy when the long (greater) saphenous vein is incompetent.[7] This has led to improved results, particularly in the control of thigh varicosities.[8,9]

INITIAL EXAMINATION

An organized examination is directed specifically at the venous system. The findings are recorded on a specialized form (Figure 12-1). Initially the patient is asked to stand for 10 minutes. This standing loads the venous system and usually precipitates symptoms. Saphenofemoral incompetence often can be identified by a cough impulse in the upper saphenous vein, but use of a continuous-wave Doppler device is more helpful. The upper saphenous vein is insonated approximately 8 cm below the inguinal ligament with the Doppler probe while pressure is applied and released over the saphenous vein in the lower thigh (Figure 12-2). Reflux of blood in the saphenous vein that occurs when the palpating hand is released indicates saphenofemoral incompetence. This finding can be enhanced by a Valsalva maneuver performed by having the patient blow against the back of his or her hand while it is

PHYSICIAN'S NAME

R	L	COMPLAINT
		COSMETIC
		NIGHT CRAMP
		EXCESSIVE TIREDNESS
		PAIN ALONG VEIN
		HOT THROBBING PAIN
		RECURRENT PHLEBITIS
		BURSTING PAIN
		OEDEMA
		DERMATITIS
		PIGMENTATION
		INDURATION
		ULCERATION

NAME ____
ADDRESS ____

DATE ____
AGE ____ PARA ____
OCCUPATION ____ B.C.P. ____

HEIGHT ____ FT. ____ INS. ____
WEIGHT ____ LBS. — GOAL ____
ALLERGIES ____
MEDICATIONS ____

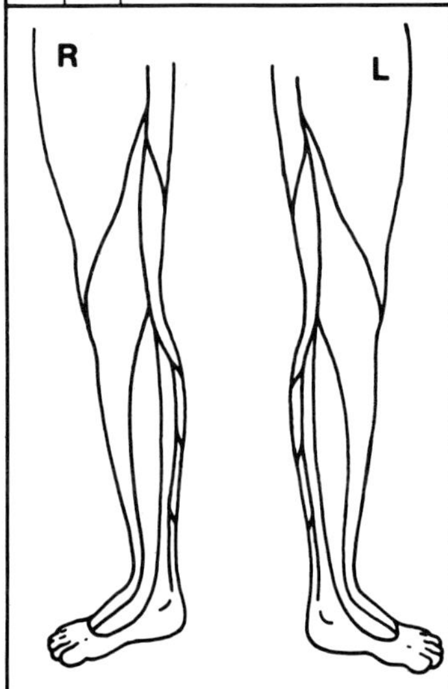

R	L	PREVIOUS MANAGEMENT
		HIGH LIGATION
		STRIP
		LOCAL TIES
		LOCAL PERFS
		SUB-FASCIAL LIGATION
		INJECTION
		COMP. SCLEROTHERAPY

VEIN INVOLVED	R	L
CAPILLARY		
SUPERFICIAL		
PERFORATING		
DEEP		
SYSTEM		
LONG SAPHENOUS		
SHORT SAPHENOUS		
COMMUNICATING VEINS		
LABIAL VEINS		
SAPHENA VARIX		
PELVIC PHLEBOGRAM		
ASCENDING "		

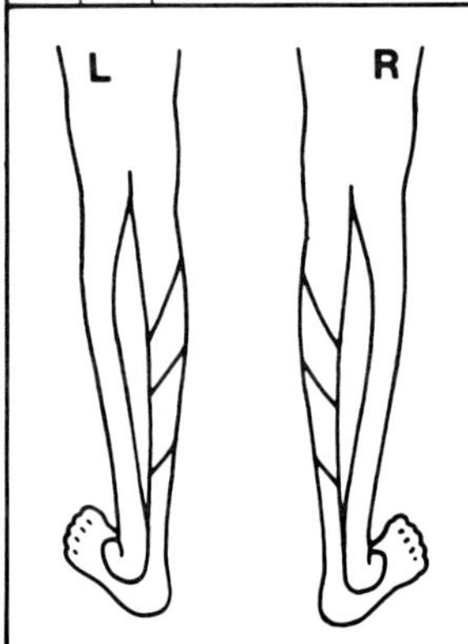

TREATED BY:

NO.	DATE	RX	RESULT

PERTINENT FACTORS	SYSTEMS	TREATMENT
FAMILY HISTORY	PULMONARY	(1) ADVISED
OBESITY	CARDIAC	(2) F.O.B.↑ 4"
PARITY	ABD.	EXERCISE
PREGNANT	G.I.	WT. LOSS
HIST. DEEP PHLEB.	HAEM	DIURETIC
HIST. LEG INJURY	PULSES R L	BK STOCKING
DIABETES	F	SPONGE PUMP
HYPERTENSION	P	
ASOD.	PT	(3) INJECT/COMP.
SUCCESSFUL ART. OR.	DP	(4) OPERATION
		DIAGNOSIS:

FIGURE 12-1. Form on which venous complaints, findings, and treatment are recorded. (Modified from Sir Patrick Dunn Hospital, Dublin, Ireland.)

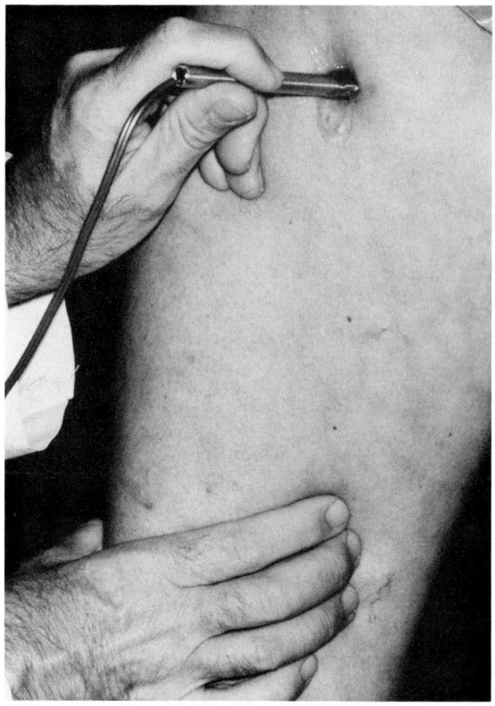

FIGURE 12-2. Use of continuous-wave Doppler probe to assess saphenofemoral reflux with release of pressure over long saphenous vein and use of Valsalva maneuver.

pressed against the mouth. It is important that the patient not move during the Valsalva maneuver because Doppler sounds indicate blood passing the probe in either direction, and movement of the leg can produce a false positive result. The short (lesser) saphenous vein is examined while the patient is standing, with notation of distention over its course in the midposterior calf and particularly at the crow's foot configuration above the lateral malleolus. Along with palpation, the Doppler probe can be used to identify the course of the vein by manually tapping the short saphenous vein near its lower end. Doppler examination is more difficult in the popliteal fossa than in the groin because of the adjacent deep venous system, but it can be helpful in identifying reflux.

The varicose veins are then examined for control or entry points and for perforators. While the patient remains standing, the veins are manually stripped of their blood. The examiner controls the vein with the fingers of one hand and uses the fingers of the other hand, moving proximally on the leg, to strip the blood from the vein. Sudden reappearance of blood filling the vein as the second examining hand moves up the leg indicates a control point or an incompetent perforator. Pressure applied at a control point may control a nest of varicosities. The anatomic perforator sites on the medial side of the lower leg are examined by palpating with the thumb, searching for tenderness, and milking away edema with repetitive pressure (Figure 12-3). Frequently, a high-pressure vein that has not been obvious

A

B

C

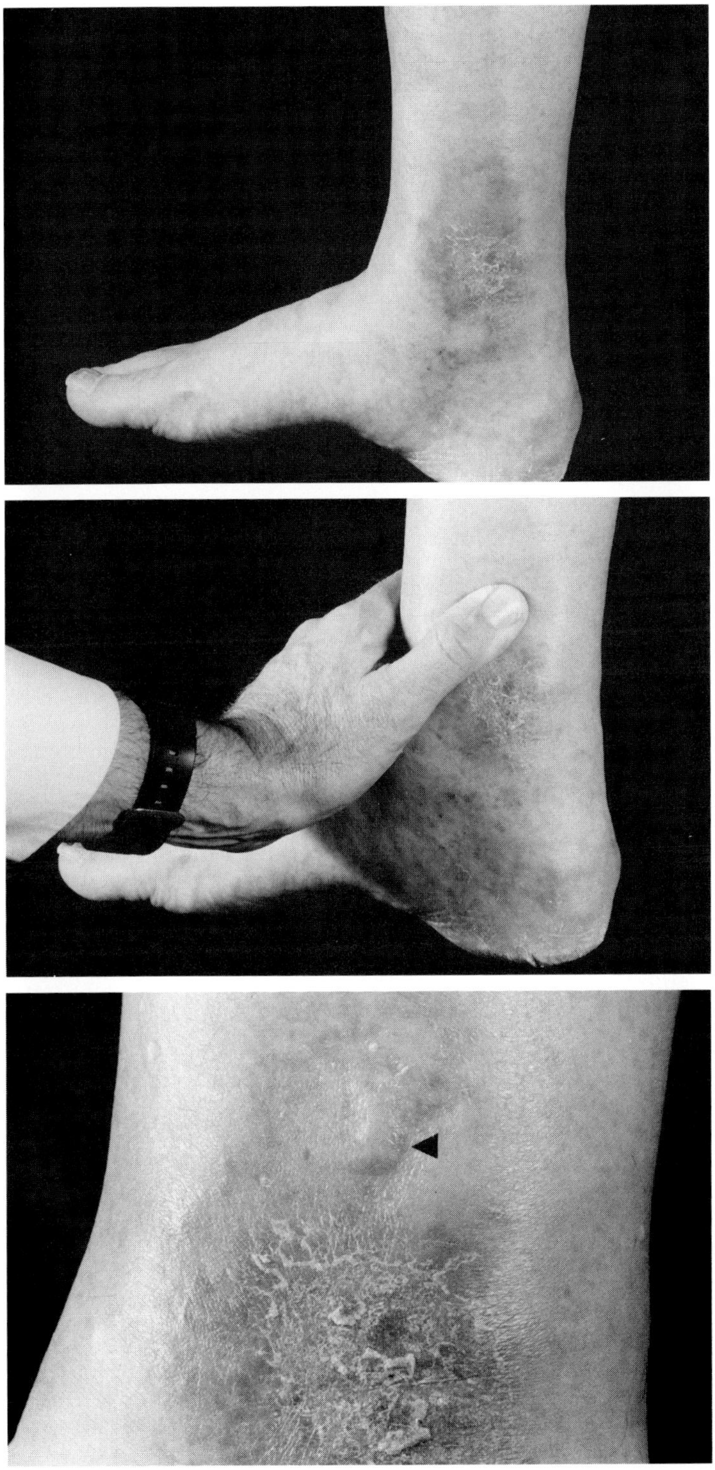

FIGURE 12-3. A, Stasis dermatitis with no visible vein. **B,** "Milking" the edema. **C,** Close-up of same area showing visible and easily palpable high-pressure vein (arrowhead) fed by Cockett perforator after "milking."

emerges from the surrounding edema when examination is done with this technique. Tender or warm areas are the most important injection sites for compression sclerotherapy. They reflect high-pressure veins and are usually venous "lakes" fed by perforators or control points. Differentiation between perforators and control points is not important because both should be treated. Edema, dermatitis, induration, and pigmentation are noted. While in a supine position, the patient is then examined for pulses and ankle pressures, if indicated, to rule out arterial disease. We do not find that the standard Trendelenburg test adds any useful information. The patient's complaints and examination are recorded on the venous form during the examination.

PREPARATION OF PATIENT

For satisfactory management, it is mandatory that the patient understand the basic principles of venous disease. Concepts of venous drainage, valves, and the calf pump need to be discussed. We stress control, not cure, of disease and spend time allaying fears of ulceration and amputation, which frequently concern the patient with venous disease. It is helpful to involve the office nurse in the discussion and to provide handouts that address many of the questions the patient may have later.

Pressure

As an integral part of treatment, all patients are fitted with a below-knee pressure-gradient stocking (30-40 mm Hg). Many patients state that they cannot tolerate a stocking, but a well-fitted stocking improves venous disease and symptoms. In fact, we often use the stocking as a "therapeutic trial" to help confirm the diagnosis of venous insufficiency. Although trained stocking fitters have improved significantly during the last 15 years, an experienced physician can often improve on a measured fit. A full range of stocking sizes kept in the office is recommended to the physician specializing in the treatment of venous disease. This supply allows the fitting of alternative stocking sizes and the stretching of the stocking by the physician to achieve a comfortable fit. The patient is instructed in the use of the stocking at the first visit (Figure 12-4). It is easiest to apply the stocking by turning it inside out and then inverting the foot portion to the heel. The patient's foot is inserted into the stocking to the heel, and the remaining stocking is everted over the foot and up the leg. The stocking should slip off the thumbs during this part of the application rather than being stretched up the leg. There should be room for one or two fingers above the stocking in the popliteal fossa with the knee bent. Frequently the stocking needs to be loosened by vigorous stretching of its cuff and ankle before application to prevent constriction of the calf and to allow it to go over the heel easily. Patient compliance is important because the stocking is worn over the bandage after compression sclerotherapy and must be well tolerated.

A

B

C

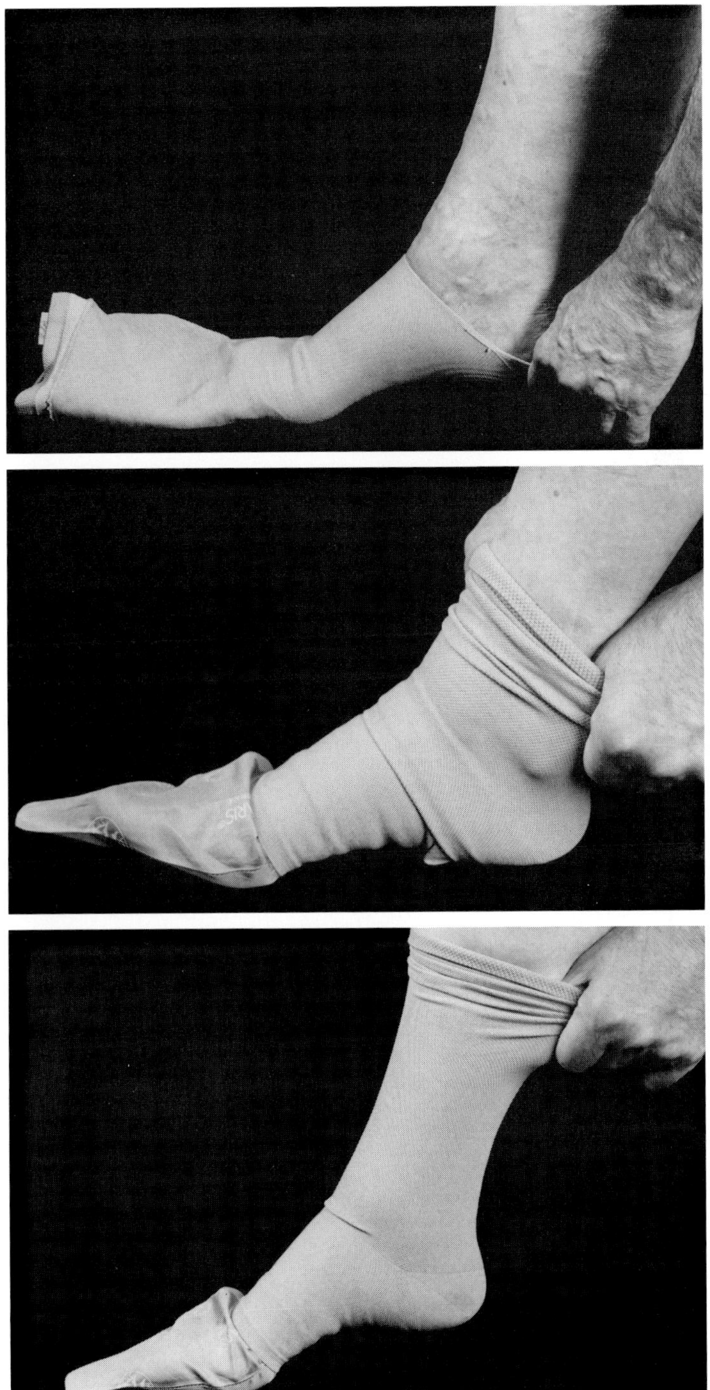

FIGURE 12-4. A, Patient's foot is inserted into foot of stocking, with the leg of stocking inside out over the foot. **B,** Stocking is eased over the heel, one layer at a time without bunching. **C,** Tension is distributed by slipping stocking off the thumbs to place stocking on the leg, rather than by stretching it upward on the leg.

Compression

If diffuse tenderness, induration, or ulceration is present on the medial lower calf, a "sponge pump" is added rather than increasing the pressure of the stocking (Figure 12-5). Initially, very few patients can tolerate stockings with a pressure gradient of 40 to 50 mm Hg. A sponge pump is made from soft, 1/2-inch latex foam rubber, measuring approximately 8 × 20 cm. The pump is rounded and beveled so that the edges do not indent the tissue, and it can be modified to apply more pressure behind the medial malleolus. The sponge pump is placed on the medial perforator area over the pressure-gradient stocking and wrapped with about one half of a 4-inch tensor bandage. The bandage is applied tightly with crisscrossing spiral wraps on the lower part of the sponge pump; as the bandage is applied upward, the pressure is reduced by spreading and easing the pressure on the wraps.

Activity

The patient is directed to walk 2 miles a day to ensure adequate deep venous outflow. If the patient has difficulty tolerating the stocking or the sponge pump, we do not proceed with high ligation or compression sclerotherapy but persist in conservative management. Patients who are unable to walk because of arthritic or cardiac problems are taught to exercise their calf against resistance. An air-mattress foot pump works well for this purpose.

COMBINED TREATMENT: FLUSH LIGATION AND COMPRESSION SCLEROTHERAPY

If the patient is comfortable for a few days with the pressure-gradient stocking and sponge pump (if indicated), we proceed with treatment.

Flush Ligation

Burnand et al.[10] have shown that an incompetent long saphenous vein may contribute more than 50% of the increase in ambulatory venous pressure at the ankle seen in venous disease, even in the presence of incompetent perforators. Approximately 60% of patients who present with large varicosities but have not had a previous saphenofemoral ligation have saphenofemoral reflux. Most of these patients undergo flush ligation of the saphenofemoral junction done on an outpatient basis and with local anesthesia. The area is explored through a 5 cm incision on the groin crease over the saphenofemoral junction, with careful ligation of all branches, with care taken not to miss collateral bypassing veins, which can cause recurrences.[11] Approximately 2 cm of saphenous vein is resected. Moderate reflux is compatible with excellent early results of compression sclerotherapy; however, in our experience these results are not lasting, particularly when thigh varicosities, often due to midthigh incompetent perforators, are present. Large thigh varicosities are easily injected at the time of flush ligation. After surgery, a 3 ml syringe is filled

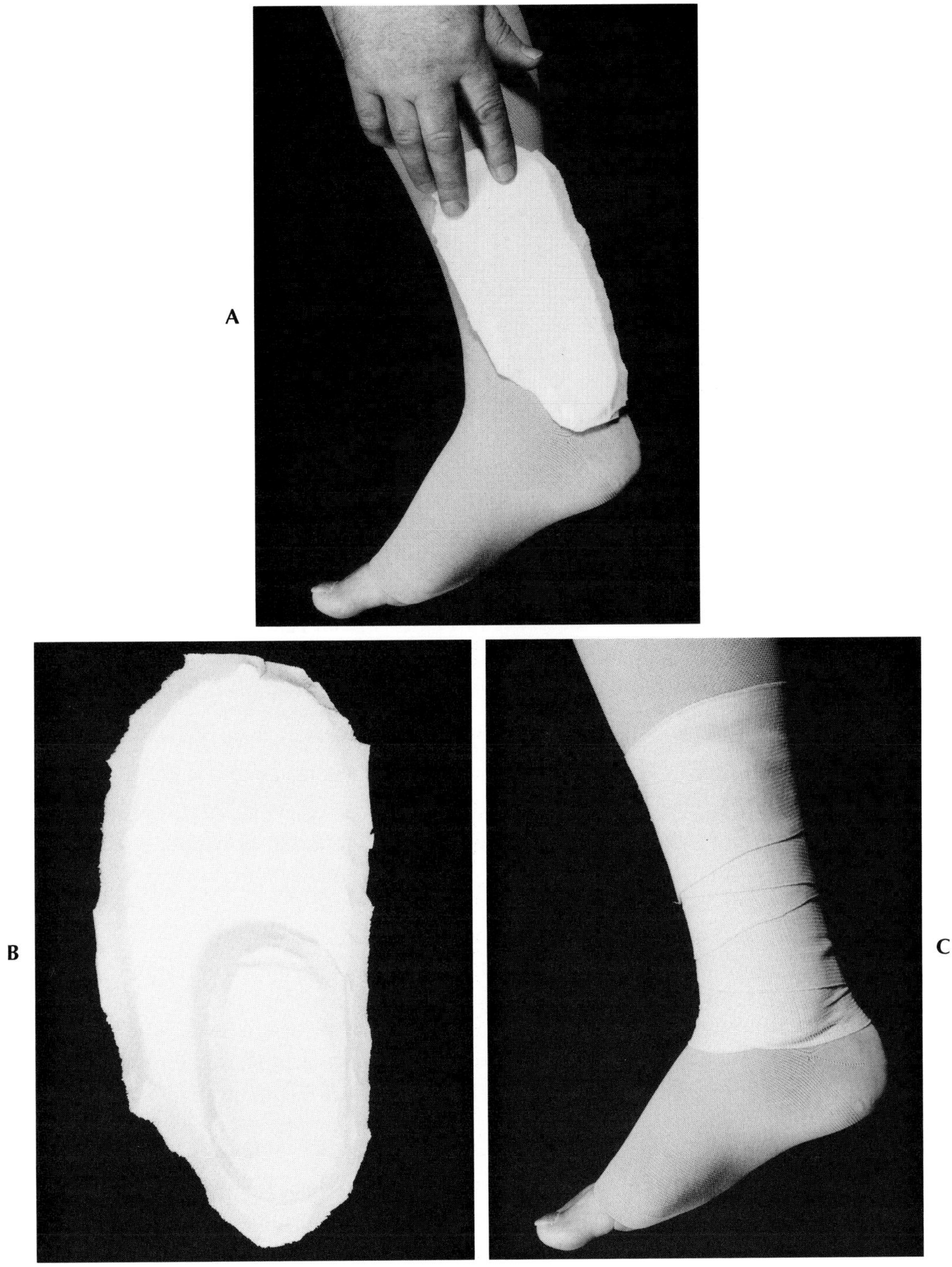

FIGURE 12-5. A, Sponge pump is made of soft ½-inch latex foam rubber sculpted to fit the area. B, Additional piece of latex foam can be used to apply more pressure behind the medial malleolus if there is an ulcer in that area. C, Four-inch elasticized bandage is applied tightly on lower part of sponge, easing the pressure above.

with 3% sodium tetradecyl sulphate, which is used to inject thigh varicosities while the patient is still in a supine position. Up to six sites are injected with 0.5 ml each from the syringe. The thigh is wrapped with a crepe or tensor bandage, with extra pressure applied over the injected area by using a latex rubber sponge or a folded abdominal dressing pad if the sponge is not available. Half of an abdominal dressing pad is placed behind the knee to prevent the bandage from piling. The pod is wrapped downward to meet the pressure gradient stocking so that the bandage is contiguous with the stocking. If an obvious large adductor canal (Dodd) perforator is present, it may be ligated at the time of flush ligation while the patient is under local anesthesia. Some patients are better treated while under general anesthesia because of anxiety or obesity or because the procedure has been done previously. Postoperatively, patients are advised to wear the pressure gradient stocking while upright and to apply additional pressure to any tender areas. They should take three or four walks each day for a total distance of at least 1 mile. It is helpful to begin a course of anti-inflammatory medication for 1 week and to prescribe a mild analgesic. Most patients are ready to return to work 3 or 4 days after surgery, and a follow-up office visit is scheduled within 7 to 10 days.

Compression Sclerotherapy

Approximately half of our patients have no significant saphenofemoral reflux or have had previous venous ligation or stripping by other practitioners and require only compression sclerotherapy. It is important that the patient understand the basic principles of venous disease and learn to master the use of the pressure gradient stocking. Therefore compression sclerotherapy is not performed at the initial visit.

Materials. An injection tray that includes prefilled syringes, precut 1/2-inch tape in 8 cm lengths, cotton fluffs, crepe bandages, sponge, adhesive elastic bandage (Elastoplast), scissors, and porous plastic tape (Micropore) is essential if the procedure is to be accomplished expediently (Figure 12-6). Syringes are prefilled with 0.5 ml of either 1% or 3% concentrations of sodium tetradecyl sulfate.* A 3% concentration is used for the large high-pressure veins, and a 1% concentration is used for the smaller veins. The different concentrations are clearly coded on the syringes with tape. We prefer 3 ml syringes with 25-gauge needles because of better tactile feedback while injecting. A standing stool is provided for the patient so that the physician can sit in a comfortable position while injecting. Applying a layer of carpeting under each end of an examining table allows it to slide over a smooth floor so it can be moved easily to the patient when it is time for the patient to lie down.

Technique. The technical steps in compression sclerotherapy can be summarized in the following way:

1. Have patient stand for 10 minutes.
2. Make multiple punctures.

**Editor's note:* Wyeth-Ayerst Laboratories (Philadelphia), the manufacturer of STS, does not advise allowing STS to remain in contact with the rubber stopper of a syringe for longer than a few hours because of degradation of the rubber (personal communication, 1992).

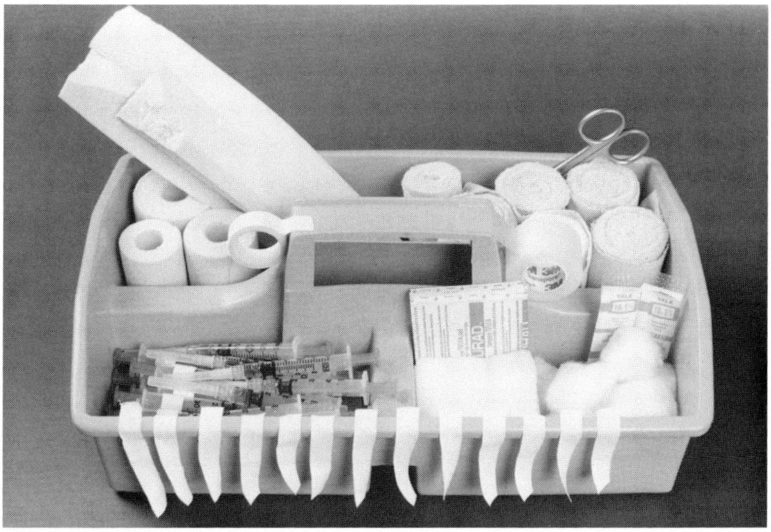

FIGURE 12-6. An organized tray expedites compression sclerotherapy.

3. Elevate the patient's leg.
4. Inject the sclerosant and trap with cotton fluffs.
5. Wrap the leg with a crepe bandage and apply latex sponge to the course of the vein.
6. Apply Elastoplast to stabilize the bandage.
7. Cover the bandage with an old nylon stocking.
8. Compression is applied through the use of a below-knee pressure-gradient stocking (30-40 mm Hg) and a 6-inch elasticized bandage or tube for the knee or thigh.

These steps are illustrated in Figure 12-7.

The patient should stand for 10 minutes to load the veins. This loading facilitates needle placement within the vein lumen. Some patients are surprisingly prone to vasovagal syncope and may be treated while sitting if the veins are large enough to palpate. The needles are introduced into the vein obliquely so that there is good tissue friction on the needle. A flash of blood into the hub of the needle indicates that the needle is in the vein lumen. Care is taken not to puncture the main saphenous trunk but rather the perforator or control point branches, if possible. The syringe is then secured to the leg with ½-inch tape.

When all the sites have been punctured, the patient lies supine on the examining table and the leg is elevated, with the foot resting on the physician's shoulder to empty the veins. The sclerosant is then injected slowly; it is trapped by digital pressure applied over cotton fluffs placed approximately 5 cm proximal to the injection site; the pressure is worked upward on the leg when possible. Assistance from the nurse is necessary at this stage. If the sclerosant extravasates, it burns severely, like a bee sting. The patient is warned of this, and the injection is stopped if

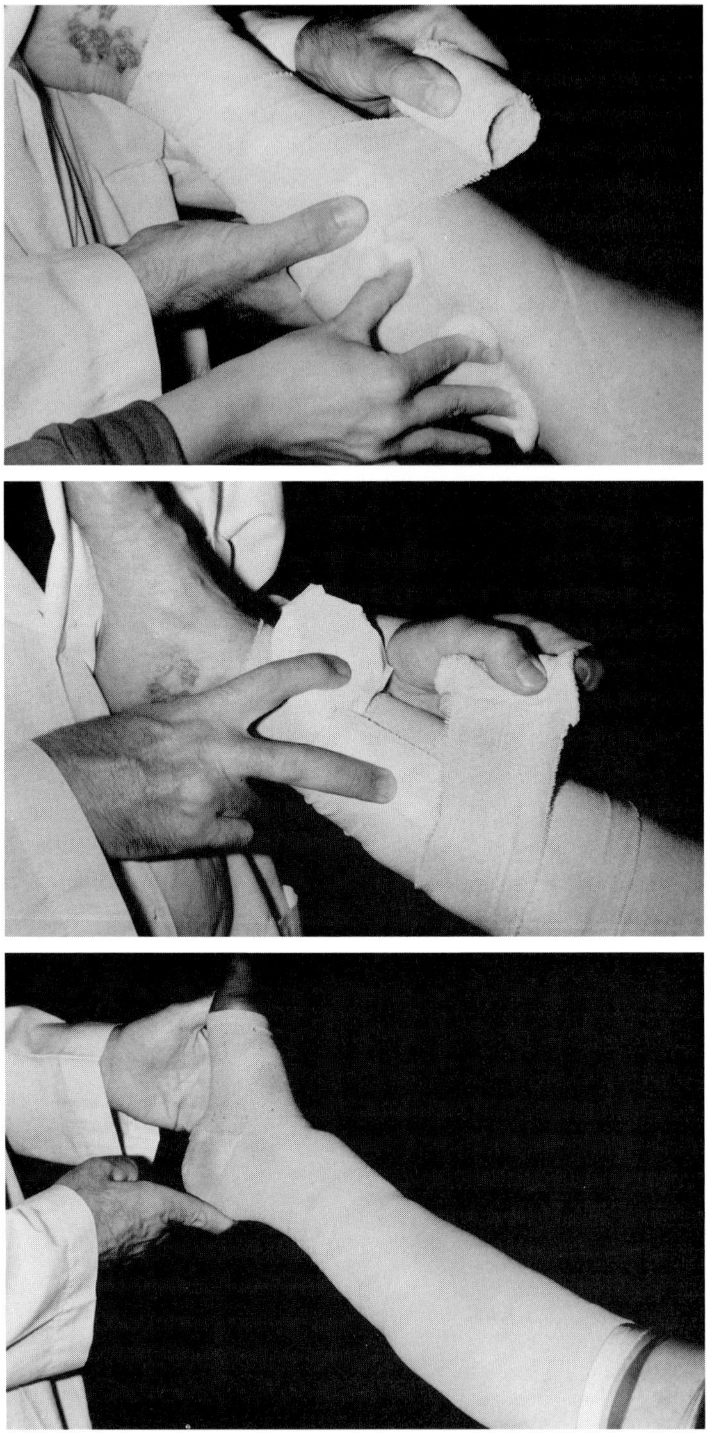

A

B

C

FIGURE 12-7. Compression sclerotherapy for large veins. **A,** After injection, sclerosant is trapped with cotton fluffs and compressed with a bandage. **B,** Precut latex sponge is applied to the course of the vein. **C,** Prefitted pressure-gradient stocking is worn over the bandage.

there is a suggestion of extravasation. Infiltration of 1% lidocaine solution controls the pain and may reduce the incidence of injection ulceration (see Chapter 15).

The needles are left in place, and the wrapping is begun in a distal to proximal direction, with syringes and needles removed as they are encountered. Leakage from the needle hole is controlled by applying a cotton fluff over the area of the vein pierced by the needle, which is slightly proximal to the skin puncture site. If there are many injection sites on the leg, it is easier to inject and wrap the lower half of the leg and then proceed with the upper half. We use a crepe bandage rather than an elasticized bandage because the former makes it much easier to control the amount of pressure applied. Precut tapered 1-inch latex sponge rubber is applied along the course of the vein, which can be seen by the outline of the cotton fluffs through the crepe bandage. The sponge is held in place with another layer of wrapping. The wrap must be applied smoothly, and the second and third layers are applied in a random fashion to support the whole wrapped area equally. The wrap should be applied firmly but not tightly. In a lean leg, tension must be reduced slightly over the anterior border of the tibia or the bandage may cause blisters or pressure symptoms such as burning. In wrapping a large leg, it may be useful to compress the sponge with a thumb as the leg is wrapped to produce more pressure locally over the course of the vein. Elastoplast is used at the top and bottom of the bandage to stabilize it, with contact with the skin avoided in order to minimize the potential for skin reaction. Bandages are covered with an old nylon stocking that is used both day and night to protect the bandage. During the day the pressure-gradient stocking is applied over the nylon stocking and slides on quite easily.

Patients are advised to reduce the tension of the bandage, particularly at the lower end, if the foot swells excessively or if the lower edge cuts in. This is accomplished by cutting the lower edge of the bandage in successive layers at the 12, 4, and 8 o'clock positions, with the cut made approximately one quarter to one third of the width of the bandage (Figure 12-8). The Elastoplast is then reapplied to produce a neat bandage with tapered pressure. Injection sites and areas of suspected extravasation are recorded on the vein chart. The foot is always cyanotic and congested when dependent, but the congestion is controlled by the pressure-gradient stocking. The patient is advised to take three or four daily walks, totaling approximately 2 miles a day, and to apply extra pressure with a sanitary napkin or similar pad over any area of tenderness. Patients who are unable to walk are advised to use an air-mattress foot pump or treadle. Analgesic or anti-inflammatory medication is not prescribed, and the patient is advised to walk if the limb feels congested. It may be necessary for the patient to get up once during the first night and take a short walk if the leg is uncomfortable. The patient removes the bandage in 3 weeks if large high-pressure veins were treated or in 10 days if smaller low-pressure veins were treated. A handout is supplied to guide the patient through this period. The patient is examined in the office 3 or 4 days after the bandage is removed. Unless there is a great deal of standing or kneeling in the patient's workplace, there should be no interruption in work schedule.

We try to minimize the number of sessions. For example, we take the opportunity to inject thigh varicosities at the time of flush ligation because bandages are

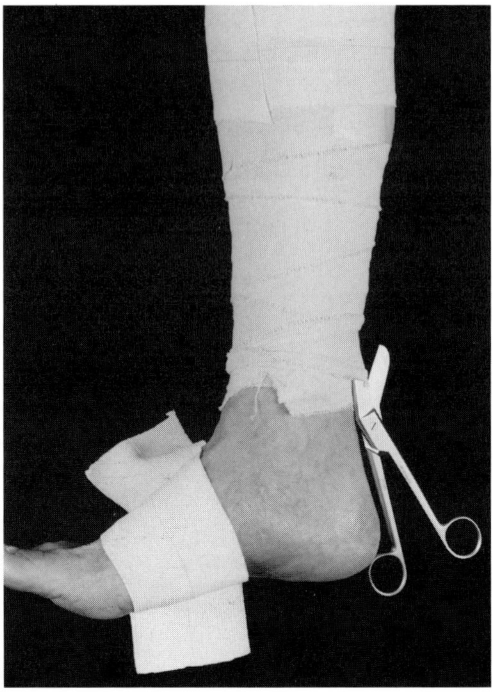

FIGURE 12-8. Without removal of the bandage, tension on the bandage can be eased by the patient by removing the lower Elastoplast and cutting the lower third of successive wraps at the 12, 4, and 8 o'clock positions, as required.

more easily tolerated if the thigh and calf are not wrapped at the same time. Varicosities of the foot also are more easily managed alone after treating the calf. A total of 150 recently completed limbs were analyzed: 78% were treated in one session; 20%, in two sessions; and 2%, in three sessions. The average number of injections per session was 6.5, 2.5, and 2, respectively.

UNUSUAL PRESENTATIONS

Varicograms are very useful in delineating the anatomy when an unusual vein in the groin is noted after flush ligation, in the thigh below the buttock, or in the popliteal area.[12,13] Gross saphenofemoral reflux after flush ligation or stripping is best treated by reoperation, with careful exploration of the origin of the saphenous vein from the femoral vein. Minor recurrence in this area can be treated by injection. Thigh perforators are sometimes difficult to treat with compression sclerotherapy. A venogram is obtained after one unsuccessful attempt and is often followed by local ligation and compression sclerotherapy. Veins draining directly from the pelvis posteriorly or laterally are best treated by ligation at their control point before injection because it is too difficult to apply effective compression in this area. Short saphenous vein incompetence is rare in the absence of long saphenous vein incompetence, but it is a significant cause of calf pain and should be considered in symptomatic venous disease. Varicograms are very helpful in delineating popliteal venous anatomy.[13] Recurrent veins found in the popliteal fossa after short saphenous ligation deserve mandatory venography. The only episode of deep phlebitis after compression sclerotherapy in our experience followed injection of recurrent varicosities in this area.

Large veins in the foot can hemorrhage, be tender, and are often disfiguring. With a few modifications, results of compression sclerotherapy are good. Bandages that incorporate the ankle may cause blisters and sometimes ulceration over the Achilles tendon because of pressure and friction. It is always necessary to protect this area when treating veins of the foot. Friction on the Achilles tendon can be reduced by covering the area with nonstick dressing (Telfa) or thin plastic wrap before bandaging. Smaller cotton fluffs are used on the foot, supplemented with a piece of ½-inch foam, custom fitted and beveled to cover the injection sites. This method reduces the bulk so that a shoe can be worn.

COMPLICATIONS

Small areas of local phlebitis occur in approximately 20% of injected limbs, particularly in the thigh and upper calf, where it is more difficult to sustain compression. If the area is more than 3 mm in diameter, the tarlike thrombus can be expressed easily by opening the skin with a No. 11 scalpel blade or aspirated with an 18-gauge needle up to 6 weeks after injection. Removal of the thrombus results in immediate relief of pain and tenderness and reduces subsequent pigmentation in the area. The area should be compressed for 3 days to avoid recurrence of phlebitis. We express or aspirate thrombi in 12% of our injected limbs. Noticeable pigmentation is present in 10% of patients at 3 months, but usually the appearance is quite acceptable at the end of a year. Oriental and East Indian patients have a greater tendency toward permanent pigmentation and should be advised of this fact.

More generalized superficial phlebitis, usually located in the thigh above the injected area, occurs in approximately 5% of limbs. This condition is treated with early application of pressure by using a sanitary napkin or folded abdominal dressing pad placed longitudinally over the area of tenderness and wrapped with a tensor bandage to give comfortable support. We use a 6-inch elasticized bandage or elasticized tube in the thigh and a 4-inch bandage in the calf for this purpose. In our treatment of several thousand limbs, there have been no occurrences of embolization and no cases requiring high ligation.

Ulceration occurs in 3% of limbs after compression sclerotherapy of large veins. Three causes should be considered: (1) extravasation (injection ulcer, Figure 12-9); (2) pressure necrosis; and (3) local hypersensitivity. Reducing the concentration of the sclerosant from 3% to 0.5% or 1% decreases the incidence of injection ulcer but has not been as effective in controlling large high-pressure varicosities in our experience. Injection ulcers may be more than 2 cm in diameter and tend to occur in the lower half of the calf. The large ones may take 3 or 4 months to heal

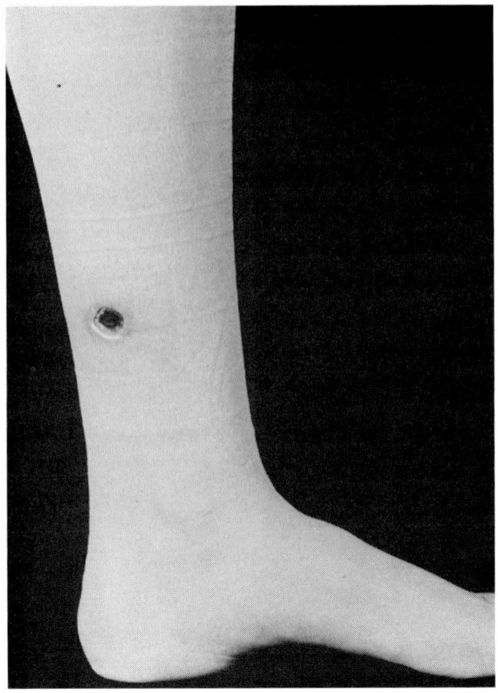

FIGURE 12-9. Injection ulcer measuring 1 cm in diameter that healed in 3 months and left a small scar. Excision would have expedited healing.

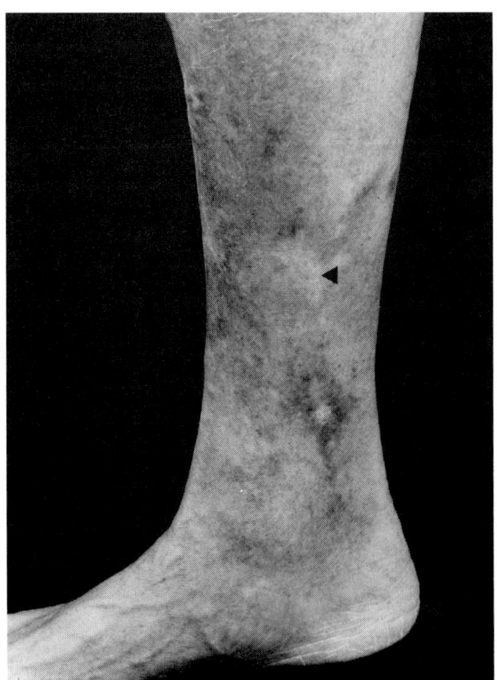

FIGURE 12-10. Scarring (arrowhead) on the leg of a 72-year-old man is seen 1 year after development of a 2.5 cm injection ulcer that could not be excised. The ulcer took 4 months to heal.

(Figure 12-10). Fortunately, they are not painful and are easily managed by placing a dry or occlusive dressing under a pressure-gradient stocking. We advise excising the large ulcers early because this practice shortens the healing time and results in a very acceptable scar. Patients with large symptomatic veins accept this complication much more easily than those with asymptomatic small reticular veins or telangiectasias for whom the cosmetic result is important. This matter should be considered in selection of the sclerosant and its concentration. Ulceration also can be caused by pressure from cotton fluffs that are too thick and firm, particularly if they are placed over the anterior subcutaneous surface of the tibia. Such ulcers tend to heal more quickly than injection ulcers do, and they do not have the characteristic depth of injection ulcers. This problem can be reduced by thinning the cotton fluffs and avoiding injection sites over the surface of the tibia. Occasionally, we have seen one or even two small ulcers at injection sites in patients who have had no apparent extravasation or undue pressure but usually have had previous courses of sclerotherapy. Such ulcers may represent local hypersensitivity to the small amount of sclerosant that leaks from the vein when the needle is removed. Frothing the sclerosant may reduce this leakage. We have seen a few cases of saphenous neuritis, one of which was permanent but localized. This complication is minimized by keeping the puncture site away from the saphenous vein and nerve.

MANAGEMENT OF INDURATION AND ULCERATION

Compression sclerotherapy is particularly applicable to the treatment of severe symptomatic disease and venous ulceration.[14] The aim is to isolate the pressure generated in the deep calf pump from the surface by obliterating the venous connecting veins and perforators. Injections should be made through normal or almost normal subcutaneous tissue and rarely adjacent to an ulcerated area.

The patient is seen and examined as described. Characteristically, venous ulcers are not painful and only slightly tender. If the ulcer is painful, there is either a significant infective component or it is a combined ulcer, associated with occlusive disease or hypertension. Ulcers on the lateral aspect of the leg are more suggestive of this condition. A few patients with badly infected stasis ulcers may require a short hospital admission for parenteral antibiotics, local debridement, and repeated applications of wet-to-dry dressings. However, hospitalization is rarely necessary, and most patients can be managed as outpatients with application of 3 × 3 inch gauze to the ulcer. The gauze is backed with a portion of abdominal padding to absorb moisture and is held in place with a nylon stocking. For additional pressure, a pressure-gradient stocking is applied over the nylon and then over the sponge pump. This dressing is changed three times a day. We find that cotton gauze, rather than the newer cellulose or synthetic materials, is better for absorption and debridement. Patients are carefully taught that pressure heals. They are instructed to walk 2 miles daily and to resume their normal activity as much as possible. It usually takes two or three follow-up office visits for the physician to be certain the patient is using the sponge pump effectively. The sponge must be sculpted to fill the concave area behind the medial malleolus, and it may be necessary to add another layer of sponge to heal an ulcer in this area (see Figure 12-5, *B*). When the ulcer is clean and relatively dry, Telfa is substituted for gauze and changed morning and evening; thus the need for the abdominal pad is soon eliminated. Patient compliance with this treatment is high. Tenderness and induration subside quickly; the patient is fully mobile and can easily monitor the progress of healing.

In an unpublished study of our experience, 100 stasis ulcers ranging from 0.5 to 8 cm in minimum diameter took 1 to 2 months to heal approximately 1 cm; they then healed at a rate of approximately 1 cm per month. Most stasis ulcers remain healed with continued use of a sponge pump or conversion to a higher grade compression stocking. Such ulcers are usually associated with obvious venous insufficiency and incompetent perforators. Patients with this type of ulcer should be treated with compression sclerotherapy and saphenofemoral ligation, if necessary. All these patients are instructed to use permanently a compression stocking with a pressure gradient of 30 to 40 mm Hg and to return temporarily to the sponge pump if the tenderness or induration recurs. The recurrence rate for stasis ulcer after compression sclerotherapy was about 3% per year after 8 years of follow-up in this group of patients in our study. The recurrence is often related to an uncontrolled perforator and responds to repeat compression sclerotherapy.

SUMMARY

Venous disease is effectively managed through combined treatment, with flush ligation used for the incompetent long saphenous vein and compression sclerotherapy used for perforating veins and major control points. Most of the long saphenous vein can be preserved, and treatment can be repeated easily when necessary. Compression sclerotherapy for large veins is not surgery-free, is not a cure, and rarely produces a "Hollywood leg." Patients with bursting pain, induration, or ulceration are ideal candidates for compression sclerotherapy, and this method is particularly applicable to patients who are elderly, obese, or at high risk for other reasons. Compression sclerotherapy, with its attendant bandaging, is well accepted by patients in North America and is an extremely useful tool in the management of venous disease.

REFERENCES

1. Homans J. The operative treatment of varicose veins and ulcers. Surg Gynecol Obstet 22:143-158, 1916.
2. Linton RR. The postthrombotic ulceration of the lower extremity: Its etiology and surgical treatment. Surgery 138:415, 1953.
3. DePalma RG. Surgical therapy for venous stasis ulcer. Surgery 76:910, 1975.
4. Sigg K. The treatment of varicosities and accompanying complications. Angiology 3:355-379, 1952.
5. Fegan WB. Continuous compression technique of injecting varicose veins. Lancet 3:109-112, 1963.
6. Hobbs JT. Surgery and sclerotherapy in the treatment of varicose veins: A random trial. Arch Surg 109:793-796, 1974.
7. McCaffery J. An approach to the treatment of varicose veins. Med J Aust 1:1379, 1969.

8. Sladen JG. Compression sclerotherapy: Preparation, technique, complications, and results. Am J Surg 146:228-232, 1983.
9. Sladen JG. Flush ligation and compression sclerotherapy in the control of venous disease. Am J Surg 152:535-538, 1986.
10. Burnand JG, O'Donnell TF, Thomas ML, Browse NL. The relative importance of incompetent communicating veins in the production of varicose veins and venous ulcers. Surgery 82:9-14, 1977.
11. Hobbs JT. Operations for varicose veins. In Rob and Smith's Operative Surgery. De Weese JA, ed. Vascular Surgery, 4th ed. St. Louis: CV Mosby and London: Butterworths, 1985, p 278.
12. Thomas ML, Bowles JN. Incompetent perforating veins: Comparison of varicography and ascending phlebography. Radiology 154:619-623, 1985.
13. Hobbs JT. Perioperative venography to ensure accurate sapheno-popliteal vein ligation. Br Med J 2:1578-1580, 1980.
14. Henry MEF, Fegan WG, Pegum JM. Five-year survey of the treatment of varicose ulcers. Br Med J 2:493-494, 1971.

Chapter 13

Role of Sclerotherapy in Greater Saphenous Vein Incompetence

Pauline Raymond-Martimbeau

As one of the two major vessels that comprise the superficial venous system, the greater (long) saphenous vein (GSV) is particularly vulnerable to incompetence, a disorder characterized by venous reflux and dilatation. Although traditionally managed surgically, GSV incompetence also may be treated by means of sclerotherapy, a nonsurgical approach in which injection of a chemical agent into the diseased vessel induces a sterile inflammatory reaction that results in fibrosis or sclerosis, thereby permanently obliterating the vein. Ideally, the vessel is reduced in diameter and reabsorbed. The technique, which is painless and nonscarring, is performed on an outpatient basis.

This chapter gives a brief review of the history of sclerotherapy and offers guidelines for preoperative evaluation and patient selection in the treatment of GSV incompetence. Sclerotherapeutic technique is described, and a discussion of postoperative management, evaluation, and potential complications is presented.

HISTORICAL OVERVIEW

Sclerotherapy of the GSV is believed to have been introduced in 1905 by Tavel, who injected a 5% phenolic acid into the GSV of a patient after surgical ligation. During the first quarter of the twentieth century, sclerotherapy was practiced mainly in Europe, sometimes in combination with surgical ligation. Unfortunately, sclerosants remained relatively toxic and often produced undesirable side effects. In 1928, brief trials of sclerotherapy were undertaken in the United States, primarily at the Mayo Clinic, but the results were disappointing, and physicians in the United States continued to favor surgery.

Modern sclerotherapy is based on progress made during the past 50 years. A key factor was the advent of improved chemical agents, including less toxic powerful sclerosants such as iodine sodium iodide and sodium tetradecyl sulfate. Several schools of thought evolved, each with its own technique. In the 1950s, Fegan[1] and his followers recommended that the injection sequence progress from bottom to top, beginning with the most distal incompetent perforating vein. Because this technique relies heavily on postoperative bandaging and compressive therapy, it is known as compression sclerotherapy. In contrast, the French school, led by Tournay, progressively expanded the concept that treatment should begin at the highest point of reflux and proceed downward. This top-to-bottom arrangement followed the logical sequence of surgical treatment. Initially, injection was performed at the junction itself, but the danger of accidentally puncturing the deep venous or arterial systems was soon recognized. Safety was increased by moving the injection site several centimeters below the saphenofemoral junction (SFJ). Digital compression of the SFJ during injection, as proposed by Chatard[2] and studied by Cloutier,[3,4] also was an important advance.

During the past 15 years, sclerotherapy has become a more exact discipline, and the results of experienced sclerotherapists now compare favorably with those of surgeons. In light of the current widespread trend toward noninvasive technology and minimally invasive techniques, sclerotherapy can be expected to gain increased popularity.

ANATOMY

On the basis of location and function, the vessels of the lower limb are divided into three main groups: (1) high-pressure deep veins, which are responsible for 90% of venous return; (2) low-pressure superficial veins, which drain blood from the skin and serve as a reservoir for blood storage; and (3) perforating veins, which link the deep and the superficial systems. In each of these groups, one-way flow is normally maintained by a series of bicuspid valves that direct the blood upward and inward. When one of these valves malfunctions, venous reflux and hypertension eventually result in varicosities. This disorder primarily affects the superficial veins because, unlike the deep vessels, they have little external support.

The two major superficial veins are the GSV, which drains much of the lower limb, and the short saphenous vein (SSV), which mainly drains the calf region. The GSV arises from the internal marginal vein in the foot, courses anteriorly toward the medial malleolus, traverses the medial portion of the tibia, following its posteromedial border, and passes behind the condyle of the femur. It then crosses the sartorius and adductor longus muscles before entering the common femoral vein at Scarpa's triangle to form the SFJ (Figure 13-1). This junction is usually crescent-shaped. Blood flow through the SFJ is regulated by a constant valve called the ostial valve, which is particularly vulnerable to malfunction (Figure 13-2). When the ostial valve is incompetent, the resulting venous reflux causes distention of the distal truncal vein; in turn, the valves of that vein become incompetent, leading to varicosity.

In a recent study of duplex ultrasonographic assessment, I found that (1) the GSV terminates in the common femoral vein at Scarpa's triangle in 91.4% of cases; (2) the SFJ is crescent-shaped in 76.2% of cases; and (3) the saphenofemoral valve

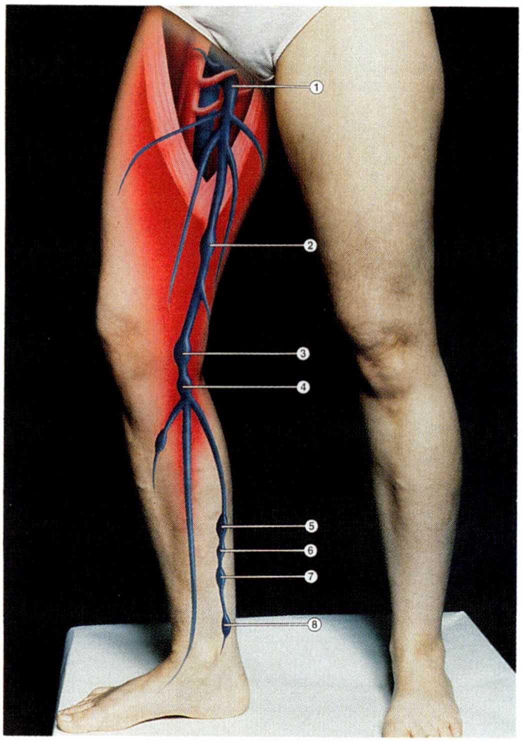

FIGURE 13-1. Anatomy of the greater saphenous vein. *1*, Saphenofemoral junction; *2*, hunterian perforator group; *3*, geniculate perforator group; *4*, Boyd perforator group; *5*, 24 cm perforating vein; *6*, Cockett III (18.5 cm); *7*, Cockett II (13.5 cm); *8*, Cockett I (6-7 cm).

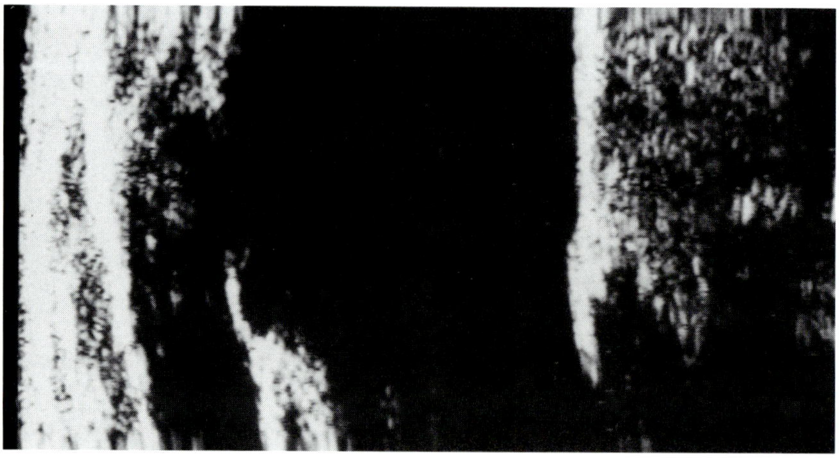

FIGURE 13-2. Duplex ultrasonographic longitudinal section shows saphenofemoral junction as crescent-shaped. Note presence of the ostial valve. (From Raymond-Martimbeau P. Phlebologia Houston '91. Dallas: PRM Editions, 1991.)

can be visualized in 82.4% of cases.[5] The GSV has a single continuous trunk in 84.3% of cases, a double trunk in 12.2%, and a triple trunk in 3.5%. Two groups of tributaries, the upper and the lower tributaries, enter the proximal segment of the GSV. The major upper tributaries, which enter the GSV near the fossa ovalis, are the superficial circumflex iliac vein, the superficial epigastric vein, and the external pudendal vein. The most important lower tributaries, which enter the GSV in the thigh, are the anterior accessory (anterior crural) saphenous vein and the posterior accessory (posterior crural) saphenous vein (also known as the Cruveilhier vein). Both groups of tributaries have a variable termination. Failure to recognize variations can lead to relapses after sclerotherapy or surgery. My study showed that the upper tributaries and the proximal segment of the GSV have a common termination in the common femoral vein in 8.4% of cases. The upper tributaries terminate in the GSV near the junction in 45.1% of cases and directly in the common femoral vein in 1.9% of cases. In the remaining cases, the upper tributaries cannot be visualized. The termination site of the lower tributaries varies from the midaspect of the thigh to Scarpa's triangle. The Giacomini vein, an anastomotic vein that links the SSV and the GSV, enters the trunk of the GSV at variable levels, ranging from near the SFJ to the knee. If the Giacomini vein enters near the SFJ, and if it is incompetent and left untreated, it can contribute to the recurrence of GSV incompetence.

In the upper third of the leg, the main trunk is joined by the anterior arch branch and the posterior arch branch (Leonardo's vein). Arteries that lie near the GSV include the external pudendal arteries at the SFJ level (Figure 13-3) and the posterior tibial artery at the distal end of the GSV. The external pudendal arteries exhibit considerable variability in their topography.

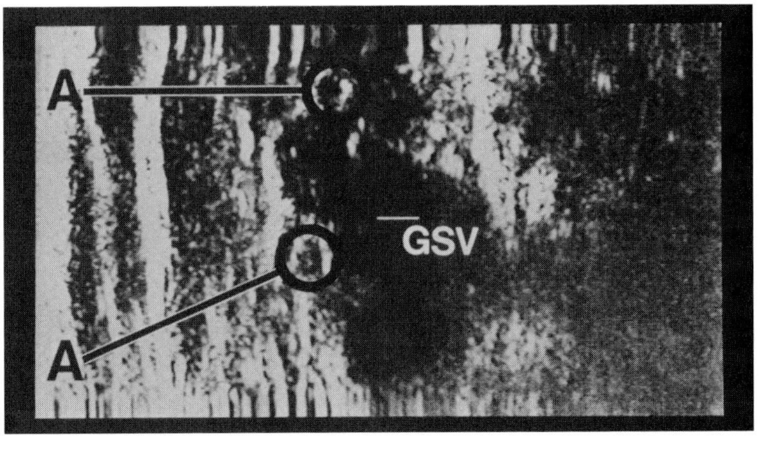

FIGURE 13-3. Duplex ultrasonographic transverse section of the greater saphenous vein (*GSV*) and pudendal arteries (*A*).

TYPES OF GREATER SAPHENOUS VEIN INVOLVEMENT*

SFJ only
SFJ + tributaries
SFJ + saphenous trunk
SFJ + saphenous trunk + single perforating vein
SFJ + saphenous trunk + multiple perforating veins
Attendant perforating vein: single or multiple
Postoperative neovascularization of GSV at SFJ
Mixed form: SSV terminating in GSV
Giacomini vein anastomosing SSV with GSV

SFJ, saphenofemoral junction; GSV, greater saphenous vein; SSV, short saphenous vein.
*At any of these levels, a stasis ulcer may be present.

CLASSIFICATION

Incompetence of the GSV can originate at one or more levels (see box), at which a stasis ulcer also may be present (Figure 13-4). In my practice, 64% of patients who present with GSV incompetence have reflux at the SFJ (Figures 13-5 to 13-7). In such cases control of incompetence at this level is a prerequisite for the treatment of more distal varicosities.

Alternatively, the SFJ may be functional, in which case GSV incompetence originates from valvular malfunction at any of the following levels: (1) the tributaries (Figure 13-8); (2) the GSV trunk; (3) one or more perforating veins (Figure 13-9); (4) the SSV; or (5) an anastomotic vein (Figure 13-10). Therefore GSV incompetence denotes a wide spectrum of disease, the development of which is progressive; such disease ranges from localized telangiectasia (Figure 13-11) or varicosity (Figure 13-12) in early cases to involvement of the entire vessel in advanced cases.

SYMPTOM COMPLEX

Incompetence of the GSV generally evolves through three stages, each of which is characterized by a different main symptom. Early mild disease is often the most painful stage because it is associated with mild venous dilatation and minimal changes in the venous wall. In more advanced disease, the patient usually complains of limb heaviness rather than pain. In complicated disease, the overall venous return is impaired and manifestations such as edema and cutaneous discoloration may be present. Patients report tiredness, tingling of the limb, and generalized malaise. At this stage pain may be absent.

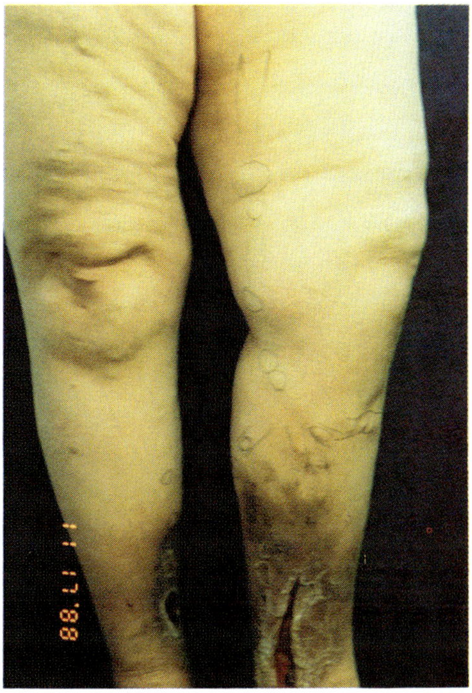

FIGURE 13-4. Bilateral saphenofemoral junction incompetence with presence of bilateral stasis ulcer.

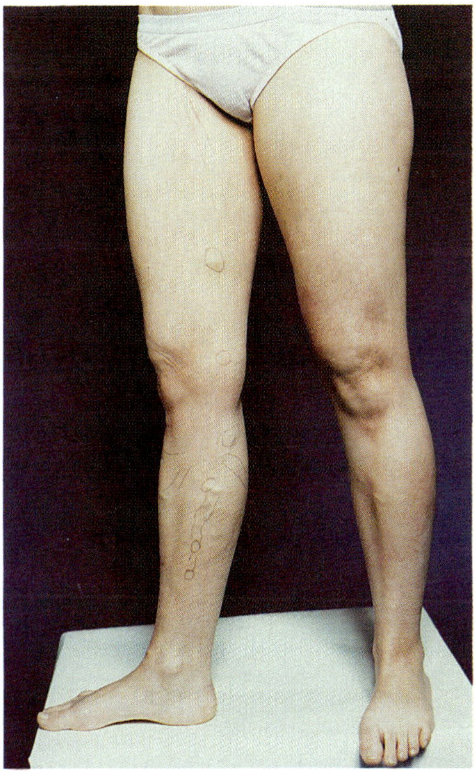

FIGURE 13-5. Saphenofemoral junction incompetence. (From Raymond-Martimbeau P. Phlebologia Houston '91. Dallas: PRM Editions, 1991.)

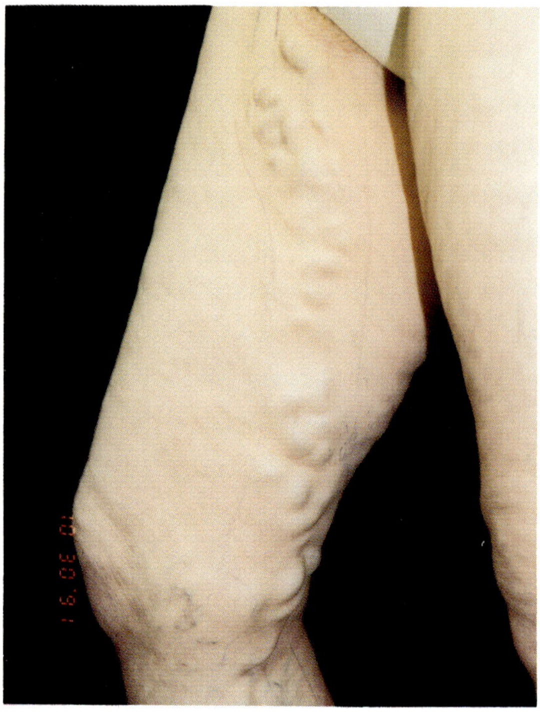

FIGURE 13-6. Saphenofemoral junction incompetence. In this case the junction is laterally located.

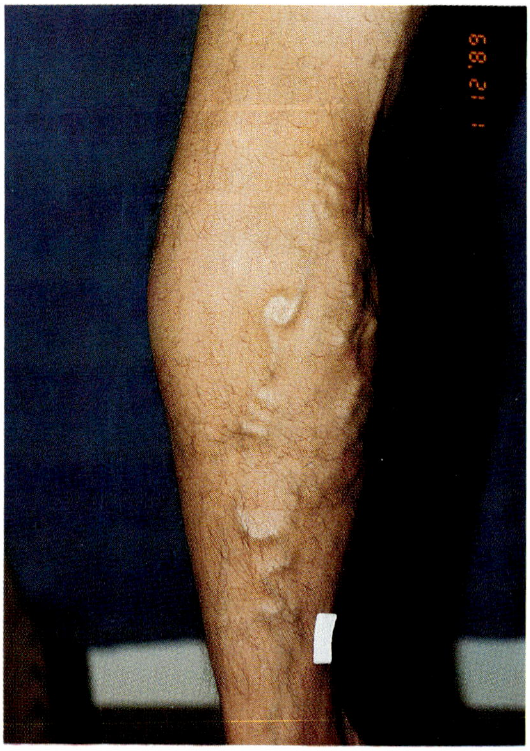

FIGURE 13-7. Saphenofemoral junction incompetence. Note location of tortuous venous dilatations in territory of the short saphenous vein.

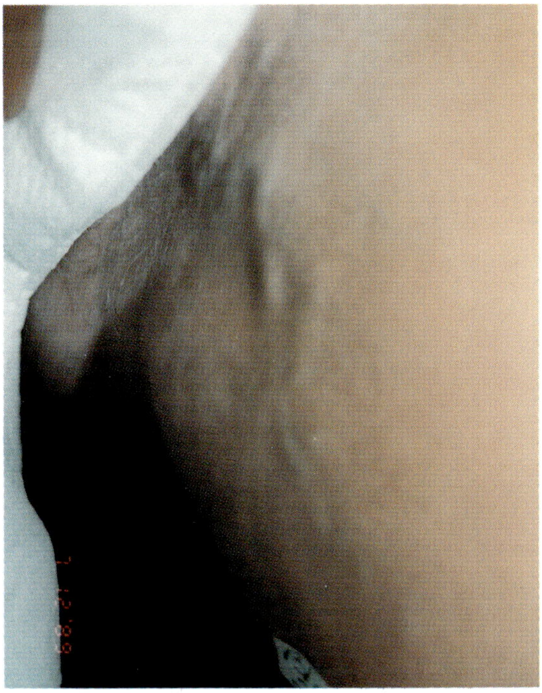

FIGURE 13-8. Greater saphenous vein's upper tributary incompetence.

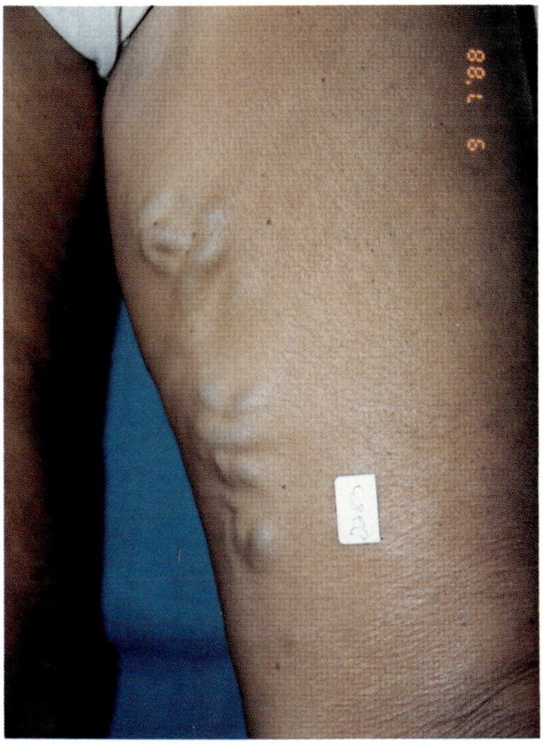

FIGURE 13-9. Perforating vein incompetence.

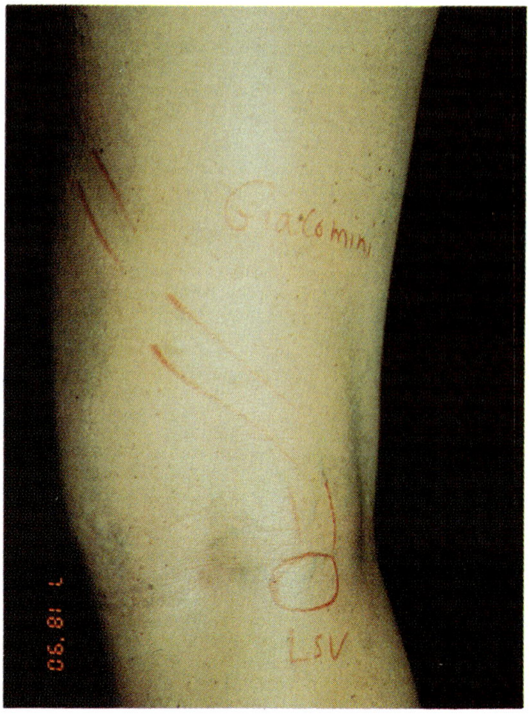

FIGURE 13-10. Short saphenous vein and anastomotic Giacomini vein incompetence.

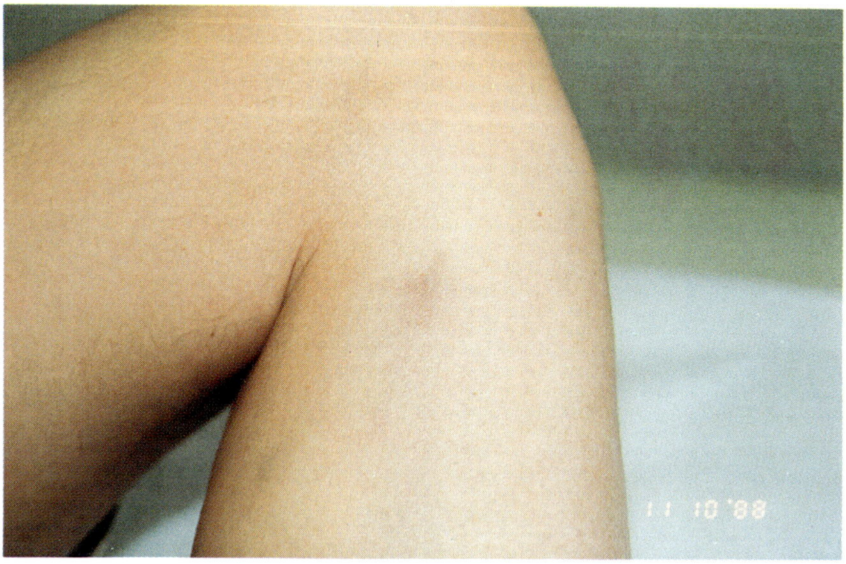

FIGURE 13-11. Saphenofemoral junction incompetence. In this case only telangiectasia at upper portion of the calf is visible.

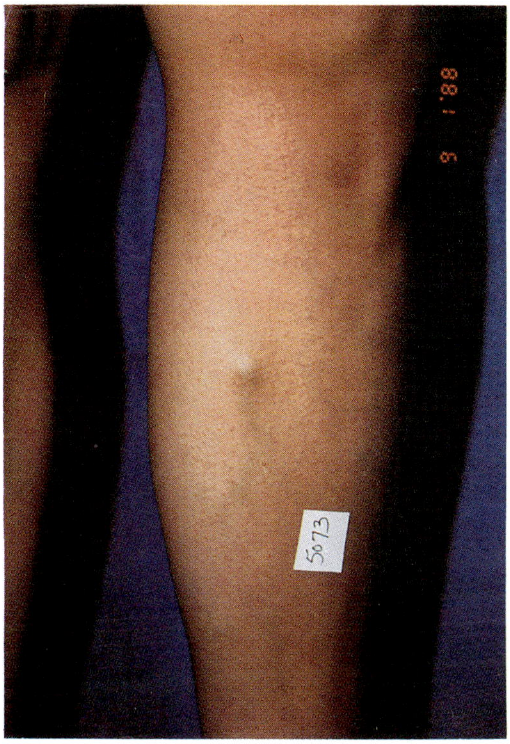

FIGURE 13-12. Saphenofemoral junction incompetence. In this case only an isolated dilatation at midportion of the leg is visible.

PREOPERATIVE EVALUATION

Clinical examination and duplex ultrasonography are the twin cornerstones of preoperative evaluation for sclerotherapy of GSV incompetence. Although clinical assessment can yield abundant information concerning the origin and extent of disease, noninvasive studies are necessary for elucidating the topologic and morphologic aspects of the superficial veins and for ruling out disease of the deep venous system.

Clinical Examination

In each case the first step is a thorough medical and surgical history, including information regarding the patient's life-style, professional activities, medications, and drug allergies. Information should include whether or not the patient has ever had deep venous thrombosis. If the patient is a woman, the number of pregnancies (if any) should be noted. The type of venous symptoms should be reported so that the stage of incompetence can be ascertained. Specifying when and under what circumstances the symptoms were first noted also is important.

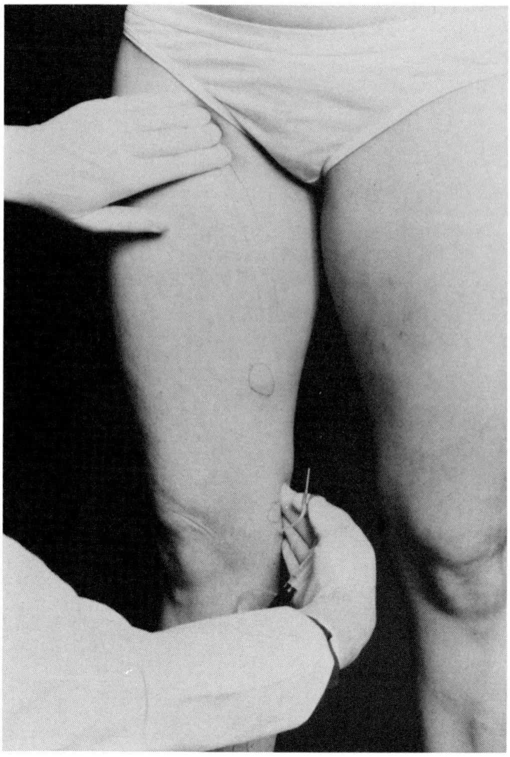

FIGURE 13-13. Schwartz maneuver in assessment of the saphenofemoral junction with patient standing.

For the physical examination, the patient should stand on a support high enough to allow the seated physician to inspect the limbs at eye level (for this purpose, I use a specially made stepped cube that measures 50 cm in height). First, the physician should determine whether the varicosities are caused by GSV or SSV incompetence or by a mixed form of incompetence. The answer is not always obvious. For evaluation of GSV incompetence, the leg should be abducted and rotated externally. The examiner should inspect the lower abdomen and the front and back of the thigh and leg. If the vein is dilated anterior to the medial malleolus, this finding can signify distention of the entire GSV trunk. The main points of reflux are identified by means of inspection, palpation, and percussion (Schwartz maneuver) (Figure 13-13). In the Schwartz maneuver, pressure is applied at a downstream site to diagnose a deficiency in upstream flow; to assess SFJ competence, percussion should be applied over the point where the GSV passes posterior to the condyle of the femur, and a finger should be placed in Scarpa's triangle to detect retrograde blood flow. The patient also can be asked to cough or perform a Valsalva maneuver while the phlebologist holds a finger on the SFJ to detect a thrill and to evaluate the presence of reflux. The points of reflux located through the Schwartz maneuver can be verified clinically through the Trendelenburg maneuver and Doppler ultrasound

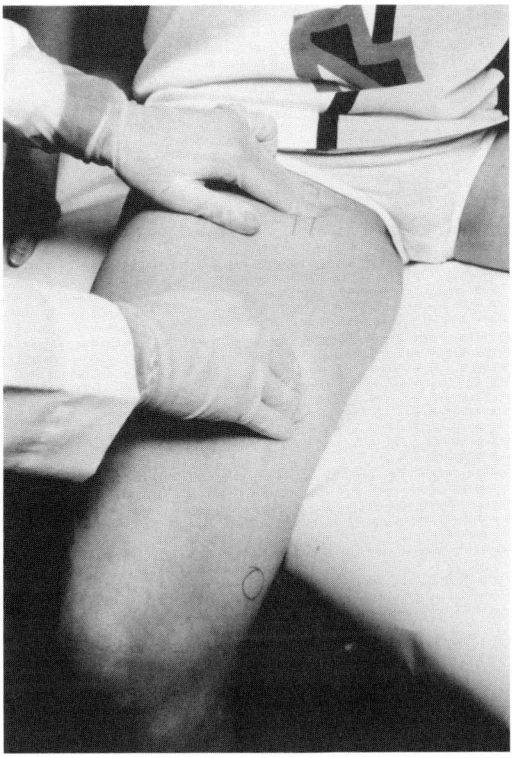

FIGURE 13-14. Schwartz maneuver in assessment of the saphenofemoral junction with patient sitting.

to confirm the highest point of incompetence. Photoplethysmography may be used to assess vein function before sclerotherapy.

The SFJ also should be examined with the patient in the sitting position and the leg abducted, rotated externally, and hanging with the knee flexed. Particular care is necessary in the case of obese patients, who are relatively difficult to examine. The position described here may be useful for such patients because it facilitates exposure of Scarpa's triangle (Figure 13-14).

Duplex Scanning

Although Doppler ultrasound examination may be sufficient for evaluating uncomplicated sites of incompetence, this technique alone is inadequate for assessing an intricate SFJ or perforating veins with an indirect trajectory. Therefore duplex scanning is performed with a high-resolution, real-time, gray-scale B-mode imager equipped with a 4, 8, or 10 MHz transducer coupled with an integrated 5 MHz pulsed Doppler probe. With the patient in reverse Trendelenburg position, the GSV and its tributaries are scanned distally and evaluated transversely and longitudinally as necessary. Important variables include luminal and parietal diameter, venous

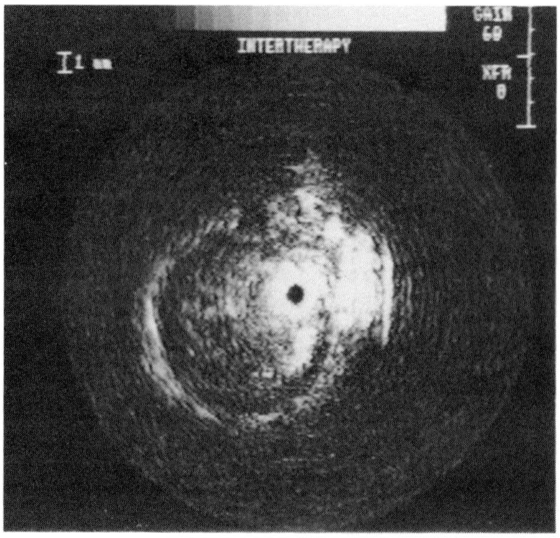

FIGURE 13-15. Intravascular ultrasound cross-sectional image from a segment of the greater saphenous vein after injection of iodine sodium iodide. Note presence of intimal thickening and intimal destruction in 12 o'clock position.

compressibility, echogenicity, direction of blood flow, and valve-leaflet motion and coaptation, particularly at the SFJ and perforator sites.

Failure to recognize variations in the termination of the upper and lower tributaries of the GSV and in the anastomotic veins to the SSV may be an important cause of relapse after sclerotherapy. The ability to pinpoint topographic and morphologic irregularities at the SFJ greatly enhances operative success. In addition, the external pudendal arteries, the common femoral vein, and the common femoral artery (all of which are subject to wide anatomic variations) must be identified to avoid puncture during sclerotherapy.

Duplex scanning also has the advantage of supplying information about perivenous tissues and extrinsic obstructing lesions. Because duplex ultrasonography is not always totally accurate, color flow Doppler imaging and/or magnetic resonance imaging may be necessary in specific cases for clarifying equivocal findings. In some cases intravenous ultrasonography with a 20 or 25 MHz transducer may be helpful to obtain even more precise data concerning the architecture of the venous wall and preoperative and postoperative venous changes (Figure 13-15).

PATIENT SELECTION

Indications

Sclerotherapy of the GSV is indicated for eradicating incompetent veins, which, if left untreated, can cause a series of progressively severe effects, including edema, dermatitis, and eventual ulceration (see Figure 13-4). Any patient with GSV incompetence is eligible for treatment, regardless of the patient's age or degree of reflux, unless contraindications are present. No incompetent vein should be ex-

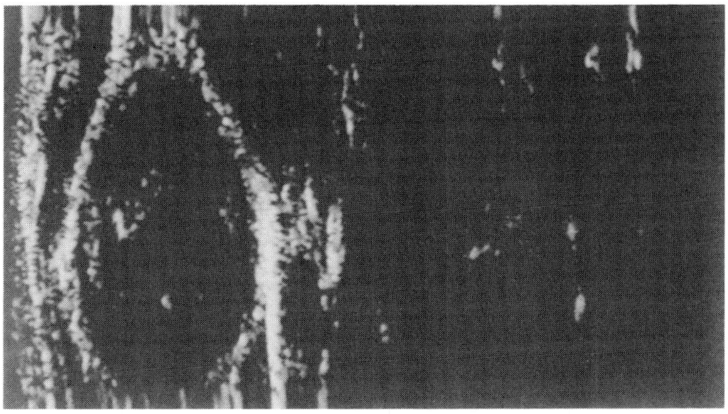

FIGURE 13-16. Duplex ultrasonographic transverse section of the incompetent greater saphenous vein shows intimal thickening.

cluded because it is deemed too large; in my experience, sclerotherapy has proved successful for veins ranging from 3.5 mm to >20 mm.

Contraindications

Sclerotherapy is inappropriate for bedridden patients or others who cannot follow the necessary postoperative exercise regimen. The technique also is inappropriate for patients with infectious disease, acute septic reactions (e.g., cellulitis, abscess, and adenitis), severe arterial occlusive disease, a history of thrombophlebitis and deep venous thrombosis, pregnant women, nursing mothers, women less than 3 months postpartum, patients with severe systemic disease (including malignancy), and those with coagulapathies (protein C and protein S deficiency). Although patients with previous thrombophlebitis and previous deep venous thrombosis are not absolutely excluded, sclerotherapy should not be considered until the signs and symptoms of the disease have abated. In patients with postphlebitic varices, sclerotherapy should be postponed until at least 6 months after the phlebitic reaction has stabilized. Allergic individuals require special consideration. Patients taking disulfiram (Antabuse) should not be treated with a sclerosant that contains alcohol; nor should persons with a history of tuberculosis or hyperthyroidism be treated with a sclerosant that contains iodine.[6]

SCLEROTHERAPY TECHNIQUE

Once the preoperative workup has confirmed the need for sclerotherapy, treatment may be initiated with or without ultrasonographic monitoring. Success depends on following a rational treatment plan.[7] Treatment consists of injecting a chemical irritant capable of traumatizing endothelium. The goals are as follows: (1) to produce a sterile, inflammatory intimal reaction (Figure 13-16) that induces a

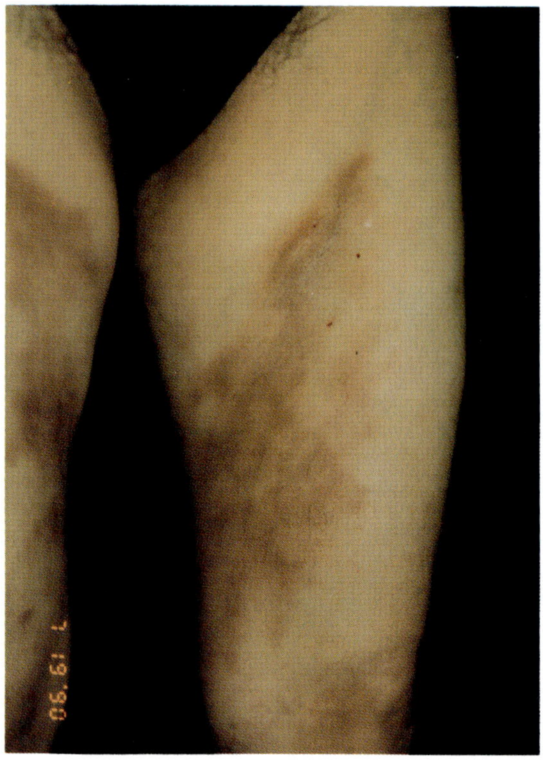

FIGURE 13-17. Permanent skin hyperpigmentation after injection of the greater saphenous vein with sodium tetradecyl sulfate.

thrombotic reaction, permitting the resulting thrombus to adhere to the venous wall; and (2) to induce a fibrotic reaction that permanently destroys the vein. In this manner the vein is transformed into a hard fibrotic cord through which blood can no longer circulate. This cord is then reabsorbed.

If the inflammatory reaction is excessive and affects all the layers of the tunica and surrounding tissue, the resulting thrombus may not be adherent, and ascending recanalization may ensue. This chemical phlebitis may extend proximally to the point of injection, inducing widespread cutaneous hyperpigmentation (Figure 13-17).

The stages that characterize a permanent, ideal sclerosing reaction (Figure 13-18) and those that indicate a failed or inappropriate sclerosing reaction (Figure 13-19) are listed in the boxes on p. 242.

Successful sclerotherapy depends on three main factors. In order of importance, they are (1) site of injection, (2) type of sclerosing agent (major rather than minor), and (3) dosage.

Failure results from injecting at a location distal to the point of reflux, attempt-

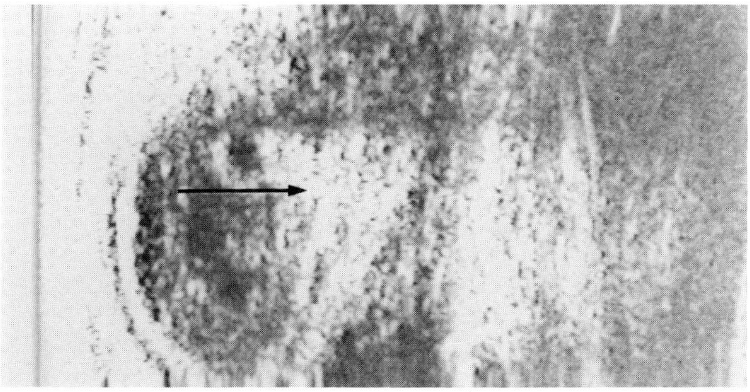

FIGURE 13-18. Duplex ultrasonographic transverse section of the greater saphenous vein after sclerotherapy. Note presence of incompressible adherent heterogeneous material (arrow) within lumen and thickening of the intima. Note presence of arteries in top portion of the vessel.

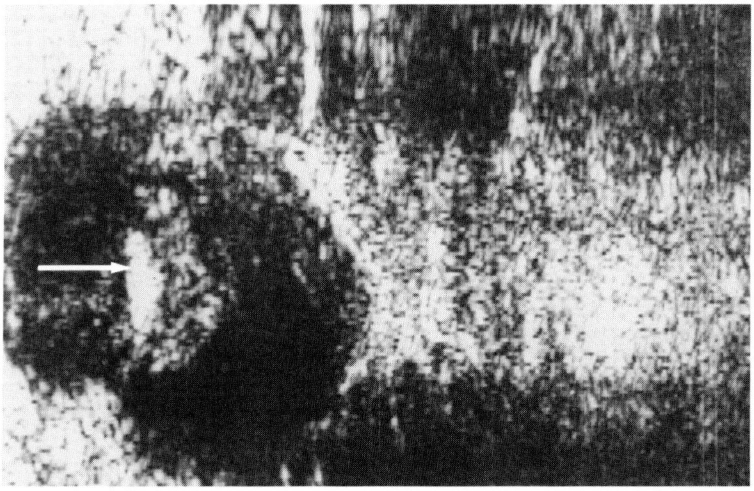

FIGURE 13-19. Duplex ultrasonographic transverse section of the greater saphenous vein shows an inappropriate sclerosing reaction: minimal intimal thickening, partial adherence of thrombus (arrow), inflammatory reaction involving surrounding tissue, and echogenic blood flow.

STAGES OF PERMANENT, IDEAL SCLEROSING REACTION

1. Endothelial trauma
2. Endothelial thickening
3. Thrombus formation
4. Thrombus adherence to site of endothelial thickening
5. Endothelial destruction
6. Reduction of venous diameter
7. Fibrous reaction, which should stop at limits of deep venous system
8. Reabsorption of vein

STAGES OF FAILED OR INAPPROPRIATE SCLEROSING REACTION

1. Minimal endothelial trauma + premature thrombus formation
2. Adventitial thickening
3. Enlargement of venous diameter
4. Inflammatory reaction involving surrounding tissue
5. Cutaneous hyperpigmentation
6. Recanalization
7. Neovascularization (telangiectasias or reticular veins)

ing to treat GSV incompetence with a minor sclerosing agent, and/or giving too strong a dose of a major sclerosing agent.

Site of Injection

The injection sequence always proceeds from top to bottom, starting at the highest point of reflux and proceeding to the next highest point until the entire GSV has been sclerosed. If the highest site of incompetence is the SFJ, it should be treated first because complete eradication of the proximal portion of the GSV is necessary to abolish venous reflux. To prevent accidental penetration of the deep venous or arterial systems, the injection should be done several centimeters below the SFJ rather than at the junction itself (Figure 13-20). The injection sequence proceeds methodically toward the most distal incompetent perforating vein, the dose being proportionally decreased as the site of injection progresses downward.

An exception is made for stasis ulcers and ruptured varices. When these conditions are present, the first step is to inject either at the closest point of reflux or into a venous dilatation near the ulcer or ruptured varices to accelerate the healing pro-

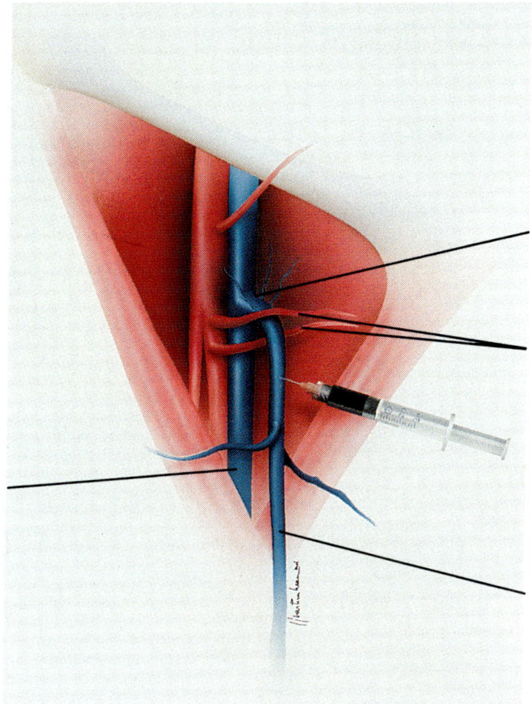

FIGURE 13-20. Injection of sclerosing agent is done below the saphenofemoral junction and away from external pudendal arteries. (From Raymond-Martimbeau P. Phlebologia Houston '91. Dallas: PRM Editions, 1991.)

cess. In these cases proper postoperative bandaging is mandatory. The second step is to inject the highest point of reflux at a later date.

Sclerosing Agent

Sclerosing agents are classified as major, intermediate, or minor according to their strength. It is extremely important that a major sclerosing agent be selected for the treatment of GSV incompetence. Only two such agents are appropriate: iodine sodium iodide (ISI) and sodium tetradecyl sulfate (STS) (see box, p. 244). The other agents are either too toxic or too weak.

It might be erroneously assumed that the use of a weaker sclerosant would provide an extra margin of safety. If administered in this setting, however, a minor agent would be swept away by the bloodstream before the desired local endothelial reaction could occur. The result would be distal sclerosis characterized by a non-adherent thrombus, which could lead to deep venous thrombosis. Use of a major sclerosant is crucial in order to produce an immediate local inflammatory reaction.

ISI is a chemical irritant that has both a strong sclerosing action and a low diffusing power. Because it is lighter than blood, it is not readily swept away from the injection site. It also has the advantage of producing pain with extravascular or

MAJOR AGENTS USED WORLDWIDE FOR SCLEROSING GREATER SAPHENOUS VEIN

Iodine, Sodium or Potassium Iodide

France:	Iodo-ioduree solution 1% to 3% (Meram Laboratory, Paris)
Switzerland:	Variglobin* 2%, 4%, 8%, 12% (Globopharm SA, Zurich)
Canada:	Sclerodine 6% (Omega Laboratories, Montreal, Quebec)
U.S.A.:	Iodine crystals USP, sodium iodide granules USP, and potassium iodide granules USP (Fisher Scientific Company, Fair Lawn, N.J.)

Sodium Tetradecyl Sulfate

France:	Trombovar 1%, 3%, 5% (Promedica, France)
Canada:	Thromboject 1%, 3% (Omega Laboratories, Montreal, Quebec)
U.S.A.:	Sotradecol 1%, 3% (Elkins-Sinn, Cherry Hill, N.J.)

*Variglobin 2%, 4%, 8%, 12% is equivalent to Sclerodine and Iodo-ioduree solution 1%, 2%, 4%, 6%.

intra-arterial injection, thereby immediately alerting the practitioner to these complications.

STS is a detergent irritant that has a strong sclerosing action and a high diffusing power; because it is heavier than blood, it is easily swept away from the injection site. It produces slight pain with intra-arterial injection but does not cause pain with extravascular injection. Therefore sodium salicylate should be added to STS so that it will produce pain when injected extravascularly.

Dosage

The dosage depends primarily on the site of injection, not solely on the size of the vein. It is important to follow a strict protocol and not be influenced by a large venous diameter. Ironically, it may take a larger dose to sclerose a small tubular GSV than a large GSV. The more endothelial damage, the easier it is to achieve sclerosis. If a large dose is injected into a large vein, the stages of sclerosing action may not occur methodically and the risk of DVT is increased. It is important to prepare the intima with a relatively low dose to ensure that satisfactory intimal thickening takes place before thrombus formation occurs.

For this treatment the physician may use either a commercial preparation of 1% to 6% ISI diluted with 0.9% sodium chloride solution or sterile water or a preparation of 1% to 5% STS. I do not consider volume to be the most important parameter. If the dose needs to be augmented to enhance the sclerosing power, it is better to increase the concentration, not the volume. The target is quite focused, and the action needs to be as local as possible; therefore increasing the volume may not greatly affect the sclerosing capability. If too great a volume of sclerosing agent is injected, the extra amount may be swept into the deep system or to distal incompetent points, where the reaction would be excessive.

SCLEROTHERAPY FOR SAPHENOFEMORAL JUNCTION INCOMPETENCE

If incompetence is isolated at the SFJ only and does not produce symptoms, the sclerotherapist should observe the progression of the disease and postpone treatment. If the incompetence produces signs and symptoms, the vein may be injected; however, care must be used because the injection must be given almost at the junction itself. As mentioned earlier, the danger of accidentally entering the arterial or deep venous system is relatively great because the relationship between the common femoral vein and the common femoral artery is variable; moreover, the number and size of pudendal arteries are variable (the inferior pudendal artery overlaps or crosses the arch of the GSV at, or close to, the SFJ). In cases in which the incompetence is isolated at the SFJ and the reflux is mild or nonexistent, the physician should start with a low dose (1 ml of 2% ISI or STS); if sclerosis does not occur, the concentration should be increased sequentially (e.g., to 1 ml of a 3% solution or 1 ml of a 4% solution).

If incompetence involves more than the junction itself, treatment is performed with the patient either standing or sitting. I have found that the standing position is associated with more extensive occlusion and a greater reduction in venous caliber, as well as less postoperative inflammation and pigmentation.[8] Moreover, surprisingly fewer vagal reactions seem to occur when the patient is standing.

Positions for Injection

If the sitting position (Figure 13-21) is chosen, the sclerotherapist remains standing while the patient is seated on the examining table with his or her leg abducted, rotated externally, and hanging with the knee flexed. The patient's leg must be very relaxed. The injection is administered 5 to 9 cm below the SFJ with a disposable standard 25-gauge, 5/8 inch needle and a 3 ml disposable plastic syringe. Digital pressure is applied at the SFJ with the left hand and is maintained for several minutes after the injection has been completed. Such pressure may be applied by an assistant (but never by the patient) in order to free the sclerotherapist's left hand to secure the needle at the injection site and to ascertain its stability.

If the standing position (Figures 13-22 and 13-23) is preferred, the patient stands on a platform with the leg abducted and rotated externally with the knee unflexed. The patient should stand perfectly still, without bending, and should look straight ahead. The patient should not touch anything because doing so may cause movement during the puncture. To ensure stability of position, the patient should apply weight to the leg to be injected. The sclerotherapist should be seated, with his or her leg and elbow secured to prevent unwanted motion during injection. The sclerotherapist should not explain or discuss the technique at this point because doing so may increase the patient's apprehension and thereby increase the likeli-

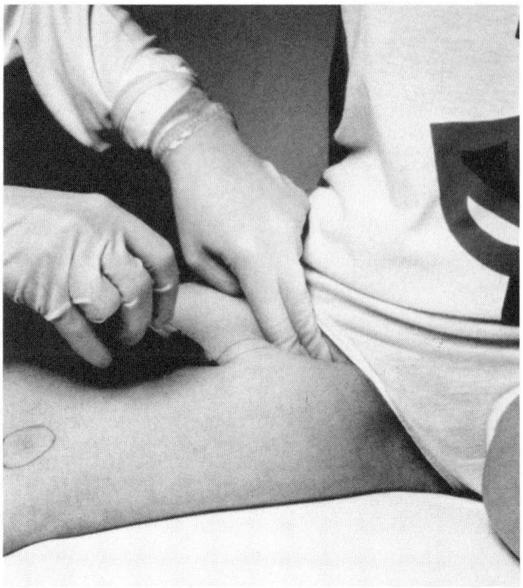

FIGURE 13-21. Injection of the incompetent saphenofemoral junction done with patient sitting.

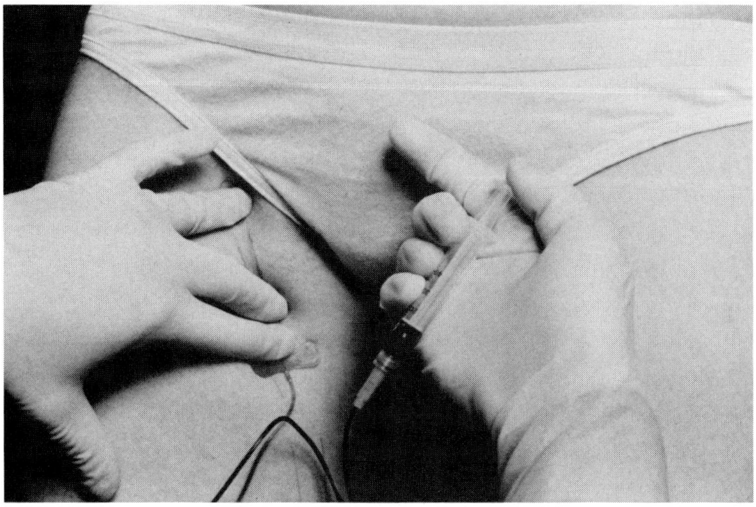

FIGURE 13-22. Injection of the incompetent saphenofemoral junction done with patient standing. Digital pressure is applied at junction with left annular finger. (From Raymond-Martimbeau P. Phlebologia Houston '91. Dallas: PRM Editions, 1991.)

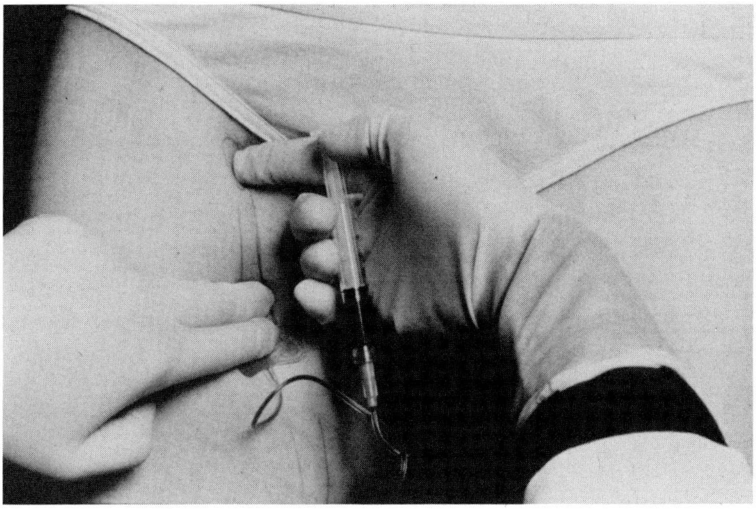

FIGURE 13-23. Injection of the incompetent saphenofemoral junction with patient standing. Digital pressure is applied at junction with right index finger.

hood of a vasovagal reaction. The injection is administered 4 to 7 cm below the SFJ with a disposable 25-gauge, ¾ inch butterfly needle with 12 inches of tubing and a 3 ml plastic disposable syringe. Digital pressure is applied in two places: (1) at the junction with either the left annular finger (see Figure 13-22) or the right index finger (see Figure 13-23), and (2) below the site of injection with the third finger of the left hand to cause sequestration and to empty the vein as much as possible, thereby allowing maximal endothelial contact with the sclerosing agent. Pressure at the junction is maintained throughout the injection and is continued for a few minutes afterward; distal pressure is released as soon as the injection is completed.

Injection Technique

In either position, before injection, the syringe should be examined for air, which reduces the degree of negative pressure and interferes with aspiration of blood. Once the injection site's depth and precise location have been confirmed by means of a percussion maneuver, alcohol is applied, and after the digital pressure is applied as described earlier, the vein is punctured briskly. The needle is generally aimed toward the torso, in the direction of the SFJ. With the patient in the standing position, the butterfly needle permits better manipulation of the syringe, allows the syringe to be oriented with the plunger facing upward, and facilitates examination of aspirated blood. When the patient is standing, ISI is preferable to STS. Because STS is heavier than blood, it tends to diffuse distally, leaving the proximal segment of the GSV unchanged.

Aspiration of a small amount of venous blood confirms proper needle placement (unfortunately, the darkness of the iodine agent may be a disadvantage for the

TABLE 13-1. Schedule and dosage of iodine sodium iodide (Sclerodine) injections for treating GSV incompetence secondary to SFJ malfunction*

Visit	Dosage	Site
1	2 ml at 3% concentration	Below SFJ
2	2 ml at 4% concentration	Below SFJ
3	2 ml at 6% concentration	Below SFJ
4	2 ml at 6% concentration 1 ml at 3% concentration	Below SFJ Midthigh level
5	2 ml at 6% concentration 1 ml at 3% concentration 1 ml at 2% concentration	Below SFJ Midthigh level Knee level

GSV, greater saphenous vein; SFJ, saphenofemoral junction.
*Data from Raymond-Martimbeau P. Two different techniques for sclerosing the incompetent saphenofemoral junction: A comparative study. J Dermatol Surg Oncol 16:626-631, 1990.

TABLE 13-2. Schedule and dosage of sodium tetradecyl sulfate injections for treating GSV incompetence secondary to SFJ malfunction

Visit	Dosage	Site
1	2 ml at 2% concentration	Below SFJ
2	2 ml at 3% concentration	Below SFJ
3	2 ml at 4% concentration OR 2 ml at 3% concentration 1 ml at 3% concentration	Below SFJ Below SFJ Midthigh level
4	2 ml at 5% concentration OR 2 ml at 3% concentration 1 ml at 3% concentration 1 ml at 2% concentration	Below SFJ Below SFJ Midthigh level Knee level

GSV, greater saphenous vein; SFJ, saphenofemoral junction.

inexperienced surgeon). The appearance of pulsatile or bright-red blood suggests that the needle has entered an artery and is an indication for immediate cessation. If the return of venous blood is not obvious, or if there is any doubt about the return, the injection should be stopped.

The injection involves three steps: (1) injecting half of the dose very slowly, (2) reaspirating the blood to confirm correct needle positioning, and (3) injecting the second half of the dose quickly to prevent spasm of the vessel, which will already be reacting to the sclerosant. The patient should be instructed to report any pain during injection because such pain can herald a serious complication. Applying digital pressure at the SFJ when injecting below the junction prevents the sclerosant from dispersing into the deep venous system and increases the local reaction.

Whichever position is used, as soon as the injection is finished, the patient should lie down while the sclerotherapist maintains digital pressure at the SFJ. The limb then is elevated to ensure optimal exposure of the SFJ to the sclerosing agent.

A selective noncircumferential compressive dressing is placed over the SFJ and should extend a few centimeters below the injection site; the dressing is left in place for 48 hours. A light compressive stocking may be applied. For daywear only, I use an 18 to 22 mm Hg pressure-gradient stocking for progressive stage II disease since injecting the highest point of reflux should lower pressure distally. For progressive stage I or stage III disease, I use a class 1 or class 2 stocking or an elastic bandage since the sclerosing reaction may be increased in these stages.

Injection Protocol

The injection protocols for ISI and STS are described in Tables 13-1 and 13-2, respectively. The protocol for ISI is similar to that reported and described by Cloutier.[3,4] Protocols for STS other than the one described here have been advocated by other authors.[9] Some experts have proposed an accelerated protocol in which the initial treatment comprises multiple injections of a major sclerosing agent into different sites of reflux.[6]

SEQUENTIAL SCLEROTHERAPY FOR OTHER AREAS OF INCOMPETENCE

After the highest point of reflux has been sclerosed flush with the common femoral vein, sclerotherapy of distal points can be started in a top-to-bottom sequential manner (Table 13-3). The injection is given at the site where the previous sclerosis ended in the GSV. It is better to obtain a short but firm sclerosis than a long, weak one.

Perineal Veins or Tributaries

When left untreated, perineal vein and upper tributary incompetence (see Figure 13-8) often leads to recurrent GSV incompetence. These veins are "sclerosensible" and require 0.5 to 0.75 ml of 0.5% to 1% STS.

Saphenous Trunk at Thigh Level

If the next highest point of incompetence is the saphenous trunk in the upper or middle third of the thigh, 1 ml of 3% ISI or STS should be injected at the limits of sclerosis and permeability; if that point is in the lower third of the thigh, 1 ml of a 2% major sclerosing agent should be used.

TABLE 13-3. Top-to-bottom sequential sclerotherapy for points of incompetence other than SFJ: Initial treatment with iodine, sodium iodide, or sodium tetradecyl sulfate*

Location	Concentration (%)	Volume (ml)
Perineal veins and tributaries	0.5-1	0.5-0.75
Saphenous trunk		
Upper or midthigh	3	1
Lower thigh	2	1
Perforating veins		
Thigh	3	1
Knee	1-2	1
Upper leg	1-1.5	1
Lower leg	1	0.5

SFJ, saphenofemoral junction.
*If SFJ is competent or sclerosed, these sites should be treated in sequence.

Perforating Veins

If the highest point of incompetence is located in a GSV-related perforator, the injection sequence should proceed methodically toward the most proximal incompetent perforating vein, with the dosage being decreased proportionally as the site of injection progresses downward.

Van Limborg[10] detailed the topography of 142 perforating veins of the leg, including 49 in the foot, 44 in the lower leg, 13 at knee level, and 36 in the thigh. However, few such veins are constant. In the upper thigh, sometimes a perforator vein is found that causes significant dilatation and reflux (see Figure 13-9). In the midthigh, the Dodd or hunterian perforators (see Figure 13-1), at the site of Hunter's canal, range from six to eight in number; as the longest perforating veins, they are often indirect and may cause significant reflux. When these thigh-level perforators are incompetent, 1 ml of a 3% major sclerosing agent should be injected as initial treatment.

At knee level, the geniculate group of perforating veins (Figure 13-24) causes a milder degree of reflux. Therefore a lower dosage is necessary for treatment at this site; 1 ml of 1% or 2% STS is normally sufficient for initiating sclerosis.

In the upper leg, the Boyd group of perforating veins (see Figure 13-1) causes a moderate degree of reflux and requires 1 ml of 1.0% to 1.5% STS. In the lower leg, the perforators of the Cockett group comprise three to four veins located on the posterior branch of the GSV (Leonardo's vein), along a vertical line depicted by Linton (see Figure 13-1). When incompetent, these perforators are very noxious to cutaneous structures and are frequently responsible for trophic problems and stasis ulcers. They are often involved in postphlebitic and posttraumatic varices, and the

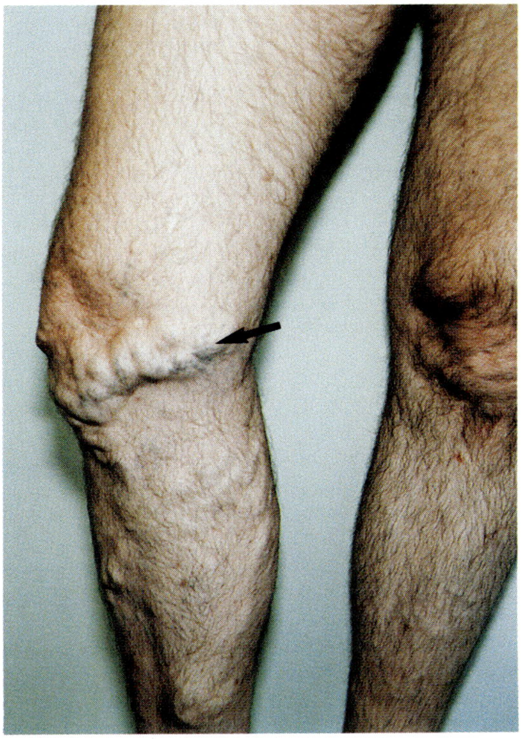

FIGURE 13-24. Primarily geniculate perforating vein incompetence (arrow).

degree of reflux can be severe in these cases. Because these veins have a short trajectory and are located distally, sclerosis should be induced with caution. Injection of 0.5 ml of a 1% major sclerosing agent should be sufficient for the initial treatment.

Occasionally, the highest point of incompetence is in small (0.5 to 2 mm) unexpected perforators not obvious through clinical or Doppler ultrasound examination. Such perforators must always be sought because they can be present all along the GSV pathway and can cause significant reflux, resulting in medium-sized distal varicosities. Their eradication is essential to ensure a successful outcome with a decreased risk of complications. Injection of 1 ml of 1.0% STS is needed to sclerose these small perforators.

I treat incompetent perforating veins by injecting the sclerosing agent into their trajectory at a 90-degree angle; small ones are injected with the patient in the standing position. This controversial approach depends on satisfactory duplex ultrasonographic monitoring and occasionally duplex guidance.

After sclerosing incompetent perforator sites, I routinely apply selective noncircumferential compressive dressings for 24 to 48 hours; this compression regimen is similar to that used after SFJ injection.

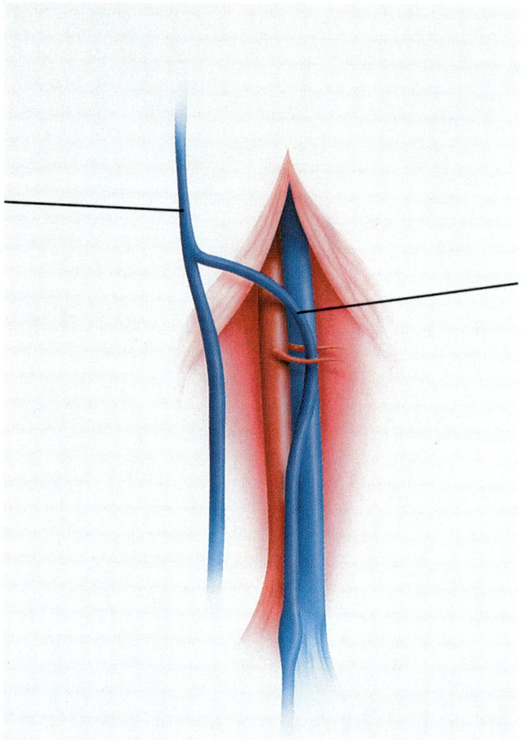

FIGURE 13-25. Termination of the short saphenous vein in the greater saphenous vein. (From Raymond-Martimbeau P. Phlebologia Houston '91. Dallas: PRM Editions, 1991.)

Mixed Incompetence

The termination point of the SSV varies considerably. When the SSV terminates in the GSV and becomes incompetent (Figure 13-25), eradication of the SSV is imperative to obtain permanent sclerosis of the GSV in order to prevent recurrence.

When an anastomotic vein (especially the Giacomini vein) (see Figure 13-10) is incompetent, eradication or permanent obliteration of this vein is essential to reduce the recurrence rate.

Postoperative Neovascularization

The highest point of incompetence may be located in vessels formed by neovascularization at the SFJ. Occlusion of these vessels is necessary to stop disease progression. These vessels are not easy to enter with a needle because they have a very thin, soft wall and do not normally cause a severe degree of reflux. Puncture should be brisk to allow intraluminal, rather than extravascular, injection. Normally, 1 ml of 1% to 3% STS is necessary. Preinjection duplex ultrasonographic monitoring is essential in these cases because vessels formed by neovascularization often have an anarchic presentation and are surrounded by small- or medium-sized arteries.

When a major sclerosant is injected in top-to-bottom fashion, a minimal number of injections and therapeutic sessions are needed for permanent obliteration of the GSV, and few adverse reactions will occur. Injecting the sites of origin according to a proper technique and protocol is often sufficient to make tortuous distal visible varicosities disappear.

POSTOPERATIVE MANAGEMENT

Compression Therapy

One of the most widely held tenets of sclerotherapy is that successful treatment of a large vein such as the GSV can only occur if the vessel remains compressed for several weeks postoperatively so that the lumen is reduced as much as possible. Some experts recommend that the compressive bandage remain in place for 3 weeks, after which the patient returns to the physician for follow-up examination and rebandaging.[11] During this period, the bandage should not be loosened or removed. Moreover, the patient should avoid any activities that may promote venous distention (i.e., hot baths, saunas, or exercises involving increased abdominal pressure).

I do not routinely use this regimen for the following reason: if the treatment is successful (i.e., the injection is performed at the highest point of reflux according to proper protocol, as described above, and closure of this point allows normalization of the distal pressure), the compromise of venous return caused by the use of strong compression might actually undermine treatment. Therefore I use compression therapy discriminatingly, prescribing light elastic support in most cases and strong compression for patients in whom the degree of immediate operative success is uncertain (i.e., those who have pain during the immediate [<5 minutes] postinjection period).

Ambulation

Postoperative ambulation is critical for preventing venous congestion. The patient should exercise after sclerotherapy. Walking, bicycling, and swimming are recommended, but high-impact activities are inadvisable.

COMPLICATIONS

Sclerotherapy of the GSV results in a minimum of complications, which may be classified as major or minor, depending on their severity. These complications and their treatment have been discussed elsewhere[12,13] and will be reviewed only briefly here.

Major Complications

Accidental intra-arterial injection is the most dreaded sequela, even among experienced sclerotherapists. Fortunately, the incidence of this complication is remarkably low. When it does occur, however, it can result in cutaneous, subcutaneous, and muscular necrosis of portions of the thigh and/or leg, as well as muscular atrophy and nerve damage necessitating eventual amputation.

During GSV sclerotherapy, the most vulnerable arterial zones are at the SFJ (site of the common femoral and external pudendal arteries) and posterior to the medial malleolus (site of the posterior tibial artery). Because intra-arterial injection causes immediate violent pain, the sclerotherapist should tell the patient to report any pain that arises during injection; if pain does occur, the injection should be stopped instantly. Prompt treatment must be instituted with heparin and corticosteroids, and a fibrinolytic agent may be given if desired.[14] Hot towels may be applied to the skin distal to the point of injection, where changes in skin coloration are occurring, to prevent arterial spasm and limit skin necrosis. Hospitalization is necessary.

Fortunately, deep venous thrombosis is also extremely rare, as are pulmonary emboli, compartmental syndrome, and gangrene. Venous thrombosis is most likely to occur in recent surgical patients and those with preneoplastic syndrome and hyperlipemia. Thrombosis is heralded by severe pain 20 to 30 minutes after injection, followed by edema involving the entire limb. At the first hint of this disorder, anticoagulants and streptokinase should be injected intravenously. Hospitalization is mandatory.

Minor Complications

Minor adverse sequelae include pain, localized urticaria, chemical phlebitis, pedal edema, and secondary telangiectasias, as well as temporary or permanent cutaneous hyperpigmentation (see Figure 13-17) and cutaneous and subcutaneous necrosis. Most of these reactions can be prevented with the use of proper technique. Most of them resolve spontaneously within a short time, and the physician rarely needs to do more than conservatively monitor the patient.

In sclerotherapy for GSV incompetence, the most frequent minor complication is induced superficial thrombophlebitis, or "chemical phlebitis," which usually results from overdosage. This condition is heralded by redness, edema, and painful induration, appearing 3 to 8 hours after injection. Treatment consists of application of local compressive dressings and elastic bandages for 5 or 6 days. Ambulation is important in preventing extension of the phlebitis; very seldom, however, does the clot spread to the deep venous system. Once the inflammation has abated, the residual intravascular hematoma should be evacuated to prevent skin discoloration. This evacuation should not be done until at least 3 weeks after the injection.

Other potential side effects during treatment with a major sclerosing agent include nausea and vomiting, a vagal reaction and loss of consciousness resulting from anxiety, a metallic taste with the administration of ISI, and visual disturbances with the use of STS. Convulsive and epileptic-type reactions also have been observed. Injection of a major sclerosant in the upper thigh can result in severe but transient pelvic and high abdominal pain. Three to eight hours after receiving excessive doses of ISI, occasional patients begin to have a toxic iodine reaction (self-limited hypersensitivity reaction characterized by flulike symptoms, fever, and shortness of breath) that disappears within 1 or 2 hours without treatment.

Sclerotherapy also can cause bruising, which usually clears up within 10 days. Venotropic agents such as gingko biloba, hamamelis, and rutin compound may help prevent ecchymoses by reducing capillary fragility.

POSTOPERATIVE EVALUATION

Follow-up visits are mandatory to assess treatment results, and duplex ultrasonography is especially important for evaluating venous changes. Within several days of injection, the vein should have been converted into a thin, irregular cord. The goal of therapy is thorough fibrosis, evidenced by a markedly reduced luminal diameter, thickened intima, and an incompressible lumen that contains a dense, echogenic, heterogeneous material.

Excessive thrombosis is the most frequent cause of recanalization after sclerotherapy. If postoperative scanning yields images of superficial thrombophlebitis (i.e., enlarged venous diameter, partial compressibility, and slight parietal changes, as well as intraluminal blood flow and only partial luminal filling with an echogenic material), the patient should be examined for proximal reflux, and further treatment will be necessary. In such cases the type and dosage of sclerosant may need to be adjusted.

Recanalization and recurrence also can be caused by failure to recognize anatomic variants involving the SFJ or SSV termination. In some cases recurrence is the result of an incompetent parietal valve within the common femoral vein.

Experience has shown that certain patients (i.e., those with a light complexion, blond hair, and blue eyes) are more "sclerosable" than others and that some veins (i.e., superficial) are more amenable to sclerotherapy than others. Surprisingly, the likelihood of a successful outcome appears to be inversely related to the degree of preoperative venous dilatation. Small-diameter tubular veins with a relatively intact endothelium are more difficult to sclerose than large-diameter vessels with thin diseased walls.

If occlusion has not been induced after the initial injection, the patient is treated according to the injection protocols described in Tables 13-1 and 13-2. Treatment sessions are spaced at intervals of between 7 and 21 days.

In some cases lack of control in recurrence is not the result of inadequate treatment but is related to an uncontrollable cause such as heredity or persistent aggravating factors. When sclerotherapy alone fails to relieve GSV incompetence, the patient may benefit from surgery or a combined approach. Neither surgery nor sclerotherapy, however, can cure the underlying venous disease, which is progressive in character. Therefore, follow-up visits are important to control further disease progression. When treatment has been completed, the patient is seen for clinical follow-up assessments at 3-, 6-, and 12-month intervals and yearly afterward.

DISCUSSION

Until recently, surgical ligation and stripping of the incompetent GSV has been the primary therapeutic approach. Because the distal dilatations of the GSV may be tortuous and not easily accessible for stripping, multiple incisions are necessary.

Potential complications include deep vein thrombosis and pulmonary embolization, arterial hemorrhage, and lymphatic disorders, as well as postoperative hematomas, paresthesias, infection, and scar formation. Occasionally, the femoral artery or vein is erroneously ligated or stripped; arterial involvement of this type can necessitate amputation. Surgical relapses may be caused by incomplete crossectomy or inaccessibility of indirect multitruncal perforating veins.

As a safe, painless, and highly effective outpatient procedure, sclerotherapy is an attractive alternative to surgical treatment of varicose veins. Unfortunately, many physicians are skeptical about sclerotherapy. They may have heard of poor results obtained with early sclerosing agents or without the use of a strict protocol; or they may have tried sclerotherapy haphazardly in a few cases, with unimpressive results, and then blamed the method for their own lack of proficiency. Critics may not realize that, during the past two decades, sclerotherapy has been transformed into a less empirical, more exact science. This transformation has been the result of improved technique and increased understanding of the mechanism of action of sclerosing agents, as well as a more rigid adherence to sound protocols. Moreover, the advent of high-technology diagnostic modalities such as duplex scanning has permitted better patient selection and assessment of injection sites, as well as the detection of early recanalization. Evolving experience has shown that practitioners can lower the incidence of adverse effects and/or recurrence by modifying their protocols.

Reported clinical experience in thousands of cases indicates that sclerotherapy of the GSV is well tolerated and that injection of a major sclerosing agent yields a successful outcome in 85% to 90% of cases.[4,8,15] The precise mechanism of various sclerosing agents has not yet been clarified, but these agents all disrupt vascular endothelium, either by cellular dehydration, maceration of intracellular cement, or direct destruction. In a recent prospective study regarding the effects of sclerotherapy on blood coagulation, injection of various doses of ISI (Sclerodine) into 26 consecutive patients with lower extremity varicosities produced no evidence of activation of blood coagulation.[16] Performed under optimal biologic conditions, this study has helped allay the fear that sclerotherapy could promote systemic fibrin formation.

Most risks and iatrogenic complications of sclerotherapy can be prevented through proper preoperative assessment, intraoperative technique and protocol, and postoperative care: intra-arterial injection can be averted with preoperative duplex ultrasound; cutaneous necrosis secondary to extravascular injection can be avoided with proper technique; phlebitis and residual pigmentation caused by overdosage can be minimized by following a sound protocol; and deep venous thrombosis resulting from incorrect dosage and/or site of injection also can be prevented with a suitable protocol.

From the patient's viewpoint, sclerotherapy is obviously the treatment of choice, and many patients simply refuse to undergo varicose vein surgery. In addition to being painless and nonscarring, sclerotherapy eliminates the need for hospitalization, general anesthesia, and intense postoperative care. The patient can return to work immediately after treatment, which has economic benefits. Furthermore, a sclerosant can treat hard-to-reach vessels (e.g., perforating veins with intricate trajectories) that would be unapproachable by a scalpel. Nevertheless, surgery and sclerotherapy are not opposed to each other but are complementary therapeutic options that may be combined in selected cases.

Whichever method is used, early and late success rates are subject to many variables, including patient age, vein size, location (proximal vs. distal), and severity and complexity of the disease. Operator experience is also a crucial factor. Moreover, in discussing optimal treatments, experts tend to underestimate the complexity of the population at risk. Ultimately, the value of different therapeutic modalities can be assessed only on the basis of prospective randomized studies in which patients are stratified according to similar disease states.

In the treatment of GSV incompetence, sclerotherapy at the SFJ is a particularly challenging procedure that remains highly controversial and is practiced by only a small number of experts. In a 6-year follow-up study, I have shown that the success rate of this procedure approaches 90% for experienced physicians.[8] Injection of the SFJ requires not only extensive sclerotherapeutic skill but also an excellent background in duplex scanning technique. Physicians who lack these qualifications are ill advised to perform sclerotherapy at this site. Before attempting the procedure, practitioners should honestly assess their capabilities. They also must realistically assess the demands of their practices to determine whether the procedure can be performed frequently enough to attain the required skill.

CONCLUSION

Sclerotherapy can be viewed as a forerunner of the minimally invasive techniques that are currently revolutionizing surgical practice. In the management of GSV incompetence, injection of the SFJ is a valuable adjunct. The technique seems well tolerated by patients, and complications are minimal when a strict protocol is followed. If sclerotherapy fails, surgery or a combined therapeutic regimen is indicated.

REFERENCES

1. Fegan G. Varicose Veins. London: William Heinemann Medical Books, 1967.
2. Chatard H. Thérapeutique. In Bassi G, ed. Les varices des membres inférieurs. Paris: Doin, 1967, p 353.
3. Cloutier G. La sclérose des crosses des saphènes internes et externes; nouvelle approche. Phlebologie 29:227-232, 1976.
4. Cloutier G. La sclérose des crosses des saphènes internes et externes avec compression. Résultats. Phlebologie 33:731-735, 1980.
5. Raymond-Martimbeau P. Duplex ultrasonography assessment of anatomical variations as a guide to sclerotherapy. In Raymond-Martimbeau P, ed. Phlebologia Houston '91. Dallas: PRM Editions, 1991, pp 48-55.
6. Vin F, Schadeck M. La Maladie Veineuse Superficielle. Paris: Masson, 1991.
7. Wallois P. The conditions necessary to achieve an effective sclerosant treatment. Phlebologie 35:337-348, 1982.
8. Raymond-Martimbeau P. Two different techniques for sclerosing the incompetent saphenofemoral junction: A comparative study. J Dermatol Surg Oncol 16:626-631, 1990.

9. Schadeck M. Sclerotherapy of the great saphenous vein. In Raymond-Martimbeau P, ed. Phlebologia Houston '91. Dallas: PRM Editions, 1991, pp 245-249.
10. Van Limborg J, Hage RW. L'anatomie systémique des veines perforantes de la jambe, en particulier des veines de Cockett. Phlebologie 35:19-28, 1982.
11. Browse NL, Burnand KG, Lea Thomas M. Diseases of the Veins. London: Edward Arnold, 1988.
12. Raymond-Martimbeau P. Complications of sclerotherapy. In Raymond-Martimbeau P, ed. Phlebologia Houston '91. Dallas: PRM Editions, 1991, pp 269-274.
13. Goldman MP. Sclerotherapy: Treatment of Varicose and Telangiectatic Leg Veins. St. Louis: Mosby–Year Book, 1991.
14. Bernard R. Emergency measures. In Raymond-Martimbeau P, ed. Phlebologia Houston '91. Dallas: PRM Editions, 1991, pp 286-287.
15. Cloutier G, Zummo M. La sclérose des crosses avec compression. Résultats à long terme. Phlebologie 39:145-148, 1986.
16. Raymond-Martimbeau P. Effects of sclerotherapy on blood coagulation: A prospective study [abstract]. J Dermatol Surg Oncol 17:91, 1991.

Chapter 14

Adverse Sequelae of Sclerotherapy Treatment of Varicose and Telangiectatic Leg Veins*

Mitchel P. Goldman

Primum non nocere—above all else do no harm. This dictum always has been a watchword in medicine and always should be considered before any form of treatment is begun. Rarely in medicine does the physician have the luxury of administering a totally benign therapy, one that has absolutely no chance of producing harm. Rather, after establishing that the treatment is truly in the best interests of the patient, one should become familiar with the potential hazards of the proposed therapy and be prepared to treat those hazards if they occur. Further, in this era of pervasive medical-legal conflicts, it is advisable to inform the patient of the various potential complications and adverse sequelae of therapy. A cognizant patient can better recognize a problem early and can more willingly participate in the necessary treatment.

Unfortunately, like any other therapeutic technique, sclerotherapy carries with it a number of potential adverse sequelae and complications. Fairly common, and often self-limiting, side effects include perivascular cutaneous pigmentation, edema of the injected extremity, a flare of new telangiectasias, pain with injection of certain sclerosing solutions, localized urticaria over injected sites, blisters or folliculitis caused by postsclerosis compression, recurrence of previously treated vessels, stress-related problems, and localized hirsutism. This chapter addresses the pathophysiology of these reactions, methods for reducing their incidence, and treatment of their occurrence.

POSTSCLEROTHERAPY HYPERPIGMENTATION

Cutaneous pigmentation is a relatively common occurrence after sclerotherapy of veins varying in size from varicose to capillary. This sequela has been reported in

*From Goldman MP. Sclerotherapy: Treatment of Varicose and Telangiectatic Leg Veins. St. Louis: Mosby–Year Book, Inc., 1991. Reprinted and updated with permission.

up to 30% of patients treated with sodium tetradecyl sulfate (STS),[1] 10% to 30% of patients treated with hypertonic saline (HS),[2-5] and 10.7%[6] to 30%[3,7] of patients treated with polidocanol (POL). A recent evaluation of patients in one practice noted a 1% incidence of pigmentation persisting after 1 year.[8] Pigmentation is usually linear in appearance along the course of the treated blood vessel. I use the term "ghost of the blood vessel" to explain to patients that such pigmentation represents a resolving vessel, not an intact one. However, in addition to linear lines of pigmentation, osmotic sclerosing solutions may produce punctate pigmentation at points of injection. This type of pigmentation may be related to the solution's mechanism of action through an osmotic gradient that produces maximal osmolality and resultant endothelial destruction at the injection site. In contrast, detergent-type sclerosing solutions destroy the treated vessel for a few centimeters along its length, producing a more linear golden-brown color (Figure 14-1).

Etiologic Factors

The etiology of postsclerotherapy hyperpigmentation is subject to much conjecture. Biegeleisen and Biegeleisen,[9] Chrisman,[10] and Chatard[11] state (without reported histologic evaluation) that such pigmentation results from a *combination* of postinflammatory hyperpigmentation (incontinence of melanin pigment) and hemosiderin deposition. However, Shields and Jansen[12] and Bodian[2] state (again without histologic confirmation) that this type of pigmentation is caused only by hemosiderin staining of the dermis. Defects in iron storage and/or transport mechanisms also have been found in a significant number of patients who developed postsclerotherapy pigmentation.[13]

Relatively few histologic studies have focused on the etiology of postsclerotherapy hyperpigmentation. Biopsy of 14 patients done 6 to 54 months after sclerotherapy treatment of varicose veins demonstrated hemosiderin without melanin incontinence.[14] A second histologic study performed after injection of varicose veins in patients with spontaneous pigmentation associated with chronic venous insufficiency was reported by Cuttell and Fox,[15] who treated seven patients with STS, using 6 weeks of compression therapy followed by an additional 2 months of wearing elastic stockings. Patients underwent biopsy both before sclerotherapy and from 10 to 23 months after sclerotherapy. Full-thickness skin biopsy specimens were stained with hematoxylin and eosin, hexamine silver, and Perls' reagent and then blindly reviewed by two histopathologists. All patients demonstrated a decrease in melanin. Dermal hemosiderin was increased in two patients, unchanged in one patient, and curiously, decreased in four patients. Cuttell and Fox concluded that "residual pigmentation following sclerotherapy of varicose veins occurs where there has been extravasation of blood at the injection site."[15]

Goldman, Kaplan, and Duffy[16] have microscopically examined this pigmentation in six patients 6 weeks to 6 months after treatment of leg telangiectasias with POL, HS, and STS. Treatment and biopsy characteristics of this study and of three

A

B

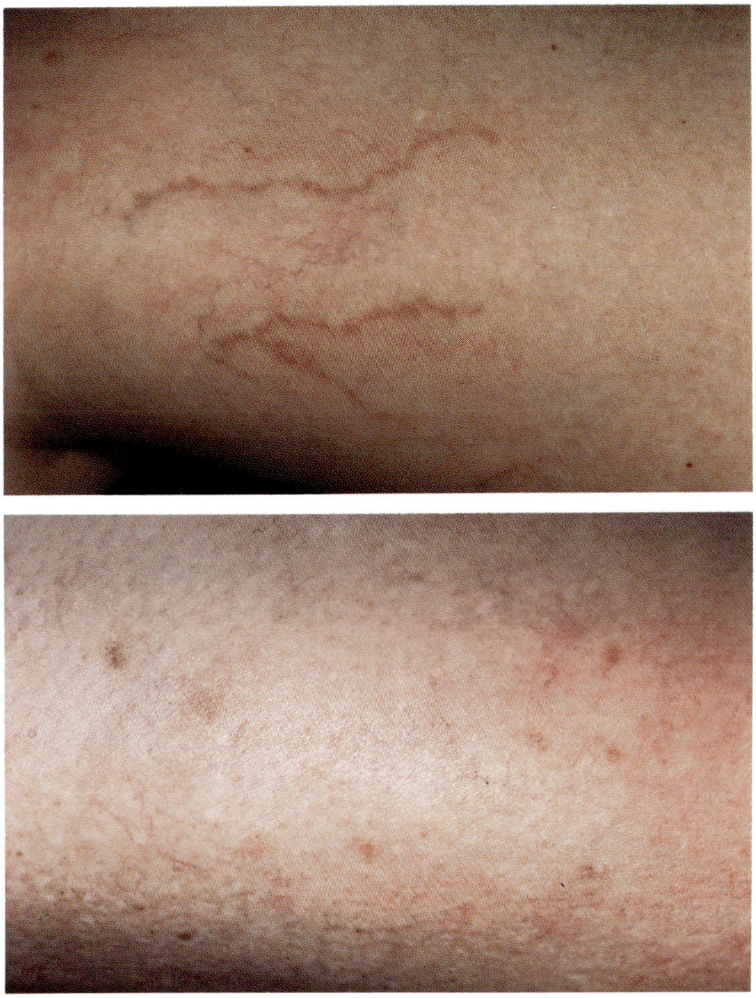

FIGURE 14-1. A, Linear pigmentation along course of a treated blood vessel 8 weeks after treatment with POL 0.5%. **B,** Punctate pigmentation 8 weeks after treatment with Sclerodex.

TABLE 14-1. Postsclerotherapy hyperpigmentation treatment characteristics

Agent/%	Race of Patient	Time of Biopsy (after injection)	Result
POL 0.25	White	6 wk	Heme
POL 0.75	White	6 wk	Heme
POL 0.75	Hispanic	6 mo	Heme
POL 0.75	White	12 mo	Heme
SM ?	White	7 yr	Heme
HS 18	White	8 mo	Heme
HS 20	White	2 mo	Heme
STS 0.5	White	5 mo	Heme
STS 0.25	Hispanic	3 mo	Heme

POL, polidocanol; SM, sodium morrhuate; HS, hypertonic saline; STS, sodium tetradecyl sulfate; heme, hemosiderin.

additional patients are listed in Table 14-1. Analysis of these patients shows that postsclerotherapy pigmentation occurred 6 to 12 weeks after treatment. There were no apparent histologic differences in the degree of pigmentation among the three sclerosing agents. In each biopsy specimen, scattered foci of golden-brown refractile pigment was noted on hematoxylin-eosin–stained specimens (Figure 14-2). Perls' reagent revealed iron deposition in the dermis. Fontana's stain demonstrated a normal pattern or melanocytes along the dermal-epidermal junction. Diapedesis of red blood cells was noted only on biopsy specimens taken from the ankle (at 6 and 8 months after injection). Interestingly, periadnexal hemosiderin was prominent in this location and in the popliteal fossae. The depth of hemosiderin ranged from 0.2 to 2.8 mm from the granular layer.[13]

Each specimen differed somewhat in the degree of dermal hemosiderin; the more darkly pigmented cutaneous lesions exhibited a greater extent of dermal hemosiderin. In this limited study there appeared to be a greater amount of hemosiderin staining in biopsy specimens taken from the ankle as opposed to the calf or thigh. In addition, darkly pigmented patients did not demonstrate melanin incontinence.

Histologic studies of postsclerotherapy pigmentation demonstrate this sequela is caused by hemosiderin deposition only.[14-16] Hemosiderin deposition predominantly occurs in the superficial dermis, although it may be present in periadnexal and middermal locations, particularly in the ankle area. This phenomenon probably takes place when red blood cells extravasate into the dermis after the rupture of treated vessels.[17] Erythrocyte diapedesis is a regular finding in chronic venous insufficiency. With that condition it is not caused by inflammatory wall alterations, but solely by a pressure rise within the cutaneous vessels.[18] Erythrocyte diapedesis also may occur after inflammation of the vessel and is commonly seen after thrombo-

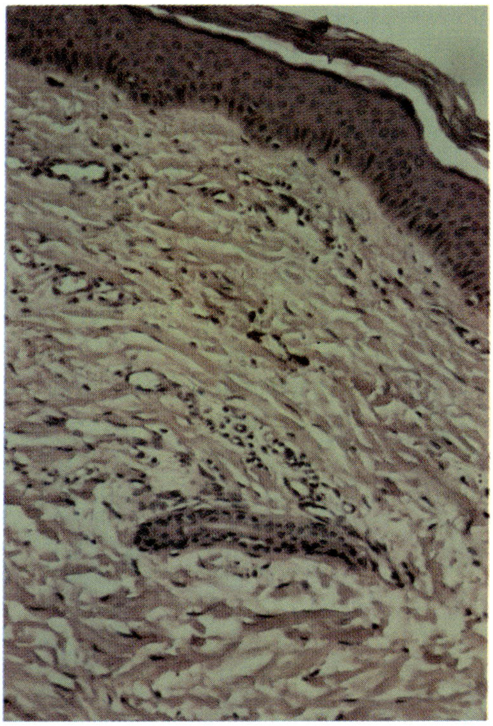

FIGURE 14-2. Section stained with hematoxylin-eosin; taken 6 months after injection with POL 0.75%. Note scattered foci of golden-brown pigment. (Original magnification ×50.) (Reprinted by permission of the publisher from Goldman MP, Kaplan RP, Duffy DM. Postsclerotherapy hyperpigmentation: A histologic evaluation. J Dermatol Surg Oncol 13:547, 1987. Copyright 1987 by Elsevier Science Publishing Co., Inc.)

phlebitis. Perivascular inflammation is presumed to promote degranulation of perivascular mast cells. Release of histamine leads to endothelial cell contraction, which results in widening of endothelial gaps through which extravasation of red blood cells can occur.[19-23]

Perivascular phagocytosis of red blood cells occurs either as intact cells or piecemeal after fragmentation by macrophages.[24,25] The intracellular fragments in the macrophage cytoplasm are further compartmentalized into hemoglobin-containing globules. These globules are referred to as secondary lysosomes. Since hemosiderin is an indigestible residue of hemoglobin degradation, it may appear as aggregates up to 100 μm in diameter.[26] Hemosiderin has a variable concentration. Iron concentrations vary from 24% to 36%.[27] Iron hydroxide contained in hemosiderin occurs in different forms with varying amounts of ferritin.[28] On unstained tissue, iron hydroxide appears golden and is 30% iron by weight. Its elimination from the area may take years—if it ever occurs.

In addition to its being insoluble, hemosiderin may directly affect cellular function. Histologic examination with x-ray fluorescence analysis of patients with varicose ulceration has disclosed an elevation of mean iron levels in periulcerated skin.[29] The authors of that analysis speculate that free radical formation resulting from local iron accumulation may cause melanocytic stimulation, thereby augmenting brown pigmentation. Indeed, multiple authors have demonstrated melanin incontinence in the presence of venous stasis, complicated by extravascular red blood cells.[30-32] Whether melanocytic stimulation plays a role in the early appearance of postsclerotherapy pigmentation is unlikely. However, this action may contribute to the persistence of pigmentation in certain patients.

Pigmentation resolves from a gradual resorption of ferritin particles from macrophage digestion. It has been hypothesized that the patient's iron storage and transport mechanisms may influence the rate of clearance of dermal hemosiderin.[33] A preliminary study of 16 patients with age-matched controls disclosed that patients who developed pigmentation had higher serum ferritin levels than those of controls. Serum ferritin has been shown to correlate with total body iron stores.[34] This finding supports the hypothesis that high total body iron stores increase the susceptibility toward hyperpigmentation. Therefore serum ferritin levels may be used to identify patients at risk for postsclerotherapy hyperpigmentation. These patients may require special attention, with meticulous microthrombectomy and increased time and extent of posttreatment compression advocated.

Regardless of its etiology, the incidence of hyperpigmentation appears to be related to multiple factors, including (1) sclerosing solution type and concentration, (2) sclerotherapy technique, (3) gravitational and other intravascular pressures, (4) innate tendency toward cutaneous pigmentation (total body iron stores and/or altered iron transport and storage mechanisms, innate enhanced histamine release/hypersensitivity, and vessel fragility), (5) postsclerotherapy treatment, (6) vessel diameter, and (7) concomitant medication.

Solution Type and Concentration

The type and concentration of the sclerosing solution affect the degree of endothelial destruction. The extent of endothelial destruction, with resulting inflammation and extravasation of red blood cells, is thought to influence the development of postsclerotherapy hyperpigmentation. Cloutier and Sansoucy[35] and Tournay[1] state that STS produces the highest incidence of pigmentation amongst sclerosing solutions. Although Goldman, Kaplan, and Duffy[16] and Duffy[3] have noted a similar incidence of pigmentation between HS and STS, Weiss and Weiss[36] have reported a 10.8% incidence of pigmentation with HS compared to a 30.7% incidence with 1% POL.

Foley[37] claims that the addition of 100 U/ml of heparin decreases the incidence of pigmentation, but in a large series of patients, Duffy[3] and Sadick[38] have not found such a decrease to occur. Sclerosing solutions reported to have the lowest incidence of postsclerotherapy pigmentation are chromated glycerin[8,35,39-41] and sodium salicylate.[8,11]

Norris, Carlin, and Ratz[42] have observed an increased incidence of pigmentation (60%) in patients treated with 1% POL compared with those treated with

0.5% POL (20%). Weiss and Weiss[36] noted a similar decrease in pigmentation between 1% POL (30.7%) and 0.5% POL (10%). Therefore excessive endothelial destruction, caused either by high concentrations of sclerosing solutions or the use of extremely caustic agents, increases perivascular inflammation. This inflammation may produce melanocytic changes in the skin or potentiate extravasation of red blood cells through endothelial disruption as previously described.

Technique

To limit the degree of intravascular pressure, larger feeding varices, incompetent varices, and points of high pressure reflux should be treated first. This approach minimizes the extent of proximal intravascular pressure, which should decrease the risk for extravasation of red blood cells. Guarde[43] has found a greater incidence of pigmentation if vessels distal to the saphenofemoral junction are treated before successful closure of the junction. Marley[44] also has reported a decreased incidence of pigmentation in his practice since he began injecting leg veins in a proximal to distal order.

Gravitational and Other Intravascular Pressures

Although it can occur anywhere on the leg, postsclerotherapy pigmentation appears most commonly in vessels treated below the knee.[11] This tendency is probably the result of a combination of increased capillary fragility and increased intravascular pressure by gravitational effects in this location. Chatard[11] also has observed an increased incidence of pigmentation when blue venulectases are treated in comparison with red telangiectasias. The explanation for this observation is unknown, but it may be related to vessel diameter. An evaluation of 113 patients treated with sclerotherapy demonstrated rare pigmentation in vessels <1 mm in diameter.[45]

Predisposition to Pigmentation

The reason that certain individuals appear to be predisposed to the development of pigmentation is unknown. Pigmentation has been reported to be more common and more pronounced in patients with dark hair and "dark-toned" skin.[9] This finding is thought to be caused by an increased incidence of postinflammatory hyperpigmentation in patients with such coloring. However, Chatard[11] has reported that pigmentation is unrelated to skin or hair color. I agree with Chatard's assessment. As described previously, iron storage and transfer mechanisms and histamine hypersensitivity also may predispose an individual to pigmentation.[33]

If histamine-induced endothelial contraction promotes extravasation of red blood cells and/or hemosiderin, histamine antagonists should prevent or limit its occurrence. The catecholamines norepinephrine and isoproterenol have been found to antagonize histamine-induced edema in canine brachial artery preparations.[46] Similarly, corticosteroids decrease the size of histamine-induced endothelial gap junctions.[47] Terbutaline also has been shown to inhibit macromolecular leakage from postcapillary venules in hamster femoral veins.[48] Cimetidine also has been noted to block histamine-induced widening of endothelial gaps in rat femoral veins.[49] Therefore patients who develop postsclerotherapy hyperpigmentation may be pretreated with one of these medications (or a combination of them) to block and/or limit histamine effects.

Vessel fragility also may indicate an innate predisposition toward pigmentation. Capillary strength has been related to both menstrual cycles and circulating estrogen.[50] Capillary fragility was measured with suction blister technique in 42 menstrual cycles in 32 nurses and found to correlate with both ovulation and menses. Decreased capillary strength occurred 3 to 5 days before menses, 2 days after menses, and during ovulation. Fragility improved with intravenous and oral administration of conjugated equine estrogen (Premarin, Wyeth-Ayerst Laboratories) in 26 postmenopausal women examined. One patient normalized her premenstrual drop in capillary strength by surreptitiously taking vitamin C.[50] However, this interesting archival study needs to be verified by additional prospective studies. Until such verification, physicians may wish to consider timing sclerotherapy treatment accordingly.

In recent years, patients taking minocycline have been found to develop postsclerotherapy pigmentation.[51,52] In one such patient, pigmentation developed after superficial ulceration. Therefore the ulcer itself with its coincidental inflammation and vascular disruption may explain the pigmentation. However, minocycline has been shown to produce pigmentation in a variety of organs and structures.[53,53a] One form of minocycline pigmentation develops in depressed acne scars or at other sites of inflammation.[54] A second form of pigmentation has been described in patients with legs exposed to ultraviolet light.[55] The pigment in minocycline hyperpigmentation has been found to be hemosiderin or some other iron-chelating compound.[56] It has been hypothesized that minocycline or a metabolite may interfere with degradation of hemosiderin through lysosomal disruption, leading to macrophage death and deposition of pigment.[57] Therefore it may be prudent to withhold minocycline therapy in sclerotherapy patients. It is clear that further studies are needed to establish such a direct relationship.

Postsclerotherapy Coagula

Finally, removal of postsclerotherapy coagula may decrease the incidence of pigmentation. Thrombi, to some degree, are thought to occur after sclerotherapy of all veins, regardless of size. Formation of thrombi takes place because it is impossible to completely occlude the vascular lumen with external pressure. The persistence of a small vascular lumen, even with maximal external pressure, has been predicted with experimental models of vein wall.[18] This effect also has been directly observed with fiberoptic varicography.[58]

Persistent thrombi are thought to produce a subacute "perivenulitis" that can persist for months.[59-61] This condition favors extravasation of red blood cells through a damaged endothelium or by increasing the permeability of treated endothelium. In addition, intratissue fixation of hemosiderin may occur.[11] Such fixation provides a rationale for drainage of all foci of trapped blood between 2 and 4 weeks after sclerotherapy. Sometimes blood can be released even 2 months after sclerotherapy.

Thrombi are best removed by gentle expression of the liquefied clot through a small incision made with a 21-gauge needle, a No. 11 blade, or a lancet (Figure 14-3). A rocking action applied around the clot may aid in its expulsion. This action should be continued until all dark blood is removed.

The art of this procedure involves finding the best location for puncture. This

A

B

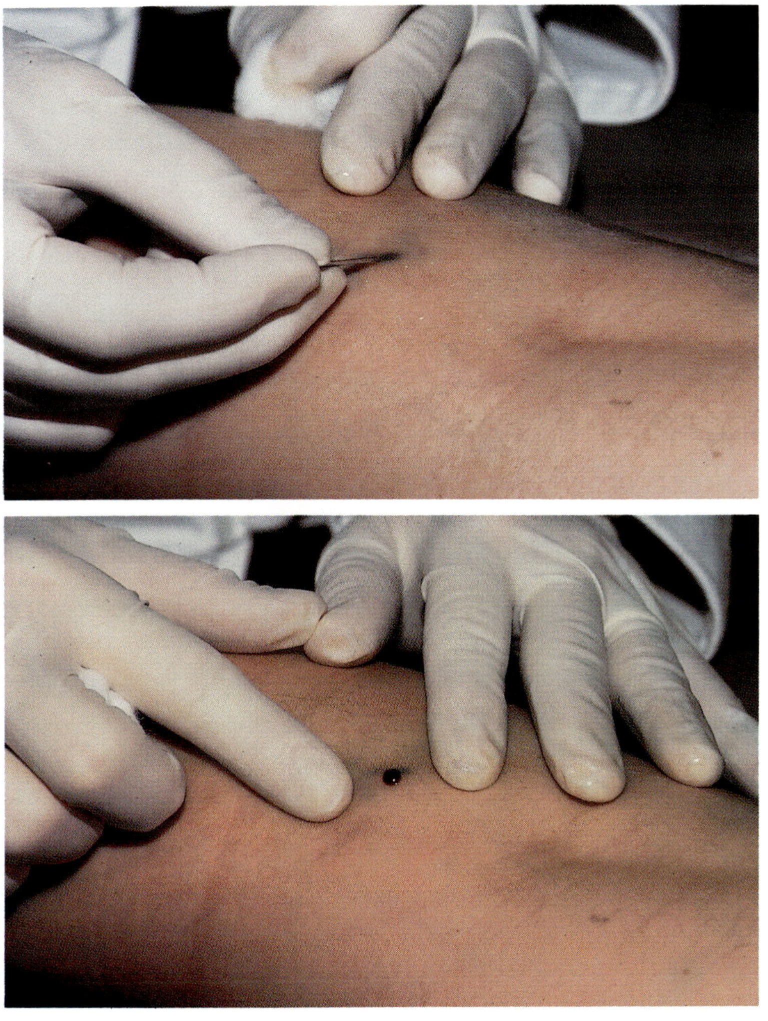

FIGURE 14-3. Method for evacuation of a thrombosis in a 1 mm diameter reticular varicose vein 2 weeks after sclerotherapy. **A,** Small incision is made. **B,** Clot is expelled. (From Goldman MP. Sclerotherapy: Treatment of Varicose and Telangiectatic Leg Veins. St. Louis: Mosby–Year Book, Inc., 1991, p 226.)

point is best perceived as a soft, fluctuating spot. If the thrombosis is located in the deep dermis, the area should be marked and 1% lidocaine can be infiltrated around the area to facilitate a less painful removal. Compression pads and/or stockings are worn by the patient for an additional 3 days to prevent further thrombosis formation and to aid in adherence of the opposing endothelial walls in order to establish effective endosclerosis.

An alternative technique for extraction of larger segments of thrombotic vein is to remove the thrombus by performing aspiration through a 16- or 18-gauge needle. This technique usually requires local infiltration of anesthetic along the course of the thrombotic vessel.

Perchuk[62] has raised the possibility of infection occurring from stab incisions. This danger was presumed to be caused by the presence of bacteria in varicose veins, a belief commonly held by physicians 40 to 50 years ago.[63,64] However, in the modern medical literature, there have been no reports of infections occurring in patients treated with stab incisions made in postsclerotherapy clots. This problem has not occurred in my practice, where this procedure is used routinely.

Duration

Despite therapeutic attempts, pigmentation often lasts from 6 to 12 months.[16] Rarely, pigmentation may last over 1 year. Georgiev[8] estimates that 1% of his patients have pigmentation lasting over 1 year, and Duffy[3] estimates that up to 10% of his patients have pigmentation for that long a period. It is important to recognize that in certain patients this pigmentation may have been present over superficial varicosities and telangiectasias before sclerotherapy was performed.[8,11] Hyperpigmentation as a result of "physiologic" diapedesis of red blood cells through fragile vessels is common in venous stasis or over varicose veins. Therefore preoperative documentation, including photographs, may be beneficial for follow-up patient visits.

Prevention

Although never formally studied, a decreased incidence of postsclerosis pigmentation appears to occur after injection treatment of deeper varicose veins. This difference may occur because sclerosis of vessels in the deeper dermis results in a more efficient reabsorption of extravasated heme, eventuating in a decreased incidence of overlying pigmentation.

To prevent the development of pigmentation, sclerotherapy should be done in a way that produces limited endothelial necrosis, not total destruction of endothelium with its resulting diapedesis of red blood cells. This effect may be achieved by meticulous technique, avoidance of excessive injection pressures, selection of appropriate solution concentration, and treatment of areas of reflux venous return in a proximal to distal manner.

Treatment

Once pigmentation has occurred, treatment is often unsuccessful. Because this pigmentation is primarily caused by hemosiderin deposition and not melanin incontinence, bleaching agents that affect melanocytic function are usually ineffective. Exfoliants (trichloroacetic acid) may hasten the apparent resolution of this pigmentation by decreasing the overlying cutaneous pigmentation, but they carry a risk of scarring, permanent hypopigmentation, and postinflammatory hyperpigmentation. However, some physicians have reported apparent success with this therapeutic modality.[65]

Effective treatments for this type of pigmentation have been reported only rarely. Chatard[11] has found that light cryotherapy performed to exfoliate the epidermis and "evict the pigment" is helpful. Cryotherapy has not been found to be useful in my practice.

Terezakis[66] has noted that the use of topical retinoic acid enhances resolution of the pigmentation. She speculates that retinoids enhance fibroblastic removal of hemosiderin. Therefore I have used topical tretinoin (Retin-A 0.1% cream, Ortho Pharmaceutical Corp., Raritan, N.J.) to treat patients who have pigmentation beyond 3 months. Although formal placebo control studies have yet to be completed, it appears that this therapy may be effective. Such therapy does not appear to have any adverse sequelae and offers the advantage of bringing the patient into active therapy.

A seemingly logical form of treatment would be chelation of the subcutaneous iron deposition. Myers[67] has described the use of a 150 mg/ml ointment of disodium ethylenediamine tetraacetic acid (EDTA) in the treatment of 10 patients with pigmentation after sclerotherapy or vein stripping or with pigmentation in chronic postphlebitic legs. He reported a consistent reduction in the shade of the pigmentation in every patient treated. Unfortunately, Myers's study was uncontrolled, and no further reports of this form of treatment have been made since its presentation in 1965. In my experience, intradermal injection of deferoxamine in an attempt to cause chelation of the hemosiderin has not proven to be uniformly beneficial.

Graduated elastic compression therapy with coadministration of the anabolic steroid stanozolol (Stromba) has been shown to decrease pigmentation from lipodermatosclerosis in 34 legs of 23 patients who also had varicose veins.[68] No change in skin pigmentation occurred when patients used graduated compression stockings alone. The authors suggest that stanozolol may exert its effect through reduction in perivascular fibrin by fibrinolytic enhancement. Unfortunately, further studies have not been published to support these claims. In addition, compression alone has been shown to improve lipodermatosclerotic skin changes, including hyperpigmentation (Partsch H, personal communication, 1992). Although it appears reasonable to advocate the wearing of graduated support stockings after treatment, further studies are clearly needed before systemic stanozolol therapy can be recommended.

Finally, laser treatment has been demonstrated to be efficacious in 45%[13] to

69%[33] of patients with pigmentation of either 12 or 6 months' duration, respectively. Hemosiderin has an absorption spectrum that peaks at 410 to 415 nm followed by a gradually sloping curve throughout the visible spectrum[69,70] (Figure 14-4). The copper vapor laser used at 511 nm in a continuous airbrush technique and the flashlamp-excited pulsed dye (FLPD) laser at 510 nm should interact relatively specifically with hemosiderin absorption spectrum. Competition from oxygenated hemoglobin (peak absorption at 577 nm) should be low. However, interaction with epidermal melanin, which has a higher absorption at these wavelengths, may be significant. These lasers are thought to produce physical fragmentation of pigment granules, which are later removed by phagocytosis. However, penetration of laser energy at 510 and 511 nm is limited to 1 mm below the granular layer.[71] Since, hemosiderin may occur up to 2.8 mm below the granular layer, nonthermal effects may result in clinical resolution. An inflammatory reaction from thermal and/or photoacoustic effects may stimulate hemosiderin absorption. Although copper vapor laser–treated pigmentation responded better than FLPD laser therapy, thermal relaxation times used in the latter laser system should be more selective. Further expanded studies should resolve this discrepancy.

The recommended treatment is "flashbulb therapy" or "chrono-therapy." Since the majority of patients will have a resolution of pigmentation within 1 year, time and photographic documentation tend to be very satisfactory for the understanding patient.

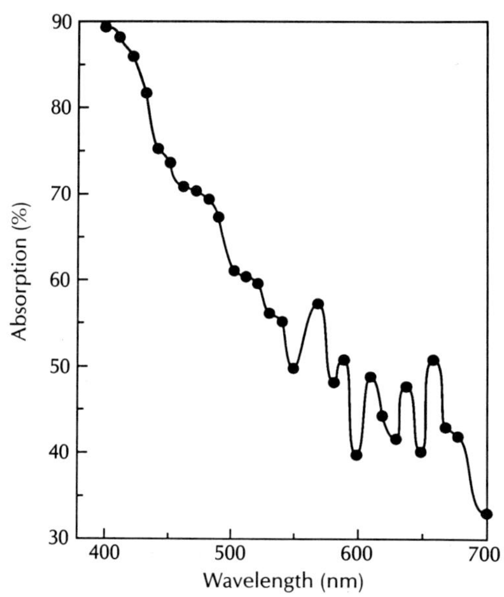

FIGURE 14-4. Absorption spectra for hemosiderin (freshly frozen, average of two determinations). (Redrawn from Wells CI, Wolken JJ. Biochemistry: Microspectrophotometry of haemosiderin granules. Nature 193:977-988, 1962.)

TEMPORARY SWELLING

Etiologic Factors

Multiple factors are responsible for swelling of a treated area. These factors include changes in the pressure differential between intravascular and perivascular space and changes in endothelial permeability. Edema is most common when varicose veins or telangiectasias below the ankle are treated. It relates both to the increase in gravitational intravascular pressure in this area and the relative sparsity of perivascular fascia at the ankle. Riddock[72] has speculated that edema is caused by an unduly prolonged reflex spasm spreading to some of the subfascial (deep) veins. Reflex vasospasm is thought to increase proximal intravascular pressures.

The extent of edema also is related to the strength of the sclerosing solutions used. This factor appears to be correlated with the degree of perivascular inflammation produced by the sclerosing solution. The by-products of inflammation, including release of histamine and various mediators, increase endothelial permeability. In addition to the degree of inflammation induced by sclerotherapy itself, the innate sensitivity of a patient's perivascular mast cells (possibly related to a history of atopia or asthma), concomitant medications that may promote or inhibit mast cell degranulation (e.g., corticosteroids, antihistamines, and nonsteroidal anti-inflammatory agents), and previous exposure sensitivity to the sclerosing agent all may contribute to edema. Duffy[3] and Goldman[7] have estimated the occurrence of pedal edema to be between 2% and 5%. They do not note a difference in the incidence of pedal edema between HS and POL use.

Edema may occur if compression is not applied in a graduated manner. It may be produced when one tries to apply localized pressure to the thigh over an injected vein with the addition of a tape dressing over or under a graduated compression stocking. If patients are informed of the possibility of a tourniquet effect being produced by the extra compression, they can be advised to remove the dressing at the first sign of edema distal to the dressing.

Prevention and Treatment

Two techniques can be used to limit temporary swelling. The first is to limit perivascular inflammation. Ankle edema occurs much less frequently if the quantity of sclerosing solution is limited to 1 ml per ankle. In addition, topical or systemic corticosteroids or systemic antihistamines may be beneficial in patients with excessive postsclerotherapy edema.

A second method for limiting the degree of pedal or ankle edema is to routinely apply a graduated pressure stocking after injection of this area. A recent study on the use of 30 to 40 mm Hg compression hosiery in the treatment of leg telangiectasia noted a significant decrease in the incidence of ankle edema when a 30 to 40 mm Hg graduated compression stocking was worn for 3 days after treatment with sclerotherapy.[73]

TELANGIECTATIC MATTING

The appearance of previously unnoticed fine red telangiectasias occurs in a number of patients after either sclerotherapy or surgical ligation of varicose veins and leg telangiectasias (Figure 14-5). This phenomenon has been termed "flares" by Arenander and Lindhagen,[74] "distal angioplasia" by Terezakis,[75] and "telangiectatic matting" by Duffy.[3] The reported incidence varies from 5%[7] to 75%.[42,74] The incidence of telangiectatic matting (TM) also was found to increase with advancing patient age.[74] The largest retrospective analysis to date (2120 patients with leg telangiectasias) reported a 16% incidence.[76] This incidence has been confirmed in a random sample of 113 female sclerotherapy patients.[36] Although most authors do not comment on a gender predisposition,[3] I have seen the development of TM in one male patient with leg telangiectasias. Because of the small number of men seeking treatment, an accurate appraisal of the gender incidence of this condition cannot be stated. TM may appear anywhere on the leg. One detailed study noted that most TM occurred on the medial ankle or medial and lateral calves.[74] However, this condition also has been reported to occur frequently on the thighs.[77]

Etiologic Factors

Probable risk factors for the development of TM in patients with leg telangiectasia include obesity, use of estrogen-containing hormones, pregnancy, and a family history of telangiectatic veins. Age and excessive standing do not appear to influence the incidence of TM.[76] Excessive postsclerotherapy inflammation also may predispose an individual to developing TM.

Postsclerosis TM was first described in the 1960s by Ouvry and Davy.[78] They observed that the incidence of matting was proportional to the degree of inflammation and thrombus formation. The etiology of TM is unknown, but it is thought to be related either to angiogenesis[3,79] or to a dilation of existing subclinical blood vessels by the promotion of collateral flow through arteriovenous anastomoses.[79,80] One or both of these mechanisms may occur. Terezakis[75] believes that TM refers to the "survival of the fittest," with new blood vessels developing after occlusion of neighboring vessels. Experimentally, there are a number of etiologic factors that can initiate or contribute to angiogenesis.

Angiogenesis. Angiogenesis is a complex process in which capillary blood vessels grow in an ordered sequence of events. Angiogenic factors act either directly on the endothelium to stimulate locomotion and mitosis or indirectly by mobilization of host helper cells (mast cells and macrophages) with release of endothelial growth factors. When a new capillary sprout grows from the side of a venule, endothelial cells degrade basement membrane, migrate toward an angiogenic source, proliferate, form a lumen, join the tips of two sprouts to generate a capillary loop, and manufacture new basement membrane.[81] Obstruction of outflow from a vessel (the end result of successful sclerotherapy) is one of the most important factors contributing to angiogenesis.[82] Initiation of angiogenesis also follows disruption of endothelial continuity or intercellular contact. This contact results in endothelial cell sprouting and migration.[83]

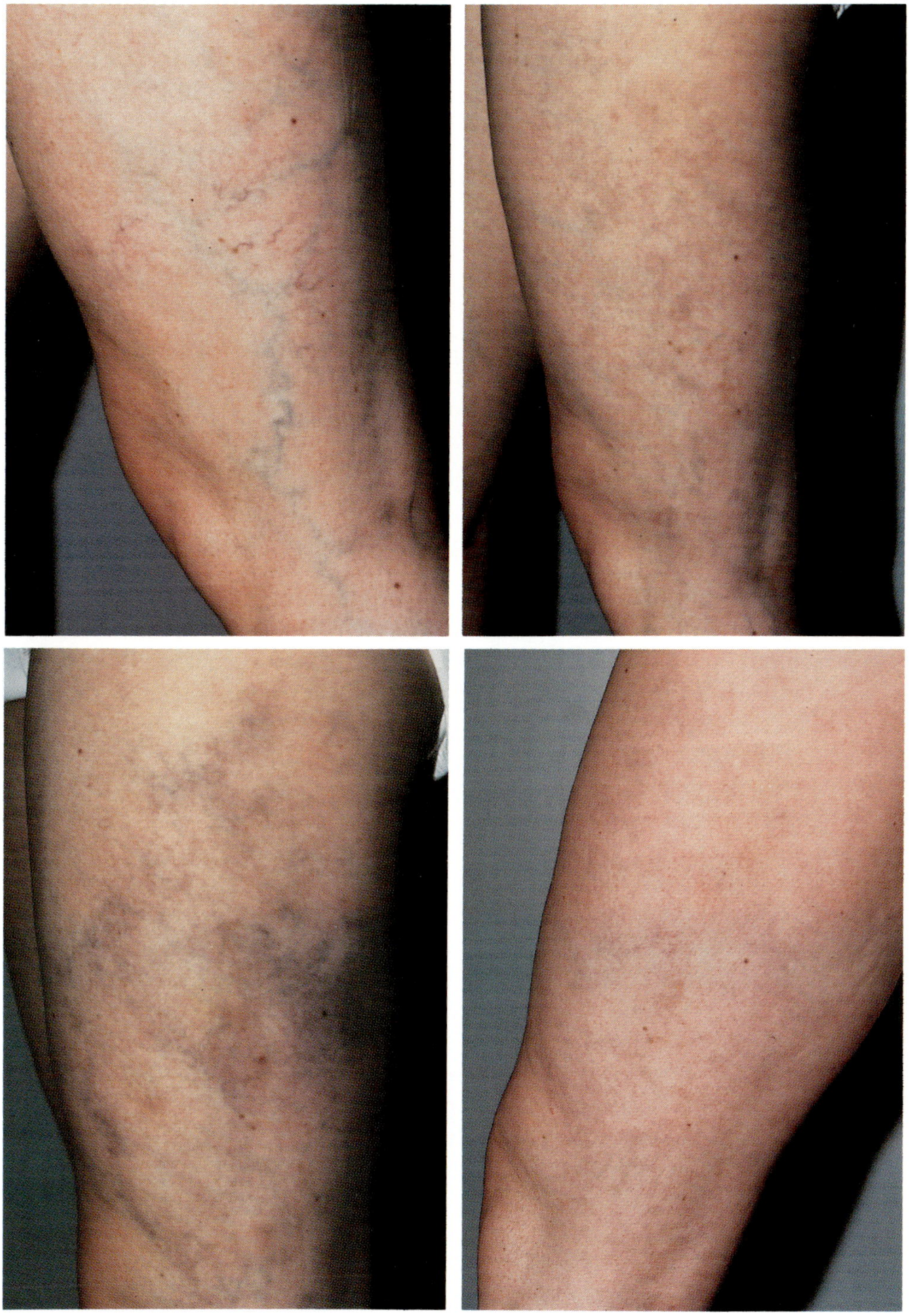

A B C D

FIGURE 14-5. Typical telangiectatic matting in a 36-year-old woman. **A,** Before sclerotherapy treatment, telangiectasias are seen on left lateral thigh. **B,** Three months after treatment of reticular veins with POL 0.75%. **C,** Six weeks after treatment of telangiectatic veins with POL 0.5%. Note development of extensive matting. **D,** Six weeks later. Note complete resolution of matting without treatment.

In addition, endothelial damage leads to the release of heparin and other mast cell factors that both promote the dilation of existing blood vessels and stimulate angiogenesis.[84,85,85a] Finally, neovascularization may be promoted by numerous other angiogenic factors, including (but not limited to) heparin-binding fibroblast growth factors,[84] tumor necrosis factor,[85,86] and platelet-derived endothelial mitogen.[87] These factors and many others are released from perivascular mast cells.[88] Thus sclerotherapy through endothelial damage promotes the release of endothelial angiogenic factors and perivascular mast cell angiogenic factors, thus providing multiple mechanisms for new blood vessel formation to occur. Indeed, it is remarkable that a greater incidence of postsclerosis TM is not seen.

Heparin has been demonstrated to (1) bind to endothelial cells and promote endothelial proliferation in vitro and (2) produce angiogenesis in vivo through an affinity for growth factors.[84] Heparin potentiates angiogenesis in vivo by stimulating endothelial cell plasminogen activator, endothelial cell chemotaxis, or both.[89] Therefore it is interesting to speculate that the high incidence of TM reported by Duffy[3] may be related to his use of heparin in the HS sclerotherapy solution. Bodian[77] has noted a 10% incidence of TM in his patients with the use of HS without the addition of heparin. Weiss and Weiss[5] have reported an 11% incidence of TM in their patient population treated with HS without heparin.

Sclerotherapy produces some degree of perivascular inflammation.[17] Inflammation may be considered as a hypermetabolic state with new vessel growth occurring as a result of increased metabolic demand.[90] In addition, mast cells are found in increased numbers in inflammatory states such as allergic contact dermatitis or delayed hypersensitivity reactions.[91] Since mast cell heparin is one factor that is responsible for capillary endothelial cell migration,[84] in an attempt to decrease angiogenic stimuli, one should try to limit the degree of inflammation as much as possible. This effect can be achieved by choosing an appropriate solution concentration for each type of vessel to be treated and by limiting the quantity of solution to an amount that will not produce excessive endothelial damage. This method was confirmed by Weiss and Weiss,[36] who found that in a random sample of 113 sclerotherapy patients, 10 patients developed TM with injection of POL 1% into vessels <1 mm in diameter. When POL 0.5% was used for subsequent treatments in these patients, none developed further areas of TM. It is interesting that cutaneous mast cells usually occur perivascularly, with a distribution ranging from 7000/mm^3 to 20,000/mm^3.[92,93] With aging, a 50% decrease in cutaneous mast cells occurs in association with a 35% decrease in subepidermal venule.[45] Thus, if TM develops from mast cell factors, its incidence should be decreased in the elderly. Chronologic aging studies might reveal interesting information.

Ouvry and Davy[78] and Mantse[94] have noted a decreased incidence of TM when the pressure of injection is minimized and the extent of dispersion of sclerosing solution is limited to 1 cm diameter with each injection. These techniques may minimize the degree of perivascular inflammation with sclerotherapy. However, these procedural cautions are discounted by Duffy,[3] who advocates the injection of up to 1.5 ml of solution through each injection site and Lary,[95] who recommends injection of up to 3 ml per injection site. Duffy[3] has reported that TM occurs in 20% to 35% of his patients. Lary[95] does not remark on the development of TM in his patients.

Estrogen may play a role in the development of TM. Indeed, it appears that there may be an increased incidence of persistent TM among patients who are taking systemic estrogen preparations.[3,36,76] Weiss and Weiss[36] have found a relative risk of 3.17 ($p < .003$) for development of TM while an individual is taking exogenous estrogen. The mechanism for promotion of TM by estrogen is speculative.

Estrogen receptors have been found in a number of tumors, including angioma of the nose, soft tissue sarcoma, breast carcinoma, endometrial carcinoma, and unilateral nevoid telangiectasia syndrome. Estrogens also have been noted to play a role in the development of vascular tissues. Spider angiomas have been reported to develop during pregnancy and resolve after delivery.[96,97] Spider nevi also are noted to occur in patients with hepatic cirrhosis associated with elevated serum estradiol.[98] In addition, Davis and Duffy[76] have reported on the virtual disappearance of leg telangiectasia and TM in a 51-year-old woman with estrogen-receptor–positive breast carcinoma after initiation of antiestrogen therapy with tamoxifen citrate (Nolvadex). However, Sadick and Niedt[99] could not demonstrate estrogen receptors in a number of biopsies from leg telangiectasias.

Thus since estrogen receptors have been implicated in the promotion of angiogenesis,[100] it may be prudent, albeit premature, to withhold estrogen therapy during sclerotherapy treatment.

Prevention and Treatment

Irrespective of the etiology of TM, since patients seek treatment in order to have leg telangiectasia eliminated, it is most important that the sclerotherapist not produce any new areas of telangiectasia. Therefore any technique that may avoid this side effect, such as limiting the injection blanch to 1 to 2 cm, should be employed. Further recommendations await future studies. Unfortunately, despite the physician's best efforts, TM will occur in a significant percentage of patients. Fortunately, TM usually resolves spontaneously over 3 to 12 months.[3,36] Rarely, TM may be permanent. Thus far, except for the pulsed dye laser,[101] TM is commonly resistant to treatment.

In the future, modifications of present treatment techniques may minimize the occurrence of TM. Experimentally, protamine blocks the ability of mast cells and heparin to stimulate migration of capillary endothelial cells.[102] Protamine also has been demonstrated to prevent the neovascularization induced by an inflammatory agent when it is applied locally. It has no effect on established capillaries that are not proliferating.[103] In addition, beta-cyclodextrin tetradeasulfate administered with cortexolone has been found to be a potent inhibitor of angiogenesis.[104] Thus preventive topical preparations or additives to the sclerosing solution may limit the development of TM.

A

B

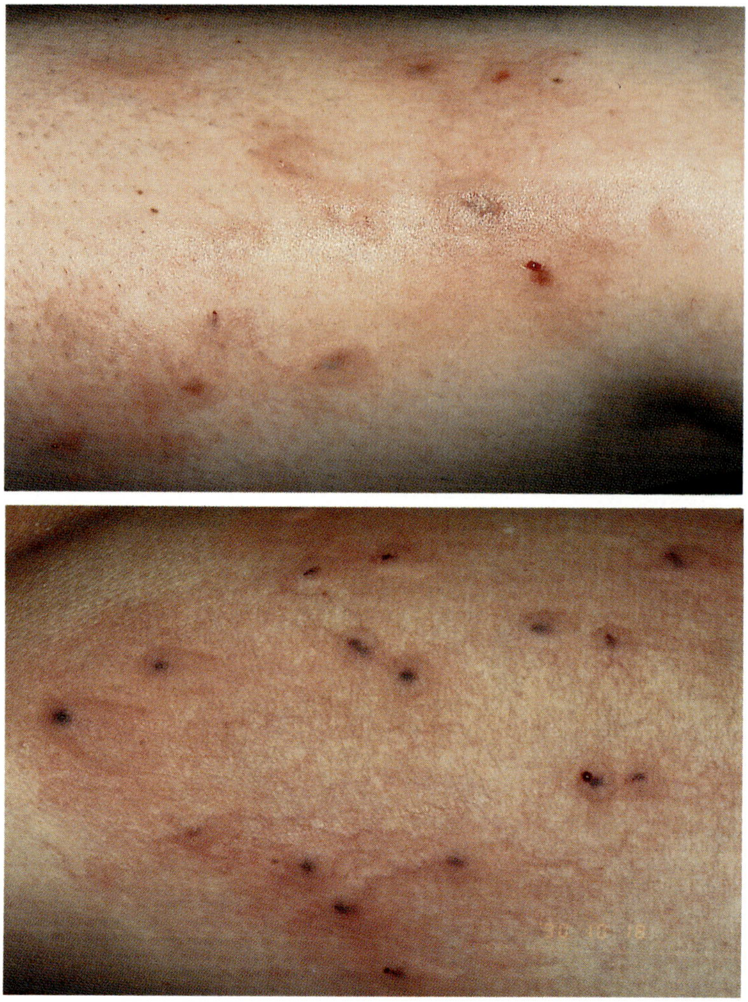

FIGURE 14-6. Urtication. **A,** Immediately after sclerotherapy with Sclerodex. **B,** Immediately after sclerotherapy with Scleremo.

LOCALIZED URTICARIA

Localized urticaria occurs after injection of all sclerosing solutions (Figure 14-6). It is usually transient, lasting about 30 minutes, and is probably the result of endothelial irritation. Localized urticaria is not likely to be an allergic response since it occurs even after injection of 23.4% unadulterated HS. It is probably related to the release of endothelial factors after these cells have been destroyed by the sclerosing solution. Alternatively, it may occur as the earliest manifestation of perivascular inflammation, again through release of endothelial- or platelet-derived factors or perivascular mast cell degranulation.

C

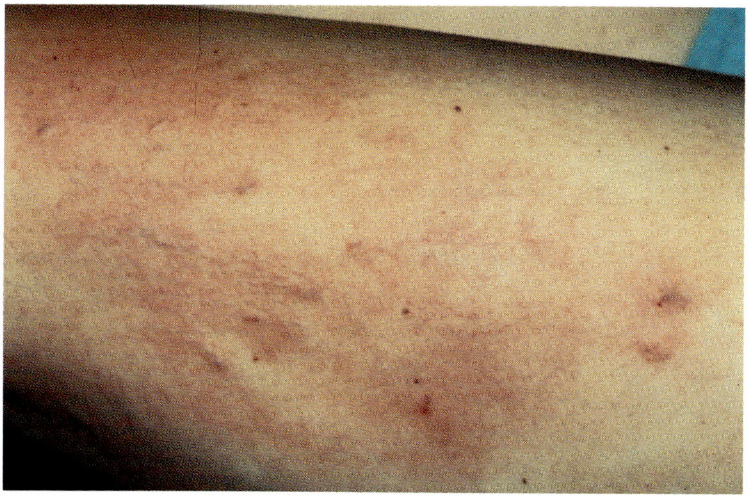

FIGURE 14-6, cont'd. C, Immediately following sclerotherapy with POL 0.5%. Note relatively increased degree of edema and erythema as compared with urtication from Sclerodex and Scleremo.

Approximately 40% of patients studied by Norris, Carlin, and Ratz[42] described temporary itching after injections with POL regardless of drug dosage. Duffy[3] has reported an almost 100% occurrence of urticaria with injection of either POL or HS-heparin-lidocaine solutions. The urtication is usually more intense when more concentrated solutions are used.[3,7] Urtication also may be more intense with repeat injection sessions, especially when POL or STS are used.

Treatment

In my experience, localized urticaria and itching may be diminished by applying topical steroids immediately after injection and by limiting the number of injections per injection site. This approach is particularly helpful for patients who will wear a graduated support stocking after treatment.

PAIN

Since many patients who seek treatment of cosmetic leg telangiectasia require several treatment sessions, each consisting of numerous injections, the physician should attempt to minimize the unpleasantness of the procedure.

Prevention

Certain affected leg areas are slightly more painful than others, especially the ankles, upper medial thighs, and medial knees. Two variables of technique that can minimize pain are the type and size of the needle used for injection and the type of sclerosing solution used.

Type and Size of Needle

Using a needle with the smallest possible diameter for injection is the most obvious way to minimize injection pain. Another factor to consider is the shape of the needle bevel. Needles, even those of the same gauge, are shaped differently and may or may not be coated with a layer of silicone. In my experience, acutely tapered needles, especially when tribeveled, and those that are silicone-coated are perceived by the patient as less painful. Finally, with some agents that are inherently painful to inject, for example, hypertonic solutions, pain can be minimized by slow infusion.[3,5] Slow injection produces a slower distention of tissue and may minimize endothelial cell separation. This method may decrease perivascular nerve stimulation.

Type of Sclerosing Solution

The second method for reducing pain is to choose the least painful sclerosing solution. Hypertonic solutions are notorious for causing pain on injection. The cramping pain that may develop after correct intravenous injection usually occurs a few minutes after injection. Weiss and Weiss[5] have reported that 72% of their patients injected with HS 23.4% experience pain that lasts less than 5 minutes; 4.5% of their patients have pain that lasts more than 5 minutes. This pain probably occurs at the time the hypertonic solution reaches the nerve fibers of the adventitia, either through the wall of the vein or through the capillaries. Subsequently, because of stimulation of sympathetic perivenous nerve fibers, an active contraction of the muscle occurs that also may produce a cramping pain.[105] In addition, vascular spasm caused by the direct effects of the hypertonic solution itself may occur.

Hypertonic solutions also produce muscle cramping after injection. With the injection of 5 to 10 ml of Heparsal (20% HS and 100 U heparin) per injection site into varicose veins, Chou et al.[106] noted that 16% of 310 patients could not tolerate the pain associated with the procedure. Duffy[3] has estimated that 82% of his patients treated with HS note moderate cramping or aching. Such discomfort can be limited somewhat by keeping the volumes injected to 0.1 ml or less per injection site and by massaging the area immediately after injection. Also, adding lidocaine to the sclerosing solution may lessen muscle cramping and allow additional injections into the same area to be done less painfully.[3,4] However, the addition of lidocaine to a hypertonic solution is associated with two problems. First, if acidified (in a multidose bottle), lidocaine is painful to inject. Therefore nonacidified lidocaine (found in single-dose "cardiac" ampules) should be used as an additive. Second, the addition of lidocaine gives the sclerosing solution the potential to produce an allergic reaction.

Chromated glycerin solutions are painful when injected and may produce a mild muscle cramping if more than 1 ml of solution is injected into a single vein.[41]

Two relatively painless solutions are POL and STS. STS has the advantage of producing pain only when it is injected into perivascular tissues, thereby providing a noticeable check on inadvertent perivascular injection. POL is painless when injected intradermally or intravenously. Therefore one does not have the sign of pain to ensure accurate placement of the sclerosing solution. In a double-blind comparison of STS, HS, and POL, patients preferred injection with POL.[107] Finally, despite optimal technique and the use of a mild sclerosing agent, posttreatment soreness for 1 or 2 weeks after injection has been noted to occur in 20% of patients.[3] With the use of nonosmotic sclerosing solutions and graduated compression stockings after treatment, I have *not* noted soreness in most patients after treatment. If patients do complain of soreness, the cause is usually found to be vessels that are thrombosed and/or inflamed. Finally, although relatively painless to inject, STS does produce a dull ache shortly after injection, but it resolves in a few minutes. POL does not produce posttreatment aching.

TAPE COMPRESSION BLISTER

The relatively uncommon cutaneous lesion, tape compression blister (Figure 14-7), occurs when a tape dressing is applied to an area of tissue movement or the

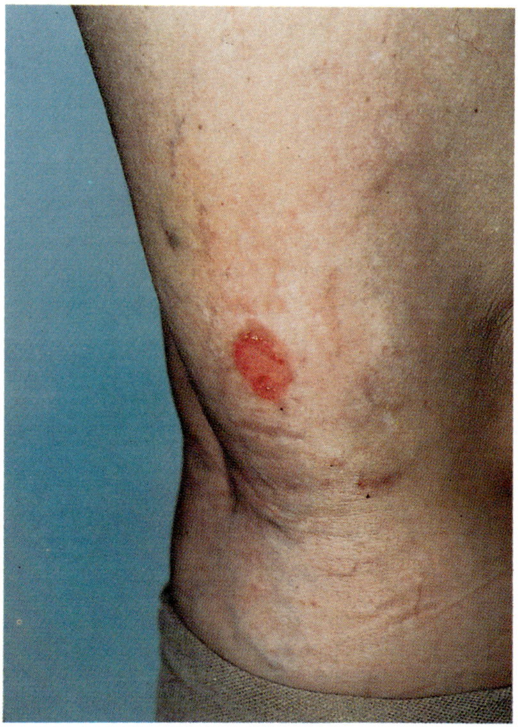

FIGURE 14-7. Superficial blister that developed 1 week after sclerotherapy treatment. Compression of treated area was produced with a foam (STD) pad overlaid with Microfoam tape and a 30 to 40 mm Hg graduated thigh-length compression stocking (shown pulled down below knee).

thin skin of an elderly patient. The blister often appears as a flaccid, fluid-filled sac overlying normal-appearing skin. It usually is not associated with induration or erythema of the adjacent skin. Common sites of occurrence are the posterior calf, medial thigh, and popliteal fossae.

Blisters may occur with the use of any tape. However, they appear more commonly when Microfoam tape (3M Medical-Surgical Division, St. Paul, Minn.) is used rather than hypoallergenic paper tape (Dermilite II; Johnson & Johnson Medical, Arlington, Tex.) over foam pads or cottonballs. This effect is probably caused by the greater adhesiveness of the Microfoam tape. In addition, Microfoam tape usually is placed over the foam dressing with a slight degree of tension, which increases the tension on both ends of the tape. Blistering is also more common in the summer months, when the weather is hotter, and in elderly patients with thinner, more fragile skin.

Blistering must be distinguished from early cutaneous necrosis, cutaneous infection, or an allergic reaction. Early cutaneous necrosis may appear as a superficial blister; in this situation the underlying and adjacent tissue usually is indurated and erythematous. Bullous impetigo may have a similar physical appearance; however, the blister usually overlies warm, erythematous skin. If not warned beforehand, the patient may think that the blister is the result of an allergy to the sclerosing solution. A detailed explanation of the cause of the blister is usually required before treatment can continue.

Prevention

If compression pads are to be used under graduated stockings in a patient who is susceptible to blistering, a Tubigrip tubular support bandage (Seton Products, Inc., Montgomeryville, Pa.) can be used over the pad to hold it in place while the stocking is being applied. Although somewhat costly, this dressing (similar to a net dressing used in burn patients) helps to prevent blister formation. It also can be used in patients with an allergy associated with tape.

Treatment

Fortunately, resolution of the blister occurs within 1 or 2 weeks without any adverse sequelae. To aid in healing and to prevent infection of the denuded skin, an occlusive hydroactive dressing such as Duoderm (ConvaTec, Princeton, N.J.) can be used. Occlusive dressings also may help to alleviate any pain associated with the blister.

TAPE COMPRESSION FOLLICULITIS

Occlusion of any hairy area can promote the development of folliculitis (Figure 14-8). When secondary alopecia of chronic venous insufficiency is not associated with their condition, men seeking treatment for varicose veins usually have hairy legs. If a tape dressing is placed over foam, or if cottonball pads are placed under a

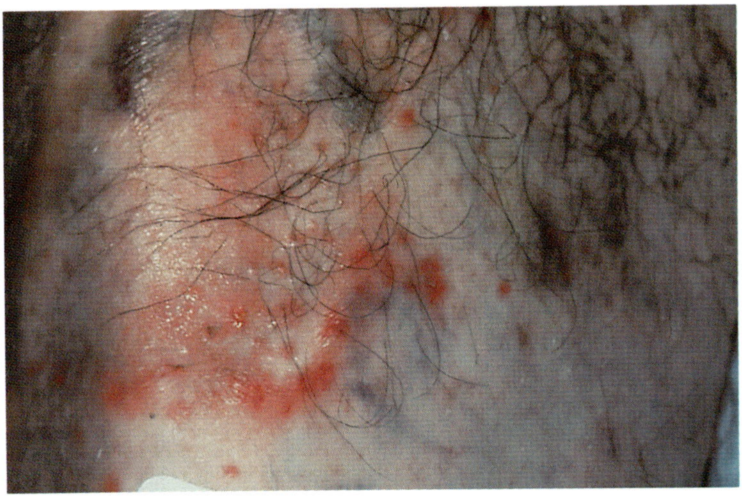

FIGURE 14-8. Folliculitis apparent 7 days after sclerotherapy. Compression of treated area was produced with foam (STD) pads overlaid with Microfoam tape. (From Goldman MP. Sclerotherapy: Treatment of Varicose and Telangiectatic Leg Veins. St. Louis: Mosby–Year Book, Inc., 1991, p 236.)

graduated compression stocking, a follicular inflammation or infection may occur. Folliculitis is more likely to occur in the summer months or when a patient is active and perspires under the dressing.

Treatment

Treatment of this type of folliculitis consists of removal of the occlusive dressing and application of topical treatment with an antibacterial soap such as chlorhexidine gluconate (Hibiclens Antimicrobial Skin Cleanser; Stuart Pharmaceuticals, Wilmington, Del.) or a topical antibiotic gel such as erythromycin 2% (Erygel Topical Gel; Herbert Laboratories, Irvine, Calif.) or clindamycin phosphate topical solution 1% (Cleocin T; The Upjohn Company, Kalamazoo, Mich.). The folliculitis usually resolves within a few days. Only rarely will systemic antibiotics be necessary.

RECURRENCE

Recurrence of sclerotherapy-treated vessels has been estimated to occur in from 20% to nearly 100% of leg telangiectasias, as noted at 5-year follow-up.[108] Recanalization of initially thrombosed leg veins is procedure-dependent. The larger the extent of intravascular thrombosis, the greater the likelihood of recanalization of the thrombosis during vascular organization.[109,110] The recanalization of injected varices without subsequent compression or with inadequate compression is caused by (1) clot contraction and the formation of sinuses that may become lined with

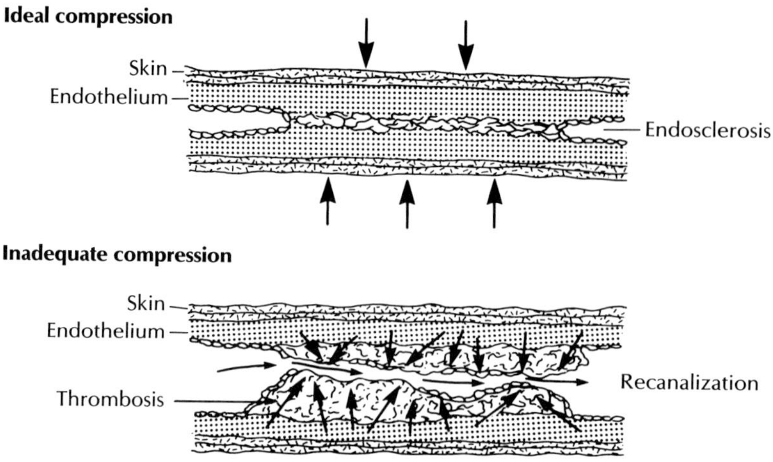

FIGURE 14-9. Diagrammatic representation of recanalization of a varicose vein through sclerotherapy-induced thrombosis. (Redrawn from Wenner L. Vasa 15:180, 1986. From Goldman MP. Sclerotherapy: Treatment of Varicose and Telangiectatic Leg Veins. St. Louis: Mosby–Year Book, Inc., 1991, p 237.)

endothelium, (2) central clot liquefaction and the formation of vascular tunnels through the thrombosis, (3) formation of vascular organization of the thrombosis and collateral vessel formation of the newly formed capillaries, and (4) formation of peripheral sinuses filled with sludged blood (Figure 14-9).[110,111] Therefore the most important factor in preventing recurrence is the limiting of intravascular thrombosis.

Treatment

Tournay[112] was the first physician to stress the importance of postinjection removal of blood clots in 1938. Since that time, the importance of draining these postsclerotherapy thrombi has been emphasized by Sigg,[113] Pratt,[114] and Hobbs.[115] Orbach[109] has advocated the routine removal of all postinjection clots, with both fluctuating and hard cords. With the patient under local anesthesia, he uses a No. 11 blade to make an incision over the vein and a von Graefe cataract knife to dissect the clot completely from the vein wall. Continuous compression is applied until resolution of the vein occurs.

With proper technique, recurrence of varicose veins only rarely occurs. A biopsy study of six patients with "recurrence" of previously treated veins demonstrated that the veins thought to have recurred were in reality new varicose veins.[116] When high recurrence rates are reported, the patients usually have been treated with minimal compression therapy.[109] For example, in one recent study of 310 patients, 83% required reinjection of a treated varicosity. These patients received only 48 hours of compression with elastic bandages.[106]

Unlike recanalization through a varicose vein cord, recanalization is not commonly achieved through a sclerosed telangiectasia. Posttreatment histologic studies have demonstrated only fibrosis in an area treated with sclerotherapy.[2]

STRESS-RELATED SYMPTOMS

Vasovagal Reflex

The vasovagal reflex is a common adverse sequela of any surgical or invasive procedure. It has been estimated to occur in 1% of patients during sclerotherapy[117] and is more common when the techniques of Fegan or Sigg are used.[118] With the latter two techniques, a 21- to 25-gauge needle is inserted into the vein while the patient is sitting or standing, and blood is allowed to flow freely from the punctured vein. Duffy,[3] who performs sclerotherapy with a 30-gauge needle and the patient in a reclining position, estimates the incidence of vasovagal reactions to be 0.001%. It is interesting to note that the percentage of men who experience this response far exceeds that of women.

Vasovagal reactions have typical clinical findings. The usual symptoms include light-headedness, nausea, and sweating. The patient also may experience shortness of breath and palpitations. Syncope rarely occurs, but it usually provokes the most concern in the physician and staff. Vasovagal reactions are most often associated with painful injection, but they may occur as a result of the patient's seeing the needle or smelling the sclerosing solution.

Prevention. The main concern in a vasovagal reaction is that the patient will fall and be injured. Therefore both the nurse and the physician should watch the patient closely for signs of restlessness and excessive perspiration. All patients should be warned to sit down if they become dizzy. When needle placement is performed on a standing patient, it is also helpful for the patient to hold onto an arm rail or other support. All such reactions are easily reversible when the patient assumes the supine or Trendelenburg position. Preventive measures include recommending that the patient eat a light meal before the appointment, allowing good ventilation in the treatment room, and maintaining ongoing communication with the patient during the procedure.

It is important that the physician recognize a vasovagal response in a patient and not assume that an allergic reaction is occurring. If epinephrine is administered subcutaneously in the mistaken belief that an anaphylactic reaction is occurring, the patient's symptoms will become both exaggerated and obscured. This result only further confuses the clinical situation and adds to the patient's apprehension regarding further treatment sessions.

Underlying Medical Disease

More serious stress-induced problems include the exacerbation of certain underlying medical diseases. For example, patients with a history of asthma may experience wheezing, which can be treated with a bronchodilator such as metaproterenol sulfate (Alupent; Boehringer Ingelheim Pharmaceuticals, Inc., Ridgefield, Conn.) (Proventil; Schering Corporation, Kenilworth, N.J.) or over-the-counter epinephrine bitartrate or with a metered-dose inhaler (Primatene; Whitehall Laboratories Inc., New York, N.Y.).

Patients with cardiovascular disease may develop angina, which is treatable with sublingual nitroglycerin tablets. Urticaria can be treated easily with an oral antihistamine, but it may be a sign of systemic allergy. Therefore it is important to carefully evaluate the use of the sclerosing agent for future treatment sessions. It is noteworthy that urticaria and periorbital edema have occurred after injection of unadulterated HS.[119] Such reactions may be related to histamine release from irritated perivascular mast cells. Finally, the triggering of frequent migraine headaches has been noted to occur as a result of sclerotherapy.[3]

Localized Hirsutism

Localized hypertrichosis that develops after sclerotherapy has been described in association with the use of multiple sclerosing agents. The etiology is thought to be an improved cutaneous oxygen content that stimulates hair growth or a long-standing, low-grade inflammatory reaction that increases vascularity. In support of this phenomenon, patients with chronic venous insufficiency have been reported to have developed localized hair growth after surgical treatment.[120]

Hair growth at the site of injection has been described in three patients treated with STS.[121] All three patients were given injections of between 1 and 6 ml of STS over the course of 5 to 10 treatment sessions. Localized hair growth developed 4 to 7 months after the last injection. The site of hair growth was related to the area of skin most damaged by venous incompetence. Weissberg[122] also has reported on the development of localized hirsutism in 1 of 62 patients. The hair growth occurred at the site of injection 1 month after treatment. It lasted 4 months and then subsided. Sclerotherapy with polyiodinated iodine also has been associated with hypertrichosis at the injection site in three patients.[116]

SUMMARY

Sclerotherapy of varicose and telangiectatic leg veins may be associated with a number of adverse sequelae, which may occur despite optimal treatment and complications. Some adverse sequelae may be preventable to a limited degree, but given a large enough number of procedures, these adverse sequelae will occur in any practice.

REFERENCES

1. Tournay PR. Traitement sclérosant des très fines varicosites intra ou sous-dermiques. Soc Fran Phlebol 19:235-241, 1966.
2. Bodian EL. Techniques of sclerotherapy for sunburst venous blemishes. J Dermatol Surg Oncol 11:696-704, 1985.
3. Duffy DM. Small vessel sclerotherapy: An overview. In Callen JP, Dahl MV, Golitz LE, et al., eds. Advances in Dermatology, vol 3. Chicago: Year Book, 1988, pp 221-240.

4. Alderman DB. Surgery and sclerotherapy in the treatment of varicose veins. Conn Med 39: 467-471, 1975.
5. Weiss R, Weiss M. Resolution of pain associated with varicose and telangiectatic leg veins after compression sclerotherapy. J Dermatol Surg Oncol 16:333-336, 1990.
6. Cacciatore E. Experience of sclerotherapy with aethoxysklerol. Minerva Cardioangiolica 27: 255-262, 1979.
7. Goldman P. Sclerotherapy of superficial venules and telangiectasias of the lower extremities. Dermatol Clin 5:369-379, 1987.
8. Georgiev M. Postsclerotherapy hyperpigmentations: A one-year follow-up. J Dermatol Surg Oncol 16:608-610, 1990.
9. Biegeleisen HI, Biegeleisen RM. The current status of sclerotherapy for varicose veins. Clin Med 83:24-36, 1976.
10. Chrisman BB. Treatment of venous ectasias with hypertonic saline. Hawaii Med J 41:406-408, 1982.
11. Chatard H. Discussion de la question de J-C Allart: Pigmentations post-sclérotherapiques. Phlebologie 29:211-216, 1976.
12. Shields JL, Jansen GT. Therapy for superficial telangiectasias of the lower extremities. J Dermatol Surg Oncol 8:857-860, 1982.
13. Goldman MP. Postsclerotherapy hyperpigmentation: Treatment with a flashlamp excited pulsed dye laser. J Dermatol Surg Oncol 18:417-422, 1992.
14. Barner FR, Holzegel K, Voigt K. Über Hyperpigmentation nach Krampfaderverödung, Phlebol u Proktol 6:54-61, 1977.
15. Cuttell PJ, Fox JA. The etiology and treatment of varicose pigmentation. Phlebologie 35:387-389, 1982.
16. Goldman MP, Kaplan RP, Duffy DM. Postsclerotherapy hyperpigmentation: A histologic evaluation. J Dermatol Surg Oncol 13:547-550, 1987.
17. Goldman MP, Kaplan RP, Oki LN. Sclerosing agents in the treatment of telangiectasia: Comparison of the clinical and histologic effects of intravascular polidocanol, sodium tetradecyl sulfate, and hypertonic saline in the dorsal rabbit ear vein model. Arch Dermatol 123:1196-1201, 1987.
18. Moreno AH, Katz AI, Gold LV. Mechanics of distention of dog veins and other thin-walled tubular structures. Circ Res 27:1069-1080, 1970.
19. Grega GJ, Svensjo E, Haddy FJ. Macromolecular permeability of the microvascular membrane: Physiological and pharmacological regulation. Microcirculation 1:325-341, 1981-1982.
20. Majno G, Palade GE, Schoefl GI. Studies on inflammation: The site of action of histamine and serotonin along the vascular tree—A topographic study. J Biophys Biochem Cytol 11:607-626, 1961.
21. Bjork J, Smedegard G. The microvasculature of the hamster cheek pouch as a model for studying acute immune-complex–induced inflammatory reactions. Int Arch Allergy Appl Immunol 74: 178-185, 1984.
22. Fox J, Galey F, Wayland H. Action of histamine on the mesenteric microvasculature. Microvas Res 19:108-126, 1980.
23. Simionescu N, Simionescu M, Palade G. Open junctions in the endothelium of the postcapillary venules of the diaphragm. J Cell Biol 79:27-44, 1978.
24. Bessis M. Living blood cells and their ultrastructure. Berlin: Springer-Verlag, 1973.
25. Leu HJ, et al. Veränderungen der transendothelialen Permeabilität als Ursache des Ödems bei der chronisch-venösen Insuffizienz. Med Welt 31:781-785, 1980.
26. Bessis M, Lessin LS, Beutler E. Morphology of the erythron. In Williams WJ, et al., eds. Hematology, 3rd ed. New York: McGraw-Hill, 1983, pp 257-259.
27. Ludewig S. Hemosiderin. Isolation from horse spleen and characterization. Pro Soc Exp Biol Med 95:514-517, 1957.
28. Richter GW. The nature of storage iron in idiopathic hemochromatosis and in hemosiderosis. J Exp Med 112:551-569, 1960.

29. Ackerman Z, Seidenbaum M, Loewenthal E. Overload of iron in the skin of patients with varicose ulcers. Arch Dermatol 124:1376-1378, 1988.
30. Chatarel H, Dufour H. Note sur la nature mixture, hématique et mélanique, des pigmentations en phlébologie. Phlebologie 36:303-306, 1983.
31. Merlen JF, Coget J, Sarteel AM. Pigmentation et stase veineuse. Phlebologie 36:307-314, 1983.
32. Kluken N, Zabel M. La pigmentation est-elle un signe caractéristique de l'insuffisance veineuse chronique? Phlebologie 36:315-320, 1983.
33. Thibault P, Wlodarczyk J. Postsclerotherapy hyperpigmentation: The role of serum iron levels and the effectiveness of treatment with the copper vapor laser. J Dermatol Surg Oncol 18:47-52, 1992.
34. Pippard MJ, Hoffbrand AV. Iron. In Hoffbrand AV, Lewis SM, eds. Postgraduate Haematology. London: Heinemann Medical Books, 1989.
35. Cloutier G, Sansoucy H. Le traitement des varices des membres inférieurs par les injections sclérosantes. Union Med Can 104:1854-1863, 1975.
36. Weiss RA, Weiss MA. Incidence of side effects in the treatment of telangiectasias by compression sclerotherapy: Hypertonic saline vs polidocanol. J Dermatol Surg Oncol 16:800-804, 1990.
37. Foley WT. The eradication of venous blemishes. Cutis 15:665-668, 1975.
38. Sadick N. Treatment of varicose and telangiectatic leg veins with hypertonic saline: A comparative study of heparin and saline. J Dermatol Surg Oncol 16:24-28, 1990.
39. Hutinel B. Esthétique dans les scléroses de varices et traitement des varicosites. La Vie Médicale 20:1739-1743, 1978.
40. Nebot F. Quelques points techniques sur le traitement des varicosites et des telangiectasies. Phlebologie 21:133-135, 1968.
41. Landart J. Traitement médical des varices des membres inférieurs. La Revue du Praticien 26: 2491-2494, 1976.
42. Norris MJ, Carlin MC, Ratz JL. Treatment of essential telangiectasia: Effects of increasing concentrations of polidocanol. J Am Acad Dermatol 20:643-649, 1989.
43. Guarde C. Personal communication, 1989.
44. Marley W. Low-dose Sotradecol for small vessel sclerotherapy. Newsletter of North Am Soc Phlebol 3(2):3-4, 1989.
45. Gilchrest BA, Stoff JS, Soter NA. Chronologic aging alters the response to ultraviolet-induced inflammation in human skin. J Invest Dermatol 79:11-15, 1982.
46. Marciniak DL, Dobbins DE, Maciejko JJ, et al. Antagonism of histamine edema formation by catecholamines. Am J Physiol 234:H180-H185, 1978.
47. Svensjo E. Pharmacological modulation of venular permeability with some antiinflammatory drugs. In Vanhoutte PM, ed. Return Circulation and Norepinephrine: An update. Paris: John Libbey Eurotext, 197-205, 1991.
48. Svensjo E, Persson CGA, Rutili G. Inhibition of bradykinin-induced macromolecular leakage from post-capillary venules by a β_2-adrenoreceptor stimulant, terbutaline. Acta Physiol Scand 101:504-506, 1977.
49. Heltianu C, Simionescu M, Simionescu N. Histamine receptors of the microvascular endothelium revealed in situ with a histamine-ferritin conjugate: Characteristic high-affinity binding sites in venules. J Cell Biol 93:357-364, 1982.
50. Clemetson CAB, Blair L, Brown AB. Capillary strength and the menstrual cycle. Ann N Y Acad Sci 93:277-300, 1962.
51. Jacoby WD. Comment 21. Schoch Letter 41:2, 1991.
52. Leffell DJ. Minocycline hydrochloride hyperpigmentation complicating treatment of venous ectasia of the extremities. J Am Acad Dermatol 24:501-502, 1991.
53. Billano RA, Ward WQ, Little WP. Minocycline and black thyroid [letter]. JAMA 249:1887, 1983.
53a. Poliak SC, DiGiovanna JJ, Gross EG, et al. Minocycline-associated tooth discoloration in young adults. JAMA 254:2930-2932, 1985.

54. Basler RSW, Kohnen PW. Localized hemosiderosis as a sequela of acne. Arch Dermatol 114: 1695-1697, 1978.
55. Ridgway HA, Sonnex TS, Kennedy CTC, et al. Hyperpigmentation associated with oral minocycline. Br J Dermatol 107:95-102, 1982.
56. Sato S, Murphy GF, Bernhard JD, et al. Ultrastructural and x-ray microanalysis observations of minocycline-related hyperpigmentation of the skin. J Invest Dermatol 77:264-271, 1981.
57. Basler RSW. Minocycline therapy for acne [letter]. Arch Dermatol 115:1391, 1979.
58. Muntlak H. Personal communication, 1989.
59. Wenner L. Sind endovarikose hamitische Ansammlungen eine Normalerscheinung bei Sklerotherapie? Vasa 10:174-176, 1981.
60. Leu HJ, Wenner A, Spycher MA. Erythrocyte diapedesis in venous stasis syndrome. Vasa 10: 17-23, 1981.
61. Orbach EJ. Hazards of sclerotherapy of varicose veins—Their prevention and treatment of complications. Vasa 8:170-173, 1979.
62. Perchuk E. Injection therapy of varicose veins: A method of obliterating huge varicosities with small doses of sclerosing agent. Angiology 25:393-409, 1974.
63. de Takats G. Problems in the treatment of varicose veins. Am J Surg 18:26, 1932.
64. Biegeleisen HI. Sclerotherapy: Clinical significance. Clin Med Surg 47:140, 1940.
65. Bernier EC, Escher E. Treatment of postsclerotherapy hyperpigmentation with trichloroacetic acid, a mild and effective procedure. Proceedings of the Second Annual International Congress of the North American Society of Phlebology. New Orleans, February 25, 1989.
66. Terezakis N. Personal communication, 1989.
67. Myers HL. Topical chelation therapy for varicose pigmentation. Angiology 17:66-68, 1966.
68. Burnand K, Clemenson G, Morland M, et al. Venous lipodermatosclerosis: Treatment by fibrinolytic enhancement and elastic compression. Br Med J 280:7-11, 1980.
69. Shoden A, Sturgeon P. Hemosiderin: I. A physio-chemical study. Acta Haematol (Basel) 23: 376-392, 1960.
70. Wells CI, Wolken JJ. Biochemistry: Microspectrophotometry of haemosiderin granules. Nature 193:977-988, 1962.
71. Anderson R. Personal communication, 1991.
72. Riddock J. Treatment of varicose veins. Br J Med 2:671, 1947.
73. Goldman MP, Beandoing D, Marley W. Compression in the treatment of leg telangiectasia. J Dermatol Surg Oncol 16:322-325, 1990.
74. Arenander E, Lindhagen A. The evolution of varicose veins studied in a material of initially unilateral varices. Vasa 7:180-184, 1978.
75. Terezakis N. Sclerotherapy treatment of leg veins. Paper presented at the summer session of the American Academy of Dermatology. San Diego, June 17, 1989.
76. Davis LT, Duffy DM. Determination of incidence and risk factors for post-sclerotherapy telangiectatic matting of the lower extremity: A retrospective analysis. J Dermatol Surg Oncol 16:327-330, 1990.
77. Bodian EL. Sclerotherapy. Semin Dermatol 6:238-248, 1987.
78. Ouvry P, Davy A. Le traitement sclérosant des telangiectasies des membres inférieurs. Phlebologie 35:349-359, 1982.
79. Merlen JF. Telangiectasies rouges, telangiectasies bleues. Phlebologie 23:167-174, 1970.
80. Biegeleisen K. Primary lower extremity telangiectasias, relationship of size to color. Angiology 38:760-768, 1987.
81. Shing Y, Folkman J, Haudenschild C. Angiogenesis is stimulated by tumor-derived endothelial cell growth factor. J Cell Biochem 29:275-287, 1985.
82. Ashton N. Corneal vascularization. In Duke-Elder S, Perkins ES, eds. The transparency of the cornea. Oxford: Blackwell Scientific Publications, 1960.
83. Haudenschild CC. Growth control of endothelial cells in atherogenesis and tumor angiogenesis. In Altura BM, ed. Advances in microcirculation, vol 9. Basel: Karger, 226-251, 1980.

84. Folkman J, Klagsbrun M. Angiogenic factors. Science 235:442-447, 1987.
85. Frater-Schroder M, Risaw W, Hallmann R, et al. Tumor necrosis factor type alpha, a potent inhibitor of endothelial cell growth in vitro, is angiogenic in vivo. Proc Natl Acad Sci USA 84:5277-5281, 1987.
85a. Ryan TJ. Factors influencing the growth of vascular endothelium in the skin. Br J Dermatol 82(Suppl 5):99-111, 1970.
86. Leibovitch SJ, Polverini PJ, Shapard HM, et al. Macrophage-induced angiogenesis is mediated by tumor necrosis factor-alpha. Nature 329:630-632, 1987.
87. Miyazono K, Okabe T, Urabe A. Purification and properties of an endothelial cell growth factor from human platelets. J Biol Chem 262:4098-4103, 1987.
88. Rothe MJ, Nowak M, Kerdel FA. The mast cell in health and disease. J Am Acad Dermatol 23:615-624, 1990.
89. Castellot JJ Jr, Kambe AM, Dobsen DE. Heparin potentiation of 3T3-adipocyte–stimulated angiogenesis: Mechanisms of action on endothelial cells. J Cell Physiol 127:323-329, 1986.
90. Barnhill RL, Wolf JE Jr. Angiogenesis and the skin. J Am Acad Dermatol 16:1226-1242, 1987.
91. Dvorak AM, Mihm MC Jr, Dvorak HF. Morphology of delayed-type hypersensitivity reactions in man. II. Ultrastructural alterations affecting the microvasculature and the tissue mast cells. Lab Invest 34:179-191, 1976.
92. Enerback L. Mast cells in rat gastrointestinal mucosa. I. Effects of fixation. Acta Pathol Microbiol Scand 66:289-302, 1966.
93. Mikhail GR, Miller-Milinska A. Mast cell population in human skin. J Invest Dermatol 43: 249-254, 1964.
94. Mantse L. More on spider veins. J Dermatol Surg Oncol 12:1022-1023, 1986.
95. Lary BG. Varicose veins and intracutaneous telangiectasia: Combined treatment in 1500 cases. South Med J 80:1105-1110, 1987.
96. Corbett DA. Discussion. Br J Dermatol 26:200, 1914.
97. Bean WB. The vascular spider in pregnancy. In Bean WB, ed. Vascular Spiders and Related Lesions of the Skin. Springfield, Ill.: Charles C Thomas, 1958, pp 59-78.
98. Pirovino M, et al. Cutaneous spider nevi in liver cirrhosis: Capillary microscopical and hormonal investigation. Klin Wochenschr 66:298-302, 1988.
99. Sadick NS, Niedt GW. A study of estrogen and progesterone receptors in spider telangiectasias of the lower extremities. J Dermatol Surg Oncol 16:620-623, 1990.
100. Saski GH, Pang CY, Wittcliff JL. Pathogenesis and treatment of infant skin strawberry hemangiomas: Clinical and in vitro studies of normal effects. Plast Reconstr Surg 73:359-370, 1984.
101. Goldman MP, Fitzpatrick RE. Pulsed-dye laser treatment of leg telangiectasia: With and without simultaneous sclerotherapy. J Dermatol Surg Oncol 16:338-344, 1990.
102. Azizkhan RG, Azizkhan JC, Zetter BR. Mast cell heparin stimulates migration of capillary endothelial cells in vitro. J Exp Med 152:931-944, 1980.
103. Taylor S, Folkman J. Protamine is an inhibitor of angiogenesis. Nature 297:307-312, 1982.
104. Folkman J, Weisz PB, Joullie MM. Control of angiogenesis with synthetic heparin substitutes. Science 243:1490-1493, 1989.
105. de Takats G, Quint H. The injection treatment of varicose veins. Surg Gynecol Obstet 50: 545-561, 1930.
106. Chou F-F, Chen M-F, Jan Y-Y. The treatment of leg varicose veins with hypertonic saline–heparin injections. J Formosan Med Assoc 83:206-210, 1984.
107. Carlin MC, Ratz JL. Treatment of telangiectasia: Comparison of sclerosing agents. J Dermatol Surg Oncol 13:1181-1184, 1987.
108. Alderman DB. Therapy for essential cutaneous telangiectasias. Postgrad Med 61:91-95, 1977.
109. Orbach EJ. The importance of removal of postinjection coagula during the course of sclerotherapy of varicose veins. Vasa 3:475-477, 1974.
110. Orbach EJ. A new approach to the sclerotherapy of varicose veins. Angiology 1:302-305, 1950.
111. Fegan WG. Varicose veins—Compression sclerotherapy [film]. Produced by Pharmaceutical Research Limited, Hereford, England.

112. Tournay R. Collections hématiques intra ou extra-veineuses dans les phlébites superficielles ou après injections sclérosantes de varices a quel moment la thrombectomie? Soc Fran Phlebol 19:339-342, 1966.
113. Sigg K. Varizenverödung am hochgelgerten Bein. Deutsches Arzteblatt—Ärztliche Mitteilungen. 69. Jahrgang, Heft 14, S. 809-818. 6. April 1972. Postverlagsort Koln.
114. Pratt D. The technique of injection and compression. Stoke Mandeville Hospital Symposium: The treatment of varicose veins by injection and compression. Oct. 15, 1971, pp 23-27.
115. Hobbs JT. The management of recurrent and residual veins. Stoke Mandeville Hospital Symposium: The treatment of varicose veins by injection and compression, Oct. 15, 1971, pp 28-31.
116. Holzegel VK. Über Krampfaderverödungen. Dermatol Wochenschr 153:137-142, 1967.
117. Winstone N. The treatment of varicose veins by injection and compression. In Proceedings of the Stoke Mandeville Symposium. Hereford, England; Pharmaceutical Research STD Ltd., 1971, p 41.
118. Browse NL, Burnard KG, Thomas ML. Diseases of the Veins: Pathology, Diagnosis, and Treatment. London: Edward Arnold, 1988, pp 242-243.
119. Duffy DM. Personal communication, 1989.
120. Schraibman IG. Localized hirsuties. Postgrad Med J 43:545-547, 1967.
121. Marks G. Localized hirsuties following compression sclerotherapy with sodium tetradecyl sulphate. Br J Surg 61:127-128, 1974.
122. Weissberg D. Treatment of varicose veins by compression sclerotherapy. Surg Gynecol Obstet 151:353-356, 1980.

Chapter 15

Complications of Sclerotherapy Treatment of Varicose and Telangiectatic Leg Veins*

Mitchel P. Goldman

Sclerotherapy, like any therapeutic technique, carries with it the potential for adverse sequelae and complications. Although relatively rare, the complications include systemic allergic reactions, localized cutaneous necrosis, arterial injection, superficial thrombophlebitis, pulmonary embolism/deep vein thrombosis, nerve damage, and air embolism. This chapter addresses the pathophysiology of these reactions, methods for reducing their incidence, and treatment of their occurrence.

SYSTEMIC ALLERGIC REACTIONS

Sclerotherapy treatment of varicose and telangiectatic leg veins is safe and effective. Fortunately, both minor and major systemic allergic reactions to sclerotherapy treatment occur only rarely.

Minor Reactions

A minor reaction such as urticaria can be treated easily with an oral antihistamine, for example, diphenhydramine (Benadryl; Parke-Davis, Morris Plains, N.J.) 25 to 50 mg by mouth, or hydroxyzine (Atarax; Roerig, New York, N.Y.) 10 to 25 mg by mouth. Rarely, it might be necessary also to administer corticosteroids if the reaction does not subside readily. A short course of prednisone, 40 to 60 mg per day for 1 week, in conjunction with the administration of a systemic antihistamine every 6 to 8 hours, would be helpful. Since suppression of the adrenal axis is not a problem with this type of short course, a tapering schedule would not be necessary.

Because of the possibility of angioedema or bronchospasm, each patient with evidence of an allergic reaction should be examined for stridor and wheezing.

*From Goldman MP. Sclerotherapy: Treatment of Varicose and Telangiectatic Leg Veins. St. Louis: Mosby–Year Book, Inc., 1991. Reprinted and updated with permission.

Auscultation should be done over the neck and chest while the patient breathes normally. With the patient in the supine and sitting positions, blood pressure and pulse should be checked to rule out orthostatic changes, hypotension, or tachycardia, which might result from the vasodilation that precedes anaphylactic shock.

Patients with a minor degree of angioedema can be treated with oral antihistamines. However, if stridor is present, an intramuscular injection of diphenhydramine should be given, and intravenous corticosteroids should be administered. In addition, a laryngoscope and endotracheal tube should be available.

Bronchospasm is estimated to occur after sclerotherapy in 0.001% of patients.[1] A patient with this reaction usually responds to the addition of an inhaled bronchodilator or intravenous aminophylline, 6 mg/kg over 20 minutes, to the antihistamine/corticosteroid regimen already described.

Coverman[2] has reported that wheezing occurred in up to 5% of patients treated with hypertonic saline. He noted that the wheezing occurring 15 minutes after sclerotherapy had been completed but it resolved spontaneously. Coverman also found that if treatment is performed with the patient sitting at a 45-degree angle, wheezing can be aborted. In most instances, wheezing is probably not an allergic reaction but a manifestation of irritation of the airways. Alternatively, wheezing may be related to rapid infusion of histamine from perivascular mast cell degranulation associated with damage from the hyperosmotic solution.

Major Reactions

Four types of potentially serious systemic reactions specific to the type of sclerosing agent used have been noted: anaphylaxis, pulmonary toxicity, cardiac toxicity, and renal toxicity. These reactions will be discussed both in a general way and separately in relation to each sclerosing solution.

Anaphylaxis is a systemic hypersensitivity response caused by exposure or, more commonly, reexposure to a sensitizing substance. Anaphylaxis is usually an IgE-mediated, mast cell–activated reaction that occurs most often within minutes of antigen exposure. Other classes of immunoglobulin such as IgG also may produce anaphylaxis.[3] Since the risk of anaphylaxis increases with repeated exposure to the antigen, the physician should be prepared for this reaction in every patient.[4]

The principal manifestations of anaphylaxis occur in areas where mast cell concentrations are highest: skin, lungs, and gastrointestinal tract. Histamine release is responsible for the clinical manifestations of this reaction. Although urticaria and abdominal pain are common signs, the three principal manifestations of anaphylaxis are airway edema, bronchospasm, and vascular collapse. Urticaria alone does not constitute anaphylaxis; it should not be treated as such because of the potential side effects of treatment with epinephrine, especially in older patients.

Initially, the signs and symptoms of anaphylaxis may be subtle. They commonly include anxiety, itching, sneezing, coughing, urticaria, and angioedema. Wheezing may be accompanied by hoarseness and vomiting. Shortly after these presenting signs have appeared, breathing becomes more difficult, and the patient usually collapses from cardiovascular failure caused by systemic vasodilation. One helpful clue for distinguishing anaphylaxis from a vasovagal reaction is heart rate. Sinus tachycardia is almost always present in anaphylaxis, whereas bradycardia or cardiac rhythm disturbances are commonplace in vasovagal reactions.

The recommended treatment for anaphylaxis is epinephrine 0.2 to 0.5 ml 1:1000 administered subcutaneously. This dose can be repeated three to four times at 5- to 15-minute intervals to maintain a systolic blood pressure above 90 to 100 mm Hg. After administration of epinephrine, an intravenous line of 0.9% sodium chloride should be established. Next, diphenhydramine hydrochloride 50 mg is given along with cimetidine 300 mg; both the intravenous fluids and oxygen are administered at 4 to 6 L/min. An endotracheal tube or a tracheostomy is necessary when laryngeal obstruction is present. For asthma or wheezing, intravenous theophylline 4 to 6 mg/kg is infused over 15 minutes. At this point it is appropriate to transfer the patient to the hospital. Methylprednisolone sodium succinate 60 mg is given intravenously, and this dose is repeated every 6 hours for a total of four doses. Corticosteroids are not used as emergency medication since their effect appears only after 1 to 3 hours. They are given 3 to 8 hours after the initial event to prevent the recurrence of symptoms. The patient with anaphylaxis should be hospitalized overnight for observation.

Allergic Reactions to Sclerosing Agents

Sodium morrhuate. Although described by the manufacturer as a natural sclerosing agent, sodium morrhuate causes a variety of allergic reactions, including mild erythema with pruritus,[5-7] generalized urticaria,[7-9] gastrointestinal disturbances with abdominal pain and diarrhea,[5,6] and anaphylaxis. It has been estimated that "unfavorable reactions" occur in 3% of patients.[10] The high number of allergic reactions associated with this product may be related to the fact that it is impossible to remove all the fish proteins that are present in sodium morrhuate. In fact, 20.8% of the fatty acid composition of the solution is unknown.[11]

Many instances of anaphylaxis have occurred a few minutes after injection of sodium morrhuate, but such reactions are noted more commonly when therapy is reinstituted after a few weeks.[7,12-14] Most of the cases described occurred before 1950. In rare instances, the anaphylaxis has resulted in fatalities,[8,10,15] many of which have not been reported in the medical literature.[5]

Pleural effusions with pulmonary edema and acute respiratory failure (appearing as adult respiratory distress syndrome) are common with esophageal injection of sodium morrhuate.[11] It has been estimated that pleural effusions occur in 46% of patients who have esophageal injection.[16] With injection into esophageal varices, the sclerosing solution rapidly enters the pulmonary circulation, causing increased permeability of the pulmonary microvasculature.[11] There have been no reports of pleural effusions associated with injection into varicose veins of the legs.

Prolonged dysrhythmia that requires permanent placement of a cardiac pacemaker has been reported in two cases.[17] This complication has been described as a direct cardiotoxic effect of sodium morrhuate.

Ethanolamine oleate. Ethanolamine oleate (Ethamolin; Reed & Carnrick, Jersey City, N.J.) is a synthetic mixture of ethanolamine and oleic acid with an empirical formula of $C_{20}H_{41}NO_3$. The minimal lethal intravenous dose in rabbits is 130 mg/kg.[9] The oleic acid component is responsible for the inflammatory action. Oleic acid also may activate coagulation in vitro by release of tissue factor and Hageman factor. Ethanolamine was first reported in the medical literature as an ideal sclerosing agent by Biegeleisen[18] in 1937. He observed no toxic effects in 500 injections. Ethanolamine is thought to involve a lesser risk of allergic reactions in comparison with sodium morrhuate or STS.[19] However, pulmonary toxicity and allergic reactions have been associated with ethanolamine oleate.

Pleural effusion, edema, infiltration, and pneumonitis have been demonstrated in human trials with injection of esophageal varices. The product manufacturer has estimated that pleural effusion or infiltration occurs in 2.1% of patients; pneumonitis, in 1.2% of patients. One study of 75 patients treated for esophageal varices disclosed abnormal chest x-ray films showing infiltration or effusion in 45 patients, an incidence of 60%.[20] These conditions usually resolve spontaneously within 48 hours.

Anaphylactic shock has been reported by the product manufacturer after injection in three cases (Product information, 1989, Glaxo Pharmaceuticals, Research Triangle Park, N.C.). Another case of a nearly fatal anaphylactic reaction during the fourth treatment of varicose leg veins with 1 ml of solution also has been reported.[21] In another case a fatal reaction occurred in a man with a known allergic disposition (Product information, 1989, Glaxo Pharmaceuticals, Research Triangle Park, N.C.). One episode of a fatal anaphylactic reaction occurred in a woman having her third series of injections.[5] This episode represented one reaction in 200 patients from that author's practice. Generalized urticaria occurred in 1 of 400 patients, and the affected patient responded rapidly to administration of an antihistamine.[22]

Acute renal failure with spontaneous recovery occurred after injection of 15 to 20 ml of Ethamolin in two women.[23] A hemolytic reaction was noted in 5 patients in a series of more than 900 patients, with injection of >12 ml of 0.5% ethanolamine oleate per patient per treatment session.[22] The patients were described as "feeling generally unwell and shivery, with aching in the loins and passage of red-brown urine. All rapidly recovered with bed rest and were perfectly normal the next day." Injections of <12 ml per treatment session have not resulted in this type of reaction.

Transient chest pain also has been reported in 13 of 23 patients treated for esophageal varices.[24] However, pyrexia and substernal chest pain are said to be common sequelae of esophageal varicosis injection with any sclerosing agent.[19]

Ethanolamine oleate also has been tested for carcinogenic activity through intradermal injection in the albino rat, and the result was no induction of tumors.[25]

Sodium tetradecyl sulfate. A synthetic detergent developed in the 1940s, sodium tetradecyl sulfate (STS) is used throughout the world as a sclerosing solution. A comprehensive review of the medical literature in multiple specialties and languages disclosed a total of 47 cases of nonfatal allergic reactions in a review of 14,404 treated patients. This review included six case reports.[26] A separate review of treatment in 187 patients with 2249 injections disclosed no evidence of allergic or systemic reactions.[27] An additional report of 5341 injections given to an unknown number of patients found "no unfavorable reaction."[28] From January to July of 1991, the Clinical Drug Safety Surveillance Group of Wyeth-Ayerst Laboratories disclosed one episode of erythema multiforme; one episode of adult respiratory distress syndrome; one episode of fever, lymphadenopathy, and rash; and three episodes of abdominal pain, nausea, vomiting, and diarrhea.[29] If reviews of more than 1000 patients are combined, the incidence of nonfatal allergic reactions is approximately 0.3%.[22,30-33]

Fegan[34] has reviewed his experience with STS in 16,000 patients. He reported 15 cases of "serum sickness, with hot stinging pain in the skin, and an erythematous rash developing 30 to 90 minutes after injection." These patients subsequently underwent additional uneventful treatment with STS after premedication with antihistamines. Ten additional patients developed "mild anaphylaxis" that required treatment with an injection of epinephrine.

The product manufacturer has noted two fatalities associated with the use of STS. One fatality occurred in a patient who was receiving an antiovulatory agent. Another death (fatal pulmonary embolism) was reported in a 36-year-old woman who was not taking oral contraceptives.

Since all reported cases of allergic reactions are of the IgE-mediated immediate-hypersensitivity type, it is recommended that patients remain in or near the office for 30 minutes after sclerotherapy when STS is used. However, patients also may develop allergic reactions hours or days after the procedure.[33,35] For example, urticaria occurred 8 hours after treatment in one patient[36] and 2 weeks after treatment in two other patients.[33] Therefore patients should be warned about the possibility of allergic reactions and how to obtain care if a reaction should occur. An additional case report of erythema multiforme was reported in a woman after her thirteenth sclerotherapy treatment.[36] The patient developed pruritus the morning after the last injection, and a generalized eruption began to appear on the legs 4 days later. This eruption was followed by fever the next day. A rapid tapering course of oral prednisone was given, and complete resolution of the rash was noted in 2 weeks. This was the first report of erythema multiforme to STS reported in the literature or to the manufacturer.[37]

In a review of 2300 patients treated throughout 16 years, four cases of allergic reactions were reported (0.17% incidence).[38] Reactions in this study were described as periorbital swelling in one patient and urticaria in three. All reactions were easily treated with oral antihistamines. It is of interest that French phlebologists advocate a 3-days-before/3-days-after treatment course with an antihistamine. Flurie has noted no episodes of allergic reactions in 500 patients treated in this manner.[39]

As of January 1990, a total of 37 reports of adverse reactions had been reported to the FDA's Drug Experience Monitoring Program. However, this information cannot be used to estimate the incidence of adverse drug reactions since there was no central reporting agency before August 1985. A review of these adverse reactions was remarkable because five cases of suspected anaphylaxis and two cases of asthma induced by injection were reported. One of the cases of anaphylaxis resulted in death (see following discussion). Numerous reports of cutaneous necrosis also were reported along with a number of other nonspecific "complications." A review of the available notes on the complications were remarkable for the poor technique and inexperience on the part of the treating physician. In addition, on review it was unclear to me whether anaphylaxis actually occurred in every reported case.

In 1990 a fatality (noted above) was reported that occurred after a test dose of 0.5 ml of STS 0.5% was given to a 64-year-old woman.[40] An autopsy performed by the Hennipin County coroner's office revealed no obvious cause of death. Subsequently, mast cell tryptase studies were performed on blood collected approximately 1 hour after the reaction, while the patient was on life-support systems. A normal tryptase level is <5 ng/ml; in experimental anaphylactic reactions induced in the laboratory, levels up to 80 ng/ml have been noted. In this patient the levels were extremely high (6000 ng/ml), which suggested that an anaphylactoid reaction had caused her death. Unfortunately, tryptase levels are experimental at this time, and it is unclear how such a high level could be obtained. Therefore it is also unclear whether fatal anaphylaxis is a significant possibility with STS.

In short, anaphylaxis has been reported only rarely.[41,42] The most common systemic reaction consists of transient low-grade fever and chills lasting up to 24 hours after treatment. This reaction also has been noted in one of my patients. Of note is that three patients with allergic systemic reactions to ethanolamine oleate had no evidence of allergy to STS.[43]

A hemolytic reaction occurred in 5 patients in a series of more than 900 patients with injection of >8 ml of STS 3%.[22] As with a similar reaction that occurred with ethanolamine oleate, patients were described as "feeling generally unwell and shivery, with aching in the loins and passage of red-brown urine. All rapidly recovered with bed rest and were perfectly normal the next day." Injections of <8 ml per treatment session did not result in this type of reaction. Intravascular hemolysis also was reported to the FDA after injection of STS into a hepatic artery feeding a hepatic tumor.

The intravenous median lethal dose (LD_{50}) in mice is 90 mg/kg.[42] The lethal volume after intravenous injection in the rat is about four to six times as high for STS as for POL in equivalent concentrations.[42]

Polidocanol. Allergic reactions to polidocanol (POL) have been reported in only four patients in a review of the world's literature with an estimated incidence of 0.01%.[26] Amblard[44] reported no allergic reactions in more than 250 patients, even in two patients who were intolerant of STS. Hoffer[45] reported no allergic reactions in more than 19,000 cases. In addition, patients who are allergic to STS or iodine have no allergic manifestations to injections of POL.[44,46,47] However, rare allergic reactions to POL have been reported, including a case of nonfatal anaphylactic shock after 1 ml of POL 2% was injected into a varicose vein during the fourth treatment session.[39,48-50] Also, Ouvry et al.[51] reported on a patient who developed generalized urticaria with cough and dyspnea after receiving 2 ml of POL 2%; the condition resolved in 30 minutes with intravenous administration of corticosteroids. Recently, three cases of anaphylaxis (nonfatal) were reported in the Netherlands. Two of the patients had received the drug for the first time.[52]

Jaquier and Loretan[53] believe that the decrease in antigenicity is the result of the absence of a benzene nucleus and a paramine group and the presence of a single free alcohol group. The product manufacturer in France recommends that this substance not be used in subjects with an allergic diathesis (e.g., asthma) (Product information and oral personal communication, 1985, Dexo SA Pharmaceuticals, France). However, the product manufacturer in Germany states that there are no contraindications that arise from the product itself (Product insert, 1986, Chemische Fabrik Kreussler & Co. GmbH, Germany). Thus allergic reactions to POL are much rarer than those reported with STS.

Like ethanolamine oleate and sodium morrhuate, POL has demonstrated a dose-dependent cardiac toxicity when injected into esophageal varices. POL has a negative inotropic effect and reduces atrioventricular and intraventricular conduction. Animal studies demonstrate a reversible, dose-dependent decrease in myocardial contractility, blood pressure, and pulse rate and a prolongation of the P-Q interval.[54] This effect may explain the etiology of heart failure in three elderly patients with severe liver failure who were given massive quantities of POL during esophageal sclerotherapy (760 mg in a 74-year-old woman; 600 mg in a 70-year-old woman; 750 mg in a 76-year-old woman).[55,56]

The LD_{50} in rabbits at 2 hours is 0.2 g/kg, which is three to six times greater than the LD_{50} for procaine hydrochloride.[57] The LD_{50} in mice is 1.2 g/kg.[58] The systemic toxicity is similar to that of lidocaine and procaine.[59]

Chromated glycerin. Chromated glycerin 72% (Scleremo) is a sclerosing solution that has a very low incidence of side effects (Product information, 1987, Laboratories E. Bouteille, 7 Rue des Belges, Limoges 8100, France).[60-62] Hypersensitivity is a very rare complication with Scleremo.[62,63] Hematuria accompanied by ureteral colic can occur transiently after injection of large doses of the solution. Ocular manifestations, including blurred vision and a partial visual field loss, with resolution in less than 2 hours have been reported by one author.[64]

An additional case has been reported of transient hypertension and visual disturbance after the injection of 12 ml of 50% Scleremo into spider and "feeder" leg veins in a fourth treatment session. These symptoms occurred 2½ hours after treatment and lasted over a 3-hour period without treatment. They may have represented a retinal spasm or an ophthalmic migraine.[65]

Polyiodide iodine. Polyiodide iodine (Varigloban; Chemische Fabrik Kreussler & Co. GmbH, Wiesbaden-Biebrich, Germany); Variglobin (Globopharm, Zurich, Switzerland); Sclerodine 6 (Omega; Montreal, Canada) is a stabilized water solution of iodide ions, sodium iodine, and benzyl alcohol. Sigg et al.[66] reported on their experience in treatment with more than 400,000 injections of Variglobin. Paravenous injections readily produced tissue necrosis. In 1975, Sigg and Zelikovski[67] reported an incidence of side effects of 1.25 per 1000 injections, 0.13 per 1000 allergic cutaneous reactions, 0.04 per 1000 instances of localized necrosis, and 1 per 1000 instances of varicophlebitis. No systemic allergic reactions were observed. Obvious contraindications to the use of polyiodide iodine are hyperthyroidism and allergies to iodine and benzyl alcohol.

Iodine solutions also may produce bronchiomucosal lesions if used in high concentration. Therefore Wenner[68] has recommended that a maximum of 5 ml of 12% solution be used in a single sclerosing session.

Hypertonic saline. In itself, hypertonic saline shows no evidence of allergenicity or toxicity. Complications that may arise from its specific use include (1) hypertension, which may be exacerbated in predisposed patients when an excessive sodium load is given; (2) sudden hypernatremia; (3) central nervous system disorders; (4) extensive hemolysis; and (5) cortical necrosis of the kidneys.[69] These complications and others led one manufacturer (American Regent Laboratories, Shirley, N.Y.) to add to its label the warning "FOR IV OR SC USE AFTER DILUTION" in bold red ink.

Dodd[70] has reported painless hematuria in five patients injected with hypertonic saline. Sometimes blood appears in the urine after one to two acts of micturition or at other times throughout the day. Usually no other ill effects are noted, and the hematuria resolves spontaneously. Hematuria probably occurs because of hemolysis of red blood cells during sclerotherapy.

Coverman[71] has described two patients injected with up to 6 ml of hypertonic saline 23.4% who developed "peculiar visual symptoms in just one eye" that were manifest as either blurred vision or an aura. No other symptoms were present, and each incidence of symptoms passed quickly and spontaneously. Coverman has speculated that these complications may have been caused by the addition of lidocaine to the hypertonic saline solution.

Heparin in hypertonic saline. Although many physicians use unadulterated hypertonic saline solutions in concentrations from 15% to 30% for the treatment of varicose and telangiectatic leg veins, the addition of heparin to the solution to prevent the theoretical risk of embolization associated with sclerotherapy has been advocated.[72] Although the necessity for heparin has been discounted in a well-controlled randomized study involving 800 patients,[73] Foley's solution (Heparsal), consisting of hypertonic saline 20% with heparin 100 U/ml and procaine 1%, is commonly used in the treatment of telangiectatic leg veins. Therefore the risk of adverse reactions to heparin should be noted.

Commercial preparations of heparin consist of straight-chain anionic polysaccharides of variable molecular weight (usually 7000 to 40,000). Heparin prepared from different tissues also appears to vary: more protamine is required to neutralize a unit of beef lung heparin than porcine mucosal heparin. Plasma lipolytic activity, antifactor Xa activity, and activated partial thromboplastin time ratios are significantly different.[74]

Fever, urticaria, and anaphylaxis occur occasionally after administration of heparin.[74-78] Necrosis has been reported in patients receiving subcutaneous heparin.[66,79-82] It usually occurred 3 to 10 days after multiple subcutaneous injections. Pruritus, local tenderness, and burning sensations associated with large, indurated erythematous plaques also were reported to occur in six patients 10 to 20 days after the beginning of administration of prophylactic doses of heparin.[83] Therefore a measurable risk of toxicity to heparin is present.

Although heparin is not a totally benign substance, there have been no reports by those who use Heparsal of any adverse reactions that could be attributed to the heparin component.[1,72,73,84] In fact, the absence of side effects has been reported when volumes of 10 to 20 ml were injected into varicose veins in a series of 310 patients.[84] Therefore, in the doses used, heparin in Heparsal may produce no significant side effects, but one must be aware of the potential dangers associated with its use.

Lidocaine in hypertonic saline. Alderman[30] and Duffy[1] have advocated the addition of lidocaine (to achieve a 0.4% final concentration) to minimize patient discomfort during injection of hypertonic saline. This addition means that the

A 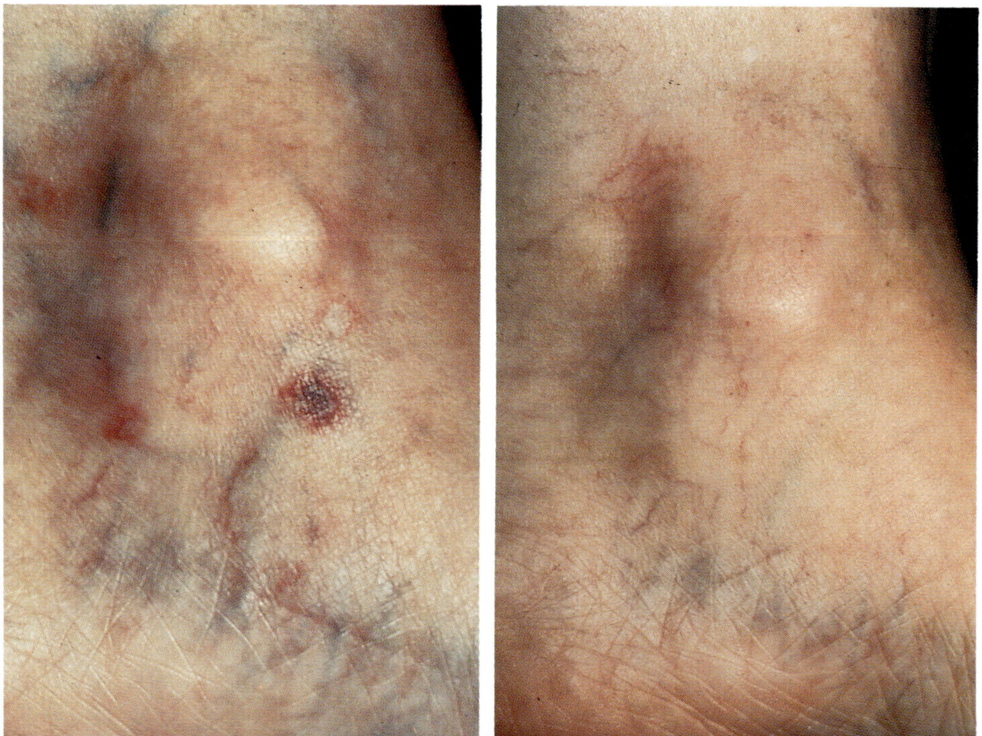 B

FIGURE 15-1. Cutaneous necrosis after injection with STS 0.25%. **A**, Condition 3 weeks after injection. **B**, Complete resolution of necrosis after 20 months.

sclerosing mixture has the potential to be allergenic. Although the most common etiologies of a previous allergic reaction to lidocaine involve psychogenic or vasovagal reactions,[85] allergic reactions may occur.

Despite the low risk of allergenicity to lidocaine, multiple allergic reactions, including anaphylaxis, have been reported.[86-93] Therefore hypertonic solution, when adulterated with lidocaine, may place the patient at risk for allergic reactions.

The amide class of anesthetics has a very low risk of allergic reaction.[94-99] Allergy is most likely caused by the methylparabens or sodium metabisulfite that is used as a preservative in the anesthetic solutions.[94,95,100-102] Therefore, to keep the allergic risk as low as possible, one should use single-dose vials of lidocaine without preservatives.

CUTANEOUS NECROSIS

Etiology

Cutaneous necrosis can occur with the injection of any sclerosing agent (Figures 15-1 and 15-2). Its cause may be the result of (1) extravasation of a sclerosing

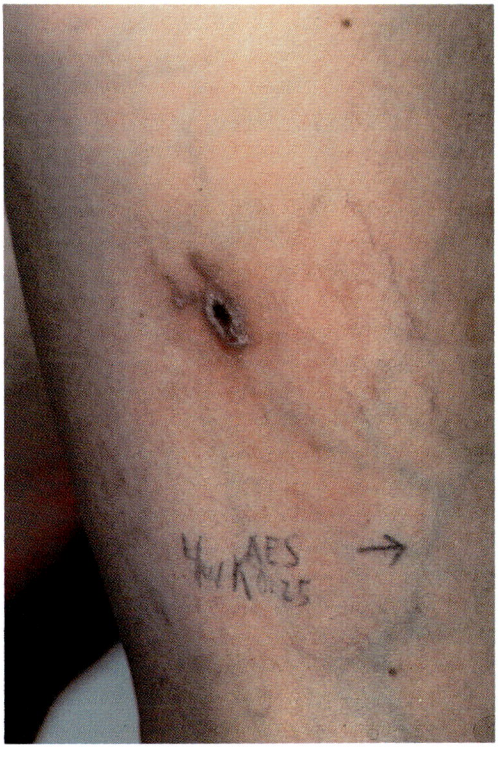

FIGURE 15-2. Cutaneous necrosis 6 weeks after sclerotherapy with POL 0.25%. Note that 2 ml of solution was injected into a feeder vein (arrow) approximately 10 cm distal to necrotic area.

solution into the perivascular tissues, (2) injection into a dermal arteriole or an arteriole feeding into a telangiectatic or varicose vein, (3) a reactive vasospasm of the vessel, or (4) excessive cutaneous pressure created by compression techniques.

Extravasation

Extravasation of caustic sclerosing solutions can directly destroy tissue. During injection of an abnormal vein or a telangiectasia, even the most adept physician may inadvertently inject a small quantity of sclerosing solution into the perivascular tissue (Figure 15-3). A tiny amount of sclerosing solution may be left in the tissue when the needle is withdrawn, and sclerosing solution can leak out of the injected vessel, which has been traumatized by multiple or through-and-through needle punctures. In rare instances, the injection of a strong sclerosing solution into a fragile vessel can lead to endothelial necrosis and rupture, producing a "blow-out" of the vessel and perivascular extravasation of sclerosing solution. Therefore injection technique is an important, but not a foolproof, factor in avoiding this complication, even under optimal circumstances.

Sclerosing solutions vary in the degree of cellular necrosis they produce. If minimal tissue necrosis is caused by a sclerosing agent, that agent may even be suitable for perivascular injection in the treatment of telangiectatic mats, the vessels of which cannot be cannulated with a 33-gauge needle.

Hypertonic saline 23.4% is a caustic sclerosing agent, as demonstrated in intradermal injection experiments. Clinically, small punctate spots of superficial epidermal damage occur at points of injection, especially when a small bleb of the solution escapes from the vein. However, subcutaneous injection of up to 1 ml of hypertonic saline 23.4% (done by mistake) in lieu of lidocaine into the neck or cheek

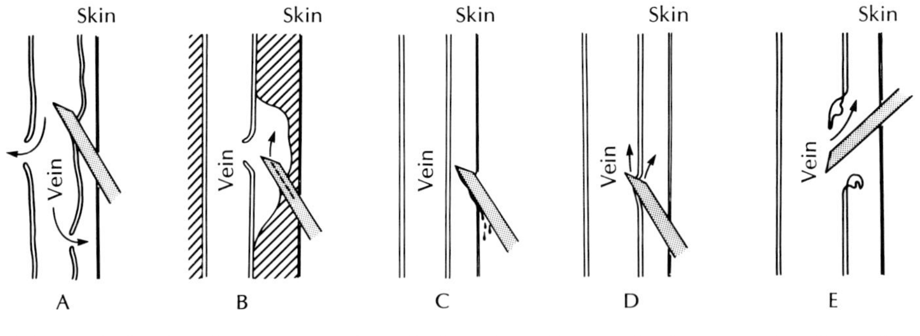

FIGURE 15-3. Mechanism for extravasation of sclerosing solution. **A,** Extravasation through multiple needle puncture holes. **B,** Extravasation from injection of solution after slight withdrawal of needle. **C,** Extravasation of solution along needle shaft. **D,** Extravasation from injection with needle bevel both in and out of vein. **E,** Extravasation through excessive destruction of vein wall. (Redrawn from Biegeleisen HI. Varicose Veins, Related Diseases, and Sclerotherapy: A Guide for Practitioners. Montreal: Eden Press, 1984. From Goldman MP. Sclerotherapy: Treatment of Varicose and Telangiectatic Leg Veins. St. Louis: Mosby–Year Book, Inc., 1991, p 241.)

has been reported to result in no adverse sequelae.[103] In such a situation, cutaneous necrosis is most likely avoided by rapid physiologic dilution of hypertonic saline. Alternatively, dermal tissue may be more resistant to the caustic effects of hypertonic solutions. However, the increasing frequency with which cutaneous necrosis occurs after extravasation of inadvertent subcutaneous injection of hypertonic saline has prompted the Department of Health and Human Services and the product manufacturer to recommend that storage of hypertonic saline be in pharmacies where all dilutions are performed just prior to dispensing. This practice would eliminate the possibility of an iatrogenic medication error outside the pharmacy.[69]

Based on experimental study, POL appears to be the sclerosing agent that is least toxic to subcutaneous tissue. Jaquier and Loretan[53] and Hoffer[46] have advocated the use of intradermal POL 0.5% in the treatment of telangiectatic leg veins smaller than the diameter of a 30-gauge needle and have reported no evidence of cutaneous necrosis. However, in sufficient concentration, POL has been reported to cause cutaneous necrosis. Solutions of POL >1.0% may produce superficial necrosis when intradermal injection is done.[53] Unfortunately, this result occurred in my practice when 0.1 ml of POL 5% solution was mistakenly injected into a leg telangiectasia that was 0.2 mm in diameter. This injection resulted in extensive overlying cutaneous necrosis, which took 8 weeks to heal. Therefore POL is not without the risk of cutaneous necrosis if a strong enough concentration is injected.

Chromated glycerin solutions have not been reported to produce cutaneous necrosis with extravasation. Duffy[104] has shown that injection of "full strength" Scleremo will not produce cutaneous necrosis when it is injected into the middle dermis. Histologic examination of Duffy's patient showed no evidence of dermal or epidermal damage.

However, even when sclerotherapy is performed with expert technique and the safest sclerosing solutions and concentrations are used, cutaneous ulceration may occur. Therefore it appears that extravasation of caustic sclerosing solutions alone is not totally responsible for this complication.

Arteriolar Injection

De Faria and Moraes[105] have observed that 1 in 26 leg telangiectasias are associated with a dermal arteriole. I hypothesize that inadvertent injection either into or near this communication is the most common cause of cutaneous ulceration.

POL has been injected intradermally to effect sclerosis of telangiectatic matting in my practice without the development of cutaneous ulceration, even with the injection of 0.5 ml of a 0.75% solution. However, I have noted the development of 3 to 6 mm diameter ulcerations in approximately 0.0001% of injections with POL 0.5% (Figure 15-4). Five consecutive ulcerations that appeared over the course of 12 months were excised. In these patients each cutaneous ulceration developed as a result of the occlusion of the feeding dermal arteriole. This occlusion produced a classic wedge-shaped arterial ulceration (Figure 15-5). Therefore it appears that this complication may be unavoidable to some extent.

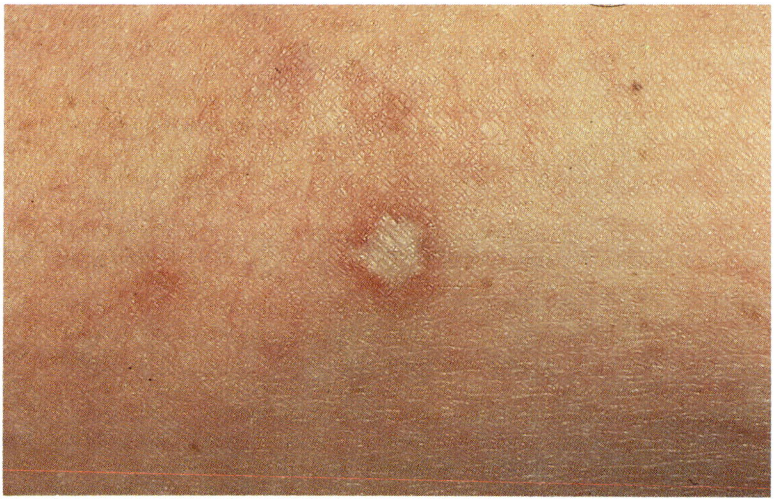

FIGURE 15-4. Porcelain-white cutaneous reaction immediately after injection with POL 0.5% in upper lateral thigh. Frank cutaneous ulceration later developed in this area. (From Goldman MP. Sclerotherapy: Treatment of Varicose and Telangiectatic Leg Veins. St. Louis: Mosby–Year Book, Inc., 1991, p 245.)

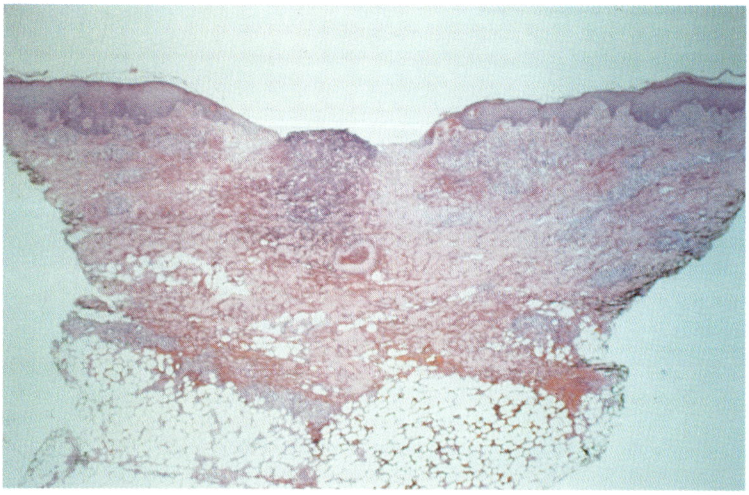

FIGURE 15-5. Low-power magnification view showing arterial ulceration and focal inflammation extending into subcutaneous fat. A thrombosed vessel, most likely an artery, is present directly under area of necrosis (hematoxylin-eosin ×25). (From Goldman MP. Sclerotherapy: Treatment of Varicose and Telangiectatic Leg Veins. St. Louis: Mosby–Year Book, Inc., 1991, p 243.)

Vasospasm

Rarely, after injection of the sclerosing solution, a porcelain-white appearance to the skin is immediately noted at the site of injection (Figure 15-6). A hemorrhagic bulla usually forms over this area within 2 to 48 hours (Figure 15-7) and then progresses to an ulcer.[106] This cutaneous reaction might represent an arterial spasm.

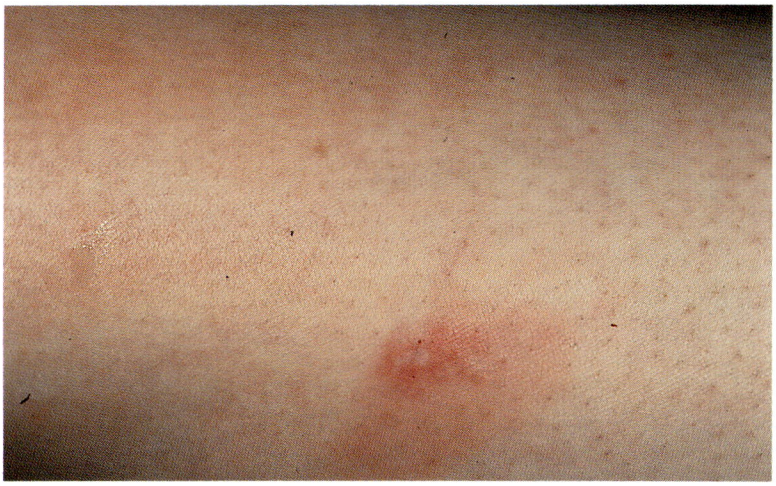

FIGURE 15-6. Porcelain-white cutaneous reaction immediately after injection with POL 0.25%. This area healed within 4 weeks without any complication. (From Goldman MP. Sclerotherapy: Treatment of Varicose and Telangiectatic Leg Veins. St. Louis: Mosby–Year Book, Inc., 1991, p 244.)

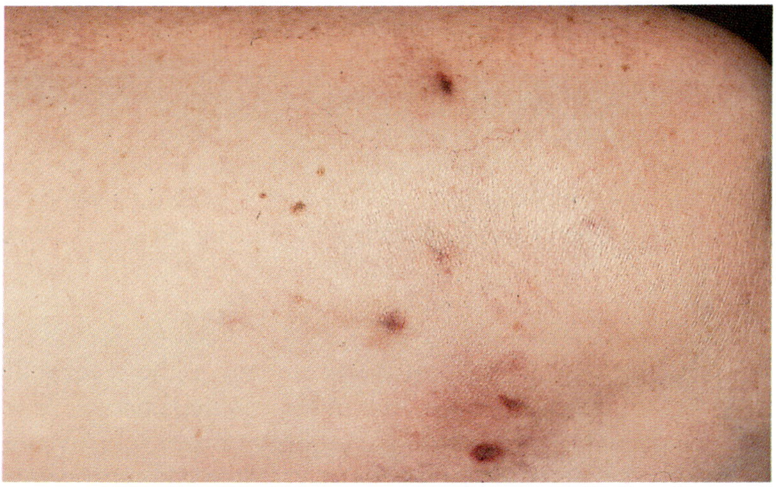

FIGURE 15-7. Hemorrhagic bulla, a macular reaction 1 week after injection with POL 0.5%. This area healed without any complication. (From Goldman MP. Sclerotherapy: Treatment of Varicose and Telangiectatic Leg Veins. St. Louis: Mosby–Year Book, Inc., 1991, p 244.)

In an attempt to reverse the spasm, I have performed vigorous massage when the white macule appears and in this way sometimes ulceration has been averted. However, the prevention of ulceration through massage alone is not always successful (see Figure 15-4). Massaging with nitroglycerin ointment 2% (generic) is an alternative method of preventing ulceration.

The major systemic action of nitrates is a direct reduction in venous smooth muscle tone.[107] Nitrates also relieve spasm of angiographically normal and diseased arteries.[108] Topical nitroglycerin ointment has been reported to be beneficial in the treatment of both dopamine extravasation and vasoconstriction necrosis.[109,110] Although more experience from other investigators needs to be reported, it seems prudent to use this technique.

Arterial spasm also may explain the development of cutaneous ulceration upstream from the injection site (see Figure 15-2). In the case illustrated in the figure, 2 ml of POL 0.25% was injected into a feeding reticular vein, as shown by the arrow. This was the only injection given to the patient in the sclerotherapy session.

Lymphatic Injection

Injection into a lymphatic vessel may lead to cutaneous necrosis. Histologic studies have disclosed evidence of lymphovenous anastomoses in humans.[111] It is possible for injection into such an anastomosis to result in necrosis of the associated lymphatic vessel and infiltration of the sclerosing solution extravascularly. If the sclerosing solution is caustic to extravascular tissues, use of the solution may result in tissue necrosis.

Excessive Compression

Finally, excessive compression of the skin overlying the treated vein may produce tissue anoxia with the development of localized cutaneous ulceration. Subcutaneous tissue flow in the leg is decreased when cutaneous pressure exceeds 20 mm Hg.[112] In addition, external pressure >30 mm Hg reduces muscle blood flow in some patients.[113] Therefore excessive compression may produce tissue ischemia. However, both of the above-mentioned studies employed indirect measurements of subcutaneous tissue flow and calf muscle blood flow and thus need to be viewed with caution. A more physiologic method for measuring the effect of compression on blood flow was recently performed through determination of femoral blood flow.[114] The authors demonstrated that in the recumbent patient, static, graduated, external compression of approximately 20 mm Hg at the ankle, reduced to approximately 10 mm Hg in the upper thigh, produces an increase in femoral flow of up to 75%. However, if calf pressures exceed 30 mm Hg when the patient is recumbent, a progressive fall in subcutaneous tissue flow and deep venous velocity occurs. Therefore it is recommended that patients not wear a graduated compression stocking of >30 to 40 mm Hg when lying down for prolonged periods.

One method of applying compression to treated veins that can be varied with patient position is using a double layer of graduated compression stockings. This practice ensures that maximal pressure over the vein is maintained while the patient is ambulatory. When the patient is recumbent, the outer stocking is removed, thereby decreasing the cutaneous pressure to 20 to 30 mm Hg at the ankle, which should prevent a reduction in cutaneous and subcutaneous blood flow.

Prevention

If extravasation of sclerosing solution occurs, the solution must be diluted immediately. Hypertonic solutions should be diluted with copious amounts of normal saline. At least 10 times the volume of extravasated solution should be injected in order to limit osmotic damage.

Detergent sclerosing solutions of adequate strength also may be toxic to tissues. Again, dilution is of paramount importance. In addition, experimental studies have shown that the addition of hyaluronidase (150 U/ml) to normal saline as the diluent significantly improves clinical outcome.[115] This preliminary report deserves further review. Finally, the optimal concentration of hyaluronidase needs to be determined.

Treatment

Whatever the cause of the ulceration, the complication must be dealt with when it occurs. Fortunately, ulcerations, when they do occur, are usually fairly small. In my practice, they average 4 mm in diameter. At this size, primary healing usually leaves an acceptable scar. Bodian,[116] who uses 23.4% hypertonic saline, notes that ulceration usually takes 3½ months to heal even when judicious wound care is given. He advocates treatment with daily application of 20% benzoyl peroxide powder (Vanoxide-HC Acne Lotion; Dermik Laboratories, Blue Bell, Pa.) under moist dressings cut to fit snugly over the ulcer. However, benzoyl peroxide is cytotoxic for newly growing epidermis. Therefore its use cannot be recommended. I have found that occlusive or hydrocolloid dressings result in an apparent decrease in wound healing time. Occlusive dressings do not speed healing of full-thickness ulcers until granulation tissue has formed. Therefore dressings such as Duoderm (Convatec, Princeton, N.J.) may be useful. Duoderm also has been shown to enhance debridement of wounds, possibly through its pectin-gelatin base. Non-gelatin, non-pectin hydrocolloid dressings act only to stimulate fibrin lysis. Thus their enhanced efficacy may be related to wound debridement, which always should be done medically or surgically to promote granulation tissue formation.

More important, occlusive dressings decrease the pain associated with an open ulcer. However, because an ulcer may take 4 to 6 weeks to heal completely, even under ideal conditions, if possible, excision and closure of these lesions are recommended at the earliest possible time. This method affords the patient the fastest healing and an acceptable scar.

ARTERIAL INJECTION

The most feared complication in sclerotherapy is inadvertent injection into an artery. Fortunately, this complication is very rare.[117-119] Five examples of arterial injection had been reported to the Medical Defense Union in Great Britain by 1985.[120] Cockett[121] has reported 18 cases, including those which were reported to the two medical protection societies in the United Kingdom over a 10-year period. However, Cockett believes that this number is too low because many cases occur but never reach the courts or the medical literature.

Arterial injection of a sclerosing solution causes the development of an embolus. This result has been confirmed experimentally in the canine femoral artery.[35] The experiments demonstrate little effect on the artery itself through injection. Spasm does not occur. The sclerosing solution acts to denature blood in smaller arteries, producing a sludge embolus, which obstructs the microcirculation. Stagnant blood flow, secondary thrombosis, and necrosis soon follow.

Occlusion of small arteries may lead to the development of a compartmental syndrome. Intracompartmental pressures of 30 mm Hg or more in humans usually produce neural deficits characterized by pain during stretching of the muscles involved, paresthesia, and then paresis and anesthesia in the sensory distribution of the nerve that courses through the affected compartment. The final result is paralysis.[36] Sensory deficit in the first web space (deep peroneal nerve) implicates anterior compartmental syndrome. Sensory deficit on the dorsum of the foot (superficial peroneal nerve) implicates the lateral compartment. The superficial posterior compartment is indicated by sensory deficit of the sural nerve distribution (lateral foot). Deep compartmental syndrome is likely if the sole of the foot is affected (posterior tibial nerve).

Unless large arteries are blocked, peripheral pulses will be intact and capillary filling can be identified easily since the compartmental pressure must be greater than 80 mm Hg to occlude large artery flow.[122] This apparent normalcy may lull the physician into a false sense of security, and the underlying compartmental syndrome may not be recognized. Intracompartmental pressures from 30 to 40 mm Hg lasting for 6 to 12 hours can cause irreversible damage to the nervous tissue caused by impairment of microcirculation.[36]

Etiology

Arterial injection occurs most commonly in the posterior or medial malleolar region, particularly during an attempt to inject the internal ankle perforating vein, specifically in the posterior tibial artery.[119,121,123,124] The patient will usually, but not always, note immediate pain. The pain slowly extends down into the foot and the outer toes during the following 2 to 6 hours. During this time arterial pedal pulses are palpable. Ten to 12 hours later, the four outer toes become white and the sole of the foot becomes painful to touch. Cutaneous blanching of the injected area usually occurs in an arterial pattern associated with a loss of pulse and progressive cyanosis of the injected area.

Another area where the artery and veins are in close proximity is the junction of the femoral artery and greater saphenous vein. A review of one sclerotherapy practice throughout 20 years disclosed two cases of accidental arterial injection in this area that required thigh amputations.[125] In this location the external pudendal artery may pass anterior or posterior to the greater saphenous vein slightly beyond the point of its connection with the femoral vein. In addition, the junction of the short saphenous vein with the popliteal vein has been demonstrated to have a tortuous and variably located satellite arteriole.[126] Because the collateral arteries vary anatomically in these locations, it may be useful to perform duplex scanning before sclerosing these vessels.

Finally, with the onset of duplex-assisted sclerotherapy, small arteries in superficial and deep aspects of the thigh and the calf have been injected inadvertently. The usual sequelae are loss of tissue and nerve damage. Color flow duplex scanning and the use of open needles for injection of these difficult areas is recommended. Obviously, a physician should be present at all times to give immediate treatment if needed.

Prevention and Treatment

Arterial injection is a true emergency. The extent of cutaneous necrosis usually is related to the amount of solution injected. Although therapeutic efforts to treat this complication are usually unsatisfactory, they should be attempted.[119] Hobbs[128] recommends that on realization of arterial injection, blood and sclerosing solution should be aspirated back into the syringe to empty the needle of solution. In addition, aspiration of the injected artery as rapidly and completely as possible may help to remove the injected sclerosing solution if the action is performed immediately. The needle should not be withdrawn, but the syringe should be replaced with one containing 10,000 U of heparin, which should be injected slowly into the artery. Unfortunately, this maneuver is difficult to accomplish since the patient is usually in considerable pain and finds it difficult to hold still.

Perhaps a more practical treatment is periarterial infiltration with procaine 3%, 1 ml, which will complex with STS and render it inactive.[123,124] The patient's foot should be cooled with ice packs to minimize tissue anoxia. Recommended are (1) immediate heparinization, to be continued for 6 days, and (2) intravenous administration of dextran 10%, 500 ml per dose, for 3 days. Intravenous administration of streptokinase also may be considered if there are no contraindications to its use. Finally, the use of oral prazosin, hydralazine, or nifedipine for 30 days should be considered. However, Cockett[121] has found that treatment delayed for more than 1 hour has no effect in limiting damage to the foot.

Recently, a favorable resolution of arterial injection occurred with injection of tissue-type plasminogen activator.[129] In this case promazine was injected into an artery. Heparin, axillary plexus blockade, and intravenous sodium nitroprusside were not successful. Brachial artery injection of tissue-type plasminogen activator (Actilyse, 50 mg over 8 hours) resulted in therapeutic efficacy. Therefore local fibrinolytic therapy should be considered if conservative treatments prove ineffective.

Given the known relationship of injection site to the development of this problem, the necessity for injecting vessels in the vicinity of the medial malleolus must be considered carefully. In this regard, there is an interesting report in the

British Medical Journal[117] about a legal case brought against a physician for performing such an injection, which resulted in a transmetatarsal amputation. The judgment was made in favor of the physician after several renowned sclerotherapists stated that if the patient would benefit from the injection it should be attempted since the risks are infrequent and the benefits are significant.

Prevention of the dreaded complication of arterial injection is best accomplished by visualization of the blood emanating from the needle. If it is pulsatile and continues to flow after the leg is horizontal, injection should not be attempted at this site. Mantse[33] has advised that when the medial malleolar area is being treated, placement of the sclerosing needle should be done while the patient is standing so that the varix will be bulged and the distance between the artery and the vein increased.

Theoretically, visualization of arteries and veins with duplex-assisted sclerotherapy should negate this risk. Indeed, newer color flow duplex imagers allow visualization of minute arteries and veins. However, a number of arterial ulcerations have occurred with this technique, even when the site of injection was the posterior calf, gastrocnemius, and saphenofemoral junctional varicose veins. Therefore no technique is fully free from this complication.

SUPERFICIAL THROMBOPHLEBITIS

Before the advent of modern-day sclerotherapy, which employs graduated compression to limit thrombosis, thrombophlebitis, both superficial and deep, occurred in a significant number of sclerotherapy patients.[130] In fact, it was commonly thought that phlebitis was so common a sequela of sclerotherapy that there was doubt about whether this form of therapy was legitimate.[131] With the use of compression therapy and the realization that many adverse effects resulted from thrombus formation in treated veins, the incidence of thrombophlebitis greatly decreased.

It is important to note that certain patients may be predisposed to the development of thrombophlebitis. Fegan[123] has stated that this complication occurs more commonly if perforator veins in the region of treatment are undiagnosed and not treated.

Etiology

One to three weeks after injection, superficial thrombophlebitis appears as a tender erythematous induration over the injected vein (Figure 15-8). Duffy[1] has estimated that it occurs in 0.5% of his patients. Mantse[33] reported an incidence of 1% in the treatment of varicose (nontelangiectatic) veins despite the use of a tensor bandage for 6 weeks. Mantse noted that the patients who developed superficial thrombophlebitis found the bandage to be too tight and reapplied it too loosely at home. In my experience this complication occurs to some degree in approximately 0.01% of patients. Severe cases, requiring treatment with compression therapy and anti-inflammatory agents, occur very rarely (less than 0.001% of patients).

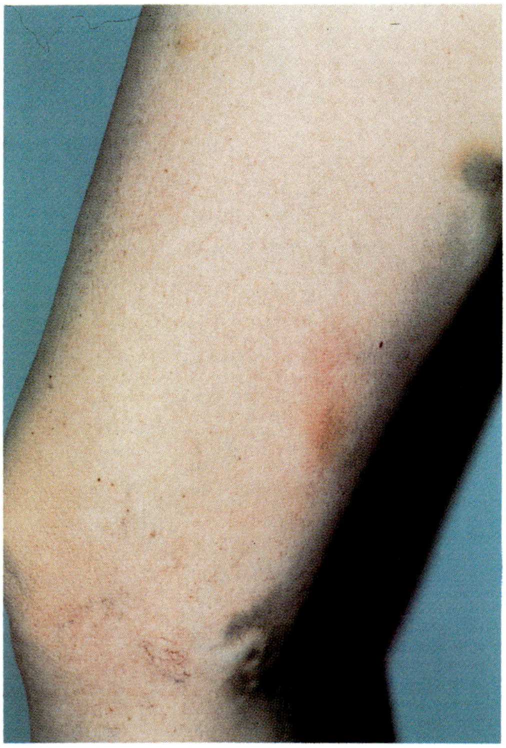

FIGURE 15-8. Superficial thrombophlebitis developed in this patient 14 days after sclerotherapy with STS 0.5%. Note ecchymosis (arrow) from compression padding and graduated-support stocking, worn for only 1 week on upper medial/posterior thigh.

Prevention and Treatment

The decreased incidence in my practice may be the result of the greater degree and length of compression used in the treatment of all injected veins. Indeed, the cause of thrombophlebitis is related in part to treatment technique. An inadequate degree or length of compression results in excessive intravascular thrombosis. Sigg[132] has noted that perivenous inflammation is observed only at those parts of the limb that are not covered by a compression dressing. Thus, to avoid this complication, one should prevent or minimize the development of postsclerosis thrombosis through the use of compression pads and compression hosiery.

However, even when appropriate compression is used over treated varicose veins, thrombosis and perivascular inflammation may occur. Ascending phlebitis in the long saphenous vein or its long tributaries that starts at the upper edge of the compression stocking is relatively common. At this point the sclerosing action continues up the abnormal vessel, even beyond what appears to be the extent of the abnormality. It is thought that the sclerosing solution destroys damaged endothelium to a greater extent than normal endothelium (Product description of Hydroxypolyethoxydodecane, May 1985). Therefore the placement of a Sorbo pad extending above the compression stocking or bandage to create a gradual transition of pressure from compressed to noncompressed vein may provide a safety margin. Also, this may prevent damage to the vein by the otherwise abrupt cutoff of the pressure stocking.

In addition to adequate compression, drainage of thrombi (after liquefication occurs) 2 weeks after sclerotherapy will hasten resolution of the otherwise slow, painful resorption process.[132]

Thrombophlebitis is a complication that should not be taken lightly. If untreated, the inflammation and clot may spread to perforating veins and the deep venous system, which leads to valvular damage and possible pulmonary embolic events. Therefore, when thrombophlebitis occurs, the thrombus should be evacuated, adequate compression should be applied, and frequent ambulation should be maintained until the pain and inflammation resolve. Aspirin or other nonsteroidal anti-inflammatory agents may be helpful in limiting both the inflammation and the pain.

PULMONARY EMBOLISM/DEEP VENOUS THROMBOSIS

Pulmonary emboli (PE) and deep vein thrombosis (DVT) very rarely occur as a complication of sclerotherapy. In the 1930s and 1940s, PE following sclerotherapy of varicose veins occurred in, at most, 0.14% of patients.[133,134] In a series of 45,000 injections given to 7500 patients, only one episode of PE was reported.[135] In 1928, Sicard reported 325,000 injections without a pulmonary infarction.[136] Linser and Vohwinkel[137] reported four cases of PE after 75,000 injections, only one of which was fatal. More recently, with the use of compression techniques in combination with sclerotherapy, this complication has become even less common. Sigg[138] has reported the occurrence of PE only once in 42,000 injections. A French vascular surgeon who treats approximately 75 sclerotherapy patients a week, amounting to 25,000 yearly injections, reported only one case of PE in 20 years.[118] Fegan[34] has reported that he has never seen conclusive evidence of DVT occurring after the injection treatment of 16,000 patients in his clinic.

The clinical diagnosis of DVT is accurate only 50% of the time as compared to fibrinogen scanning.[139] Venous Doppler examination has a 30% to 96% accuracy, depending on the experience of the investigator.[140-142] Likewise, impedance phlebography has a 40% accuracy.[142] Therefore the incidence for the development of DVT after sclerotherapy treatment may be low. To more accurately evaluate incidence, 13 patients undergoing compression sclerotherapy with Fegan's technique were studied with continuous-screening ascending venography. Not more than 1 ml of 3% STS was injected, with the total amount not exceeding 5 ml. Patients were seen in follow-up 1 week later for comparison venography. No patients developed radiographic evidence of DVT.[143]

Etiology

The cause of DVT, with or without PE after sclerotherapy, is unclear. The three major factors responsible for DVT were first elucidated more than 100 years ago by Virchow: (1) endothelial damage, (2) vascular stasis, and (3) changes in coagulability.[144] Sclerotherapy treatment always produces the first two factors. Changes in coagulability are related to the unique properties of sclerosing solutions and any predisposing factors of the patient.

Chemical endophlebitis produced by sclerotherapy should anchor the thrombus to the site of injection. Histologic examination of treated varicose veins has demonstrated that firm thrombosis occurs only on the abnormal endothelium. Nonadherent thrombosis occurs on normal endothelium.[145] Therefore the most logical explanation for the development of emboli is damage to the deep venous system by migration of sclerosing solution or a partly attached thrombosis into deep veins from superficial veins as a result of either injection of excessive volumes of sclerosing solution or physical inactivity after injection.[146]

An additional possibility concerns injection of tributary communicating veins, which may directly communicate with the deep venous system. In this situation inadequate compression or injection of even 0.5 ml of sclerosing solution may force early clots into the deep circulation with muscle contraction. Ascending venography and digital subtraction phlebography performed on 15 women with leg telangiectasias demonstrated spread of 0.7 ml of contrast medium from the telangiectatic branches into the saphenous system in eight patients.[147] Two of the eight patients had telangiectasia as the only perceptible abnormality. Therefore it is possible that up to 13% of patients with superficial varicose and telangiectatic veins are at risk for spread of sclerosing solution directly into the deep venous system. This finding further emphasizes the importance of limiting injection volumes.

Amount of Injection

Through radiography, the circulation and direction of blood flow in varicose veins has been determined to be stagnant or reversed (away from the heart) so that the chemically induced thrombus is forced distally toward the smaller branching veins.[148] However, cinematographic studies have documented that a small amount of sclerosing solution entered the deep circulation after injection of between 0.5 and 1 ml of solution into a superficial varicosity in seven of 15 injections given to nine subjects.[149] Fortunately, no adverse effects were noted in these patients, who were treated with POL 2%. The lack of adverse effects was probably related to rapid compression and ambulation of treated individuals and to the resulting rapid dilution of the sclerosing agent within the deep venous system. In addition, venographic evaluation of injection of 0.5 to 1 ml of sclerosing solution in 15 patients with incompetent perforating veins failed to demonstrate extension of radiocontrast media into the deep venous system.[143] However, DVT and embolic episodes usually occur 4 to 28 days after the sclerotherapy treatment session.[133] Therefore longer follow-up is necessary. Although DVT and PE have been reported to occur with injection of large quantities of sclerosing solution (12 ml) in a single site,[150] two case reports of these complications occurring with injection of <0.5 ml of POL 1% have been published.[151] In the latter cases, the veins injected were leg telangiectasias. In addition, Reid and Rothine[22] reported that the injection of 0.5 to 1 ml of sclerosing solution above the midthigh resulted in a presumed thrombus at the saphenofemoral junction and pulmonary emboli. Consequently, they recommended that injections not be given above the midthigh.

Therefore it is important to limit the quantity of sclerosing solution per injection site to ensure that the agent will remain within the superficial system and to rapidly stimulate blood flow in the deep venous system after sclerotherapy through compression and muscle movement.

Finally, an additional study involving the use of impedance plethysmography and Doppler ultrasonic examination was performed before and after sclerotherapy done with the classic Fegan technique in the treatment of 67 legs.[152] This study showed that there were no alterations in deep venous blood flow at 1 and 2 weeks after injection treatment. This finding confirmed the clinical experience that sclerotherapy done with the Fegan technique is highly unlikely to be complicated by the development of DVT.

Inappropriate Compression

The inappropriate tourniquet effect of an excessively tight wrap in the thigh has been noted as a rare cause for the development of DVT.[153] In the case described, occlusion of deep venous flow resulted in popliteal vein thrombosis. This condition resolved with conservative treatment. The adverse effects of nongraduated compression emphasize the importance of properly fitted graduated support stockings in sclerotherapy treatment.

Hypercoagulable States

A number of primary and secondary hypercoagulable states can be ruled out through an appropriate patient history and a review of systems in the presclerotherapy treatment evaluation (see box, p. 313). The prevalence of inherited thrombotic syndromes in the general population is 1 in 2500 to 5000, but it increases to 4% in patients with a history of thrombosis.[154] A discussion of all hypercoagulable states is beyond the scope of this chapter, but the most common states will be addressed. The reader is referred to review articles on this important subject.[154-156]

Oral Contraceptive Agents

The mechanism for thromboembolic disease in women who use oral contraceptives is multifactorial. Both estrogens and progestogens have been implicated in promoting thrombosis despite low-dose therapy.[157-159] All studies have indicated that the increased risk occurs while the preparations are actually being taken and perhaps for 1 week or longer after discontinuation.[160,161] The highest rates of

CONDITIONS AND FACTORS ASSOCIATED WITH HYPERCOAGULABLE STATES*

Primary Hypercoagulable State

Deficiency in inhibitors of coagulation
Antithrombin III deficiency
Protein C deficiency
Protein S deficiency
Disorders of fibrinolytic system
Plasminogen deficiency
Plasminogen activator excess
Dysfibrinogenemias
Vascular damage (homocystinuria)
Platelet damage (paroxysmal nocturnal hemoglobinuria)
Lupus anticoagulant

Secondary Hypercoagulable State

Abnormalities of coagulation and fibrinolysis
Pregnancy
Malignancy
Nephrotic syndrome
Oral contraceptives
Estrogen/progestin supplementation
Inflammatory bowel disease
Infectious diseases
Secondary syphilis
Psittacosis
Platelet abnormalities
Myeloproliferative disorders
Diabetes mellitus
Hyperlipidemia
Paroxysmal nocturnal hemoglobinuria
Lupus anticoagulant
Heparin-associated thrombocytopenia
Stasis or aberrant blood flow
Varicose veins
Congestive heart failure
Immobilization
Obesity
Advanced age
Perioperative state
Polycythemia vera, sickle cell disease
Dehydration
Paraproteinuria
Endothelial damage
Intravenous catheters
Intravenous solutions
Intravenous drug abuse
Vasculitis
Behçet's disease
Thromboangiitis obliterans

*Data from Thomas JH. Pathogenesis, diagnosis and treatment of thrombosis. Am J Surg 160:547-551, 1990; Samlaska CP, James WD. Superficial thrombophlebitis II. Secondary hypercoagulable states. J Am Acad Dermatol 23:1-18, 1990.

thromboembolism occur with higher levels of estrogen.[157-160,162] Some studies show an increase of elevenfold.[161,163] However, a detailed review of the statistical methodologies of these studies did not prove a *definite* risk.[164] Yet it seems prudent to examine the available literature on this topic.

It has been estimated that oral contraceptives are responsible for one case of superficial thrombophlebitis or DVT per 500 women users per year.[165] This estimate of hypercoagulability may be low since an examination of plasma fibrinogen chromatography has demonstrated a 27% incidence of silent thrombotic lesions in 154 new contraceptive users of either mestranol 100 μg or ethinyl estradiol 50 μg.[166] Oral contraceptive users as a group have numerous alterations in their coagulation system that promote a hypercoagulable state. These include hyperaggregable platelets, decreased endothelial fibrinolysis, decreased negative surface charge on vessel walls and blood cells,[167] elevated levels of procoagulants, reduced red cell filterability,[168] increased blood viscosity secondary to elevated red blood cell volume,[169] and decreased levels of antithrombin III.[170-172] Any of these factors, alone or in combination, may predominate in women taking oral contraceptives. The extent of this derangement in the hemostatic system determines whether thrombosis will occur. When endothelial damage is initiated with sclerotherapy in this population, an increased incidence of thrombosis may occur.

The most important factors preventing clot propagation are antithrombin III and vascular stores of tissue-type plasminogen activator (t-PA).[170,173-175] Antithrombin III levels have been demonstrated as 20% lower in some women taking oral contraceptive agents.[173] Of women using oral contraceptive agents who have thromboembolic events, 90% have a twenty-five–fold decrease in releasable t-PA.[170,173,174] An abnormally low plasminogen activator content in the vein walls is found in 51.6% of users. Therefore a certain subgroup of women taking birth control pills are at particular risk for thromboembolic disease.

In addition, increased distensibility of peripheral veins may occur with the use of systemic estrogens and progestins.[176] This change may promote valvular dysfunction and a relative stasis in blood flow that add to the hypercoagulable state. Since it is almost impossible, and also impractical, to determine which women are at risk, it seems prudent to recommend that patients consider discontinuing this medication before sclerotherapy treatment.

Tamoxifen. For several reasons, including prevention of breast cancer in high-risk populations, adjunctive treatment of breast cancer, and possibly treatment or prevention of osteoporosis, tamoxifen (Nolvadex; ICI Pharma, Wilmington, Del.) is not an uncommon medication in patients who also present for sclerotherapy and/or surgical treatment. An unusual and poorly understood complication of Tamoxifen use is the development of thrombophlebitis and DVT. This complication may occur in up to 1% of treated patients.[177,178] Evaluation of various coagulation parameters and factors, including sex hormone–binding globulin, antithrombin III fibrinogen level, platelet count, protein C, and fibrinopeptide A, have been normal.[178-181] Therefore, until more is known about this theoretical predisposing factor to thrombosis, the physician should take note of patients taking Tamoxifen.

Pregnancy

As early as 1579, it was common medical practice not to tamper with varicose veins in a pregnant patient.[182] However, some physicians advocate removal of varicose veins to prevent postpartum venous thrombosis.[183] These authors report a lack of complications to both mother and infant with this practice, even though treatment spanned the first through the eighth month of gestation. However, in addition to the possible effects on the fetus resulting from passage of sclerosing solution through the placental barrier, the potential for stimulating thrombosis exists.

Endothelial cell damage, presumably caused by sclerotherapy, releases tissue plasminogen activator to promote coagulability on the already formed clot, which invariably occurs in the immediate postsclerotherapy period.[184] In addition, coexistent hypercoagulability may promote excessive (uncontrolled) thrombosis.

The hypercoagulable state in the immediate antepartum period is largely responsible for the development of superficial thrombophlebitis and DVT in 0.15% and 0.04% of patients, respectively.[185] Even more important is the immediate postpartum period, during which the incidence of superficial thrombophlebitis and DVT is 1.18% and 0.15%, respectively.[185] DVT developed by postpartum day 2 in 50% of patients. This complication may have been caused by the rapid decrease in coagulation factors at partum that normalizes in most patients on postpartum day 3.[186] However, additional factors must play a role since an additional 21% developed DVT between 2 and 3 weeks postpartum. It is interesting to note that two thirds of the patients who developed postpartum DVT had varicose veins. The age of the mother also was linked to venous thrombosis, with the rate changing from approximately 1 in 1000 in women younger than 25 years of age to 1 in 200 in women older than 35.[162]

During pregnancy there is an increase in most procoagulant factors and a reduction in fibrinolytic activity. Decreased fibrinolytic activity is probably related to a decrease in circulating plasminogen activator.[187] In addition, a 68% reduction in protein S levels has been measured during pregnancy and in the postpartum period.[188] Protein S levels do not return to normal until 12 weeks postpartum. These changes are necessary to prevent hemorrhage during placental separation. Therefore sclerotherapy should be avoided until coagulability returns to normal 6 weeks postpartum.

Inherited Factor Deficiency

Another subgroup of patients is at an increased risk for DVT. Protein C and protein S are two vitamin K–dependent substances that are important anticoagulant factors in the prevention of thrombosis. Protein S is a cofactor for activated protein C on factor Va. It has been estimated that the prevalence of deficiency of heterozygous protein C may occur from 1 in 300 to 1 in 60 healthy adults in the United States.[189] Over 95% of these subjects are asymptomatic and have no history of thrombotic disease. However, the deficiencies may predispose these individuals to the development of DVT. Seventy-five percent of patients homozygote for protein S deficiency will develop venous thrombosis before age 35.[190] It has been speculated that damaged endothelium in combination with protein S deficiency may be necessary for symptomatic thrombosis to occur.[191] Therefore patients who exhibit excessive thrombosis as a result of sclerotherapy and patients who have a family history of thrombotic disease should be screened for deficiencies of protein C and protein S before treatment.

Antithrombin III deficiency occurs in between 1 in 2000 and 1 in 5000 in the general population.[192,193] Acquired antithrombin III deficiency may occur in association with liver disease and the use of oral contraceptives.

Defects in the fibrinolytic system, specifically plasminogen, may occur in up to 10% of the normal population.[194] Although by themselves such defects involve little risk of thrombosis, abnormal plasminogen may predispose an individual to thrombosis.

Lupuslike anticoagulants are present in 16% to 33% of patients with lupus erythematosus, but they also are associated with a variety of autoimmune disorders.[195-197] Thirty to fifty percent of patients with lupuslike anticoagulants develop a thrombosis.[197,198]

Prevention and treatment. Because of the potentially lethal nature of excessive thrombosis, all attempts should be made to minimize its occurrence. The quantity of sclerosing solution should be limited to 0.5 to 1 ml per injection site to prevent leakage of the solution into the deep venous system.[124] Other techniques that will minimize damage to the deep venous system include rapid compression of the injected vein with a 30 to 40 mm Hg pressure-gradient stocking followed by immediate ambulation or calf movement of the injected extremity and frequent ambulation thereafter to promote rapid dilution of the solution from the injected area. When these recommendations were followed, Fegan[199] reported no cases of DVT or pulmonary emboli in 13,352 patients if the sclerosing solution quantity was limited to 0.5 ml and rapid compression was used.

Fegan[123] has stated that STS is rapidly inactivated by the blood and that it is a hemolytic agent, not a thrombotic agent. Therefore he considers thrombosis to be an extremely rare complication associated with the use of this sclerosing agent. However, Fegan does recommend against treatment with STS in women who are taking oral contraceptive agents because of a theoretical increase in thromboembolic events.

Foley[200] has advocated the addition of heparin, 100 U/ml, to hypertonic saline to prevent the theoretical possibility of embolization associated with "microthrombus formation" in sclerotherapy. However, a well-controlled, randomized study of 800 patients treated with and without heparin in the sclerosing solution noted no evidence of embolization and no difference in the incidence of thrombophlebitis or microthrombosis requiring puncture evacuation.[169]

NERVE DAMAGE

Because of their close proximity to veins, the saphenous and sural nerves may be inadvertently injected with solution during sclerotherapy. Injection into a nerve is reported to be very painful; if continued, it may cause anesthesia and even a permanent interruption of nerve function.[201]

Occasionally, a patient may complain of an area of paresthesia in the treated leg. This sensation is probably caused by perivascular inflammation extending from the sclerosed vein to adjacent superficial nerves. Steps to limit inflammation, including the use of nonsteroidal anti-inflammatory medications and high-potency topical steroids, may hasten resolution of this minor annoyance. However, this complication may take 3 to 6 months to resolve.[34]

AIR EMBOLISM

When the air-block[202,203] or the foam technique is used to inject the sclerosing solution, the possibility of air embolism is raised. The danger is that if enough air enters the heart at one time, the result might be vascular collapse. In addition, if air enters a cerebral vascular artery, a cerebral vascular infarction may occur. However, it is more likely that transient ischemic symptoms will occur with this injection technique.

The introduction of small amounts of air into the venous system does not lead to clinical air embolism.[202,203] It appears that small amounts of air are absorbed into the bloodstream before it enters the pulmonary circulation. It has been estimated that 480 ml of air would need to be put into the venous system within 20 to 30 seconds to cause death in a person weighing 60 kg.[204] Such an event has never been reported in the medical literature, and it has not occurred in a series of 297 cases in which the air-block technique was used.[202]

SUMMARY

Like any other invasive procedure, sclerotherapy of varicose and telangiectatic leg veins may be associated with certain complications. However, such complications are rare, and to some extent they may be avoidable. All patients should be evaluated and cautioned about the possible complications before treatment is begun. A summary of the complications that can occur with commonly used sclerosing agents is presented in Table 15-1.

TABLE 15-1. Summary of complications associated with use of sclerosing agents

Agent	Active Ingredient	Allergic Reaction	Necrosis	Pain
Sodium morrhuate*	Fatty acids in cod liver oil	Occasional	Frequent‡	Moderate
Sotradecol*	Sodium tetradecyl sulfate	Rare	Occasional‡	Mild
Ethamolin*	Ethanolamine oleate	Occasional	Rare‡	Mild
Polidocanol†	Hydroxypolyethoxy-dodecane	Very rare	Very rare‡	None
Hypertonic saline	10%-30% Saline	None	Occasional‡	Moderate
Sclerodex†	10% Saline and 5% dextrose	Very rare	Rare	Mild
Scleremo†	1.11% Chromated glycerin	Very rare	Very rare	Moderate
Variglobin†	Iodide, sodium iodine	Very rare	Frequent‡	Moderate

*Approved for use by the Food and Drug Administration.
†Not approved for use in the U.S.A.
‡Concentration-dependent, especially with extravasation.

REFERENCES

1. Duffy DM. Small vessel sclerotherapy: An overview. In Callen JP, et al., eds. Advances in Dermatology, vol 3. Chicago: Year Book Medical Publishers, Inc., 1988, pp 221-240.
2. Coverman M. Personal communication, 1991.
3. Beall GN, Casaburi R, Singer A. Anaphylaxis—Everyone's problem (Specialty Conference). West J Med 144:329-337, 1986.
4. Wasserman SI. Anaphylaxis. In Middleton E, Reed CE, Ellis EF, eds. Allergy: Principles and Practice, 2nd ed. St. Louis: CV Mosby, 1983, pp 689-699.
5. Shelley J. Allergic manifestations with injection treatment of varicose veins: Death following injection of monoethanolamine oleate. JAMA 112:1792-1794, 1939.
6. Schmier AA. Clinical comparison of sclerosing solutions in injection treatment of varicose veins. Am J Surg 36:389-397, 1937.
7. Zimmerman LM. Allergic-like reactions from sodium morrhuate in obliteration of varicose veins. JAMA 102:1216-1217, 1934.
8. Lewis KM. Anaphylaxis due to sodium morrhuate. JAMA 107:1298, 1936.
9. Meyer NE. Monoethanolamine oleate: A new chemical for obliteration of varicose veins. Am J Surg 40:628-629, 1938.
10. Dick ET. The treatment of varicose veins. N Z Med J 65:310-313, 1966.
11. Monroe P, Morrow C, Millen JE. Acute respiratory failure after sodium morrhuate esophageal sclerotherapy. Gastroenterology 85:693-699, 1983.
12. Dale ML. Reaction due to injection of sodium morrhuate. JAMA 108:718-719, 1937.
13. Ritchie A. The treatment of varicose veins during pregnancy. Edinburgh Med J 40:157-165, 1933.
14. Probstein JG. Major complications of intravenous therapy of varicose veins. J Missouri Med Assoc 33:349-353, 1936.
15. Dodd H, Oldham JB. Surgical treatment of varicose veins. Lancet 1:8-10, 1940.
16. Kilby A, Saks B, Dietrich P. Abnormal chest roentgenograms following endoscopic injection sclerosis of esophageal varices. Hepatology 2:709, 1982.
17. Perakos PG, Cirbus JJ, Camara S. Persistent bradyarrhythmia after sclerotherapy for esophageal varices. South Med J 77:531-532, 1984.
18. Biegeleisen HI. Fatty acid solutions for the injection treatment of varicose veins: Evaluation of four new solutions. Ann Surg 105:610-615, 1937.
19. Hedberg SE, Fowler DL, Ryan LR. Injection sclerotherapy of esophageal varices using ethanolamine oleate: A pilot study. Am J Surg 143:426-431, 1982.
20. Hughes RW Jr, Larsch DE, Viggiano TR. Endoscopic variceal sclerosis: A one-year experience. Gastrointest Endosc 28:62-66, 1982.
21. Foote RR. Severe reaction to monoethanolamine oleate. Lancet 2:390-395, 1944.
22. Reid RG, Rothine NG. Treatment of varicose veins by compression sclerotherapy. Br J Surg 55:889-895, 1968.
23. Maling TJB, Cretney MJ. Ethanolamine oleate and acute renal failure. N Z Med J 82:269, 1975.
24. Harris OD, Dickey JD, Stephenson PM. Simple endoscopic injection sclerotherapy of esophageal varices. Aust N Z J Med 12:131-135, 1982.
25. Shubik P, Hartwell JL. Survey of compounds which have been tested for carcinogenic activity. Washington, D.C.: U.S. Department of Health, Education, and Welfare, Public Health Service, 1969.
26. Goldman MP, Bennett RG. Treatment of telangiectasia: A review. J Am Acad Dermatol 17: 167-182, 1987.
27. Steinberg MH. Evaluation of Sotradecol in sclerotherapy of varicose veins. Angiology 6:519-532, 1955.
28. Nabatoff RA. Recent trends in the diagnosis and treatment of varicose veins. Surg Gynecol Obstet 90:521-528, 1950.
29. Minicozzi P [Wyeth-Ayerst Laboratories]. Personal communication, 1991.
30. Alderman DB. Surgery and sclerotherapy in the treatment of varicose veins. Conn Med 39: 467-471, 1975.

31. Wallois P. Incidents et accidents au cours du traitement sclérosant des varices et leur prévention. Phlebologie 24:217-220, 1971.
32. Mantse L. A mild sclerosing agent for telangiectasias. J Dermatol Surg Oncol 11:855, 1985.
33. Mantse L. The treatment of varicose veins with compression sclerotherapy: Technique, contraindications, complications. Am J Cosmet Surg 3:47-53, 1986.
34. Fegan G. Varicose veins: Compression sclerotherapy. London: Heinemann Medical, 1967.
35. Mubarak SJ, Owen CA, Hargens AR, et al. Acute compartment syndromes: Diagnosis and treatment with the aid of the wick catheter. J Bone Joint Surg 178(60-A):1091-1095, 1978.
36. Shick LA, Laing K. Possible allergic reaction to agent used in sclerotherapy. Clin Cases Dermatol 4:2-5, 1992.
37. Ruane N [Wyeth-Ayerst Laboratories]. Personal communication, 1991.
38. Fronek H, Fronek A, Saltzbarg G. Allergic reactions to Sotradecol. J Dermatol Surg Oncol 15:684, 1989.
39. Passas H. One case of tetradecyl-sodium sulfate allergy with general symptoms. Soc Fran Phlebol 25:19-26, 1972.
40. Clinical Case 1. Presented at the Third Annual Meeting of the North American Society of Phlebology. Phoenix, Feb. 21, 1990.
41. Schneider W. Contribution à l'historique du traitement sclérosant des varices et à son étude anatomo-pathologique. Soc Fran Phlebol 18:117-130, 1965.
42. Reiner L. The activity of anionic surface active compounds in producing vascular obliteration. Proc Soc Exper Biol Med 62:49-54, 1940.
43. Dingwall JA, Lin W, Lyon JA. The use of sodium tetradecyl sulfate in the sclerosing treatments of varicose veins. Surgery 23:599-601, 1948.
44. Amblard P. Our experience with Aethoxysklerol. Phlebologie 30:213-215, 1977.
45. Hoffer AE. Aethoxysklerol (Kreussler) in the treatment of varices. Minerva Cardioangiologica 20:601-604, 1972.
46. Hartel S. Complications and side effects of sclerotherapy. Z Arztl Fortbild (Jena) 78:331-332, 1874.
47. Heberova V. Treatment of telangiectasias of the lower extremities by sclerotization: Results and evaluation. Czechoslovakia Dermatol 51:232-235, 1976.
48. Eichenberger H. Results of phlebosclerosation with hydroxypolyethoxydodecane. Zentralbl Phlebol 8:181-183, 1969.
49. Jakobsen BH. Aethoxysklerol: A new sclerosing agent for varicose veins. Ugeskr Laeger 136: 532-534, 1974.
50. Feuerstein W. Anaphylactic reaction to hydroxypolyaethoxydodecon. Vasa 2:292-294, 1973.
51. Ouvry P, Chandet A, Guillerot E. First impressions of Aethoxysklerol. Phlebologie 31:75-77, 1978.
52. Stricker BH, van Oijen JA, Kroon C, et al. Anaphylaxis following use of polidocanol. Nederlands Tijdschiff voor Geneeskunde 134:240-242, 1990.
53. Jaquier JJ, Loretan RM. Clinical trials of a new sclerosing agent, Aethoxysklerol. Soc Fran Phlebol 22:383-385, 1969.
54. Thies E, Lange V, Iven H. Cardiac effects of polidocanol, a sclerotherapeutic drug—experimental evaluations. Chirurgisches Forum 192:313-316, 1982.
55. Imperiali G, Terruzzi V, Spotti D. Heart failure as a side effect of polidocanol given for esophageal variceal sclerosis. Endoscopy 18:207, 1986.
56. Paterlini A, Salmi A, Buffoli F. Heart failure and endoscopic sclerotherapy of variceal bleeding. Lancet 2:1241, 1984.
57. Siems KJ, Soehring K. Die Ausschaltung sensibler Nerven duren peridurale und paravertebrale Injektion von Alkylpolyathylenoxydathern bei Meerschweinchen. Arzneimittel Forsche 2:109-111, 1952.
58. Soehring K, Scriba K, Frahm M. Beitrage zur Pharmakologie der alkylpolyathylenoxyd-Derivate I: Untersuchungen über die acute und subchronische Toxizität bei verschiedenen Tierarten. Arch Int Pharmacodyn 87:301-320, 1951.

59. Soehring K, Frahm M. Studies on the pharmacology of alkylpolyethyleneoxide derivatives. Arzneimittel Forsche 5:655-662, 1955.
60. Shields JL, Jansen GT. Therapy for superficial telangiectasias of the lower extremities. J Dermatol Surg Oncol 8:857-860, 1982.
61. Moreno AH, Katz AI, Gold LV. Mechanics of distention of dog veins and other thin-walled tubular structures. Circ Res 27:1069-1080, 1970.
62. Nguyen VB. Sclérotherapie des varices des membres inférieurs étude de 522 cas. La Saguency Médical 23:134-145, 1976.
63. Ouvry P, Davy A. Le traitement sclérosant des telangiectasies des membres inférieurs. Phlebologie 35:349-359, 1982.
64. Wallois P. Incidents et accidents de la sclérose. In Tournay R, ed. La Sclérose des Varices, 4th ed. Paris: Expansion Scientifique Française, 1985, pp 297-319.
65. Zimmet SE. Letter to the editor. J Dermatol Surg Oncol 16:1063, 1990.
66. Sigg K, Horodegen K, Bernbach H. Varizen-Sklerosierung: Welches ist das wirksamste Mittel? Deutsches Arzteblatt 34/35:2294-2298, 1986.
67. Sigg K, Zelikovski A. Kann die Sklerosierungotherapie der Varizen oben Operation in jedem Fall wirksam sein? Phlebol Proktol 4:42-54, 1975.
68. Wenner L. Anwendung einer mit Athylalkahol modifizierten Polijodidjonenlosung bei sklerose-resistenten Varizen. Vasa 12:190-192, 1982.
69. Helenek M [American Regent Laboratories, Inc.]. Personal communication, 1990.
70. Dodd H. The operation for varicose veins. Br Med J 2:510, 1945.
71. Coverman M. Personal communication, 1989.
72. Barner FR, Holzegel K, Voigt K. Über Hyperpigmentation nach Krampfaderverödung. Phlebol u Proktol 6:54-61, 1977.
73. Cuttell PJ, Fox JA. The etiology and treatment of varicose pigmentation. Phlebologie 35:387-389, 1982.
74. Anticoagulants. In Bennett R, ed. AMA Drug Evaluations, 5th ed. Chicago: American Medical Association, 1983, pp 821-822.
75. Zinn WJ. Side reactions of heparin in clinical practice. Am J Cardiol 14:36-38, 1964.
76. Gervin AS. Complications of heparin therapy. Surg Gynecol Obstet 140:789-796, 1975.
77. White PW, Sadd JR, Nensel RE. Thrombotic complications of heparin therapy, including six cases of heparin-induced skin necrosis. Ann Surg 190:595-608, 1979.
78. Dukes MNG, ed. Meyler's Side Effects of Drugs: An Encyclopaedia of Adverse Reactions and Interactions, 9th ed. Amsterdam: Excerpta Medica Foundation, 1980.
79. O'Toole RD. Heparin: Adverse reaction. Ann Int Med 79:759, 1973.
80. Hume M, Smith-Petersen M, Fremont-Smith P. Sensitivity to intrafat heparin. Lancet 1:261, 1974.
81. Hall JC, McConahay D, Gibson D. Heparin necrosis: An anticoagulation syndrome. JAMA 244:1831-1832, 1980.
82. Shelley WB, Ayen JJ. Heparin necrosis: An anticoagulant-induced cutaneous infarct. J Am Acad Dermatol 7:674-677, 1982.
83. Tuneu A, Moreno A, de Moragas JM. Cutaneous reactions secondary to heparin injections. J Am Acad Dermatol 12:1072-1077, 1985.
84. Chou F-F, Chen M-F, Jan Y-Y. The treatment of leg varicose veins with hypertonic saline–heparin injections. J Formosan Med Assoc 83:206-210, 1984.
85. DeShago RD, Nelson HS. An approach to the patient with a history of local anesthesia hypersensitivity: Experience with 90 patients. J Allergy Clin Immunol 63:387-394, 1979.
86. Kennedy KS, Cave RH. Anaphylactic reaction to lidocaine. Arch Otolaryngol Head Neck Surg 112:671-673, 1986.
87. Promisloff RA, Dupont DC. Death from ARDS and cardiovascular collapse following lidocaine administration. Chest 83:585, 1983.
88. Aldrete JA. Sensitivity to lidocaine. Anaesth Intensive Care 7:73-74, 1979.

89. Gill C, Michaelides PL. Dental drugs and anaphylactic reactions: Report of a case. Oral Surg 50:30-32, 1980.
90. Chin TM, Fellner MJ. Allergic hypersensitivity to lidocaine hydrochloride. Int J Dermatol 19:147-148, 1980.
91. Ravindranathan N. Allergic reaction to lidocaine: A case report. Br Dent J 111:101-102, 1975.
92. Lehner T. Lidocaine hypersensitivity. Lancet 1:1245-1246, 1971.
93. Fischer MM, Pennington JC. Allergy to local anaesthesia. Br J Anaesth 54:893-894, 1982.
94. de Jong RH. Local anesthetics, 2nd ed. Springfield, Ill.: Charles C Thomas, 1977.
95. Swanson JG. Assessment of allergy to local anesthetic. Ann Emerg Med 12:316-318, 1983.
96. de Jong RH. Toxic effects of local anesthetics. JAMA 239:1166-1168, 1978.
97. Incaudo G, Schatz M, Patterson R. Administration of local anesthesia to patients with a history of adverse reaction. J Allergy Clin Immunol 61:339-345, 1978.
98. Thomas RM. Local anesthetic agents and regional anesthesia of the face. J Assoc Military Dermatol 8:28-33, 1982.
99. Fregert S, Tegner E, Thelin I. Contact allergy to lidocaine. Contact Dermatitis 5:185-188, 1979.
100. Covino BG, Vassallo HG. Local Anesthetics: Mechanisms of Action and Clinical Use. New York: Grune & Stratton, 1976.
101. Eriksson E. Illustrated Handbook of Local Anesthesia, 2nd ed. Philadelphia: WB Saunders, 1980.
102. Baker JD, Blackmon BB. Local anesthesia. Clin Plast Surg 12:25-31, 1985.
103. Eaglestein W. Inadvertent intracutaneous injection of hypertonic saline (23.4%) in two patients without complication. J Dermatol Surg Oncol 16:878-879, 1990.
104. Duffy DM. Personal communication, 1992.
105. de Faria JL, Moraes IN. Histopathology of the telangiectasias associated with varicose veins. Dermatologia 127:321-329, 1963.
106. Wenner L. Sind endovarikose hamitische Ansammlungen eine normale Scheinung bei Sklerotherapie? Vasa 10:174-176, 1981.
107. Dinkler JA, Cohen BE. Reversal of dopamine extravasation injury with topical nitroglycerin ointment. J Plast Reconstr Surg 84:811-813, 1989.
108. American Medical Association. AMA Drug Evaluation, 6th ed. Chicago: The Association, 1986, pp 463, 502.
109. Franks AG. Topical glyceryl trinitrate as adjunctive treatment in Raynaud's disease. Lancet 1:76-77, 1982.
110. Ross M. Dopamine-induced localized cutaneous vasoconstriction and piloerection. Arch Dermatol 127:586-587, 1991.
111. Chavez CM. The clinical significance of lymphatico-venous anastomoses. Vasc Dis 5:35-47, 1968.
112. Chant ADB. The effects of posture, exercise, and bandage pressure on the clearance of 24Na from the subcutaneous tissues of the foot. Br J Surg 59:552-555, 1972.
113. Campion EC, Hoffman DC, Jepson RP. The effects of external pneumatic splint pressure on muscle blood flow. Aust N Z J Surg 38:154-157, 1968.
114. Lawrence D, Kakkar V. Graduated, static, external compression of the lower limb: A physiological assessment. Br J Surg 67:119-121, 1980.
115. Zimmet SE. Therapeutic interventions in the prevention of extravasation necrosis. XI World Congress of the Union Internationale de Phlébologie, Montreal, 1992.
116. Bodian EL. Sclerotherapy. Semin Dermatol 6:238-248, 1987.
117. From our Legal Correspondent: Hazards of compression sclerotherapy. Br Med J 3:714-715, 1975.
118. Goldstein M. Les complications de la sclérotherapie. Phlebologie 32:221-228, 1979.
119. Oesch A, Stirnemann P, Mahler F. Das akute Ischamiesyndrom des Fusses nach Varizenverödung. Schweiz Med Wochenschr 114:1155-1158, 1984.

120. MacGowan WAL. Sclerotherapy: Prevention of accidents: A review. J R Soc Med 78:136-137, 1985.
121. Cockett FB. Arterial complications during surgery and sclerotherapy of varicose veins. Phlebology 1:3-6, 1986.
122. Matsen FA, Mayo KA, Krugmire RB, et al. A model compartmental syndrome in man with particular reference to the quantification of nerve function. J Bone Joint Surg 59A:648-653, 1977.
123. Fegan WG. The complications of compression sclerotherapy. The Practitioner 207:797-799, 1971.
124. Orbach J. A new look at sclerotherapy. Folia Angiologica 25:181-185, 1977.
125. Benhamou AC, Natali J. Les accidents des traitements sclérosant et chirurgical des varices des membres inférieurs: A propos de 90 cas. Phlebologie 34:41-51, 1981.
126. de Somer-Leroy R, Wang A, Ouvry P. Echographie du creux poplite recherche d'une artériole petite saphène avant sclérotherapie. Phlebologie 44:69-78, 1991.
127. Reference deleted in proofs.
128. Hobbs JT. Personal communication, 1991.
129. Bounumeaux H, Schneider P-A, Huber-Saüteur E. Severe ischemia of the hand following intra-arterial promazine injection: Effects of vasodilatation, anticoagulation, and local thrombolysis with tissue type plasminogen activator. Vasa 19:68-71, 1990.
130. Garber N. A criticism of present-day methods in the treatment of varicose veins. S Afr Med J 21:338-349, 1947.
131. Ogilvie WH. Some applications of the surgical lessons of war to civil practice. Br Med J 1:619-623, 1945.
132. Sigg K. The treatment of varicosities and accompanying complications. Angiology 3:355-379, 1952.
133. Smith L, Johnson MA. Incidence of pulmonary embolism after venous sclerosing therapy. Minn Med 31:270-272, 1948.
134. Natali J, Marmasse J. Enquête sur le traitement chirurgical des varices. Phlebologie 15:232-284, 1962.
135. Barber THT. Modern treatment of varicose veins. Br Med J 1:219-220, 1930.
136. Kern MM, Angle LW. The chemical obliteration of varicose veins: A clinical and experimental study. JAMA 93:595, 1929.
137. Linser P, Vohwinkel H. Moderne Therapie der Varizen, Hämorrhoiden und Varicocele. Stuttgart: Ferdinand Enke, 1942.
138. Sigg K. Zur Behandlung der Varizen der Phlebitis und ihrer Komplikationen. Hautarzt 1-2: 443-450, 1950.
139. Kakkar VV, Howe CT, Nicolaides AN, et al. Deep vein thrombosis of the leg. Am J Surg 120:527-530, 1970.
140. Evans DS, Cockett FB. Diagnosis of deep-vein thrombosis with ultrasonic Doppler technique. Br J Med 28:802-804, 1969.
141. Milne RM, Gunn AA, Grifiths MT, Ruckley CV. Postoperative deep venous thrombosis. A comparison of diagnostic techniques. Lancet 2:445-447, 1971.
142. Borrow M, Goldson H. Postoperative venous thrombosis. Evaluation of five methods of treatment. Am J Surg 141:245-251, 1981.
143. Stevenson IM, Seddon JA, Parry EW. The occurrence of deep venous thrombosis following compression sclerotherapy. Angiology 27:311-321, 1976.
144. Virchow R. Cellular pathology as based on physiological and pathological histology. London: Churchill, 1860.
145. Schneider W, Fischer H. Fixierung und bindegewebige Organisation artifizieller Thromben bei der Varizenverödung. Dtsch Med Wochenschr 89:2410-2412, 1964.
146. Atlas LN. Hazards connected with the treatment of varicose veins. Surg Gynecol Obstet 77: 136-140, 1943.

147. Bohler-Sommeregger K, Karnel F, Schuller-Petrovic S, Santler R. Do telangiectases communicate with the deep venous system? J Dermatol Surg Oncol 18:403-406, 1992.
148. McPheeters HO, Rice CO. Varicose veins–The circulation and direction of venous flow. Surg Gynecol Obstet 49:29-33, 1929.
149. Muller JHA, Petter O, Kostler H. Kinematographische Untersuchungen bei der Varizenverödungstherapie. Z Arztl Fortbild (Jana) 78:345-346, 1984.
150. d'Addato M. Gangrene of a limb with complete thrombosis of the venous system. J Cardiovasc Surg 7:434-440, 1966.
151. Goor W, Leu HJ, Mahler F. Thrombosen in tiefen Venen und in Arterien nach Varizensklerosierung. Vasa 16:124-129, 1987.
152. Williams RA, Wilson SE. Sclerosant treatment of varicose veins and deep vein thrombosis. Arch Surg 119:1283-1285, 1984.
153. Tretbar LL, Pattisson PH. Injection-compression treatment of varicose veins. Am J Surg 120: 539-541, 1970.
154. Thomas JH. Pathogenesis, diagnosis and treatment of thrombosis. Am J Surg 160:547-551, 1990.
155. Samlaska CP, James WD. Superficial thrombophlebitis II. Secondary hypercoagulable states. J Am Acad Dermatol 23:1-18, 1990.
156. Schafer AI. The hypercoagulable states. Ann Int Med 102:814-828, 1985.
157. Kaplan NM. Cardiovascular complications of oral contraceptives. Ann Rev Med 29:31-40, 1978.
158. Durand JL, Bressler R. Clinical pharmacology of the steroidal oral contraceptives. Adv Int Med 24:97-126, 1979.
159. Stooley PD, Tonascia JA, Tockman MS, et al. Thrombosis with low-estrogen oral contraceptives. Am J Epidemiol 102:197-208, 1975.
160. Vessey M, Mant D, Smith A, Yeates D. Oral contraceptives and venous thromboembolism: Findings in a large prospective study. Br J Med 292:526, 1986.
161. Helmrich SP, Rosenberg L, Kaufman DW, et al. Venous thromboembolism in relation to oral contraceptive use. Obstet Gynecol 69:91-95, 1987.
162. Seigel DG. Pregnancy, the puerperium and the steroid contraceptive. Milbank Mem Fund Q 50(Suppl 2):15-23, 1972.
163. Boston collaborative drug surveillance program: Oral contraceptives and venous thromboembolic disease, surgically confirmed gallbladder disease, and breast tumours. Lancet 1:1439-1440, 1973.
164. Realini JP, Goldzieher JW. Oral contraceptives and cardiovascular disease: A critique of the epidemiologic studies. Am J Obstet Gynecol 152:729-798, 1985.
165. Stadel BV. Oral contraceptives and cardiovascular disease. N Engl J Med 305:612-618, 1981.
166. Alkjaersig N, Fletcher A, Burstein R. Association between oral contraceptive use and thromboembolism: A new approach to its investigation based on plasma fibrinogen chromatography. Am J Obstet Gynecol 122:199-211, 1975.
167. Srinivasan S, Solash J, Redner A, et al. The alteration of surface charge characteristics of the vascular system by oral contraceptive steroids. Contraception 9:291-303, 1974.
168. Oski FA, Lubin B, Buchert ED. Reduced red cell filterability with oral contraceptive agents. Ann Int Med 77:417-419, 1972.
169. Sadick N. Treatment of varicose and telangiectatic leg veins with hypertonic saline: A comparative study of heparin and saline. J Dermatol Surg Oncol 16:24-28, 1990.
170. Dreyer NA, Pizzo SV. Blood coagulation and idiopathic thromboembolism among fertile women. Contraception 22:123-136, 1980.
171. Sagar S, Thomas DP, Stamatakis JD, Kakkar VV. Oral contraceptives, antithrombin-III activity, and postoperative deep-vein thrombosis. Lancet 1:509-511, 1976.
172. von Kaulla E, von Kaulla KN. Oral contraceptives and low antithrombin-III activity. Lancet 1:36, 1970.

173. Pizzo SV. Venous thrombosis. In Koepke JA, ed. Laboratory Hematology, vol 2. New York: Churchill Livingstone, 1984.
174. Miller KE, Pizzo SV. Venous and arterial thromboembolic disease in women using oral contraceptives. Am J Obstet Gynecol 144:824-827, 1982.
175. Astedt B. Thrombosis and oral contraceptives: Possible predisposition. Br Med J 4:631-634, 1973.
176. Goodrich SM, Wood JE. Peripheral venous distensibility and velocity of venous blood flow during pregnancy or during oral contraceptive therapy. Am J Obstet Gynecol 90:740-744, 1964.
177. Lipton A, Harvey HA, Hamilton RW. Venous thrombosis as a side effect of tamoxifen treatment. Cancer Treat Rep 68:887-889, 1984.
178. Fisher B, Costantino J, Redmond C, et al. A randomized clinical trial evaluating tamoxifen in the treatment of patients with node-negative breast cancer who have estrogen-receptor–positive tumors. N Engl J Med 320:479-484, 1989.
179. Jordan VC, Fritz NF, Tormey DC. Long-term adjuvant therapy with tamoxifen: Effects on sex hormone–binding globulin and antithrombin III. Can Res 47:4517-4519, 1987.
180. Love RR, Surawicz TS, Williams EC. Antithrombin III level, fibrinogen level, and platelet count changes with adjuvant tamoxifen therapy. Arch Intern Med 152:317-320, 1992.
181. Auger MJ, Mackie MJ. Effects of tamoxifen on blood coagulation. Cancer 61:1316-1319, 1988.
182. Paré A. Cited by Ritchie A. The treatment of varicose veins during pregnancy. Edinburgh Med J 40:157-164, 1933.
183. Hamilton HG, Pittam RF, Higgins RS. Active therapy of varicose veins in pregnancy. S Med J 42:608-612, 1949.
184. Finley BE. Acute coagulopathy in pregnancy. Med Clin North Am 73:723-743, 1989.
185. Aaro LA, Johnson TR, Juergens JL. Acute deep venous thrombosis associated with pregnancy. Obstet Gynecol 28:553-559, 1966.
186. Beller FK. Thromboembolic disease in pregnancy. In Gailv & Anderson, eds. Thromboembolic Disorders. New York: Harper & Row, 1968.
187. Bonnar J, McNicol GP, Douglas AS. Fibrinolytic enzyme system and pregnancy. Br Med J 3:387-389, 1969.
188. Comp PC, Thurnau GR, Welsh J, Esmon CT. Functional and immunologic protein levels are decreased during pregnancy. Blood 68:881-885, 1986.
189. Miletich J, Sherman L, Broze G Jr. Absence of thrombosis in subjects with heterozygous protein C deficiency. N Engl J Med 317:991-996, 1987.
190. Engesser L, Brockmans AW, Briet E, et al. Heredity protein S deficiency: Clinical manifestations. Ann Int Med 106:677-682, 1987.
191. Rick ME. Protein C and protein S: Vitamin K–dependent inhibitors of blood coagulation. JAMA 263:701-703, 1990.
192. Collen D, Schetz J, de Cock F, et al. Metabolism of antithrombin III (heparin cofactor) in man: Effects of venous thrombosis and of heparin administration. Eur J Clin Invest 7:27-35, 1977.
193. Odegaard OR, Abildgaard U. Antithrombin III: Critical review of assay methods. Significance of variations in health and disease. Haemostasis 7:127-134, 1978.
194. Towne JB. Hypercoagulable states and unexplained vascular graft thrombosis. In Bernhard VM, Towne JB, eds. Complications in Vascular Surgery. St. Louis: Quality Medical Publishing, 1991, pp 101-117.
195. Espinoza LR, Hartmann RC. Significance of the lupus anticoagulant. Am J Haematol 22: 331-337, 1986.
196. Tabechnik-Schor NF, Lipton SA. Association of lupus-like anticoagulant and nonvasculitic cerebral infarction. Arch Neurol 43:851-852, 1986.
197. Shi W, Krilis SA, Chong BH, et al. Prevalence of lupus anticoagulant and anticardiolipin antibodies in a healthy population. Aust N Z J Med 20:231-236, 1990.
198. Mueh JR, Herbst K, Rapaport SI. Thrombosis in patients with the lupus anticoagulant. Ann Int Med 92:156-159, 1980.

199. Fegan WG. Continuous compression technique of injecting varicose veins. Lancet 2:109-112, 1963.
200. Foley WT. The eradication of venous blemishes. Cutis 15:665-668, 1975.
201. Browse NL, Burnand KG, Lea Thomas ML. Diseases of the Veins: Pathology, Diagnosis, and Treatment. London: Edward Arnold, 1988, pp 242-243.
202. Orbach EJ. Sclerotherapy of varicose veins: Utilization of intravenous air block. Am J Surg 66:362-366, 1944.
203. Orbach EJ. Clinical evaluation of a new technic in the sclerotherapy of varicose veins. J Inter Coll Surg 11:396-402, 1948.
204. Richardson HF, Coles BC, Hall GE. Experimental air embolism. Can Med J 36:584-588, 1937.

PART FOUR

Complex Problems Involving Varicose Veins

Chapter 16

Treatment of Varicose Veins Associated With Congenital Vascular Malformations

J. Leonel Villavicencio

Dilated venous trunks in the extremities are present in several pathologic entities. The treatment of the problem varies considerably, depending on the cause and magnitude of the clinical manifestations, type of varicosities present, and condition of the patient. To treat varicose veins properly, an accurate diagnosis of the cause of the varicosities must be made. Varicose veins of the extremities are most often observed in the following pathophysiologic entities:

1. Genetic, primary, or essential varicose veins appear early in life, sometimes during childhood. Usually a strong family history of varicosities is present. Telangiectasia, venous lakes, and venules are skin blemishes that have a striking familial tendency.
2. Postthrombotic, secondary, or acquired varicose veins appear as sequelae of deep venous thrombosis. The clinical manifestations are usually severe and vary widely, depending on the extent and location of initial damage to the deep venous system as well as on the degree of obstruction and incompetence of perforating veins.
3. Congenital abnormalities of the vascular system with or without congenital arteriovenous fistulas often involve other tissues (i.e., muscle, nerves, bone, and skin). Some malformations are predominantly arterial, whereas others are venous, lymphatic, or a combination of the three. Varicosities are either part of the syndrome or may develop as a consequence of arteriovenous shunting.
4. In acquired iatrogenic, or traumatic, arteriovenous fistulas, varicose veins are secondary to venous hypertension. Hemodynamic effects on the venous system depend on the location, size, and duration of the arteriovenous fistula.

Each of the four types of varicose veins described requires a distinct and specific type of treatment. The cause must be recognized to establish the appropriate form of therapy.

COMMON CONGENITAL VASCULAR MALFORMATIONS ASSOCIATED WITH VARICOSE VEINS

The presence of varicose veins has been recognized in several congenital malformations of the vascular system. Even though congenital malformations are present in a relatively small percentage of patients attending a vascular clinic, the severity of the clinical manifestations and the magnitude of the problem are challenging. Management of varicose veins associated with congenital malformations of the vascular system requires knowledge of the pathophysiology involved, common sense, and experience.

The most common vascular malformations presenting with varicose veins are Klippel-Trenaunay syndrome (KTS), Parkes-Weber syndrome, and Maffucci syndrome. Hemangiomas may or may not be present with these syndromes. The presence of these hemangiomas, however, usually requires careful assessment of their size, nature, location, and associated symptoms. Management depends on the patient's age, the histologic nature of the lesion, and the severity of the patient's symptoms. Hemangiomas are frequently found in the Maffucci syndrome and less often in Parkes-Weber syndrome or KTS. On occasion, a hemangioma may thrombose spontaneously and as a result produce acute symptoms that require surgical intervention.

The clinical syndrome that was described by Klippel and Trenaunay[1] in 1900 was a congenital vascular anomaly with capillary port-wine stain, varicose veins, and limb hypertrophy occurring in association. Almost 15,000 cases have been reported since 1900, but confusion still exists with regard to nomenclature, cause, and management of this clinical entity.[2] A condition akin to KTS was described by Parkes-Weber[3] in 1907. In 1918 he reported a similar but clinically distinct group of patients with varicose veins, limb hypertrophy, and arteriovenous communications.[4] This report was the first description of the clinical condition subsequently known as Parkes-Weber syndrome.

Although clinically similar, the differences between KTS and Parkes-Weber syndrome are probably a matter of degree. The clinical distinction hinges on the absence of clinically detectable arteriovenous fistulas in KTS which are present in Parkes-Weber syndrome. The natural history of congenital arteriovenous fistulas and their sequelae highlight their importance in Parkes-Weber syndrome and has made their management the natural focus of treatment. The absence of clinically detectable arteriovenous fistulas in KTS has left the management of this condition without a clear focus. However, recent investigations with radioactive isotopes have allowed the detection of previously subclinical arteriovenous fistulas.[5,6] The findings of arteriovenous fistulas in a small percentage of patients with KTS further blur the distinction between the two syndromes. As experience with KTS has grown, it has become evident that this condition may be associated with angiomatous involvement of other organ systems, including the eye, gastrointestinal tract, bladder, and external genitalia.[7-10] Dargeon[11] described a child with a bladder hemangioma who also had unilateral lower extremity hypertrophy and a port-wine skin malformation. Kuffer et al.[12] reported the association of visceral angiomas and thrombocytopenia in KTS. Hendry and Vinnicombe[13] reviewed 31 patients with bladder hemangiomas; 10 patients (31%) were younger than 20 years, and two of them had KTS. Of patients with KTS, 3% to 6% suffer from bladder hemangioma.

Involvement of the lymphatic system also is frequently described.[14,15] In addition, KTS has been reported in association with Sturge-Weber syndrome, in which a vascular stain is present on the upper face and ipsilateral leptomeninges.[16,17] It seems likely that these clinical syndromes may have a common cause and may be regional manifestations of the same genetic disorder.[18]

The cause of KTS is controversial. Servelle[14] stated that the changes seen in this syndrome were the sequelae of obstruction. He based his assumptions on venographic demonstration of venous obstruction. On the other hand, Baskerville et al.[19] reported that most patients had no impairment of venous drainage and suggested that a mesodermal abnormality occurring during fetal development led to the maintenance of microscopic arteriovenous fistulas, which resulted in the clinical syndrome. More recently, a theory was advanced suggesting that KTS was the result of either (1) a half chromatid mutation of the zygote before fertilization or (2) an early surmatic mutation that allows survival of the cells by mosaicism but produces a lethal gene preventing its transmission. The sporadic occurrence of KTS, its equal sex incidence, the variation and severity, and the relative rarity of generalized involvement is consistent with this theory. Genetic mutation could account for the spectrum of diseases known as KTS, Parkes-Weber syndrome, and Sturge-Weber syndrome.

The surgical management of KTS and Parkes-Weber syndrome has been extensively discussed and is the subject of controversy. In the presence of active arteriovenous fistulas in a severely symptomatic patient, the decision to intervene surgically is less subject to controversy than in a patient whose main clinical manifestations are giantism and sequelae of chronic venous hypertension. Servelle[14] operated on 786 patients with KTS since 1945. He found that elongation of limbs was invariably noted. Varicose veins were present in 36% of the cases, and a cutaneous port-wine stain was present in 32% of these patients. It is interesting that, based on his venographic studies, Servelle demonstrated anomalies of the popliteal veins in 51% of his cases, the superficial femoral vein in 16%, the popliteal and femoral veins in 29%, and the iliac veins in 3%, with inferior vena cava involvement in only 1% of his cases. Servelle considered that deep venous obstruction was the primary cause and that surgery directed to the abnormal superficial varicosities could worsen the patient's condition by increasing the outflow obstruction. Other authors also have cautioned against surgery on this basis.[20,21]

DIAGNOSIS

Diagnosis begins with a careful clinical examination. The presence of giantism and varicose veins associated with a port-wine stain malformation is strongly suggestive of the diagnosis of KTS. I have noted considerable variation in the extension and location of the port-wine stain. It may occupy the entire length and usually the lateral aspect of one or more limbs, or it may be present only in isolated areas of the

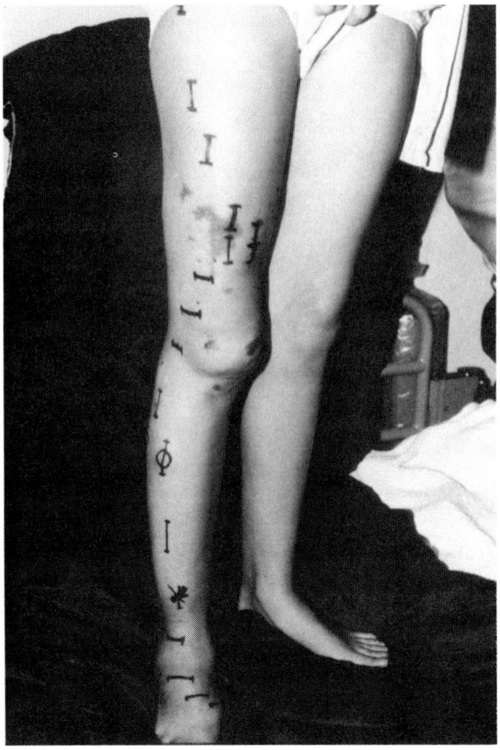

FIGURE 16-1. Port-wine stain malformation in Klippel-Trenaunay syndrome may occupy entire length of lateral aspect of the extremity or, as shown here, may be present only in isolated areas of the limb. Large hemangioma is noticeable over anterior aspect of the knee. Other hemangiomas are present over the ankle and dorsum of the foot. This patient has a patent deep venous system demonstrated through phlebography.

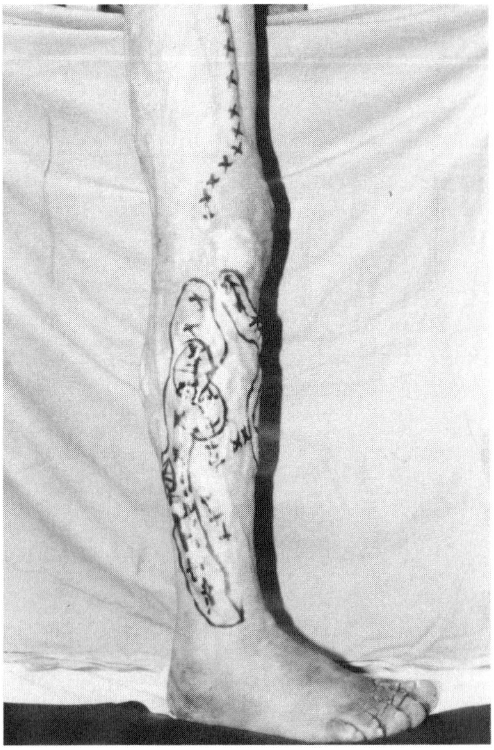

FIGURE 16-2. Lateral venous collector, a remnant of a fetal vein, can be observed in this male patient. Large aneurysmal dilatations were present along the course of the collector in the leg. Notice typical lymphatic stasis verrucosis on dorsum of the toes. Valveless lateral vein drained into the external iliac vein. Deep venous system was noted as patent through both noninvasive and phlebographic studies.

extremity (Figure 16-1). A lateral marginal venous collector, which is a remnant of a fetal vein, often can be observed in these patients (Figure 16-2).

Patients in whom the diagnosis of KTS or Parkes-Weber syndrome is suspected must undergo a number of invasive and noninvasive vascular assessments. Bidirectional Doppler examination is used to assess deep venous reflux, competence of the saphenofemoral and saphenopopliteal junctions, reflux into the abnormal marginal vein, and perforator incompetence. Strain gauge plethysmography is used to assess venous outflow and capacitance. To assess the importance and contribution of the large lateral collecting vein to the venous outflow, strain gauge plethysmography readings need to be repeated with compression of the large lateral collector shortly before the thigh cuff deflates. A pattern of venous obstruction is observed if the lateral vein collector plays an important role in the venous outflow when occluded by compression. Photoplethysmography is used to measure venous refilling time and provide an index of venous reflux. Duplex scanning and color flow Doppler studies in patients with KTS also assist in the noninvasive evaluation of the deep venous system and its anomalies.

Both ascending and descending phlebography as well as selective varicography are also useful. Varicography aids in localizing the point of entrance of the lateral collector into the deep venous system (Figure 16-3). The phlebographic technique in

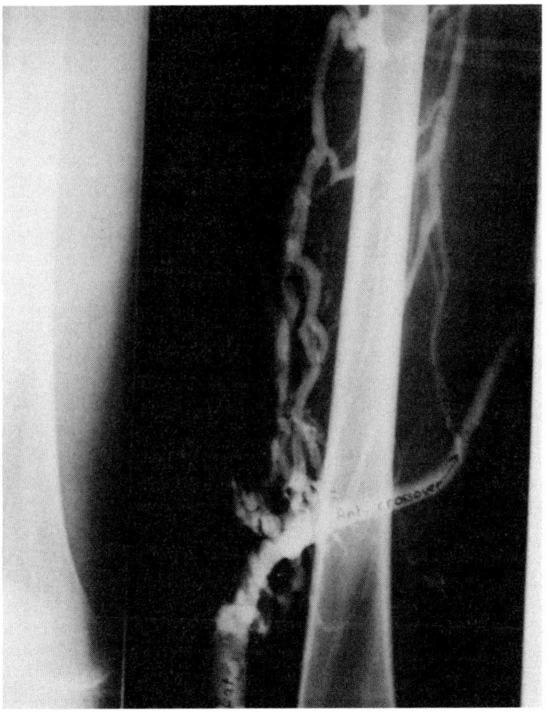

FIGURE 16-3. Varicography is extremely useful in localizing entrance point of lateral collector into the deep system and in demonstrating the anatomy of the area. Large lateral collector is seen crossing over to medial side to drain into greater saphenous vein. A thinner, plexiform venous channel continues to drain part of lateral flow into iliac venous system. A faint femoral vein is seen in background. A second injection with elastic compression of the superficial system showed a normal superficial femoral vein.

KTS usually requires modification. When poor deep venous filling is encountered despite the injection of large volumes of contrast media (>200 ml), the procedure must be repeated after compression of the large superficial venous system.

Serial arteriography or digital arteriography is done to search for arteriovenous fistulas. Both CT and MRI scanning have been used in selective patients to assess the extent of the venous malformation. The MRI studies, which enhance the diagnosis of atresia of the inferior vena cava or the pelvic veins, have been very useful in demonstrating the presence of intrathoracic chest hemangiomas. In patients with suspected Parkes-Weber syndrome, angiography may demonstrate the presence of arteriovenous connections to guide the interventional radiologist in embolization of active arteriovenous communications. Surgical ligation of most of the arterial branches of the main arterial trunks of the extremities, as described by Malan and Vollmar, is now rarely performed.

MANAGEMENT

Klippel-Trenaunay Syndrome

Compression therapy with elastic hosiery, leg elevation, and sclerotherapy have been the only forms of management offered to patients with KTS. These methods are valuable and should be used in all patients. However, some patients present with severe symptoms that do not respond to conservative treatment. In this group of patients, surgical treatment must be considered. Surgical excision of the large superficial varices in KTS has been condemned because it is believed that deep venous obstruction frequently results and aggravates venous hypertension. However, surgery must be considered and planned on the basis of both the patient's symptoms and noninvasive investigations. When duplex scanning or phlebographic studies demonstrate a patent deep venous system, my associates and I have performed extensive excision of superficial venous dilatations, including the large lateral venous collector, with ligation and division of large incompetent perforators routinely present in these patients (Figure 16-4). If hypoplasia and/or obstruction of the deep venous system is observed, the procedure may be beneficial. The most common symptoms necessitating operation are frequent and copious bleeding from skin varicosities, nonhealing venous ulceration, gross deformity, pain and edema, recurrent thrombophlebitis, and thrombosis of hemangiomas.

In 614 operated cases, Servelle[14] found the following deep venous anomalies: (1) compression of the popliteal vein in 71% of the cases, with a perivenous sheet involving the whole length of the vein in 15% of the patients; (2) agenesis or hypoplasia of the popliteal vein in approximately 7% of the cases; (3) compression of the femoral vein in 54% of cases, with a complete perivenous sheet in 2% of the patients; and (4) hypoplasia and complete agenesis of the femoral vein in 40% and 3% of the cases, respectively. Servelle recommended venolysis and resection of all the compressing fibrous bands along the entire length of the vein. He reported that the veins are restored to almost normal caliber after this operation. However, we have not had the opportunity to confirm Servelle's observation.

Preoperative marking. Preoperative marking (Figure 16-5) is the single most

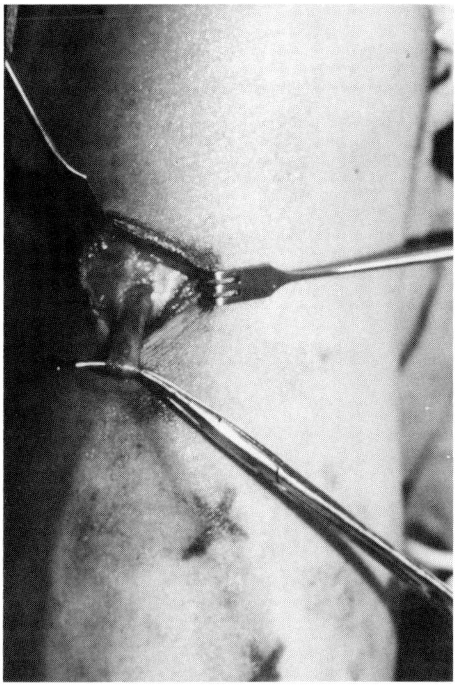

FIGURE 16-4. Large incompetent perforator (7 mm) is shown clearly in this intraoperative photograph of a patient with Klippel-Trenaunay syndrome. Considerable palliation of symptoms is achieved after numerous perforators have been divided. Venous hypertension is ameliorated, ulcers are healed, and varicosities are eliminated.

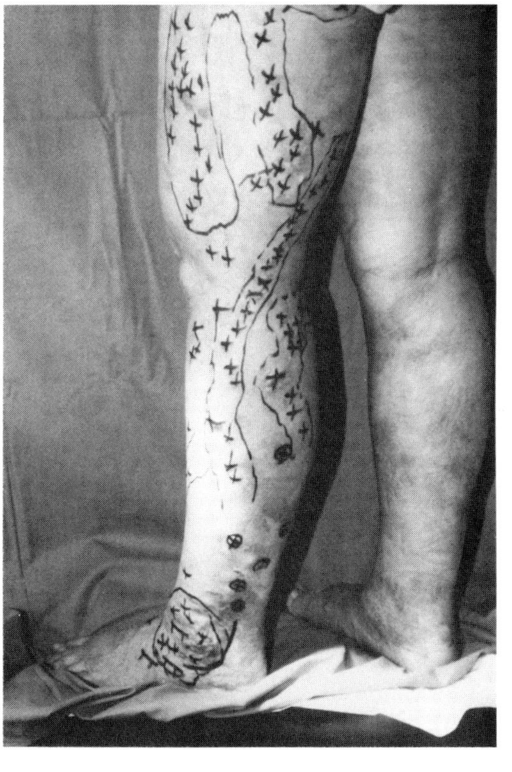

FIGURE 16-5. Preoperative marking is the single most important step in surgical management of varicose veins. Marking should be done by the operating surgeon. Inadequate preoperative marking increases the chance of surgical failure.

important technical step in surgery of the superficial venous system. The examiner must have experience, skill, and a thorough knowledge of anatomy, physiology, and pathophysiology. Both a careful physical examination and a Doppler examination should be performed. Inadequate preoperative marking is not usually listed as a causative factor in recurrent varicose veins. However, an improperly and carelessly marked extremity represents an invitation for recurrence.

Preoperative marking must be performed as follows:

1. The patient must have the extremity washed with antiseptic soap and water for at least the 3 days immediately preceding surgery.
2. The extremity and pubis (if groin exploration is contemplated) should be carefully shaved before marking. This is especially important in hairy patients.
3. Marking should be done before the administration of any preanesthetic medication. Tracing the veins requires the patient to stand on a platform under a good source of illumination and to be completely awake.
4. Marking should be done with a water-resistant marker so that it will not come off during skin preparation.
5. After the veins have been marked, the patient is advised to wear pajama pants and to avoid direct contact of one extremity with the other, which may lead to ink smearing.
6. Each surgeon develops his or her own technique for marking by using keys, clues, different signs, and tracings to identify perforators and clusters of veins. For this reason surgery must be performed by the surgeon who marks the patient (in teaching centers, the senior surgeon must be present during marking and must assist the resident or fellow with the operation). An effort should be made to locate the point of entrance of the lateral venous collector into the deep system since this point varies considerably. My associates and I have had patients in whom this drainage occurs at the level of the external iliac vein and others in whom the lateral collector drains either into the saphenous vein or into the femoral vein (Figure 16-6).

We have followed the surgical policy of selective segmental excision of the pathologic superficial venous system with division and ligation of incompetent perforating veins. This policy must be followed for all patients in whom evidence of unimpaired deep venous outflow is available. General anesthesia is used in all cases. A pneumatic tourniquet has been employed in 50% of our patients in whom extensive and large varicosities were present. The procedure involves the segmental resection of the lateral collecting vein and ligation at its point of communication with the deep venous system. Segmental excision is safer than stripping because of the large size of the vein and its tributaries. Indeed, venous aneurysms have been encountered in most patients. These require local excision to prevent excessive intraoperative bleeding (Figure 16-7). Once the large incompetent perforators have been divided, the clusters of veins can be excised through small incisions. Whenever possible, crochet-hook excision of the superficial clusters of varicose veins can be done to diminish postoperative scarring, even though this aspect of the management is not of particular concern to patients suffering from KTS. Only 1 of 14 patients

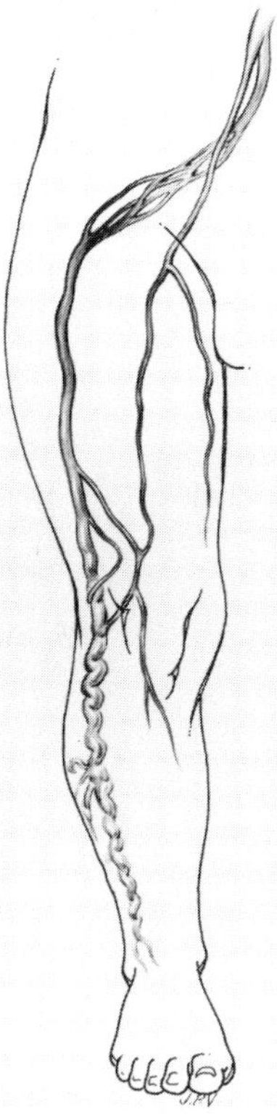

FIGURE 16-6. Lateral collector, a remnant of a fetal vein, is shown draining into the internal iliac vein through that vessel's parietal tributaries. Several degrees of deep venous hypoplasia may or may not be present. When deep venous aplasia is present and the superficial system is the main venous outflow, removal of the abnormal lateral vein may produce acute venous insufficiency, with cases of phlegmasia cerulea dolens and venous gangrene being reported.

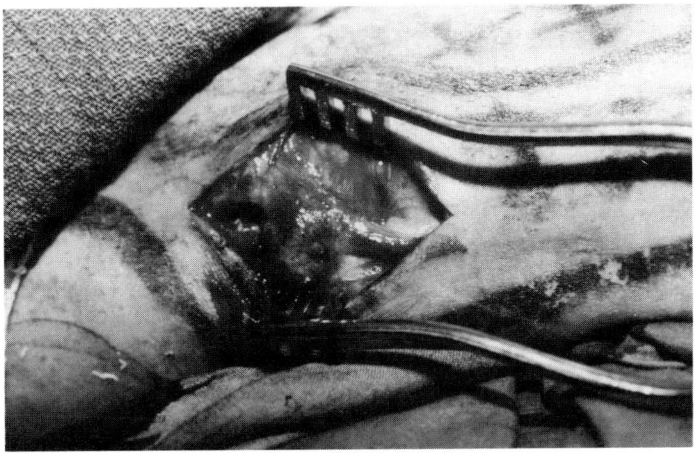

FIGURE 16-7. Large venous aneurysm encountered during surgery for varicose veins in Klippel-Trenaunay syndrome. Aneurysm was in communication with an incompetent perforator. Since stripping of venous segments in this disease may lead to profuse bleeding, segmental excision with direct exposure of the large dilatations should be done.

operated on for KTS was found to have incompetence of the long saphenous system. This patient underwent long saphenous stripping to a point just below the knee. Superficial venous clusters and venous dilatations can be excised easily in the bloodless field provided by the pneumatic tourniquet. Cavernous hemangiomas or superficial hemangiolymphangiomas have been excised in 25% of our patients (Figure 16-8). In those patients with extensive abnormalities, it is wise to have surgery staged over two or three sessions to achieve satisfactory results. Staging was performed in 11 of 14 of our cases. In the postoperative period, external compression with elastic hosiery is strongly recommended.

Sclerotherapy plays an important role in the management of KTS and should begin 2 months after surgery, once the postoperative ecchymosis has disappeared. This form of treatment must be used in association with surgery in patients with intractable symptoms.

If the principles of management delineated for patients with KTS are followed, an excellent functional outcome should be expected. Surgery is largely a containment exercise to palliate symptoms. No claims of cure are made. No patient's condition, however, has worsened as a result of excision of the superficial veins. When the management guidelines described here were followed, no patient had recurrent varicorrhage, all ulcerations healed, and the patient's index of satisfaction, ranging from 0 (unsatisfied) to 4 (very satisfied), has been 3 to 4.

Surgery for varicose veins in patients with the Parkes-Weber syndrome should not be attempted until the interventional radiologist has completed the treatment of

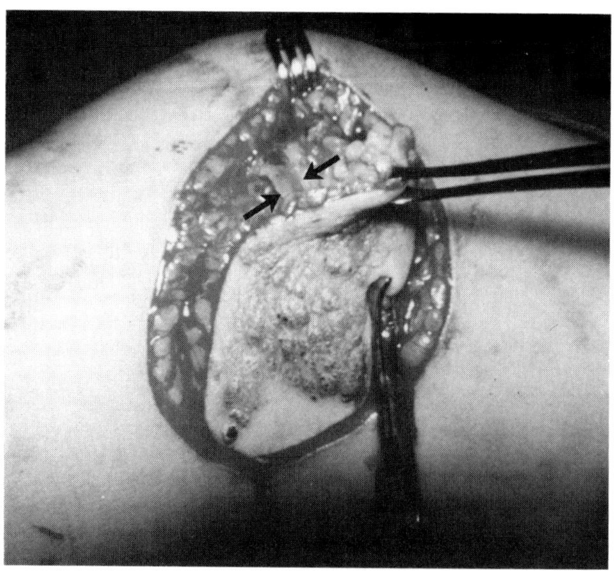

FIGURE 16-8. Cavernous hemangiomas or hemangiolymphangiomas have been excised in 25% of our patients with Klippel-Trenaunay syndrome. This intraoperative photograph shows en bloc excision of a large hemangiolymphangioma that had bled repeatedly. Note large venous perforator draining the lesion (between arrows).

the arteriovenous communications by percutaneous catheter embolization. Often the elimination of active arteriovenous communications produces sufficient palliation so that the management of the superficial varicosities can be attempted with judicious sclerotherapy. However, sclerotherapy will not produce good long-term results if points of reflux remain. In such cases ligation and division of the large incompetent perforators, followed by sclerotherapy, is the treatment of choice and should provide considerable palliation. Sclerotherapy should not be considered in any patient in whom active arteriovenous fistulas are demonstrated. The practice of injecting a sclerosing agent into arterial communications carries too high a risk, and it may be accompanied by arterial thrombosis, necrosis, and catastrophic consequences.

Maffucci Syndrome

Maffucci syndrome is a congenital nonfamilial syndrome that includes both dyschondroplasia (enchondromas) and hemangiomatosis. It is a rare disease, with only 200 cases reported in the past 140 years. Recurrent bleeding, pain, and limb disfigurement may lead to vascular consultation. Affected individuals have hemangiomas at birth, and skeletal deformities may be noted later. The diagnosis of Maffucci syndrome is made after clinical, radiologic, and pathologic evidence of hemangiomatosis and enchondromas has been collected. Patients with this syndrome frequently have phlebectasia and hemangiomas. Both conditions may be treated by excision. However, larger lesions should be treated only after careful evaluation of the arterial and venous anatomy. Maffucci syndrome is rare, but diagnosis of this condition must be considered in the evaluation of patients with congenital hemangiomas so that the presence of potentially malignant enchondromas will not be missed. We have treated four patients during the last 20 years who presented with signs and symptoms consistent with Maffucci syndrome. All of them complained of pain and heaviness of the involved extremity. All had hemangiomas at birth, skeletal deformities, and enchondromas. In three patients, the arterial inflow was evaluated with arteriography; in one patient, MRI was used. Two patients had excision of hemangiomas, and one had sclerotherapy and compression therapy. All had bone biopsies performed, and none of the enchondromas or the soft tissue lesions demonstrated malignant transformation. Three patients had their arterial inflow evaluated with arteriography. Evidence of arteriovenous fistulas was demonstrated in one patient (Figure 16-9). There was one episode of acute thrombosis of a chest hemangioma, which was documented by CT scanning. CT and MRI scanning were useful in our series to evaluate the nature, extent, and vascularity of vascular and bony lesions. Three of the four patients were children; throughout follow-up ranging from 2 to 20 years, no evidence of malignant degeneration of enchondromas or soft tissue lesions was found. In the older patient, no malignancy was noted; however, the extension and complications resulting from that patient's disease process were so severe as to be life-threatening. Malignant degeneration with sarcomatous transformation of the hemangiomas and enchondromas occurs in almost 20% of patients with Maffucci syndrome.[22] These tumors are of mesodermal origin, with the

A 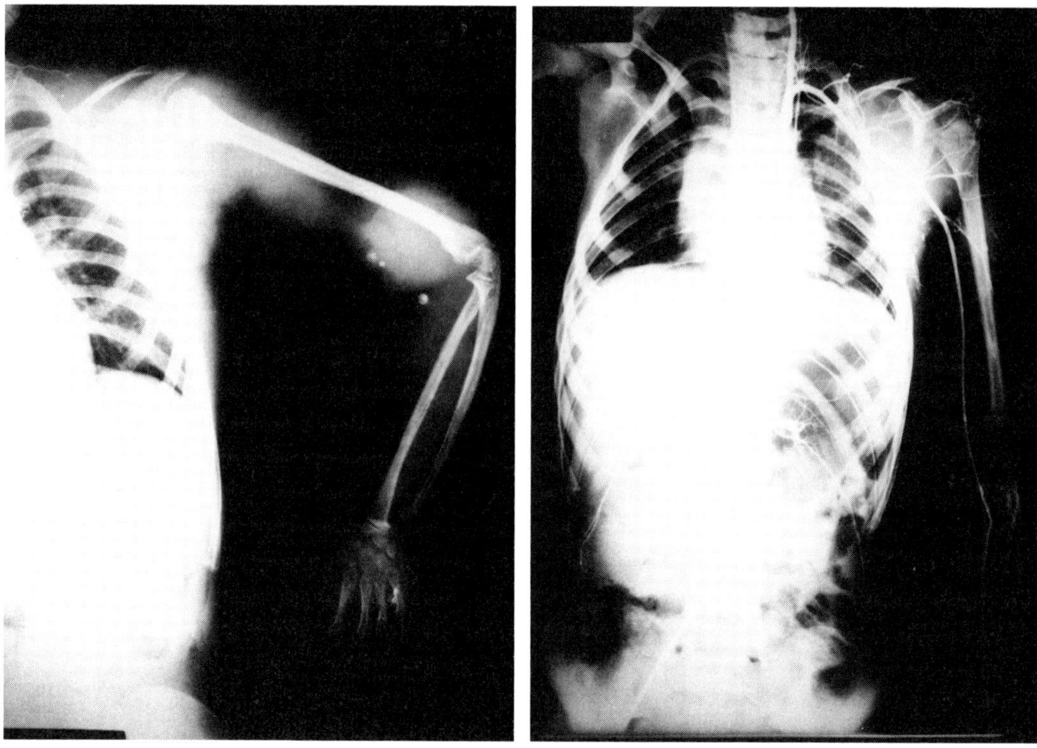 B

FIGURE 16-9. Radiographic studies of a patient with Maffucci syndrome. A, This photograph, taken 5 minutes after arteriography, shows phlebolyths and marked osteoporosis with thinning of bone cortex. Note static venous flow where contrast material remained for long periods of time. True phlebectasia was observed in phlebographic studies performed. Some dilatations are hemangiomatous masses. B, Arteriogram of same patient. Note small arteriectatic lesions on shoulder area. These lesions corresponded to small areas of arteriovenous fistulas that responded well to embolization. Resection of hemangiomas under pneumatic tourniquet ischemia resulted in palliation of this patient's malformation.

majority being chondrosarcomas. Other malignancies include hemangiosarcomas, lymphangiosarcomas, fibrosarcomas, gliomas, ovarian tumors, and carcinoma of the pancreas.[23]

Benign tumors also have been found in patients with Maffucci syndrome; these include pituitary adenomas, ovarian thecomas, uterine tumors, and multiple fibromas.[24]

Because of the potential for associated malignancies, such as malignant transformation of enchondromas and hemangiomas, biopsies should be performed on suspicious lesions. With soft tissue lesions that are accessible, excisional or incisional biopsy should be done because of the excessive and uncontrollable bleeding that may result from needle biopsy.

Management of Maffucci syndrome is palliative. Definitive therapy for vascular lesions is surgical. In an attempt to reduce the size of the hemangiomas, radiation has been used. However, the benefits of this method are questionable. Tumor shrinking with sclerotherapy has been used either alone or with surgical excision.

Management of bony abnormalities is important during the adolescent period. Procedures for decreasing normal growth in the patient's unaffected leg may be performed to prevent marked scoliosis and limb asymmetry. Amputation, a course of last resort, may be necessary to relieve the patient of the inconvenient, swollen, and cumbersome extremity. With massive deformities or malignant transformation, disarticulation and wide resection may be indicated.[25] Disarticulation has not been necessary in our series.

SUMMARY

Surgery of the superficial veins in patients with KTS has been condemned because it was believed to result in the frequent occurrence of deep venous obstruction. However, our series did not demonstrate this effect. Superficial vein surgery may have been unsuccessful in the past for a number of reasons, the most obvious of which is the initial presence of venous obstruction. In such a situation, severe venous stasis results. Adequate demonstration of a hemodynamically sound deep venous system is a crucial prerequisite to superficial venous surgery. In addition, superficial surgery sometimes has been inappropriately directed toward removal of the long and short saphenous systems. We found varicosities of the saphenous vein in only 1 of 14 operated cases; therefore we recommend selective saphenous vein surgery only in those patients shown to have overt saphenous vein dilatation, tortuosity, and incompetence. In 13 of our 14 patients, the greater saphenous vein was surprisingly healthy looking in radiographic studies and was found to be competent through Doppler examination. Last, all patients had demonstrable perforator vein incompetence, often in communication with the large lateral collector vein. Perforator ligation and division should be an integral part of the treatment program. Because of the large diameter of the incompetent perforator veins (see Figures 16-4 and 16-7), stripping of any vein in patients with KTS should not be done because of the risk of profuse bleeding. Instead, segmental excision is the procedure of choice. Patients with intractable symptoms who have a patent deep venous system should be treated with an aggressive surgical policy directed toward the elimination of deep reflux to the superficial system and the excision of the dilated venous clusters. Management of the severe lymphatic anomalies and gross deformities often observed in patients with KTS should be an integral part of the management of this challenging syndrome, and excisional therapy should be considered to alleviate the heaviness of the affected limbs.

REFERENCES

1. Klippel M, Trenaunay P. Du noevus variqueux et osteo-hypertrophique. Arch Gen Med (Paris) 185:641-672, 1900.
2. McKusick KA. Mendelian Inheritance in Man: Catalogues of Autosomal Dominant, Autosomal Recessive and X-Linked Phenotypes, 6th ed. Baltimore: Johns Hopkins University Press, 1983.
3. Parkes-Weber F. Angioma formation in connection with hypertrophy of limbs and hemihypertrophy. Br J Dermatol 19:231-235, 1907.
4. Parkes-Weber F. Hemangiectatic hypertrophy of limbs—Congenital phlebarteriectasis and so-called congenital varicose veins. Br J Child Dis 15:13-17, 1918.

5. Bollinger A, Vogt B, Luthy E, Hegglin R. Flow measurement in patients with multiple arteriovenous fistulae of the extremity. Helv Med Acta 33:76-87, 1976.
6. Haimovici H, Sprayregen S. Congenital microarterio-venous shunts: Angiographic and Doppler ultrasonographic identification. Arch Surg 121:1065-1070, 1986.
7. O'Connor PS, Smith JL. Optic nerve variant in the Klippel-Trenaunay-Weber syndrome. Ann Ophthalmol 10:131-137, 1978.
8. Gloviczki P, Hollier L, Telander RL. Surgical implications of Klippel-Trenaunay-Weber syndrome. Ann Surg 197:353-362, 1983.
9. Hall BD. Bladder hemangiomas in the Klippel-Trenaunay-Weber syndrome. N Engl J Med 285: 1032-1033, 1971.
10. Tjaden BL, Buscema J, Haller JA, Rock JA. Vulvar congenital dysplastic angiopathy. Obstet Gynecol 75:552-554, 1990.
11. Dargeon HW. Tumors of Childhood. New York: Paul B. Hoeber, 1960, p 367.
12. Kuffer FR, Starzynski TE, Girolami A, et al. Klippel-Trenaunay syndrome, visceral angiomatosis and thrombocytopenia. J Pediatr Surg 3:65-72, 1968.
13. Hendry WF, Vinnicombe M. Hemangioma of the bladder in children and young adults. Br J Urol 43:309, 1971.
14. Servelle M. Klippel-Trenaunay syndrome. Ann Surg 197:365-373, 1985.
15. Baskerville PA, Ackroyd JS, Lea Thomas M, Browse NL. The Klippel-Trenaunay syndrome: Clinical radiological hemodynamic features and management. Br J Surg 72:232-236, 1985.
16. Stewart G, Farmer G. Sturge-Weber and Klippel-Trenaunay syndromes with absence of inferior vena cava. Arch Dis Child 65:546-547, 1990.
17. Furakawa T, Igata A, Toyokura Y, Ikeda S. Sturge-Weber and Klippel-Trenaunay syndrome with nevus of ota and ito. Arch Dermatol 102:640-645, 1970.
18. Happle R. Lethal genes surviving by mosaicism. A possible explanation for sporadic birth defects involving the skin. J Am Acad Dermatol 16:899-906, 1987.
19. Baskerville PA, Ackroyd JS, Browse NL. The etiology of the Klippel-Trenaunay syndrome. Ann Surg 202:624-627, 1985.
20. Lindenhauer SM. The Klippel-Trenaunay syndrome. Ann Surg 162:303-314, 1965.
21. Vollmar J, Vogt K. Angiodysplasie und Skeletsystem. Chirurg 47:205, 1976.
22. Schwartz HS, Zimmerman NB, Simon MA, et al. The malignant potential of enchondromatosis. J Bone Joint Surg 69A:269-274, 1987.
23. Johnson JL, Webster JR, Sippy HI. Maffucci's syndrome (dyschondroplasia with hemangiomas). Am J Med 228:864-866, 1960.
24. Lewis RJ, Ketchum AS. Maffucci's syndrome: Functional and neoplasm significance. Case report and review of the literature. J Bone Joint Surg 55A:1465-1467, 1973.
25. Sun TS, Swec RG, Shives TC, Unni KK. Chondrosarcoma in Maffucci's syndrome. J Bone Joint Surg 67A:1214-1219, 1985.

Chapter 17

Varicose Veins and Venous Ulceration: Rationale for Conservative Treatment

Gregory L. Moneta and John M. Porter

An examination of the potential relationship between venous ulceration and varicose veins requires consideration of a number of issues, the first of which is the definition of varicose veins. Next, the prevalence of varicose veins in patients with venous ulceration must be determined and accompanied by a careful evaluation of the evidence that varicose veins themselves contribute to the ulcerative process and are not merely another manifestation of abnormal venous hemodynamics that lead to the development of a venous ulcer. In addition, the circumstances under which treatment specifically directed toward varicose veins will lead to prevention, healing, or decreased rate of recurrence of venous ulceration need to be determined. Finally, if a relationship does exist between varicose veins and venous ulcers, various therapies available for treating coexisting varicose veins and venous ulceration must be considered to select optimal treatment for the individual patient.

DEFINITION

Unfortunately, the basic definition of what constitutes a varicose vein is controversial. Most practicing physicians regard any large, tortuous superficial vein as a varicose vein, regardless of the process leading to venous dilation. From this perspective a tortuous superficial vein resulting from an intrinsic defect in the vein wall, a primary varicosity, and one arising as a result of abnormal deep venous hemodynamics, a secondary varicosity, are both considered varicose. It is interesting that the definition of varicose veins given by the World Health Organization is: "a sacular dilatation of the veins which are often tortuous." Tortuous dilated veins secondary to previous venous thrombosis or congenital or acquired arteriovenous fistulas are specifically excluded from this definition of varicose veins.[1]

Clearly dilated and tortuous superficial venous channels often are found in patients with previous deep venous thrombosis and either concurrent or prior venous ulceration. Since these dilated superficial veins may contribute to the formation of a venous ulcer, their treatment also will be addressed in this chapter. Therefore, despite the World Health Organization definition, for purposes of the present discussion, we will consider any tortuous dilated superficial vein as a varicose vein, regardless of whether it developed primarily or followed prior deep venous thrombosis. Such a definition is obviously more realistic for the clinician who is evaluating a patient with coexisting dilated, tortuous superficial veins and a venous ulcer. As will be discussed below, however, the use of this definition does not obviate the need to distinguish primary from secondary varicose veins; nor does it diminish the necessity to determine the relative contributions of superficial and communicating vein insufficiency and deep venous insufficiency to the formation of a venous ulcer.

HISTORY

An association between varicose veins and venous ulcers was a recurring theme in the writings of early Greek, Egyptian, and Roman physicians. Celsus (25 BC-AD 50), Galen (AD 130-200), and Aeties (AD 502-574) described bandages for the treatment of venous ulcers.[2-4] In addition, the use of both avulsion and cautery to eliminate varicose veins accompanying venous ulcers was advocated by these early writers. Indeed, it appears that up until the eighteenth century most physicians believed that varicose veins always accompanied venous ulceration. Eighteenth century physicians, however, began to discard the idea that varicose veins were an absolute prerequisite to venous ulceration. Bell[5] and Baynton[6] made no references to varicose veins as a cause of venous ulceration in their discussions of leg ulcers. Spender[7] noted that venous ulcers could occur in the absence of varicose veins provided that the patient's deep veins were damaged by an episode of venous thrombosis. By 1916, Homans[8] clearly recognized the varying etiologies of venous ulceration. He divided venous ulcers into those associated with leg varicose veins (and "cured by the removal of these veins") and the more intractable "postphlebitic" venous ulcer.[9]

Currently, it is clear that venous ulceration may occur with and without associated superficial varicosities. In clinical reports of patients with venous ulcers, the incidence of coexisting varicose veins varies from 30% to 67% (Table 17-1).

TABLE 17-1. Associated superficial venous varicosities in patients with venous ulcers

Author	Year	No. of Patients	% With Varicosities
Mayberry et al.[10]	1991	113	32
Gooley and Sumner[11]	1988	15	67
Kitahama et al.[12]	1982	65	33
Cranley[13]	1975	1300	30
Healey et al.[14]	1978	18	67

ETIOLOGY OF VENOUS ULCERS

A complete discussion of the complex pathophysiology of venous ulceration is presented in Chapter 3. In short, alterations in cutaneous microcirculatory physiology accompany the formation of a venous ulcer. Pericapillary fibrin deposition, alterations in fibrinolysis and/or plasminogen activation, and microcirculatory leukocyte trapping (with associated cutaneous capillary and lymphatic destruction) all appear to interact in a complex and incompletely defined manner to produce local conditions conducive to ulcer formation.[15-18] Although the precise microcirculatory events leading to venous ulceration have not been determined, there is general agreement that persistent elevation of ambulatory venous pressure is the driving force leading to the microcirculatory changes associated with venous ulceration.

Elevated ambulatory venous pressure (AVP) and shortened venous recovery time (VRT) are clearly associated with an increased incidence of concurrent or past venous ulcer. Nicolaides and Zukowski[19] have demonstrated a virtual absence of venous ulceration in patients with ambulatory venous pressures less than 40 mm Hg. Conversely, patients with an AVP greater than 80 mm Hg are quite likely to have suffered from venous ulceration.

Most patients with venous ulceration have pronounced deep venous valvular insufficiency associated with elevated AVP and shortened VRT. However, severe reflux in the superficial venous system alone may be associated with a markedly elevated AVP and decreased VRT with a normal deep venous system.[20,21] Although it is clear that the large majority of patients with venous ulcers or marked lipodermatosclerosis have both deep and superficial venous reflux, an appreciable minority do not have detectable deep venous insufficiency.[11,20,22,23] The logical conclusion is that isolated abnormalities of superficial and/or perforating veins must be capable of inducing the microcirculatory changes required to produce a venous ulcer without participation of an abnormal deep venous system.

A number of studies suggest that venous ulceration may occur in the absence of detectable deep venous insufficiency. Burnand[24] has demonstrated that incompetent calf perforating veins may be present in patients with normal deep venous hemodynamics. Dodd and Cockett[25] noted an association between leg ulcers and incompetent calf perforating veins and varicose veins in certain patients with phlebographically normal deep veins. Sturrup[26] also has described a subset of patients with venous ulcers who, when standing with a thigh tourniquet, empty their superficial veins with exercise, implying normally functioning deep veins (Perthes' test). More recently Hoare et al.[20] described 20 patients with venous ulceration and longstanding severe varicose veins who were found to have normal deep venous systems through photoplethysmography, AVP measurements, and Doppler ultrasound. All patients, however, had severe reflux of either their greater or lesser saphenous vein. Moore et al.[21] reported that 10% of their patients with severe venous stasis changes were noted to have isolated superficial venous incompetence on the basis of continuous wave Doppler examinations.

The problem with these observations is the inability to distinguish in a quantitative fashion perforating and superficial venous incompetence and to determine the relative importance of reflux in the perforating and superficial venous systems with respect to eventual venous ulceration. There is in fact no well accepted method for determining and quantitating reflux in perforating veins. Physical examination, continuous wave Doppler studies, thermography, and venography all have been found to have either low sensitivities or high false positive rates when compared to the accepted "gold standard" of obvious perforating vein back-bleeding at the time of subfascial ligation.[27] Certainly, however, patients with venous ulceration and apparent isolated superficial venous incompetence may have perforating vein incompetence that contributes to their venous ulceration.

The suggestion that varicose veins themselves may cause venous ulceration also is complicated by the observation that 72% of patients with varicose veins and no signs of lipodermatosclerosis and/or ulceration do not have greater or lesser saphenous vein insufficiency.[28] Venous insufficiency, if present at all in such patients, appears to be limited to branches of the greater or the lesser saphenous vein. Conversely, almost all patients with venous ulcers and concurrent varicosities have saphenous or deep venous insufficiency.[10-12,15]

In our view, consideration of the preceding discussion leads to the following conclusions:

1. Varicose veins can be present with or without deep venous insufficiency and with and without greater or lesser saphenous vein insufficiency.
2. Varicose veins are not required for formation of a venous ulcer.
3. Patients with varicose veins and venous ulcers almost always have deep venous insufficiency.
4. The uncommon patient with venous ulceration, varicose veins, and no detectable deep venous insufficiency will virtually always have incompetence of the greater or lesser saphenous veins.
5. Perforating vein insufficiency currently cannot be reliably detected and quantitated.
6. Therefore patients with venous ulcers and apparent isolated greater or lesser saphenous vein insufficiency may have undetected coexisting perforating vein insufficiency.

We therefore believe that there is no evidence that varicose veins themselves, in the absence of deep venous or greater or lesser saphenous vein insufficiency, lead to venous ulceration. The obvious exception is direct pressure necrosis by a varicosity on the overlying skin, which is not a true lipodermatosclerotic ulceration.

TREATMENT OF VENOUS ULCERATION

For a long time compression therapy has been the standard treatment for venous ulceration. Our patients with venous ulceration are treated exclusively with a strict regimen of ambulatory compression through the use of elastic compression stockings. Our policy is to disregard the presence of branch varicosities in the treatment of patients with venous ulcers. Such patients are, however, evaluated through AVPs and VRTs in an effort to identify apparent isolated greater or lesser saphenous vein insufficiency. To date, patients with isolated superficial venous insuf-

PROTOCOL FOR TREATMENT OF VENOUS ULCERS*

1. Initial bedrest
2. Systemic antibiotics for cellulitis or infection
3. 30 to 40 mm Hg below-knee graduated elastic compression stockings
4. Daily soap-and-water cleansing of ulcer
5. Dry gauze dressing under stocking
6. Treatment of stasis dermatitis with corticosteroid ointment
7. Continued use of graduated elastic compression stockings after healing

*Oregon Health Sciences University, Portland, Ore.

ficiency and lipodermatosclerosis but not venous ulceration and isolated greater or lesser saphenous vein insufficiency have been identified in our practice. However, patients with isolated superficial venous insufficiency apparently constitute 5% to 20% of the venous ulcer population in the experience of others.[13,20]

Over the last 15 years we have treated 113 patients with venous ulcers, 32% of whom had associated superficial varicosities, with the method summarized in the accompanying box.[10] An initial period of bedrest is prescribed until ankle edema resolves as much as possible. In recent years the availability of home health care has greatly diminished the necessity for hospitalization. A brief course of intravenous or oral antibiotics along with local wound care (gentle soap and water scrubs followed by dry gauze dressings changed every 8 hours) also is used during the period of bedrest if periulcer cellulitis or obvious invasive infection, suggested by severe pain in the ulcer, is present.

Edema usually resolves in a few days. The patient then is fitted with an elastic compression stocking and allowed to ambulate. A 30 to 40 mm Hg pressure-gradient below-knee stocking is preferred. The patient is issued two pairs of stockings so that a clean pair is available each day. Wound care is continued with soap and water washing of the ulcer daily. A corticosteroid ointment, such as hydrocortisone or triamcinolone in white petrolatum, is applied to areas of stasis dermatitis but not to the ulcer itself. In fact, no additional medications are ever applied to the ulcer. Dry gauze is placed over the ulcer and changed at least twice daily. The gauze is held in place by a nylon stocking to allow the elastic compression stocking to be placed without disturbing the dressing. We also have found stocking application devices, such as the Medi-Butler (medi USA, Elk Grove, Ill.) (Figure 17-1), to be quite helpful in allowing elderly patients to apply their stocking without assistance.

Despite the perception that patients are noncompliant with the use of elastic compression stockings, among our patients we noted 90% compliance. Complete healing of the venous ulcer occurred in 97% of patients who were compliant with the use of stockings. In only 55% of the small number of noncompliant patients did

A 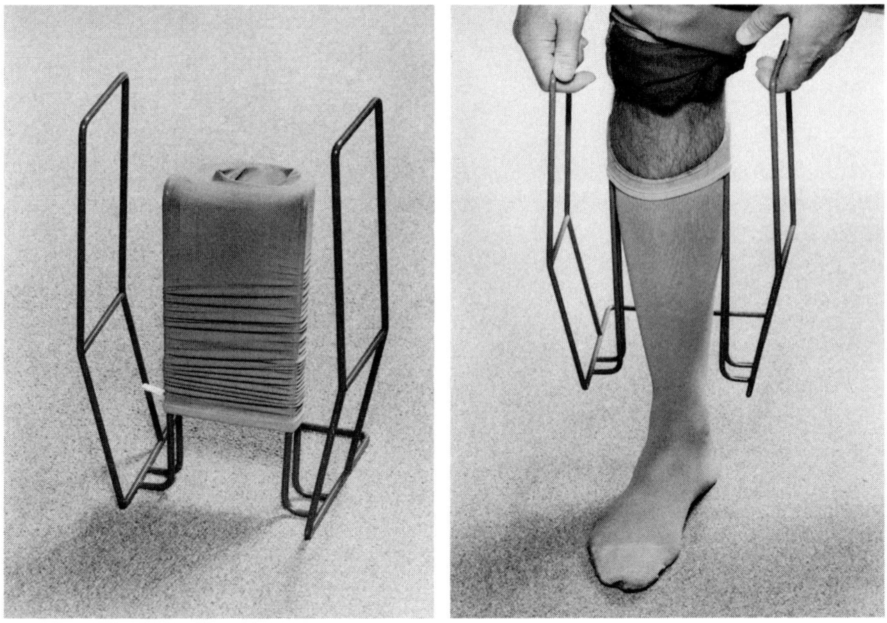 B

FIGURE 17-1. Medi-Butler device for application of elastic compression stockings. Once stocking is loaded (A), the patient merely steps into stocking and pulls it up to apply it to the leg (B).

the ulcer heal. Seventy-nine percent of patients having long-term follow-up (n = 73, with mean follow-up of 30 months) remained compliant with the recommendation of lifelong use of stockings. Sixteen percent of these compliant patients developed a recurrence of their venous ulcer, a 29% 5-year life-table recurrence rate. All patients who discontinued the use of elastic stockings after initial healing had recurrence of venous ulcers by 36 months (Figure 17-2). Similar results can be obtained by using compression therapy with various paste boots, so-called Unna's boot.[29] However, a cost analysis shows that, at least in our hospital, treatment with elastic compression stockings is considerably less expensive.[30]

Our results with compression therapy of venous ulceration with elastic compression stockings are at least as good as those obtained with subfascial ligation of communicating veins (Table 17-2). We do not believe that removal of superficial varicosities and/or stripping of an incompetent saphenous system is a mandatory adjunct to effective treatment of venous ulceration. We continue to reserve sclerotherapy or surgical excision of superficial varicosities to indications of cosmesis, hemorrhage, pain in the varicosity itself, and diffuse aching in the extremity that occurs at the end of the day in a leg with hemodynamically normal or nearly normal deep veins.

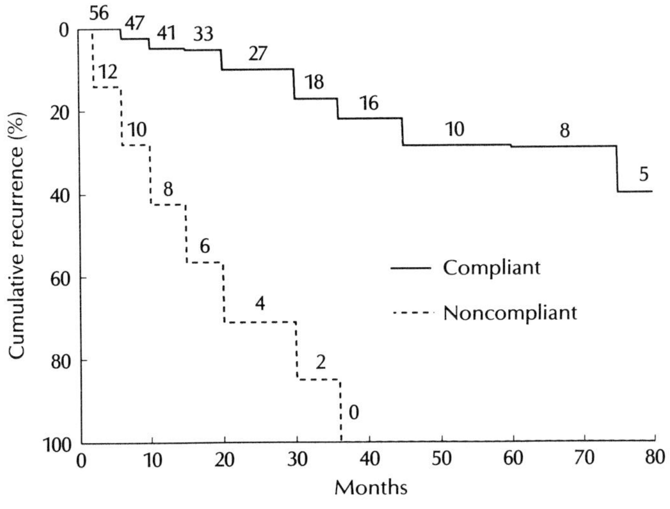

FIGURE 17-2. Life-table recurrence of venous ulceration in patient with healed venous ulcers who were either compliant or noncompliant with the recommendation for continued use of elastic compression stockings. Number of patients at risk in each time interval is printed above graph. Five-year recurrence rate for compliant patients was 29%. All noncompliant patients had recurrence by 36 months ($p = 0.0001$; chi-square). (From Mayberry JC, Moneta GL, Taylor LM Jr, et al. Fifteen-year results of ambulatory compression therapy for chronic venous ulcers. Surgery 109:575, 1991.)

TABLE 17-2. Long-term recurrence of venous ulceration after subfascial ligation of communicating veins*

Author	Year	No. of Patients	Total Recurrence (%)	Stockings Worn Postoperatively
Thurston and Williams[31]	1973	89	13	Yes
Bowen[32]	1975	55	32	Yes
Burnand et al.[33]	1976	41	55	?
DePalma[34]	1979	53	6	Yes
Hyde et al.[35]	1981	109	24	Yes
Negus and Friedgood[36]	1983	77	13	Yes
Johnson et al.[37]	1985	37	41 (3 yr)†	?
			51 (5 yr)†	?
Cikrit et al.[38]	1988	27	22	Yes

*Modified from Mayberry JC, Moneta GL, Taylor LM Jr, et al. Fifteen-year results of ambulatory compression therapy for chronic venous ulcers. Surgery 109:575, 1991.
†Life-table recurrence.

ADDITIVE SUPERFICIAL AND DEEP VENOUS REFLUX AND VENOUS ULCERS

It has been noted that the results of deep venous reconstructions may be better in patients who also undergo removal of incompetent superficial veins. Ferris and Kistner[39] reported that in patients undergoing valvuloplasty or venous segment transpositions, 58% who also had interruption of their perforating veins had normal postoperative ambulatory venous pressures. AVP was normal in only 11% of patients with deep venous reconstructions who had untreated perforating veins. It has been hypothesized that in a significant number of patients the combination of deep and superficial incompetence may be required to produce a venous ulcer. In an effort to identify these patients and to quantitate venous reflux at varying locations in the superficial and deep veins, investigators have begun using duplex ultrasound to measure reflux volumes or peak velocities.

Quantitative duplex-derived measurements of forward flow in lower extremity veins was reported by Strandness and his group in 1988.[40] These and other investigators subsequently have applied duplex technology to quantify venous reflux in patients with and without the sequela of chronic venous insufficiency.[41,42]

Duplex evaluation of venous reflux is performed with the patient in an upright and non–weight-bearing position with respect to the leg undergoing examination. To allow for application of standard compression, a pneumatic cuff is placed on the thigh and leg and connected to an automatic inflator. The site to be examined is insonated with duplex ultrasound just cephalad to the cuff. The cuff is inflated to a predetermined level for 3 seconds. Then it is rapidly deflated (in <0.5 second). Venous reflux in response to cuff deflation is recorded with the duplex scanner. With this technique, Vasdekis et al.[42] have determined that a total peak reflux volume flow of >10 ml/second correlates well with the presence of venous ulceration and/or lipodermatosclerosis. It is interesting that this correlation appears to hold regardless of whether the reflux is present in the deep or the superficial venous system, or both.[42] Since many patients with venous ulceration have detectable reflux in both the deep and the superficial system, it may be that a critical level (>10 ml/sec) of total reflux exists.

The clinical implication of duplex localization of venous incompetence is that if total reflux were reduced to <10 ml/second, either through removal of incompetent superficial veins and associated varicosities or by various forms of deep venous reconstruction, the patient's propensity to develop venous ulceration would be reduced. Duplex quantification of total venous reflux may provide a method for identifying patients with superficial venous insufficiency, varicose veins, and venous ulceration who are most likely to benefit from obliteration of the greater or the lesser saphenous vein and associated varicosities either by surgery or sclerotherapy. Although this hypothesis has not been formally tested, some clinicians already are incorporating duplex quantification of superficial and deep venous reflux into their vascular laboratory evaluation of patients with varicose veins and venous ulcers.[23] Raju and Fredericks[43] also have noted that total venous reflux appears to be a better predictor of severely symptomatic venous insufficiency than single measurements of

AVP or VRT. Whether obliteration of superficial veins selectively identified by duplex scanning as contributing significantly to overall venous reflux will reduce the recurrence rate of a healed venous ulcer awaits the result of a carefully designed clinical trial.

CONCLUSION

Available data suggest that superficial varicosities themselves do not lead to venous ulceration, although associated superficial venous incompetence may serve as the primary source of, or an important contributing component to, the venous reflux necessary for formation of a venous ulcer. If superficial venous insufficiency can be implicated as an important contributing factor to venous ulceration in selected patients, and if such patients can be reliably identified, obliteration of incompetent superficial veins and associated varicosities in patients with venous ulcers may be indicated. However, since we have not identified isolated superficial venous incompetence to be a clinical problem in our patients with venous ulcers, we continue to recommend conservative treatment of venous ulceration with compression stocking therapy. Thus far no other form of therapy has proven superior in the large majority of patients with venous ulcers.

REFERENCES

1. Prerovskly I. Diseases of the Veins. Geneva: World Health Organization, WHO-PA 10964 [internal communication].
2. Celsus AC. Of Medicine in Eight Books. Grieve J, trans. London: Wilson & Durham, 1756.
3. Galen C. Claud: Galeni Opera Omnia. In Kühn CG, ed. Lipsiac: Office Library C Cnobochii, 1821-1833, 22 volumes.
4. Anning ST. Historical aspects. In Dodd H, Cockett FB, eds. The Pathology and Surgery of Veins of the Lower Limb. Edinburgh: Livingstone, 1956.
5. Bell B. Treatise on the Theory and Management of Ulcers. Edinburgh: C Elliot, 1779.
6. Baynton T. A New Method of Treating Old Ulcers of the Legs. Bristol: Emery & Adams, 1799.
7. Spender JK. A Manual of the Pathology and Treatment of Ulcers and Subcutaneous Diseases of the Lower Limbs. London: Churchill, 1866.
8. Homans J. The operative treatment of varicose veins and ulcers, based upon a classification of these lesions. Surg Gynecol Obstet 22:143, 1916.
9. Homans J. The etiology and treatment of varicose ulcers of the leg. Surg Gynecol Obstet 24:300, 1917.
10. Mayberry JC, Moneta GL, Taylor LM Jr, et al. Fifteen-year results of ambulatory compression therapy for chronic venous ulcer. Surgery 109:575, 1991.
11. Gooley NA, Sumner DS. Relationship of venous reflux to the site of venous valvular incompetence: Implications for venous reconstructive surgery. J Vasc Surg 7:50, 1988.
12. Kitahama A, Elliott LF, Kerstein MD, et al. Leg ulcer: Conservative management or surgical treatment. JAMA 247:197, 1982.
13. Cranley JJ. Venous stasis [letter]. Surgery 77:730, 1975.
14. Healey PJM, Healey EH, Wong R, et al. Surgical management of the chronic venous ulcer: The Rob procedure. Am J Surg 137:556, 1978.
15. Browse NL, Burnand KG. The cause of venous ulceration. Lancet 2:243, 1982.
16. Leach RD, Browse NL. Effect of venous hypertension on canine hind limb lymph. Br J Surg 72:275, 1985.

17. Thomas PRS, Nash GB, Dormandy JA. White cell accumulation in the dependent legs of patients with venous hypertension: A possible mechanism for trophic changes in the skin. Br Med J 296:1693, 1988.
18. Bollinger A, Pfister G, Hoffman U, et al. Fluorescence microlymphography in chronic venous incompetence. Int Angiol 8:23, 1989.
19. Nicolaides AN, Zukowski AJ. The value of dynamic venous pressure measurements. World J Surg 10:919, 1986.
20. Hoare MC, Nicolaides AN, Miles CR, et al. The role of primary varicose veins in venous ulceration. Surgery 92:450, 1982.
21. Moore DJ, Himmel PD, Sumner DS. Distribution of venous valvular incompetence in patients with the post-phlebitic syndrome. J Vasc Surg 3:49, 1986.
22. Young J, Moneta GL. Severe primary varicose veins. Postgrad Vasc Surg 1:134, 1990.
23. Schanzer H, Pierce EC II. A rational approach to surgery of the chronic venous stasis syndrome. Ann Surg 195:25, 1982.
24. Burnand KG. The relative importance of incompetent communicating veins in the production of varicose veins and venous ulcers. Surgery 82:9, 1977.
25. Dodd H, Cockett FB. The Pathology and Surgery of the Veins of the Lower Limb, 2nd ed. London: Churchill Livingstone, 1976, p 248.
26. Sturrup H. Ulcus Cruris. Copenhagen: Arne Front-Hansens Forlag, 1950.
27. Nicolaides AN, Sumner DS. Investigation of Patients with Deep Vein Thrombosis and Chronic Venous Insufficiency. Nicosia, Cyprus: Med-Orion Publishing, 1991, pp 50-56.
28. Hanrahan LM, Kechejian J, Cardts PR, et al. Patterns of venous insufficiency in patients with varicose veins. Arch Surg 126:687, 1991.
29. Hendricks WM, Swallow RT. Management of stasis leg ulcers with Unna's boots versus elastic support stockings. J Am Acad Dermatol 12:90, 1985.
30. Chitwood RW, Moneta GL, Porter JM. Nonoperative management of chronic venous insufficiency. In Strandness DE Jr, van Breda A, eds. Vascular Diseases: Surgical and Interventional Therapy. New York: Churchill Livingstone (in press).
31. Thurston OG, Williams HTG. Chronic venous insufficiency of the lower extremity: Pathogenesis and surgical treatment. Arch Surg 106:537, 1973.
32. Bowen FH. Subfascial ligation (Linton operation) of the perforating leg veins to treat post-thrombophlebitic syndrome. Am Surg 41:148, 1975.
33. Burnand K, O'Donnell T, Thomas ML, et al. Relation between postphlebitic changes in the deep veins and results of surgical treatment of venous ulcers. Lancet 1:936, 1976.
34. DePalma RG. Surgical therapy for venous stasis: Results of a modified Linton operation. Am J Surg 137:810, 1979.
35. Hyde GL, Litton TC, Hull DA. Long-term results of subfascial vein ligation for venous stasis disease. Surg Gynecol Obstet 153:683, 1981.
36. Negus D, Friedgood A. The effective management of venous ulceration. Br J Surg 70:623, 1983.
37. Johnson WC, O'Hara ET, Corey C, et al. Venous stasis ulceration: Effectiveness of subfascial ligation. Arch Surg 120:797, 1985.
38. Cikrit DF, Nichols WK, Silver D. Surgical management of refractory venous stasis ulceration. J Vasc Surg 7:473, 1988.
39. Ferris EB, Kistner RL. Femoral vein reconstruction in the management of chronic venous insufficiency. Arch Surg 117:1571, 1982.
40. Moneta GL, Bedford G, Strandness DE Jr. Duplex assessment of venous diameters, peak velocities and flow patterns. J Vasc Surg 8:286, 1988.
41. van Bemmelen PS, Bedford G, Beach K, et al. Quantitative segmental evaluation of venous valvular reflux with duplex ultrasound scanning. J Vasc Surg 10:425, 1989.
42. Vasdekis SN, Clarke H, Nicolaides AN. Quantification of venous reflux by means of duplex scanning. J Vasc Surg 10:670, 1989.
43. Raju S, Fredericks R. Hemodynamic basis of stasis ulceration—A hypothesis. J Vasc Surg 13:491, 1991.

Chapter 18

Pelvic and Vulvar Varices: Pelvic Congestion Syndrome

Abraham Lechter

HISTORICAL BACKGROUND

In the past, vulvar and pelvic types of varicose veins were poorly understood; hence their treatment was not rational. With the advent of vascular radiology, ascending and descending phlebography of pelvic and gonadal veins became possible. In 1954, with publication of the classic work by Guilhem and Baux,[1] exploration and invasion of these veins began. These vessels were visualized mainly from below in an upward direction; thus the data were inconclusive (see box, p. 354).

From 1965 through 1968, reports from Ahlberg, Bartley, and Chidekel[2-4] of Scandinavia furnished substantial information about exploration of gonadal veins from above in a downward direction.

In 1975, Craig and Hobbs[5] described the pelvic congestion syndrome. Laparoscopy, popular in the 1970s and 1980s, became instrumental in the diagnosis and clarification of the cause of this syndrome. The laparoscopic approach is the most useful tool for differentiating nonvascular or somatic pathologic conditions from vascular pathologic conditions, specifically varicocele of the gonadal system.

However, as recently as 1991, the medical school of Walter Reed Hospital in Washington, D.C., advocated the internal iliac vein theory of pelvic and vulvar veins.[6,7] At our institution, my colleagues and I studied 225 gonadal vein phlebograms, of which 75% included iliac injection. We have rarely observed a spilling or dumping of dye into the vulva or upper thigh with iliac vein injection. As Hobbs[8] has aptly said, the iliac system is only the "middleman" in the whole picture.

On September 14, 1984, we performed the first operation of bilateral gonadal vein resection through a long median incision and using a transperitoneal approach. Since then, 250 operations for varices of pelvic origin and vulvar veins have been performed with a retroperitoneal approach; in addition, 28 operations for pelvic congestion syndrome were performed with this approach. Exceptional cases included three instances of chronic pelvic pain with associated somatic and vascular pathology in which hysterectomy and gonadal resection were simultaneously per-

EVOLUTION OF CONCEPT OF PELVIC VARICES

1. Segmental pelvic varices without direct connection to the saphenous vein were commonly noted.
2. Before elective removal, such varices were studied by varicography, which might show the leakage point at the superficial or deep system through a perforator vein. (The cases described as pelvic varices in this chapter did not show the entrance of contrast material into any vein.)
3. High-pressure escape points from the pelvis into the vulva, labia, and upper thigh, constituting a true pelvic varicocele, were suspected, and positive diagnostic phlebography of gonadal veins confirmed the clinical impression.
4. Excellent surgical results obtained by bilateral resection of gonadal veins and ligation of communications to uterine veins, followed by varicectomy with sparing of the saphenous system, further confirmed the nonsaphenous cause of pelvic varices.

formed using a transperitoneal approach. Of these 278 operations, 260 included bilateral ligation and excision of both gonadal veins; some of the failures of the early cases could be attributed to unilateral operations of the gonadal system. Both gonadal systems should be operated on, even if the pathologic condition is restricted to one leg or to one side of the vulva.[9-12]

The first operations for pelvic congestion syndrome were performed in 1986. Only 28 such procedures have been done by our group in 5 years. Despite excellent results, gynecologists in Colombia and in Europe still consider this treatment a highly controversial issue.[13] More information is needed to successfully approach the problem of pelvic congestion syndrome.

PELVIC VARICES AND GONADAL VEINS

The concept of high back pressure as the cause of varicose veins in the legs was proposed by Trendelenburg in the first decade of the twentieth century and by Dodd and Cockett in the 1940s, relating to their work on the saphenofemoral junction and perforating veins in the leg, respectively. There are, however, varicose veins in the leg that cannot be explained by back pressure. The purpose of this chapter is to present our findings, collected during a 7-year period, from the study and treatment of patients who had high-pressure escape points located in pelvic and abdominal veins.

This group comprised 250 patients included in a prospective study from September 1984 to September 1991. All were women aged 31 to 49, with a mean age of 40. All patients had multiple full-term pregnancies (2 to 14 pregnancies), with an average of four deliveries. Their symptoms included pain and often incapacitating heaviness in the thighs and legs. Premenstrual and menstrual pelvic, vulvar, and thigh pain also was present. In addition, pain in the lateral areas of the legs and feet was noted. No trophic changes were observed.

A

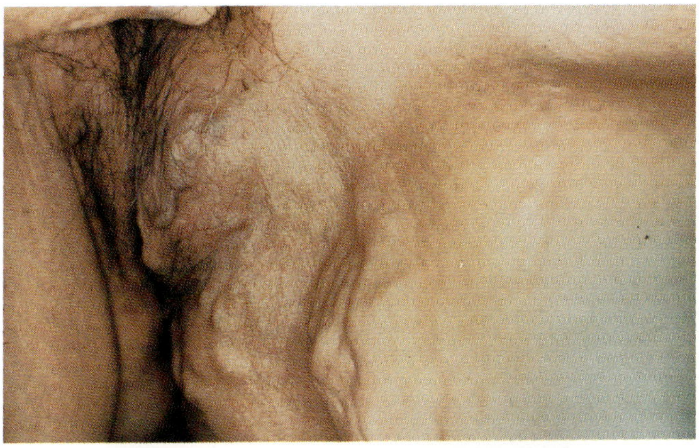

B

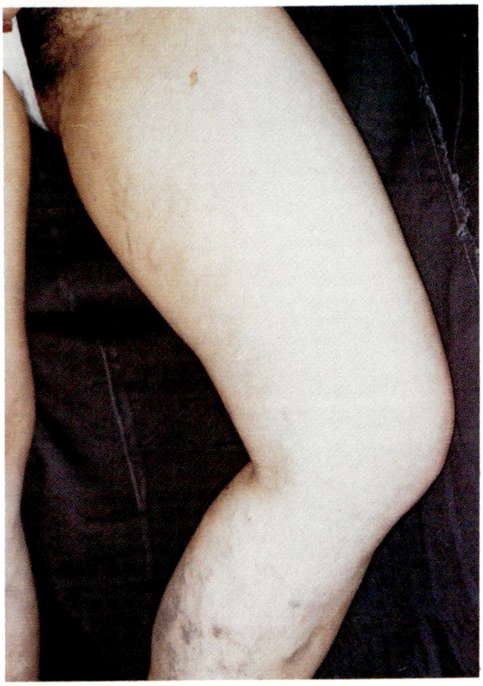

FIGURE 18-1. A, Varicose veins beginning at root of thigh at union of external border of labia with inner face of thigh. **B,** Varicosities cascade down to leg; they are superficial, deep blue, or violaceous.

Physical examination of these patients showed the following characteristics:

1. Saphenous veins were "not open," and the saphenofemoral junction was not obviously incompetent, as determined by palpation or Doppler examination.
2. Vulvar varices were frequently present (180 of 250 cases).
3. Varicose veins began at the root of the thigh at the union of the external border of the labia and the inner area of the thigh (Figure 18-1).

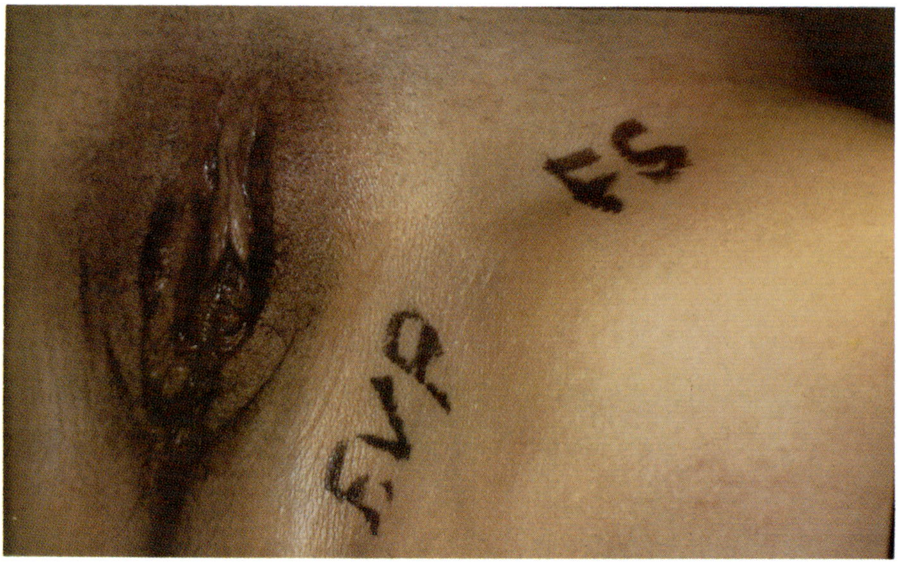

FIGURE 18-2. Two fossae observed when patient lies recumbent with thigh and knee flexed and slightly abducted. Pelvic fossa (*FVP*); saphenous fossa (*FS*).

4. Two fossae appeared when the patient was recumbent and the thigh was flexed to 45 degrees and slightly abducted (Figure 18-2). The long adductor muscle tendon was prominent and separated the two depressions. The external depression was the saphenous fossa. The inner one was the pelvic fossa, in which varicose extensions of the pelvic veins appeared.
5. The course of the varices did not follow the saphenous system. Typically, it crossed the posterior or anterior area of the thigh to the lateral leg, foot, and popliteal fossa.
6. Small veins often cascaded down the posterior and lateral areas of the thigh and leg. These very superficial veins were usually deep blue or violaceous. They were fragile, prone to ecchymosis and hematomas, and difficult to surgically remove.

Vascular Radiology

Diagnosis is confirmed with invasive phlebography. We rely on direct visualization of pelvic and vulvar veins via the gonadal veins. The ovarian vein has been demonstrated through color flow imaging.[14]

Fifteen cases were assessed with standard ascending phlebography, and the results were normal. Varicography performed on 25 patients failed to show the site of varicose vein entry into the saphenous or deep venous systems through perforator veins. Of 250 patients, 225 underwent phlebography of the gonadal veins accom-

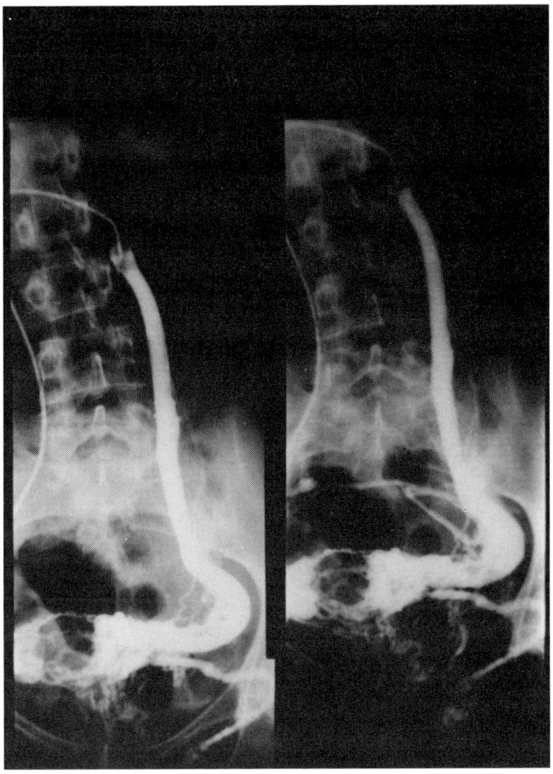

FIGURE 18-3. Dilatation of left gonadal vein followed by plexiform varices in pelvis.

plished with the Seldinger technique. With this technique, a catheter inserted under fluoroscopic control reaches the right gonadal vein through the vena cava or the left gonadal vein through the left renal vein; contrast medium is injected intermittently. Both gonadal veins were studied in 160 of the 225 patients. The left gonadal vein was almost always catheterized. Although initially the orifice of the right gonadal vein in the vena cava was difficult to enter, more experience allowed location of this orifice in 80% of the attempts.

A recent anatomic study revealed variations in the termination of gonadal veins in 22% of cases.[15] Such variations may explain some failures in gonadal phlebography. General findings within our patient group included the following:

1. Dilatation of the utero-ovarian veins with valvular incompetence.
2. Plexiform varicose veins in the pelvis, involving the uterine, vesical, and broad ligament veins (Figure 18-3).
3. Varices in the vulva and vagina. "Leaking" of contrast material that resulted in filling of varicose veins in the inner and posterior aspects of the thigh (Figure 18-4). This effect has been described as "dumping." We have dem-

onstrated such dumping to knee level by filling varices in this area with injection into the gonadal vein (Figure 18-5). Schobinger[16] has reported examples of dumping from the gonadal veins to varices at the ankle and foot.

4. Drainage of the internal pudendal vein, the obturator veins, and, more rarely, the inferior gluteal vein to the hypogastric vein; drainage of the round ligament vein to the broad ligament veins and of the external pudendal vein to the femoral vein.
5. Filling of the contralateral side in all cases but in varying degrees. Crossflow explains varices on one side and gonadal insufficiency on the other (Figure 18-6). This situation was present in 11% of our cases.
6. A consistent pattern shows reflux from gonadal veins filling broad ligament veins descending into the vulva and thigh via the obturator, internal pudendal, inferior gluteal, and round ligament veins. Of the last 180 phlebographic studies completed, 140 showed bilateral dilatation and reflux of gonadal veins; 15 studies demonstrated dilatation and reflux only on the left side and 25 only on the right side.
7. Examination of common, external, and internal iliac veins showed competence. The pattern of iliac injection (Figure 18-7) is different from that of gonadal injection, with 95% of iliac veins being competent.

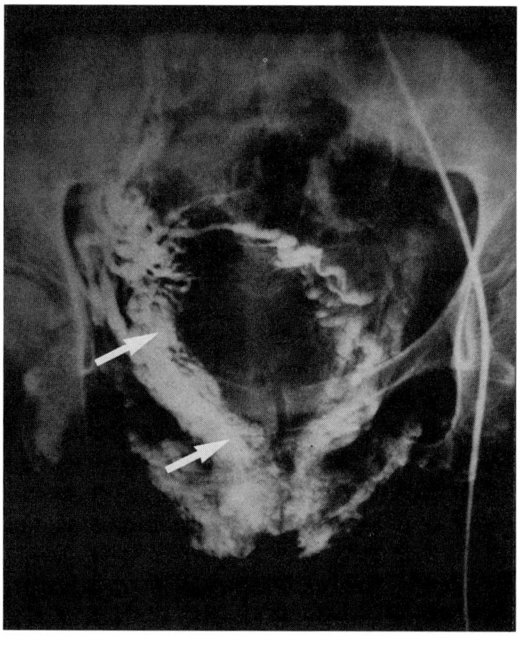

FIGURE 18-4. Vulvar phase of right gonadal phlebography demonstrating filling of vulvar varices via internal pudendal (upper arrow) and obturator (lower arrow) veins. Note filling of both pelvic systems due to pelvic cross-communication and reflux.

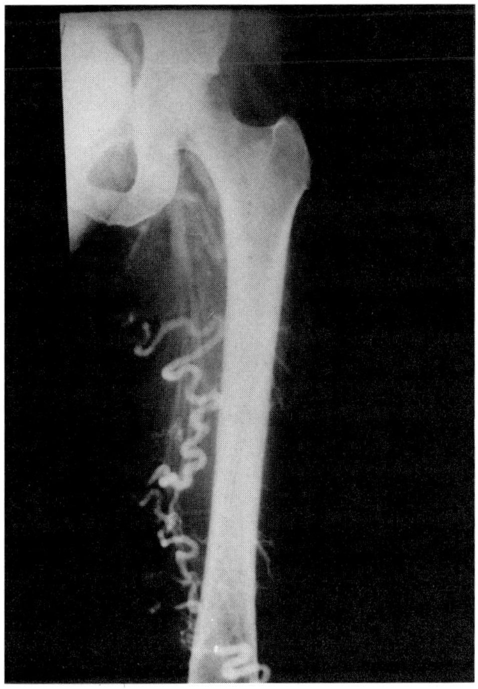

FIGURE 18-5. Dumping from gonadal vein to knee level.

A 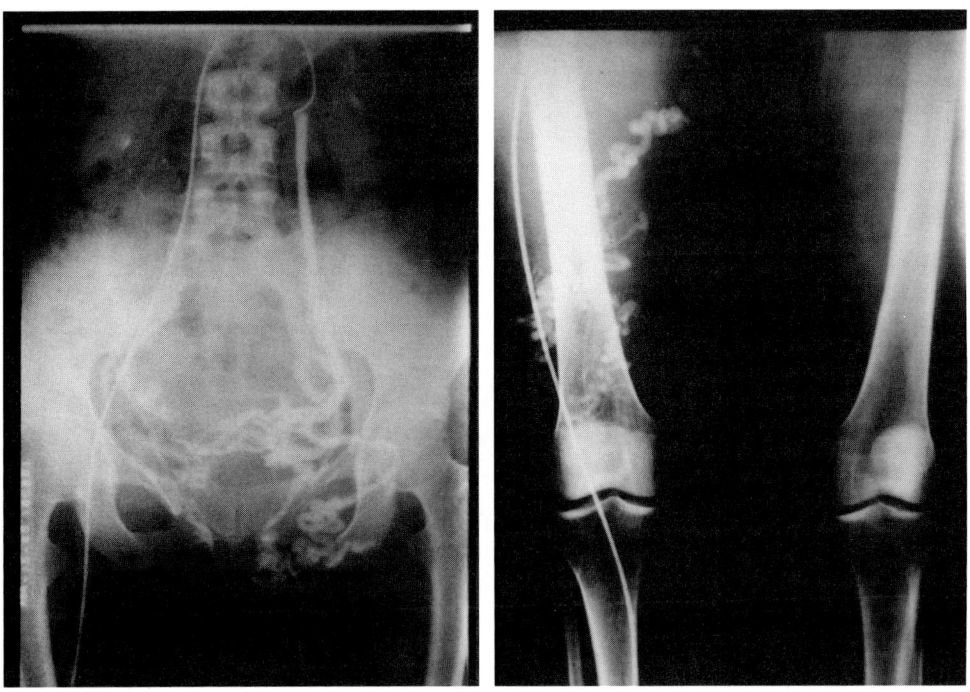 B

FIGURE 18-6. A, Injection in left gonadal vein filling veins in right pelvic and vulvar areas. B, Varices in right leg filled from injection in left gonadal vein.

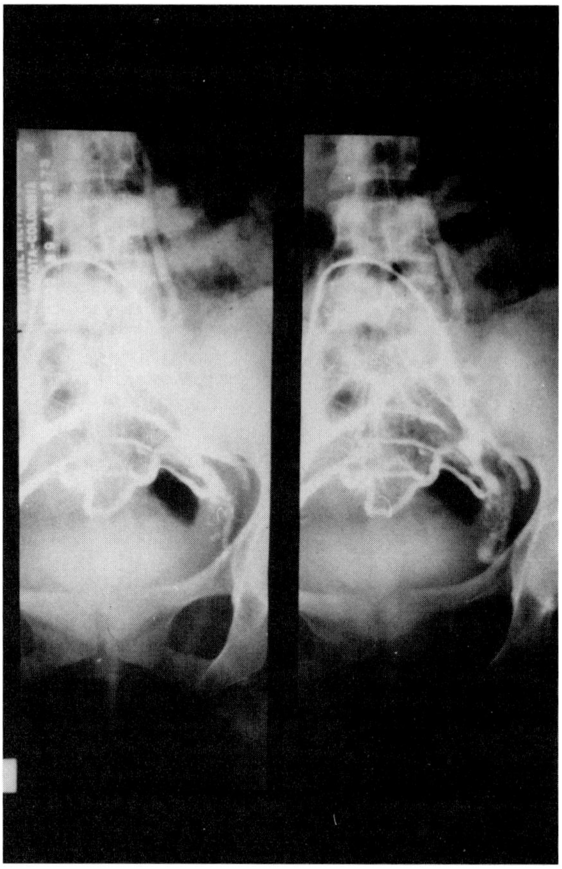

FIGURE 18-7. Pattern of iliac injection. System is competent with no dumping noted.

Surgical Treatment

Gonadal veins are exposed through a curved, almost transverse 6 cm incision located anterior and medial to the anterior iliac spine. Extensive muscle splitting exposes the retroperitoneal space. The gonadal vein is usually attached to peritoneal fat (Figure 18-8). Because the gonadal vein is large and fragile, it is dissected carefully for a few centimeters, ligated, and divided. Hemostats are not used to clamp the vein because they may tear the vessel, producing severe hemorrhage. The ovarian vein is handled with utmost care through the use of atraumatic vascular forceps, and ligatures are passed around and securely tightened above and below the dissected gonadal vein. A careful search for other gonadal veins is performed since at this level the ovarian vein may be double or triple.[15] If a duplication is left unligated, the varicocele may recur. The lower ligature is left long, and dissection of the vein continues into the pelvis (Figure 18-9). As dissection progresses downward, the gonadal vein opens, in an umbrella-like fashion, in front of the ovary. Individual ligations are not done because they are difficult, bloody, and time-consuming. In-

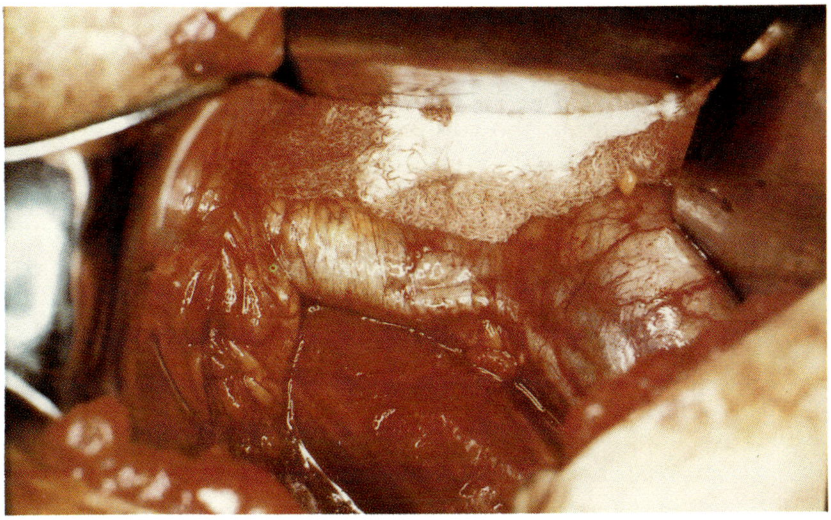

FIGURE 18-8. Dilated right gonadal vein exposed extraperitoneally. Note distal bifurcation of main trunk, psoas muscle, and retroperitoneal fat.

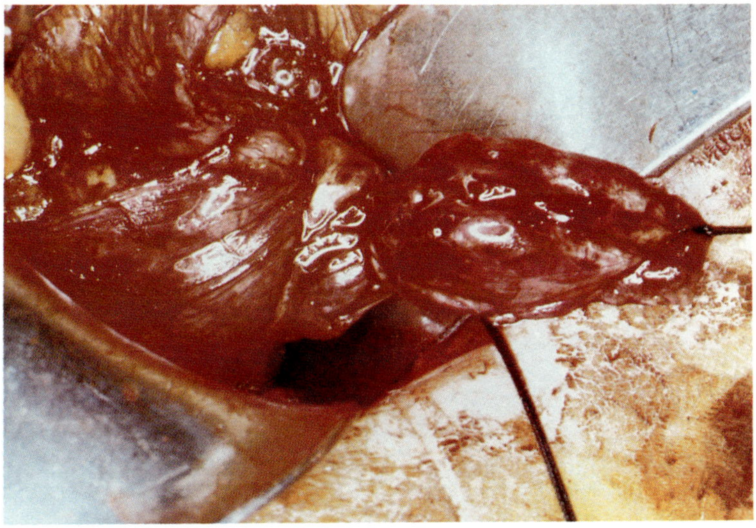

FIGURE 18-9. En bloc dissection and ligature of gonadal vein into pelvis anterior to ovary.

stead, en bloc dissection and ligature are performed at the ovary. At this point, as many as 11 branches usually are found and ligated en masse. A transfixion ligature is applied proximally, near the severed stump.

Muscles and skin are closed in the usual manner. Next, the contralateral gonadal vein is ligated and resected. This step should always be done to avoid failures in the treatment of pelvic and vulvar veins since both gonadal systems communicate freely across the pelvis in the midline. The second part of the operation consists of varicectomy of the vulvar veins (Figure 18-10) and removal of leg veins through small transverse incisions done with the hemostatic technique. Excision of more superficial veins is performed by traction and forcipressure (varicectomy). Alternatively, sclerotherapy can be performed postoperatively. The skin is closed with 5-0 monofilament sutures, and elastic pressure is applied.

Surgical Data and Results

A total of 250 patients presented for treatment. Bilateral gonadal vein ligation was performed in 232 patients (92.8%) (Table 18-1). Unilateral ligations were done in the remaining patients: right gonadal vein resection in 12 patients (4.8%) and left gonadal vein resection in 6 patients (2.4%). During our earliest surgical experience, in 1984 and 1985, we performed ligation and resection of gonadal veins of the affected side. Currently, we believe that because of cross-communications of pelvic veins and cross-reflux into the vulva and thigh, both gonadal veins should be

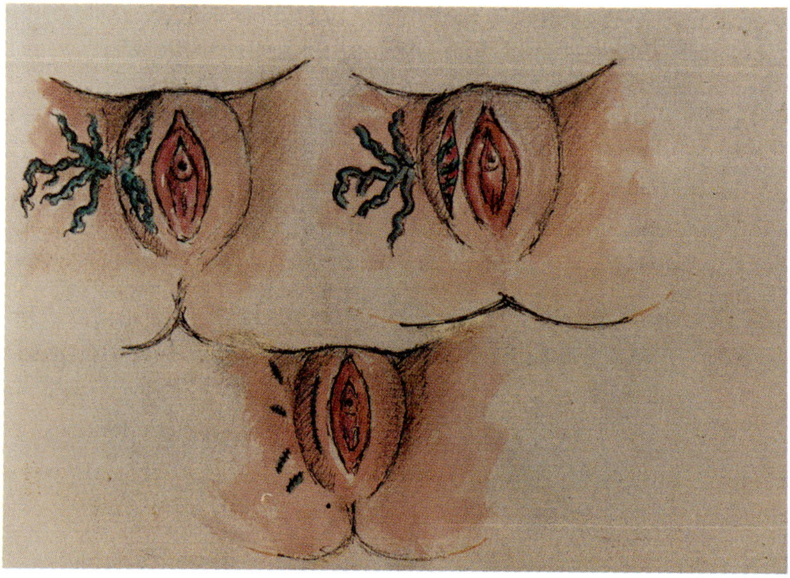

FIGURE 18-10. Varicectomy of vulvar veins. Upper left: varices in pelvic fossa and vulva; upper right: vertical incision in labia to dissect and resect varices; lower center: varicectomy completed in vulva and pelvic fossa with skin sutures shown.

interrupted. The last 220 patients in our study group had bilateral treatment. Of 40 patients (16%) with saphenous insufficiency, 25 patients (10%) had unilateral insufficiency and 15 (6%) had bilateral insufficiency. The operation was always completed by treating both conditions, pelvic and saphenous. A total of 50 patients (20%) had previous saphenous vein surgery. Among 25 patients (10%), one or more pregnancies followed this surgery and pelvic varices recurred. Recurrent varices after adequate saphenous surgery (12 of our own cases) may be treated by gonadal vein resection. Complementary sclerotherapy should be performed on small veins for cosmetic reasons. Most patients (90%) request this additional procedure.

Of the 250 patients, 215 showed excellent results and 25 had good results. A total of 240 patients (96%) had very satisfactory outcomes (Figure 18-11). Eight patients had fair outcomes, and two patients showed no improvement, even though gonadal veins were ligated (both unilateral) and varicose veins were removed (Figure 18-12).

TABLE 18-1. Treatment of pelvic varices in 250 surgical cases, Sept. 1984-Sept. 1991

	No. of Patients	% of Patients
Bilateral resection of gonadal vein	232	92.8
Right gonadal vein resection	12	4.8
Left gonadal vein resection	6	2.4
Vulvar varicectomy	180	72
Leg varicectomy (thigh, leg, foot)	250	100
Postoperative sclerotherapy	209	90

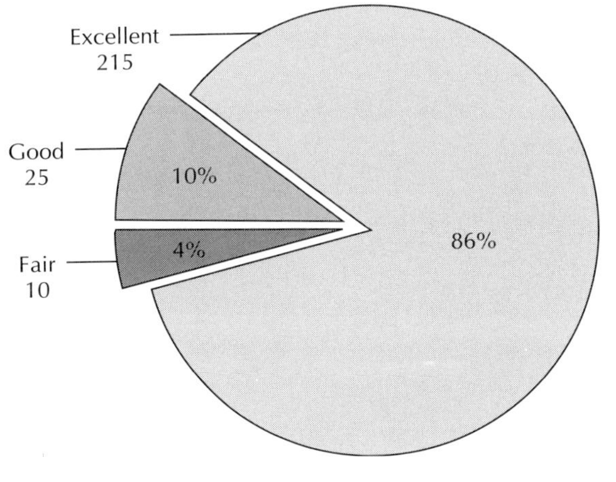

FIGURE 18-11. Results of treatment of pelvic varices in 250 surgical cases (Sept. 1984-Sept. 1991).

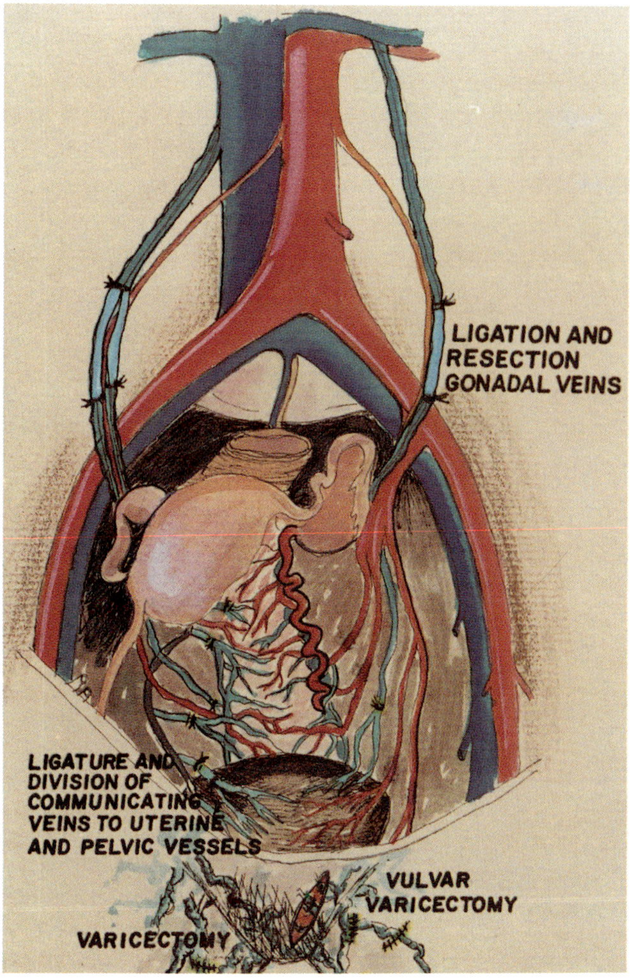

FIGURE 18-12. Artist's view of complete operation for treatment of pelvic varices and gonadal veins. Bilateral gonadal resection and ligation with vulvar and leg varicectomy are shown.

Discussion

Pelvic veins have been the subject of observation for many years. Lea Thomas et al.[17] described veins that appear during pregnancy in the vulva, labia, and on the medial and posterior thigh. The cause was proposed to be from reflux through the internal pudendal and obturator veins from the high-pressure internal iliac vein into the thin-walled vulvar and inner thigh veins which dilate during pregnancy and occasionally do not disappear. This change was believed to give rise to premenstrual symptoms of vulvar and thigh congestion and pain. Varicectomy was advised as treatment.[18,19]

Craig and Hobbs[5] demonstrated the association of pelvic congestion syndrome and vulvar varices. They advocated vulvar venography to demonstrate drainage into the internal iliac vein via the obturator and internal pudendal veins for visualization of pelvic varicosities in the vesical plexus and broad ligaments. Sumner[20] stated, "Vulvar veins may persist postpartum giving rise to varicosities that extend from the posteromedial thigh down the back of the leg to the posterior and lateral aspect of the thigh and popliteal fossa. They can become congested and painful, especially before the onset of menstruation." Vulvar and leg varicectomy was advised by Craig and Hobbs[5] as treatment.

By performing phlebographic studies in late pregnancy, Kerr et al.[21] showed complete compression of the inferior vena cava and iliac veins against the lumbar spine and psoas muscle, with venous return provided by ascending lumbar and azygous systems and ovarian veins draining the uterus. In 1918, Ivanissevich advanced the theory that varicoceles in males were produced by retrograde flow in the left spermatic vein and described his operation. Interest in the study of pelvic venous circulation increased after the publication of the classic work by Guilhem and Baux[1] in 1954.

Intrauterine phlebography provides considerable information on pelvic pathology and the course of gonadal veins.[22-25] Excellent reviews on pelvic congestion syndrome published by Hobbs,[26] and Langeron and Quehen,[27] and many others have aided our understanding of pelvic congestion pain. Retrograde injection techniques, especially selective catheterization of the gonadal vein,[2-4,28] are reliable and successful methods of identifying the anatomy and pathology of these vessels. Ahlberg et al.[4] found that ovarian veins are larger than spermatic veins because of distention of their walls during pregnancy and menses. This dilatation may persist when involution is not complete after pregnancy.

From a review of the literature and confirmation through our experience, we recommend bilateral resection of gonadal veins with ligation of their communications to uterine veins. This procedure interrupts high-pressure reflux into vulvar and thigh veins. The operation represents a radical treatment of varicoceles in females. High ligation should be complemented by complete resection of distal dilated varices, including treatment of insufficiency of the saphenofemoral junction if present. In keeping with this concept, vulvar, thigh, and leg varices should be eliminated at the same time.

PELVIC CONGESTION SYNDROME

The pelvic congestion syndrome is always associated with chronic pelvic pain (pelvagia). It is an elusive and frustrating problem, particularly when no somatic pathologic condition is found. In such a situation, the patient is then labeled as "psychosomatic" and referred to a specialist in emotional or behavioral problems or to a pain clinic. The emotional impact of pain on the patient may be alleviated by anesthesiologists or psychologists; however, if an organic condition persists, pain resurfaces and a vicious cycle occurs.[29,30]

As a final option, the treating physician frequently resorts to performing a hysterectomy of a normal uterus. This method often fails to relieve the patient's pain. It is believed that approximately 70,000 hysterectomies are performed annually in the United States to alleviate chronic pelvic pain. Although the percentage of normal tissue in this group is unknown, it is believed to be high. Of women referred to the pelvagia clinic at the Naval Hospital in San Diego, 14% had previously undergone hysterectomy and salpingo-oophorectomy with poor results.[31]

Our interest in pelvic congestion syndrome arose from talks with John Hobbs in 1985 about the publication of his article on this syndrome in 1976.[32,33] Our experience covers a 5-year period, from 1986 through 1991. A group of gynecologists was briefed on the coexistence of pelvic varicocele and pelvic pain. They were persuaded not to perform hysterectomies in patients with pelvic varicocele because hysterectomy involves close contact with the uterine body and cervix, resulting in ovarian varicoceles and dilated veins of the broad ligament. Instead, bilateral gonadal vein ligation and resection was suggested for these patients. The steps taken to approach the problem were as follows:

1. Rule out and, if present, treat all organic causes of chronic pelvic pain, such as endometriosis, adhesions, inflammation, tumors, and urinary or rectal pathology.
2. Perform a careful psychologic and/or psychiatric examination.
3. Always perform laparoscopy for positive diagnosis of pelvic varicocele. Gonadal phlebography is rarely required.
4. For optimum results, perform a complete and bilateral gonadal vein ligation and resection.

Twenty-eight patients with pelvic congestion syndrome were treated previously for organic problems or had received psychiatric care. Approximately half of these patients developed relapses from their treatments. Of the 28 patients, 5 had hysterectomies. All patients were women, ages 24 to 42 years, multiparous (two to four pregnancies), and sexually active. Table 18-2 shows the clinical profile of these patients. This group is distinct from those previously described, who had pelvic varices, varicose legs, or vulvar veins. All patients suffered from varying degrees of chronic pelvic pain, often incapacitating and at times reflecting to the lower back, buttocks, vulva, and upper thighs. To visualize the varicocele, laparoscopy was performed on all patients. Tilting the lower end of the table and having the patient perform a Valsalva maneuver enhanced the varicocele. Only three patients required gonadal vein phlebography to confirm a tentative diagnosis of varicocele by laparoscopy.

Veins at the root of the thigh and vulval area often became painful and dilated premenstrually and after coitus. Vulval symptoms were present in 50% of patients. The most common symptom, except for pelvic pain, was dyspareunia, which was present in 75% of patients. This troublesome condition caused anxiety and depression and was associated with increased marital problems. The frustration originating from dyspareunia is probably the most distressing manifestation of pelvic congestion syndrome and leads to secondary frigidity. Approximately half of these

TABLE 18-2. Pelvic congestion syndrome: Clinical profile of 28 patients before undergoing bilateral gonadal vein resection

Signs and Symptoms	No. of Patients
Chronic pelvic pain	28
Dyspareunia	20
Vulval symptoms	14
Psychosomatic symptoms	12
Premenstrual syndrome	12
Leg symptoms and varices	10
Vulval varices	9
Dysmenorrhea	8
Urinary symptoms	5
Posthysterectomy	5
Rectal symptoms	3

patients were incapacitated for several days by premenstrual symptoms and/or dysmenorrhea. One third of this group had vulvar or leg varices with related symptoms. No concomitant varicectomy of vulvar or leg veins was performed with gonadal vein surgery in these 28 patients. Of particular interest were the five patients who had undergone previous hysterectomies for various causes; they all had large varicoceles. Two of these patients had very large dilated veins, both on the right side.

This group of 28 patients, referred to us by gynecologists, were seen and operated on between May 1986 and November 1991. All but three of them underwent laparotomy, hysterectomy, and bilateral gonadal vein ligation. Three patients had retroperitoneal dissection of gonadal veins, resection of a segment of 5 to 8 cm of the right and left ovarian veins down to the ovary, and ligation of the upper and lower stumps.

Surgery was followed by an uneventful recovery, with no complications. Both the patients and the physicians were highly pleased with the results. In 20 patients, the outcome was excellent; in 8 patients, the results were good, with minor postoperative complaints. To our surprise, patients who had suffered symptoms for 10 years had no further pelvic pain, dyspareunia, or premenstrual symptoms after surgery. Even the emotional characteristics of some patients improved after relief from the pain and other symptoms.

In light of the excellent surgical results we have been able to achieve, we will continue to perform this surgery in well-chosen cases. We recommend that physicians who have patients with chronic pelvic pain associated with varicocele perform bilateral gonadal vein resection and ligation.

REFERENCES

1. Guilhem P, Baux R. La Phlebographie Pelvienne par Voies Veineuse, Osseuse et Utérine. Paris: Masson et Cie, 1954.
2. Ahlberg NE, Bartley O, Chidekel N. Right and left gonadal veins: An anatomical and statistical study. Acta Radiol 4:593-601, 1966.
3. Chidekel N. Female pelvic veins demonstrated by selective renal phlebography with particular reference to pelvic varicosities. Acta Radiol 7:198, 1968.
4. Ahlberg NE, Bartley O, Chidekel N. Retrograde contrast filling of the left gonadal vein. A roentgenologic and anatomical study. Acta Radiol 3:385, 1965.
5. Craig O, Hobbs JT. Vulvar phlebography in the pelvic congestion syndrome. Clin Radiol 25:517, 1975.
6. Gomez ER, Villavicencio JL, Coffey JM, Rich NM. Pathogenesis and surgical management of varicose veins of the vulva and upper thigh: The internal iliac venous insufficiency syndrome. In Veith FJ, ed. Current Critical Problems in Vascular Surgery, vol 2. St. Louis: Quality Medical Publishing, 1990, pp 141-142.
7. Le Page PA, Villavicencio JL, Gomez ER, Sheridan MN, Rich NM. The valvular anatomy of the iliac venous system and its clinical implications. J Vasc Surg 14:678-683, 1991.
8. Hobbs JT. Personal communication. Vienna, 1990.
9. Lechter A. Pelvic varices: Treatment. J Cardiovasc Surg 26:111, 1985.
10. Lechter A, Alvarez A. Pelvic varices and gonadal veins. In Negus D, Jantet G, eds. Phlebology 1985. London: John Libbey, 1986, pp 225-228.
11. Lechter A, Alvarez A, Lopez G. Pelvic varices and gonadal veins. Phlebology 2:181-188, 1987.
12. Lechter A, Lopez G, Franco CA, Martinez C, Camacho J. New concepts in the clinical, radiological and surgical aspects of varices of pelvic origin [abstract]. Vienna: Fifth European American Venous Symposium, 1990.
13. Schraibman IG, Hobbs JT. Pelvic congestion syndrome and ligation of ovarian veins [letter]. Br J Hosp Med 44:14, 1990.
14. Richardson G, Beckwith TC, Sheldon M. Ultrasound assessment in the treatment of pelvic varicose veins. Fort Lauderdale: Third American Venous Forum, 1991.
15. Lechter A, Lopez G, Martinez C, Camacho J. Anatomy of the gonadal veins: A reappraisal. Surgery 109:735-739, 1991.
16. Schobinger RA. Ilio-femoral dumping syndrome [abstract]. Vienna: Fifth European American Venous Symposium, 1990.
17. Lea Thomas M, Fletcher EWL, Andress MR, Cockett FB. The venous connections of vulvar varices. Clin Radiol 18:313, 1967.
18. Dodd H, Payling-Wright H. Vulval varicose veins in pregnancy. Br Med J (Clin Res) 1:831-832, 1959.
19. Dixon JA, Mitchell WA. Venographic and surgical observations in vulval varicose veins. Surg Gynecol Obstet 131:458-464, 1970.
20. Sumner DS. Venous dynamics varicosities. Clin Obstet Gynecol 24:743-761, 1981.
21. Kerr MG, Scott DB, Samuel E. Studies of the inferior vena cava in late pregnancy. Br Med J 1:532, 1964.
22. Topolanski-Sierra R. Am J Obstet Gynecol 76:44, 1958.
23. Chidekel N, Edlundh KO. Transuterine phlebography with particular reference to pelvic varicosities. Acta Radiol 7:1, 1968.
24. Jaramillo R, Mejia A, Morales H. Flebografía pélvica y varicocele del ligamento ancho. Tribuna Medica 4:1-19, 1965.
25. Mayall RC, Dias Garcia Mayall AC, Moreira Jannuzzi JC. Varices pelviennes de la femme. Phlebologie 36:191-195, 1983.
26. Hobbs JT. Treatment of vulval and pelvic varices. In Bergan JJ, Yao JST, eds. Venous Disorders. Philadelphia: WB Saunders, 1991, pp 250-257.

27. Langeron P, Quehen E. Les algies pelviennes chez la femme. Ann Chir 19-20:1096-1108, 1966.
28. Helander CG, Lindbom A. Varicocele of the broad ligament: A venographic study. Acta Radiol 53:97, 1960.
29. Beard RW, Reginald PW, Pearce S. Pelvic pain in women. Br Med J 293:1160-1162, 1986.
30. Beard RW, Highman JH, Pearce S, Reginald PW. Diagnosis of pelvic varicosities in women with chronic pelvic pain. Lancet 2:946, 1984.
31. Reiter RC. Alteraciones somáticas ocultas en mujeres con dolor pélvico crónico. In Pitkin RM, Scott JR, eds. Clínicas Obstétricas y Ginecológicas, vol 1. Apdo: McGraw-Hill Interamericana de México, 1990, pp 155-160.
32. Hobbs JT. The pelvic congestion syndrome. Practitioner 216:529-540, 1976.
33. Hobbs JT. The pelvic congestion syndrome. Br J Hosp Med 43:200-206, 1990.

PART FIVE

Telangiectatic Leg Veins

Chapter 19

Treatment of Telangiectasias

Paul K. Thibault

Lower limb telangiectasias are visible, ectatic dermal veins measuring 0.1 to 1 mm in diameter.[1-4] Initially telangiectasias appear as faint erythematous lines, but with time they become progressively more dilated, tortuous, and elevated above the skin surface and turn blue. Recently the term "venulectasia" has been used to describe larger blue telangiectasias measuring 1 to 2 mm in diameter.[5] Invariably telangiectasias are closely associated with either dilated subcutaneous reticular veins or varicose veins[6] (Figure 19-1). Frequently a family history of similar abnormally dilated lower limb veins is noted,[4] but this factor is not invariable. Polygenetic inheritance from maternal or paternal lines is the probable mode of transmission of the susceptibility to form telangiectasias, with hormonal influences (particularly estrogen) being pivotal in the ultimate expression of the disorder. Hence telangiectasias are more common in women; their onset frequently is precipitated by the hormonal surges of menarche and pregnancy. The most common time of presentation for treatment is between the ages of 30 and 50 years, but with the modern trend of emphasizing physical attractiveness, presentation as early as 15 years and as late as 75 years is not unusual. It is uncommon for men to seek treatment for lower limb telangiectasias.

Unattractive or disfiguring visual appearance is the most common presenting symptom of patients with telangiectasias. However, mild to severe pain is also a well-recognized symptom.[5,7] Because the most common reason for requesting treatment is to achieve cosmetic improvement, it is essential that effective treatment be relatively free of adverse sequelae.

HISTORICAL BACKGROUND

In 1934 Biegeleisen[6] described a microinjection technique for treating telangiectasias. He used sodium morrhuate (a mixture of sodium salts of the saturated and unsaturated fatty acids present in cod liver oil), but frequently complications

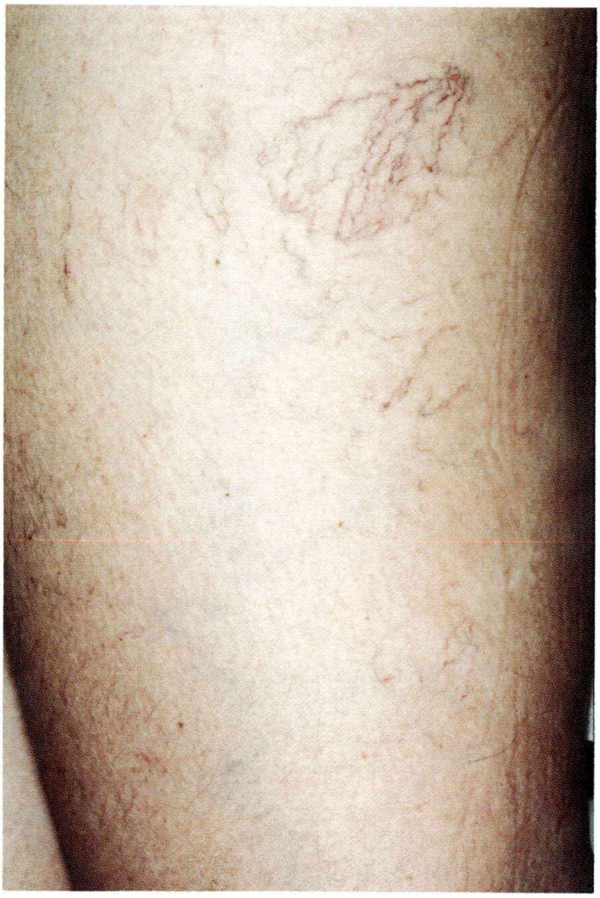

FIGURE 19-1. Lateral thigh telangiectasias with associated dilated blue subcutaneous reticular veins.

occurred, for example, cutaneous ulceration, pigmentation, and allergic reactions including anaphylaxis. It became clear that there was an obvious need for a mild sclerosing agent free of adverse local and systemic effects.

In 1925 Jausion had recommended chromated glycerin as a sclerosing agent for varicose veins, but because of the mild action of this agent it was eventually discarded for that purpose. However, in France the high safety profile of chromated glycerin for injection of small veins was recognized, and in the 1950s this agent became the most commonly used substance for the treatment of telangiectasias in that country.[8]

Polidocanol was developed in the 1950s as a topical, local, and epidural anesthetic, but its use as an anesthetic was discontinued when it was found to sclerose small-diameter blood vessels through intravascular or intradermal injection. The use of polidocanol as a therapeutic sclerosant for varicose veins was first described by Eichenberger[9] in 1969. Because of its relatively low incidence of adverse effects, polidocanol eventually was popularized as a safe sclerosant for treatment of telangiectasias by Ouvry et al.[10] Foley[11] and Alderman[12] described their experiences with the use of hypertonic saline solution in concentrations of 18% to 20%. The use of hypertonic saline with and without additives soon became popular with North American dermatologists influenced by the absence of antigenicity of unadulterated hypertonic saline solution when compared with other agents.[13]

Sodium tetradecyl sulfate (STS) was first described in 1946,[14] and it was popularized by Fegan[15] for the treatment of varicose veins. However, STS caused an unacceptable incidence of cutaneous ulceration and pigmentation when the commercially produced 1% solution was used for the injection of small veins.[16] Consequently, polidocanol (in Europe) and hypertonic saline solution (in North America) were preferred for the treatment of telangiectasias. Recently, with the correct dilution of STS ranging from 0.1% to 0.2%, this sclerosant has been widely used for treating telangiectasias.

Although steady progress has been made in using sclerotherapy as a therapeutic modality for telangiectasias, other forms of treatment, namely, electrosurgery and laser photocoagulation, have been used but have not achieved acceptance because of ineffectiveness and adverse sequelae. Electrotherapy of telangiectasias was first used in the early 1900s, but the electrical current required to desiccate cutaneous vessels resulted in dermal necrosis with varying degrees of scarring. Since 1975, various lasers have been used in photocoagulation of lower limb telangiectasias, but enthusiasm for this method has been dampened by the relative ineffectiveness of laser surgery compared with sclerotherapy. Also, laser therapy has been associated with adverse sequelae, including hypopigmentation, hyperpigmentation, cutaneous necrosis, and pain. However, certain lasers have been shown to be safe and effective for fine red telangiectasias <0.1 mm in diameter.[17] A complete discussion of laser treatment of leg veins is beyond the scope of this chapter. Hence the remainder of this chapter deals exclusively with sclerotherapy of telangiectasias.

HISTORY AND EXAMINATION

The patient who presents with telangiectasias first should have a directed history and examination. Important information to obtain in the history includes age of onset, possibility of aggravation by past pregnancies, and whether the condition is stable or deteriorating. It is important to note whether the patient's chief complaint is predominantly cosmetic or pain-related because this factor may significantly influence the patient's expectations regarding treatment outcomes and consequently affect treatment decisions. History taking should focus on whether the patient has had any bleeding disorders, episodes of superficial thrombophlebitis or deep venous thrombosis, and previous treatment, including surgery and sclerotherapy. Past and present use of hormonal contraceptives and hormonal replacement therapy, cigarette consumption, and allergy to any medications also should be noted. A thorough family history will provide valuable information as to the potential severity of the telangiectasia.

Examination of the lower limbs is best performed with the patient standing on a platform in front of the physician. Good lighting is essential for a systematic inspection of each aspect of the leg from the groin to the toes. The patterns of telangiectasias and their relationships to underlying reticular and varicose veins must be noted. It is important to remember that patients with cosmetic symptoms associated with lower limb telangiectatic veins may have incompetence of the major superficial veins (long or short saphenous veins). In a study of patients presenting with cosmetic symptoms related to lower limb superficial veins, duplex evaluation of limbs with telangiectasias without clinical evidence of associated varicose veins revealed a significant incidence of incompetence in the long or short saphenous veins[18] (Table 19-1). It is uncommon, however, for telangiectasias to be associated with deep venous incompetence. Therefore after physical examination, further diagnostic evaluation with Doppler ultrasound, plethysmography, or duplex imaging should be considered if there is clinical suspicion of incompetence of the long or short saphenous systems.

Finally, clinical photographs should be taken to document the pretreatment state of all affected areas. This step is essential to assess progress during treatment and to clarify whether adverse sequelae (e.g., telangiectatic matting) have occurred as a result of treatment. A high standard of photography is required, and color transparencies are the preferred medium. Good results normally will be achieved by using a 35 mm, single-lens reflex camera with a macrolens combined with a macroflash unit. The background for photographs should be plain and uncluttered. For color photographs a neutral background, such as light blue, is recommended. Progress photographs taken during treatment are necessary only to document unusual or adverse effects.

At the time of initial consultation, the patient should be informed fully about the treatment, the expected outcome, and the nature and likelihood of any adverse effects. This information should be made available to the patient in the form of a comprehensive information leaflet or brochure that the patient can refer to during

TABLE 19-1. Venous incompetence according to clinical classification*

	Telangiectasias Only (N = 83)	Telangiectasias and Varicose Veins (N = 314)	Varicose Veins Only (N = 84)
Average age (yr)	39.7	41.4	42.5
Superficial incompetence (%)	22.9	49.0	66.7
Deep incompetence (%)	0	1.6	1.2
Perforator incompetence (%)	1.2	10.6	13.1

*Modified from Thibault P, Bray A, Wlodarczyk J, et al. Cosmetic leg veins: Evaluation using duplex venous imaging. J Dermatol Surg Oncol 16:612-618, 1990.

treatment. Patients with cosmetic symptoms related to telangiectasias often have high expectations regarding ultimate outcome, and a realistic goal should be agreed on between patient and physician before treatment is begun.

THE SCLEROTHERAPY ROOM

Since a visit to the sclerotherapist can be a traumatic experience for some patients, a relaxing environment is essential. A warm and neutral decor and soothing background music will assist in relaxing the anxious patient and, in turn, will aid the sclerotherapist in performing his or her work efficiently.

The patient is placed in the supine position on a table that is positioned in the room so that the sclerotherapist can move around it easily. Such placement will assist in minimizing the need to reposition the patient and help to avoid placing the patient in awkward and uncomfortable postures. Good lighting is essential, with well-placed overhead fluorescent lighting that provides shadow-free illumination and obviates the need for additional accessory floor lights that can become unnecessary obstacles. Fluorescent lighting also is superior to incandescent lighting for highlighting the blue colors of reticular veins. Overhead "operating" spotlights have been recommended,[19] but such lights are expensive and generate heat within the room, making it uncomfortable for both the patient and the sclerotherapist.

A stool is situated on either side of the treatment table. In general, sclerotherapy of small veins should be performed with the sclerotherapist in the sitting position, which allows the physician to rest his or her arms on the sides of the table for greater steadiness. Either the table or the stool should be readily adjustable in height to optimize the position of the patient relative to the physician. A Mayo stand should be easily accessible to the sclerotherapist, especially if a nurse is not assisting. The stand is equipped with sclerosant solutions, needles, syringes, compression pads, gauze swabs, alcohol solution, and emergency drugs.

TREATMENT PLAN

The presence of telangiectasias should not be considered in isolation from the larger veins into which they drain. If one disregards treatment of reticular veins and proceeds directly to microsclerotherapy of telangiectasias, early recurrence will be noted in most instances because of persisting pressure from proximal sources of superficial venous reflux. Therefore sclerotherapy of telangiectasias should follow a systematic plan, consisting of the following steps: (1) treatment of associated long or short saphenous vein incompetence (if present), (2) treatment of branch varicosities (if present), (3) sclerotherapy of associated reticular veins, and (4) microsclerotherapy of telangiectasias. Steps 1 and 2 are discussed in Chapters 8, 10, 11, 12, and 13 and therefore will not be discussed here.

Treatment of Reticular Veins

The distinction between reticular and varicose veins is arbitrary. In this chapter reticular veins are defined as those abnormally dilated subcutaneous veins that are blue, measure 1 to 3 mm in diameter, and are directly associated with telangiectasias. These reticular veins, which are not in direct communication with high-pressure reflux from incompetent main trunks (long or short saphenous veins) or incompetent perforating veins, are seen most commonly over the posterolateral aspects of the thigh and the lateral aspects of the calf. In general, they appear to drain toward the popliteal fossa, with the associated telangiectasias radiating away from the knee (see Chapter 20).

Order of Treatment

As with sclerotherapy of varicose veins, the order of treatment should proceed from proximal to distal, from areas of reflux downstream, and from larger caliber veins to smaller caliber veins.[8,19] A good method is to begin giving injections at the proximal posterior thigh with the patient lying prone and to proceed distally toward the ankle before changing the patient to the lateral position. Once again injections are commenced from proximal to distal points. Next, the anterior and medial aspects of the leg are treated similarly. By using this systematic approach, abnormal veins will not be neglected. Knowing which veins to inject comes with experience, but good lighting will assist in determining the sometimes subtle connections between the cosmetically symptomatic telangiectasias in the dermis and associated abnormally dilated reticular veins in the subcutaneous tissues.

Normally only one limb is treated in a single session, with the number of treatments required determined by the extent and severity of venous dilatation. However, the maximum dose of sclerosing solutions allows complete treatment of reticular veins in one limb to be performed in one or two sessions in approximately 90% of patients.[20] Two different approaches may be used if telangiectasias are extensive and require more than one treatment. The first approach is to treat the reticular veins and associated telangiectasias in one or more adjacent areas in the same session and to leave some untreated until the next session. The second approach is to treat all the reticular veins in the limb in one session and approximately 1 month later to inject the residual telangiectasias.[16] The latter approach often results in fewer injections because many of the telangiectasias fade, either partially or completely, after the source of venous hypertension arising from the reticular veins has been removed.

Injection of Reticular Veins

Two milliliters of sclerosant solution is drawn up in a high-quality, 3 ml plastic disposable syringe fitted with either a 27-gauge or 30-gauge needle, depending on the physician's preference. When injected, the sclerosant should flow easily with a smooth, low-pressure action on the plunger. The advantage of the 27-gauge needle in reducing the plunger pressure is countered by the disadvantage of a slightly more painful skin puncture. Alternatively, a 30-gauge needle is preferred if a slow injection flow rate is required or if the patient is more sensitive to pain or feels anxious. The most common mistake in technique is to transect the vessel on needle insertion.

Therefore it is helpful to bend the needle to an angle of 30 to 50 degrees with the bevel up, so that on insertion the bevel will remain pointing upward.

There are two methods of vessel cannulation for reticular veins. The first method is similar to that for injection of telangiectasias, which will be described later. The second method (preferred by many, particularly those who are developing expertise in this field) is to insert the needle slowly but deliberately and to withdraw blood into the hub of the needle (this can be done with both 27-gauge and 30-gauge needles) in order to ensure that the needle bevel is located in the vein lumen before injection. With this method, tissue tension can be achieved by using the dorsal aspect of the nondominant index finger to stretch the patient's skin toward the syringe, which is rested on the pulp of the index finger and distal interphalangeal joint of the middle finger of the nondominant hand (Figure 19-2). If an awkward location (e.g., around the anterior aspect of the knee) prevents adequate tissue tension from being achieved by this method, digital pressure by an assistant may be required. The physician's arms are steadied by either resting them on the treatment table or, if this is not possible, by gentle pressure of the physician's elbow on the region of the physician's anterior superior iliac spine.

The volume of sclerosant injected depends on ease of flow, concentration of the sclerosant, and diameter of the vein. In general, no more than 0.5 ml should be injected at any one site. Frequently the endpoint of injection is reached when the physician detects a slight increase in resistance to the flow of the solution, denoting vessel spasm. During injection the physician observes the direction of flow of the sclerosant as the solution replaces blood in the vein. The physician should stop

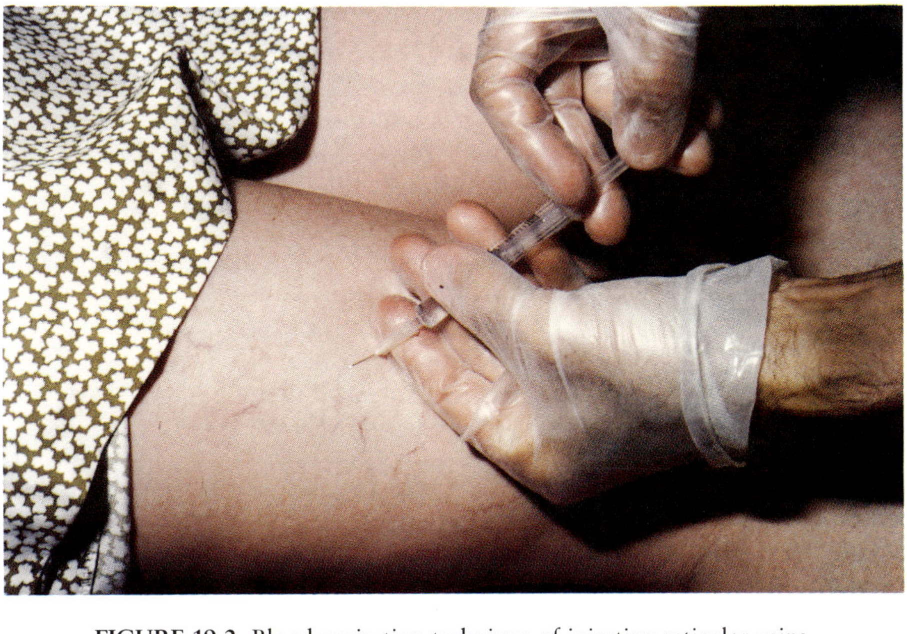

FIGURE 19-2. Blood aspiration technique of injecting reticular veins.

injecting when the desired length of vein has been treated. The maximum length of a reticular vein that can be treated with one injection is approximately 10 cm when a detergent solution is used. If osmotic solutions are used, more injections may be required because of the more localized effect produced.

During and immediately after injection, the reticular vein undergoes spasm. Within several minutes the vessel and the surrounding skin become erythematous, indicating adequate endothelial damage. This inflammation is more apparent with polidocanol than with STS, hypertonic saline solution, or chromated glycerin. If associated telangiectasias become inflamed during treatment of reticular veins, this result indicates passage of sclerosant into the telangiectasias, and no further treatment of the telangiectasias is required. However, highly concentrated solutions should not be injected into telangiectasias because this method will result in a higher incidence of postsclerotherapy pigmentation and cutaneous ulceration. Immediately after injection, pressure is applied to the injected veins by using cotton balls with pieces of paper tape stretched firmly over them. Patients usually remark that this method helps to relieve any postinjection pain. Unless the patient has a sensitivity to paper tape, the cotton balls are left in place for 24 to 48 hours.

Microinjection of Telangiectasias

The technique of microinjection of telangiectasias is covered in detail in Chapters 20 and 21. However, a few important points will be described here. As noted earlier, microinjection of telangiectasias can be performed when reticular veins are treated or, alternatively, 4 to 6 weeks later to allow for resolution of venous hypertension from the reticular veins. The order of treatment is identical to that of reticular veins, that is, injection is started proximally and proceeds distally until one particular aspect of the leg has been completed.

Magnifying loupes with powers from 2 to 3.5 magnification are recommended for obtaining good results. Before injection, the skin is wiped with alcohol. This step changes the refraction coefficient of the skin, making the telangiectasias more visible by indirect lighting. Alcohol also causes some dilatation of the telangiectasias. Disposable 3 ml plastic syringes are used, again filled with 2 ml of sclerosant. All injections are made with a 30-gauge needle, which may need to be changed after three or four injections if it becomes dull. Needles of finer gauge (32- or 33-gauge) can be used for very fine vessels, such as those that occur in telangiectatic matting, but these needles are not disposable, are expensive, and dull rapidly.

The physician should be seated in a comfortable position with his or her arms supported as described for injecting reticular veins. Tissue tension can be achieved by using the three-point technique of stretching the patient's skin between the physician's index finger and thumb of the nondominant hand and the fifth digit of the dominant hand, which is holding the syringe (Figure 19-3). Alternatively, two-point tension between the index finger and thumb of the nondominant hand with tension applied diagonally across the line of injection often suffices (Figure 19-4).

The needle should be bent to an angle of 30 to 50 degrees to prevent transec-

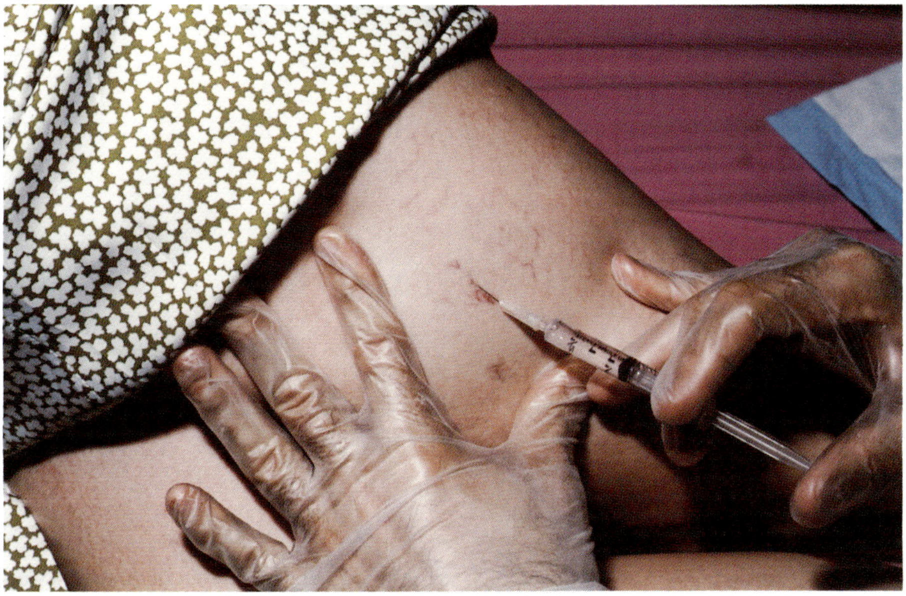

FIGURE 19-3. Three-point tension technique of injecting telangiectasias.

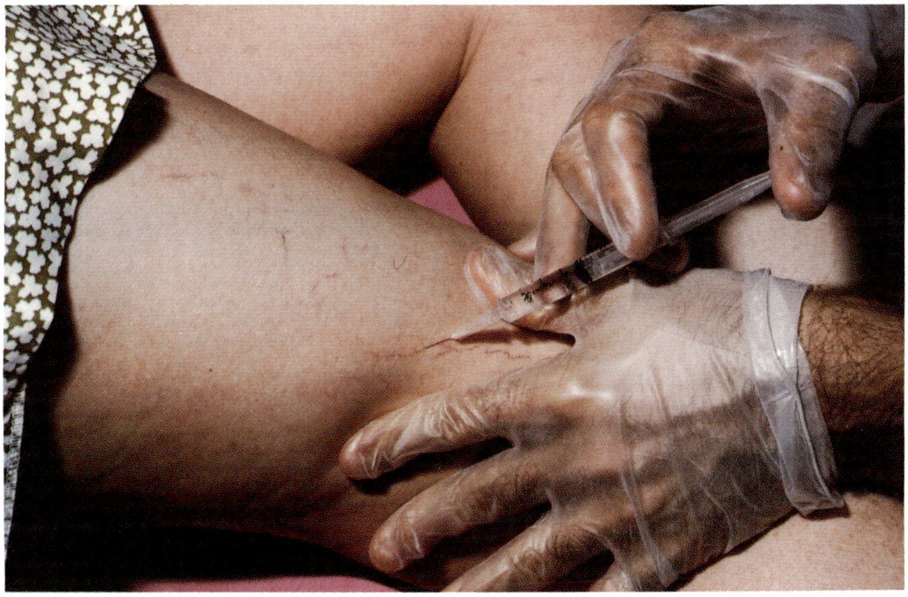

FIGURE 19-4. Two-point tension technique of injecting telangiectasias.

tion of the vessel. With the physician's dominant hand held steady, the needle tip is rested on the skin surface with the tip initially just piercing the epidermis. A gentle thrust is then made toward the vessel lumen to cannulate the telangiectatic vessel. The feel for this movement develops with experience, and with practice telangiectasias even smaller than the diameter of the needle can be cannulated reliably.[6]

The injection of sclerosant should be slow and limited to a maximum area of approximately 5 square cm. Excessive sclerosant concentration or injection pressure is manifested by perivascular blanching followed by acute severe erythema around the telangiectasia. The injection should be stopped at the first indication of extravasation. After one area has been treated, cotton balls fixed with paper tape are applied to the injection sites.

The air-block technique for injecting telangiectasias, in which a small volume of air is injected ahead of the sclerosant, has been recommended by some sclerotherapists.[2,12] This technique has the advantage of ensuring that the needle tip is located in the vein lumen. In addition, it has been hypothesized that replacement of blood by air results in maximum irritation of the endothelium by the sclerosant. However, this method is usually unnecessary since sclerosant flows in a laminar fashion in vessels <4 mm in diameter,[8] and the experienced physician acquires the "feel" of knowing when the needle tip is located correctly. The air-block technique may be useful for the novice, however, especially when hypertonic saline is being injected because it destroys all cells within its osmotic gradient and therefore is more likely to cause cutaneous necrosis when injected extravascularly.[13]

SCLEROSING AGENTS

The purpose of sclerotherapy is to produce endothelial damage that results in permanent endofibrosis and clinical obliteration of the vessel. The ideal sclerosant would have a highly specific mechanism of action, would be free of adverse effects when used for this purpose, and would not produce allergic reactions. Although many agents have been used in treating telangiectasias, thus far none have completely satisfied the criteria for the ideal sclerosant.

The sclerotherapist should have a sound knowledge of the mechanism of action and the adverse effects of all available solutions in order to select the sclerosant that will optimize results in each patient. The following agents are commonly used in the treatment of telangiectasias.

Osmotic Agents

Osmotic agents exert their effect by dehydrating endothelial cells through osmosis, which results in endothelial destruction. They are hypertonic solutions, and their effect is dependent on the existence of an osmotic gradient. Because osmotic agents are rapidly diluted in the bloodstream, they lose their potency within a short distance of injection and are less effective in the treatment of veins larger than 3 to 4 mm in diameter.[13]

Hypertonic saline solution. Hypertonic saline is the most commonly used osmotic agent. The advantages of hypertonic saline are its low cost, ready availability, lack of allergenicity of unadulterated solutions, and rapid clinical effect.[11,12,21] It also has been reported to cause less telangiectatic matting compared with polidocanol.[22] The significant adverse effects of hypertonic saline relate to its nonspecific action of destroying all cells within its osmotic gradient.[13] Therefore extravascular injection is liable to cause cutaneous ulceration, which also can occur with intravascular injection via diffusion through a damaged endothelium. Diffusion of hypertonic saline through the vein wall also results in irritation of adventitial nerves, causing postinjection pain and transient muscle cramping. Therefore injection technique, concentration, and volume are particularly important when this agent is being used.

Attempts have been made to reduce postinjection pain from hypertonic saline by the addition of local anesthetics such as procaine.[11] However, this practice appears to be counterproductive because the local anesthetics are acidic (and therefore contribute to transient pain on injection) and have known allergenicity, the very properties that proponents of hypertonic saline wish to avoid. The addition of heparin to hypertonic saline in an attempt to prevent thrombosis in larger vessels and to reduce the incidence of thrombophlebitis and postsclerotherapy pigmentation has been found to be of no therapeutic benefit in treating telangiectasias.[23] Concentrations of hypertonic saline used to treat telangiectasias range from 11.7% to 23.4%, the latter being the standard concentration available for use as an abortifacient. The incidence of postinjection pain, muscle cramping, cutaneous ulceration, and postsclerotherapy pigmentation is proportional to the concentration of solution used.[23]

Hypertonic glucose saline solution. Sclerodex (Omega; Montreal, Canada), a mixture of dextrose 250 mg/ml, sodium chloride 100 mg/ml, propylene glycol 100 mg/ml, and phenylethyl alcohol 8 mg/ml, is an osmotic agent used in Canada for the treatment of telangiectasias.[24] The addition of dextrose allows for a reduction of the sodium chloride concentration and osmolarity, which supposedly lessens the pain associated with injection of a more concentrated sodium chloride solution without a reduction in efficacy. The addition of dextrose also may explain its reportedly decreased incidence of postsclerotherapy pigmentation.[13,24] Nevertheless, as with hypertonic saline particular care needs to be taken with injection technique.

Chromated Glycerin

A chemical irritant, Scleremo (72% chromated glycerin) exerts its effect via a direct toxic action on endothelial cells. It has a very mild action and is useful only in sclerosing telangiectasias <0.5 mm in diameter. Use of this agent as a sclerosant has not been approved in the United States or Australia. Postsclerotherapy pigmentation and cutaneous necrosis are rare with this agent, and its use is recommended in those patients who have shown increased sensitivity to other sclerosants. The disadvantages of chromated glycerin are its high viscosity, which results in the solution dripping from the needle tip, and pain on injection. Both of these drawbacks can be overcome partially by dilution with lidocaine.[25] However, this results in a proportional reduction in effectiveness of a solution that already has a very mild action.

Detergent Solutions

Detergent solutions include sodium morrhuate, ethanolamine oleate, STS, and polidocanol. These agents act specifically on venous endothelium. They induce sclerosis by damaging the endothelium via interference with cell membrane lipids. They exert their effect along the vessel until either diluted or inactivated by serum surfactants.[13] Only STS and polidocanol are widely used for the treatment of telangiectasias. Table 19-2 gives the approximate equivalent concentrations of STS and polidocanol required for the treatment of lower limb veins. Because of their different mechanisms of action, it is difficult to compare concentrations of detergent solutions with hypertonic saline and Scleremo. However, in the dorsal rabbit ear vein, polidocanol 1% is equivalent to hypertonic saline 23.4%.[13,26] Scleremo is approximately equivalent in potency to polidocanol 0.25%.[25] Other factors apart from vein diameter need to be considered in selecting the concentration of solution. Patients younger than 25 years of age generally require weaker solutions to achieve effective sclerosis. Also, care should be taken with elderly patients and cigarette smokers because they may have coexisting diminished cutaneous perfusion. The area to be treated also influences the choice of concentration. Slightly lower concentrations are required on the medial distal thigh and around the ankles; slightly higher concentrations are needed for treating the lateral and posterior thighs and calves.

Sodium tetradecyl sulfate. STS is commonly used in concentrations of 0.10% to 0.50% to sclerose lower limb telangiectasias. Concentrations of 0.25% to 0.50% are used to treat reticular veins, and concentrations of 0.10% to 0.20% are used for microinjection of telangiectasias. The appropriate concentrations are achieved by diluting the available strengths of 1% and 3% with normal saline. Isotonic normal saline is used in preference to hypotonic sterile water to minimize pain on injection.

Injection of STS results in immediate vessel spasm, which aids hemostasis after needle withdrawal. When the correct dilution is used, there is a transient blanching of the vessel followed by mild erythema. Although STS has a predictable and

TABLE 19-2. Approximate equivalent concentrations of STS and polidocanol required for effective sclerosis of increasing caliber of lower limb vein

Vein Caliber (mm)	STS Concentration (%)	Polidocanol Concentration (%)
0.1-0.5	0.1	0.25
0.5-1	0.2	0.5
1-2	0.3	0.75
2-3	0.5	1
3-5	0.75	2
5-7	1	3

constant effect within the same caliber and type of vein at the same level or area of the leg, there can be variation in sensitivity of effect among patients. Younger patients with veins that have been present for a relatively short time appear to require lower-strength solutions compared with older patients with long-standing venous dilatation. In addition, I have observed that cigarette smokers appear more sensitive to solution concentration, possibly as a result of chronic endothelial damage and increased endothelial permeability caused by carbon monoxide and nicotine.[27] This increased sensitivity is likely to be directly proportional to the number of cigarettes smoked per day. Systemic reactions to STS, including allergy and anaphylaxis, are extremely rare in the treatment of telangiectasias.[28]

The main disadvantage of STS is the pain it causes for several minutes after injection, especially when reticular veins are being treated. This pain usually is relieved by applying pressure to the injection sites by using cotton balls held firmly in place with paper tape. The 0.10% to 0.20% solutions used for microinjection cause minor discomfort comparable to that caused by equivalent concentrations of undiluted Scleremo but less than the pain caused by polidocanol. Cutaneous ulceration has been commonly reported when STS is used for the treatment of telangiectasias.[16,24] These high rates of cutaneous ulceration always have occurred when excessive concentrations were used for microinjection. Reiner[14] showed that cutaneous necrosis after intradermal injection of STS in rabbits was concentration-dependent, with 0.313% solution producing no necrosis and 1.25% solution producing necrosis. In the microinjection of telangiectasias, STS rarely causes cutaneous necrosis when diluted to 0.25%.

Polidocanol. Polidocanol is used in concentrations of 0.25% to 2% to sclerose lower limb telangiectasias. Concentrations of 1% to 2% are used to treat reticular veins, and concentrations of 0.25% to 0.75% are used for microinjection of telangiectasias. Polidocanol is available in standard concentrations of 0.5%, 1%, 2%, 3%, and 5%. Other concentrations are achieved by diluting with normal saline.

Compared with STS, polidocanol causes less vessel spasm and more erythema, resulting in increased bleeding after needle withdrawal. In part, this effect may be a result of the addition of alcohol 5% to the solution as a preserving agent and for enhancement of its solubility. Like STS, polidocanol has a predictable effect within the same caliber of vein and area of the leg, but variation in effect between patients occurs. Systemic reactions to polidocanol when used in the treatment of telangiectasias have been rare.[28]

Because of its inherent local anesthetic properties, polidocanol causes less pain after intravascular injection compared with STS. Cutaneous ulceration is uncommon when concentrations of 0.25% to 1% are used, but it does occur with solutions over 1%.[29] Experimental evidence in the dorsal rabbit ear vein[25,26] indicates that polidocanol is a weaker agent than STS in producing effective endosclerosis of telangiectasias.

POSTSCLEROTHERAPY COMPRESSION

Initially described by Orbach[30] and Sigg[31] in the 1950s and popularized by Fegan[15] in the 1960s, a period of continuous compression of varicose veins after injection is now considered essential in producing long-term sclerosis. A number of theoretical reasons have been suggested to explain why continuous compression improves results in the treatment of telangiectasias.[32] First, adequate compression may result in direct apposition of the treated vein walls to produce a more effective sclerosis. Second, compressing the treated vessel decreases the extent of thrombus formation, helping to prevent recanalization of the treated vessel and decreasing the incidence of superficial thrombophlebitis and postsclerotherapy pigmentation. It also has been speculated that thrombus formation contributes to angiogenesis and the development of telangiectatic matting.[33] Therefore it is possible that postsclerosis compression reduces the incidence of this complication.

The optimum cutaneous pressure required to achieve these theoretical benefits in the treatment of telangiectasias has yet to be defined. The benefits of graduated compression hosiery in reducing superficial ambulatory pressures and aiding the optimal unidirectional flow of blood toward the heart have been well documented.[34] However, Allan[35] has shown that a presence of 80 mm Hg is required to empty blood from cutaneous capillaries in the standing position at a point 5 cm above the medial malleolus. Unfortunately, this degree of pressure results in cutaneous ischemia, especially with recumbency.[32] Therefore a compromise is made by using submaximal graduated compression, which achieves satisfactory patient compliance yet improves effectiveness of treatment and reduces the incidence of postsclerotherapy pigmentation and telangiectatic matting.

Graduated compression stockings exerting a pressure of 35 to 40 mm Hg at the ankle are more effective than bandaging in the treatment of varicose veins.[36] In the treatment of telangiectasias, Goldman et al.[37] have shown that the incidence of postsclerotherapy pigmentation is greatly decreased when graduated compression stockings exerting a pressure of 30 to 40 mm Hg are used for 3 days after treatment. The same researchers concluded that this degree of compression did not improve effectiveness of sclerosis in thigh telangiectasias or in vessels with diameters <0.5 mm. Theoretically, the effectiveness of compression by graduated stockings could be improved by the addition of a second stocking for daytime use, resulting in an effective pressure equal to or slightly higher than the sum of the individual stocking pressures.[38,39]

The importance of treating reticular veins before microsclerotherapy of telangiectasias has been emphasized earlier. Reticular veins, like varicose veins, are abnormally dilated subcutaneous veins, but they are not in direct communication with high-pressure reflux from incompetent main trunks (long or short saphenous veins) or incompetent perforating veins. Continuous compression for 3 weeks is recommended in the treatment of varicose veins.[40,41] While postsclerosis compression also is recommended in the treatment of reticular veins, empirically it can be assumed that shorter durations of compression will be adequate. I have found the following protocol to be adequate: 5 to 7 days of continuous graduated compression with a class 2 (30 to 40 mm Hg) or class 3 (40 to 50 mm Hg) compression stocking, followed by a 7-day period of wearing the stocking during the daytime.

REFERENCES

1. de Faria JL, Moraes IN. Histopathology of the telangiectasia associated with varicose veins. Dermatologica 127:321-329, 1963.
2. Bodian EL. Techniques of sclerotherapy for sunburst venous blemishes. J Dermatol Surg Oncol 11:696-704, 1985.
3. Wokalek H, Vanscheidt W, Martay K, et al. Morphology and localization of sunburst varicosities: An electron microscopic and morphometric study. J Dermatol Surg Oncol 15:149-154, 1989.
4. Goldman MP, Bennett RG. Treatment of telangiectasia: A review. J Am Acad Dermatol 17:167-182, 1987.
5. Weiss RA, Weiss MA. Resolution of pain associated with varicose and telangiectatic leg veins after compression sclerotherapy. J Dermatol Surg Oncol 16:333-336, 1989.
6. Biegeleisen HI. Telangiectasia associated with varicose veins: Treatment by a micro-injection technique. JAMA 102:2092-2094, 1934.
7. Bouthillier P. Les algies des varices dermiques. Phlebologie 2:14, 1949.
8. Ouvry PA. Telangiectasia and sclerotherapy. J Dermatol Surg Oncol 15:177-181, 1989.
9. Eichenberger H. Resultate der Varizenverödung mit Hydroxypolyäthoxy dodecan. Zbl Phlebol 8:181-183, 1969.
10. Ouvry P, Chandet A, Guillerot E. First impressions of Aethoxysklerol. Phlebologie 31:75-77, 1978.
11. Foley WT. The eradication of venous blemishes. Cutis 15:665-668, 1975.
12. Alderman DB. Therapy for essential cutaneous telangiectasia. Postgrad Med 61:91-95, 1977.
13. Goldman MP. A comparison of sclerosing agents: Clinical and histologic effects of intravascular sodium morrhuate, ethanolamine oleate, hypertonic saline (11.7%), and Sclerodex in the dorsal rabbit ear vein. J Dermatol Surg Oncol 17:354-362, 1991.
14. Reiner L. The activity of anionic surface active compounds in producing vascular obliteration. Proc Soc Exp Biol Med 62:49-54, 1946.
15. Fegan WG. Continuous compression technique of injecting varicose veins. Lancet 2:109-112, 1963.
16. Tretbar LL. Injection sclerotherapy for spider telangiectasias: A 20-year experience with sodium tetradecyl sulphate. J Dermatol Surg Oncol 15:223-225, 1989.
17. Goldman MP, Fitzpatrick RE. Pulsed dye laser treatment of leg telangiectasia: With and without simultaneous sclerotherapy. J Dermatol Surg Oncol 16:338-344, 1990.
18. Thibault P, Bray A, Wlodarczyk J, et al. Cosmetic leg veins: Evaluation using duplex venous imaging. J Dermatol Surg Oncol 16:612-618, 1990.
19. Goldman PM. Polidocanol (Aethoxysklerol) for sclerotherapy of superficial venules and telangiectasias. J Dermatol Surg Oncol 15:204-209, 1989.
20. Goldman MP. How many treatments are necessary to sclerose varicose and telangiectatic leg veins? J Dermatol Surg Oncol 17:62, 1991.
21. Bodian EL. Sclerotherapy: A personal appraisal. J Dermatol Surg Oncol 15:156-161, 1989.
22. Weiss RA, Weiss MA. Incidence of side effects in the treatment of telangiectasias by compression sclerotherapy: Hypertonic saline vs. polidocanol. J Dermatol Surg Oncol 16:800-804, 1990.
23. Sadick NS. Sclerotherapy of varicose and telangiectatic leg veins: Minimal sclerosant concentration of hypertonic saline and its relationship to vessel diameter. J Dermatol Surg Oncol 17:65-70, 1991.
24. Mantse L. A mild sclerosing agent for telangiectasias. J Dermatol Surg Oncol 11:9, 1985.
25. Martin DE, Goldman MP. A comparison of sclerosing agents: Clinical and histologic effects of intravascular sodium tetradecyl sulphate and chromated glycerin in the dorsal rabbit ear vein. J Dermatol Surg Oncol 16:18-22, 1990.
26. Goldman MP, Kaplan RP, Oki LN, et al. Sclerosing agents in the treatment of telangiectasia. Arch Dermatol 123:1196-1201, 1987.
27. Kjeldson K, Astrup P, Wanstrup J. Ultrastructural intimal changes in the rabbit aorta after a moderate carbon monoxide exposure. Atherosclerosis 16:67-82, 1972.

28. Goldman MP. Complications and adverse sequelae of sclerotherapy. In Goldman MP, ed. Sclerotherapy: Treatment of Varicose and Telangiectatic Leg Veins. St. Louis: Mosby–Year Book, 1991.
29. Jaquier JJ, Loretan RM. Clinical trials of a new sclerosing agent, Aethoxysklerol. Soc Franc Phlebol 22:383-385, 1969.
30. Orbach EJ. A new approach to the sclerotherapy of varicose veins. Angiology 1:302-305, 1950.
31. Sigg K. The treatment of varicosities and accompanying complications. Angiology 3:355-379, 1952.
32. Goldman MP. Compression in the treatment of leg telangiectasia: Theoretical considerations. J Dermatol Surg Oncol 15:184-188, 1989.
33. Ouvry PA, Davy A. The sclerotherapy of telangiectasia. Phlebologie 35:349-359, 1982.
34. Christopoulos D, Nicolaides AN, Belcaro G, et al. The effect of elastic compression on calf muscle pump function. Phlebology 5:13-19, 1990.
35. Allan JC. The micro-circulation of the skin of the normal leg, in varicose veins and in the post-thrombotic syndrome. S Afr J Surg 10:29-40, 1972.
36. Scurr JH, Coleridge Smith P, Cutting P. Varicose veins: Optimum compression following sclerotherapy. Ann R Coll Surg Engl 67:109-111, 1985.
37. Goldman MP, Beaudoing D, Marley W, et al. Compression in the treatment of leg telangiectasia: A preliminary report. J Dermatol Surg Oncol 16:322-325, 1990.
38. Partsch H. Improvement of venous pumping in chronic venous insufficiency by compression on pressure material. Vasa 13:58-64, 1984.
39. Cornu-Thenard A. Réduction à un edeme veineux par bas élastiques. Unique on superposes. Phlebologie 38:159-168, 1985.
40. Batch AJG, Wickremesinghe SS, Gannon M, et al. Randomised trial of bandaging after sclerotherapy for varicose veins. Br Med J 281:423, 1980.
41. Tolins SH. Treatment of varicose veins: An update. Am J Surg 145:248-252, 1983.

Chapter 20

Painful Telangiectasias: Diagnosis and Treatment

Robert A. Weiss and Margaret A. Weiss

Telangiectatic leg veins have been described as venous spiders, sunburst veins, starburst veins, venous plexuses, dilated venules, venous blemishes, dilated venules and venulectasias, superficial or minor varicosities, essential cutaneous telangiectasias, vanity veins, and cosmetic veins.[1] Despite the cosmetic significance implied by this terminology, all these terms describe the type of telangiectatic networks that may cause physical symptoms of pain and discomfort. Over 50% of patients presenting for treatment of these "spider veins" have aching associated with them.[2] These symptomatic veins are best categorized as arborizing networks (according to the Redisch and Pelzer classification[3]). They are actually combinations or networks of telangiectasias (0.1 to 1 mm) and venulectases (1 to 2 mm). Painful telangiectasias on the leg usually are grouped; they are rarely present as simple individual vessels or spider angiomata with a central arteriole. More important, symptomatic telangiectasias and venulectases commonly are associated with slightly larger blue veins, which have been termed feeders, reticular veins, or minor varicose veins. These small blue veins may be tributaries of the saphenous system or part of a superficial venous system that is separate from either of the saphenous systems, described as the "lateral subdermic venous system" by Albanese et al.[4]

This chapter discusses common locations and patterns of painful telangiectasias, their intricate association with reticular veins (often comprising the lateral venous system), the type and location of symptoms, and the best approach for eliminating symptoms.

CLASSIFICATION AND ANATOMY

In order to diagnose and treat painful telangiectasias in a logical way, a precise classification is helpful (see box, p. 390). A discussion of painful telangiectasias includes telangiectasias (type I), venulectases (type II), and associated blue reticular

REVISED VESSEL CLASSIFICATION*

Type I

Telangiectasia, "spider veins"
0.1-1 mm diameter
Usually red (rarely may be cyanotic)

- Type IA
  - Telangiectatic matting
  - <0.2 mm diameter network, bright red

Type II

Venulectasia (usually protrudes above skin surface, distinguished from telangiectasia by deeper color and larger diameter)
1-2 mm diameter
Violaceous, cyanotic

Type III

Reticular veins ("minor" varicose veins, "feeder" veins)
2-4 mm diameter
Cyanotic to blue

Type IV

Nonsaphenous varicose veins (primary varicosity of saphenous tributary usually related to an incompetent perforator)
3-8 mm diameter
Blue to blue-green

Type V

Saphenous varicose veins (varicosities associated with reflux at saphenofemoral or saphenopopliteal junction or major perforators of saphenous system causing enlargement of long or short saphenous vein)
Usually >8 mm in diameter
Blue to blue-green

*Data from Goldman MP. Sclerotherapy treatment for varicose and telangiectatic leg veins. In Coleman WP, Hanke CW, Alt TH, Asken S, eds. Cosmetic Surgery of the Skin. Philadelphia: BC Decker, 1991, pp 197-211; Duffy DM. Small vessel sclerotherapy: An overview. In Callen JP, Dahl MV, Golitz LE, et al., eds. Advances in Dermatology, vol 3. Chicago: Year Book, 1988, pp 221-242.

Note: This simplified classification eliminates the mixed telangiectasia/varicose category. Since most patients have a combination of multiple varicose vein types, a description of type I in association with type II or type III varicosities is simpler. Classifying varicose veins in this way allows for a more straightforward treatment plan.

veins (type III). In this discussion of painful telangiectasias, it is assumed that the major primary varicose veins of type IV and type V have been treated or are absent.

On a smaller scale, groups of reticular veins, venulectases, and telangiectasias may be subject to forces of stretch and increased venous pressure similar to those that produce major varicosities. A disturbance of normal venous physiology with back pressure and reverse flow or reflux through incompetent valves results in transmission of pressure through reticular veins into venules, causing their expansion into telangiectasias and venulectases.

Arborizing networks of telangiectasias have been shown to be dilated cutaneous venules with intrinsic connections to underlying larger veins of which they are direct tributaries.[5,6] Valves are found throughout the postcapillary venous system regulating flow within the smallest of venules.[7] Thus increased venous pressure is transmitted in a cascade effect; conducted pressure causes increased diameter and incompetence of venous valves from reticular veins to telangiectasias. Recently, this effect has been confirmed through Doppler ultrasound demonstration of audible reflux in lateral thigh reticular veins associated with telangiectasias in 319 of 400 patients who presented for treatment without associated saphenous varicosities.[8] Similar findings were reported by Tretbar,[9] who concluded that when telangiectasias are large enough for flow to be perceived (>1 mm), they are hemodynamically connected to the adjacent blue veins.

Pain associated with telangiectasias may be a consequence of stretching caused by pressure transmitted during reflux through reticular veins and venulectases. In a detailed discussion of symptoms caused by varicose veins, Lofgren[10] has stated that "the largest varicosities sometimes cause no complaints; other veins of small caliber may give rise to surprising discomfort." One theory to explain this phenomenon is that compliance of smaller veins may be greater than that of larger ones, with more distensibility and greater stretch resulting in more stimulation of neural pain receptors under a given pressure. Larger varicose veins develop intramural fibrosis with time, and this change may prevent rapid stretching.[11] In vitro studies of viscoelastic properties of varicose veins demonstrate limited stretch potential of larger varicose veins.[12] Smaller veins such as postcapillary venules may not develop intramural fibrosis, and this situation may allow dilatation two to four times in diameter with pressure. Such dilatation may correlate with the patient's reporting a feeling of "vein breaking." Alternatively, pain in telangiectasias or venulectases may occur with prolonged standing as a direct consequence of slow dilatation through pressure. The potentially increased diameter as a percentage of normal diameter is much greater for venules than for major veins.

LATERAL SUBDERMIC VENOUS SYSTEM

Originally described by Alfonso R. Albanese,[4] the lateral subdermic venous system consists of veins that are the size of reticular veins at a depth just below the dermis, longitudinally traversing the lateral thigh and calf and often having complex

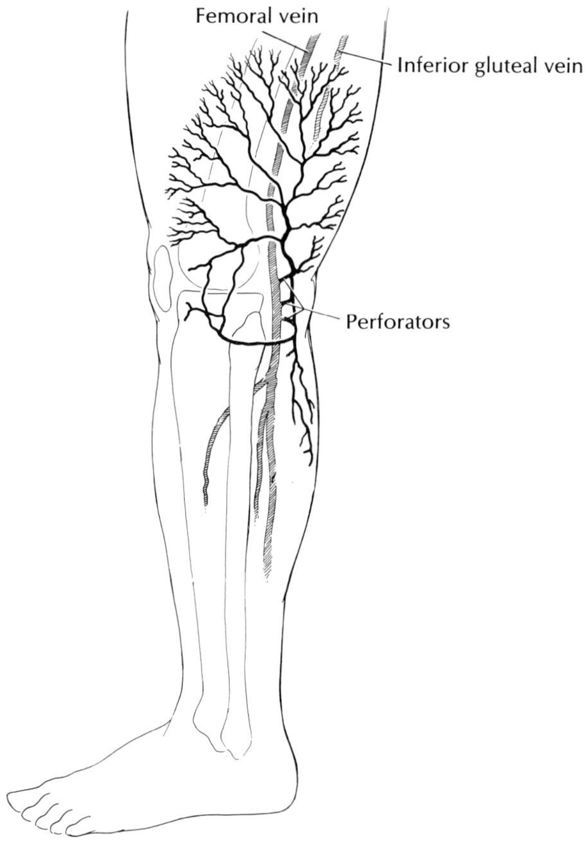

FIGURE 20-1. In the lateral subdermic venous system (Albanese venous system), vein size may range from 3 mm to >1 cm. These veins longitudinally traverse the lateroposterior thigh and lateroposterior calf, often having several direct communications with the deep venous system near the lateral knee. They are often responsible for painful telangiectatic webs seen on the thigh or calf. Reflux is often noted over the sites identified as perforators. An 8 to 10 MHz Doppler probe allows reflux to be heard clearly and loudly through distal compression release or proximal compression. Inferior gluteal vein is shown as a possible tributary to the lateral venous system.

communications at the lateral knee (Figure 20-1). This system may become varicose even in the absence of saphenous system varicosities. Small perforating veins connect the lateral venous system to the deep femoral vein or the popliteal vein, thus serving as the primary source of reflux that propagates the varicosity. Occasionally the lateral system communicates with and is enlarged by reflux through the inferior gluteal vein.

Reflux in lateral thigh reticular veins has been traced by Doppler ultrasound to points near the lateral knee[8] or the upper calf.[3] We believe that these points correlate with the previously described perforators of the lateral venous system.[4] The location of these perforators indicates that reflux through them must be of sufficient pressure to occur against gravity. This pressure is responsible for telangiectatic bridges seen on the upper lateral and posterior thigh. Retrograde reflux in reticular veins has been reported.[9] Proposed mechanisms include changes in pressure and shifts in flow with occlusion of veins during sitting.

From correlation with Doppler ultrasound findings, we believe that reflux through small perforators at the lateral knee into the lateral venous system accounts for the vast majority of painful telangiectatic groups on the lateral half of the thigh and the upper calf in patients without reflux at the saphenofemoral junction, saphenopopliteal junction, or "major" perforators associated with the saphenous system. In our experience these lateral minor varicosities are noted initially when the individual is at a younger age (teens through thirties), typically several decades before the onset of major varicosities. This earlier onset may be explained through an examination of venous system embryology of the leg.

Based on studies by Hochstetter,[13] it is known that, during the earliest stages of formation of the venous system of the leg, the predominant system is a network of superficial veins from which the lateral venous system is derived. The deep venous system then develops in a rudimentary way, with the superficial external saphenous vein being dominant, connected by small perforators to the deep system. When the deep venous system becomes predominant, the external saphenous vein disintegrates at the thigh, but not without leaving a few thigh perforators intact. Albanese et al.[4] speculated that, in areas where the superficial veins do not involute, superficial embryonic veins remain and may become easily and prematurely varicosed.[2] This change occurs for two reasons: (1) because of their superficial location, these veins are poorly supported by surrounding connective tissue, and (2) direct transfacial perforators continue to connect these veins with the deep venous system.

Albanese et al.[4] concluded that when a network of easily varicosed veins occurs on the lateral thigh, it should be considered a developmental defect. With intact lateral knee perforators serving as a direct source for transmission of high pressure from the deep venous system accompanied by a lack of structural support, reticular veins may become stretched and distended easily. The term "minor varicose vein" is fully justified for these lateral thigh reticular veins. A recent Doppler study of the distribution of varicose veins by Goren and Yellin[14] confirmed the presence of a distinct group of nonsaphenous varicosities on the lateral aspect of the thigh and calf that represented the lateral venous system.

The great importance of heredity as a factor in the development of thigh reticular varicose veins was confirmed by a recent epidemiologic study of Japanese women.[15] A separate category of web-type varicosities describing intradermal venectasia, often located on the thigh or knee, was included in this study. Such varicosities most closely correlated with reticular veins associated with telangiectasias and venulectases. It is remarkable that these reticular varicosities did not increase in frequency with age, as did the saphenous types, indicating that pre-existing factors were most important.

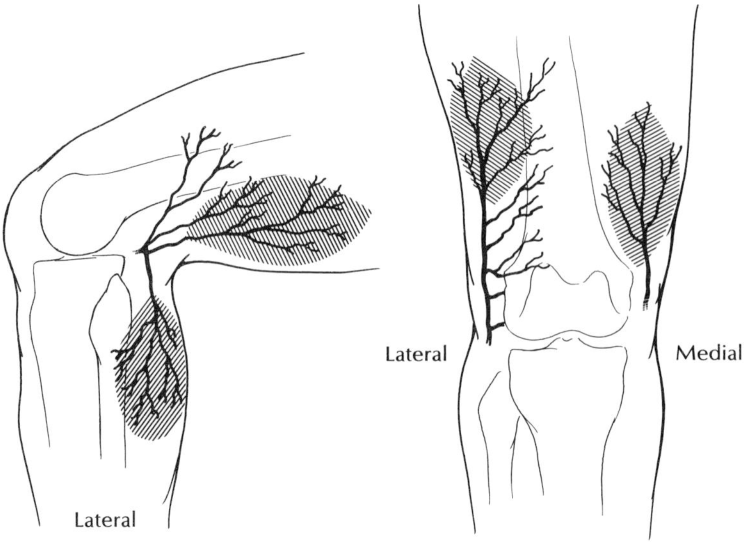

FIGURE 20-2. Regions where painful groups of telangiectasias and venulectases are most likely to occur are shown by shaded areas. Patients most often complain of focal burning, throbbing, and aching in these regions. Lateral view shows posterior distribution of pain of the lateral venous system associated with telangiectatic webs. Prolonged sitting often produces pain in the posterior thigh, whereas prolonged standing often causes pain in the calf. The anteroposterior view shows less common sites of painful telangiectatic webs on the lateral and medial thigh above the knee. A reticular vein with reflux audible through Doppler ultrasound often is associated with these regions of pain.

DISTRIBUTION

Although painful telangiectasias and venulectases may appear anywhere on the leg they are most likely to occur in certain regions (Figure 20-2). These areas include the lateral and posterior calf, medial and posterior lower thigh, lateral thigh, and ankle. Although the lateral thigh location usually is responsible for a bridge of telangiectasias and venulectases with cosmetic significance (Figure 20-3), causing the patient to seek treatment, our personal observations in treating 4500 patients indicate that extension onto the upper calf often is responsible for painful symptoms. It is presumed that the latter is caused by the greater effect of gravity during standing. Most of our patients report discomfort along the lateral to posterior calf during standing. The location of pain may be perceived to change during sitting; patients may then relate pain to telangiectatic groups localized on the posterior thigh.

As a general rule, painful telangiectasias occur either at or below the knee. One exception is the medial thigh, where a group of telangiectasias can be observed in association with a reticular vein coursing near the greater saphenous vein

A

B

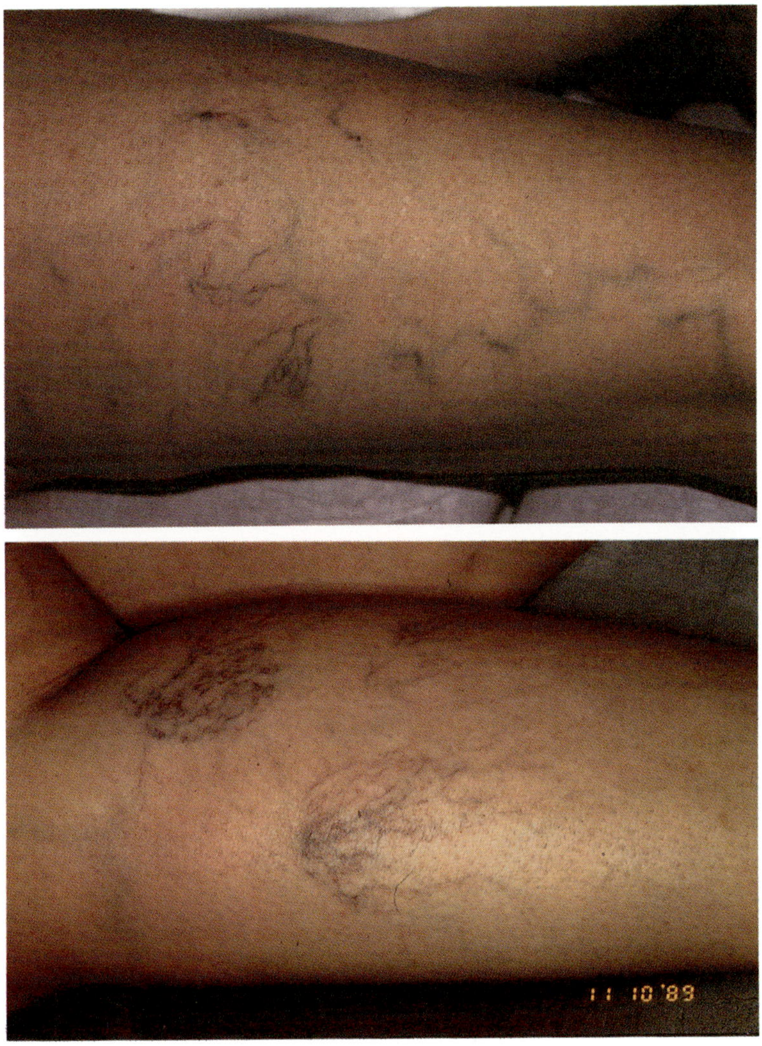

FIGURE 20-3. A, Typical lateral thigh location for a bridge of telangiectasias and venulectases associated with a reticular vein having no symptoms. B, Reticular vein extension onto upper calf leading to a group or web of telangiectasias and venulectases responsible for symptoms of focal burning.

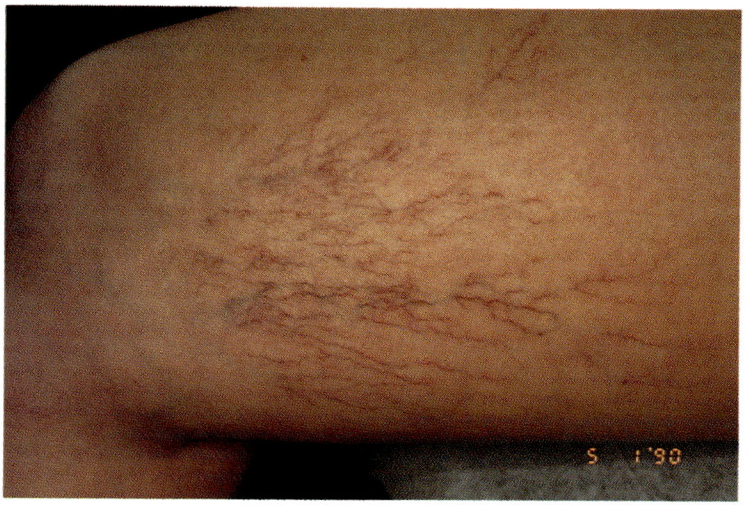

FIGURE 20-4. On the medial thigh, a group of telangiectasias is seen in association with reticular veins that course near the greater saphenous vein. Great caution must be observed in treatment of reticular veins in this region. Telangiectatic matting following treatment often occurs here.

(Figure 20-4). Occasionally patients report symptoms from telangiectasias in the medial thigh. However, most painful telangiectasias, in the absence of saphenous and major perforator varicosities, are associated with reticular veins of the lateral subdermic venous system. Finally, large varicosities connected to the saphenous system feed into reticular veins and cause pain in associated telangiectasias.

SYMPTOMS

Until recently, groups of telangiectasias were not thought to be a common cause of significant leg pain. A sensation of burning discomfort, associated with hot[16] or warm[17] weather, was the main symptom described. Tretbar[18] reported that "although treatment has not been offered to patients for relief of symptoms in the legs, a number of patients have nevertheless reported subjective improvement of aches and pains." Similarly, the association of leg pain with telangiectasia has been made by many of our patients only after telangiectasia, treated initially for cosmetic reasons, completely resolved and the patients subsequently noticed how good their legs felt.

After this initial correlation by patients, we became interested in the details of the therapeutic benefits of sclerotherapy for the relief of pain associated with telangiectasia and venulectasia. Many of our patients with occupations involving long periods of standing have complained of muscle fatigue and aching or localized pain over groups of telangiectasias and/or venulectases, and they received only slight relief by wearing support hose. In order to quantitate the effectiveness of sclerotherapy to relieve leg pain and discomfort, 350 patients were surveyed by mailed questionnaire.[2] This survey detailed the frequency and types of reported symptoms and the level of improvement following a high degree of visual resolution.

Of the patients responding to the survey, approximately 53% (114 of 214) had associated symptoms with their telangiectasias and/or venulectases. For all symptoms combined, the overall reported relief of pain following treatment was 85% (p <0.001). The most common symptom was a sensation of fatigue accompanied by a dull, generalized achiness. The second most common symptom was pain at the precise site of a group of venulectases or telangiectasias. A symptom of burning was found frequently in a region of telangiectasias and/or venulectases located at or near the site. Another frequently reported symptom was throbbing or pulsating pain along the leg, usually occurring laterally but not directly associated with a specific group of telangiectasias or venulectases.

Night cramps were reported, and they were improved by sclerotherapy. Edema of a region or engorgement of a telangiectatic group was exacerbated by prolonged standing, but this condition could be reversed by sclerotherapy. Most patients experienced several symptoms. Frequently these symptoms were exacerbated during menses. A small percentage of our patients experienced pain or swelling only during menses.[19] Leg symptoms reported by women have been attributed to the distention of the vein walls induced by hormonal changes of the menstrual cycle.[20]

Many of the symptoms reported for telangiectasias were identical to those reported for larger varicosities. These symptoms include a dull aching of the leg, particularly after prolonged standing, during menses, or as a result of the hormonal changes of pregnancy.[21] According to the Basel study III, approximately 25% of patients with major varicose veins experienced symptoms such as heaviness, swelling, cramps, pain or aching, and restless legs.[22] Estimations of intermittent pain in larger varicosities have been as high as 50%.[23]

Although there are many causes of leg pain, such as arthritis and tendonitis, several clues may be helpful in determining whether leg pain is caused by webs of telangiectasias or venulectases. A dull, throbbing ache or a sensation of heaviness in the legs that occurs at the end of the day but is not noticeable on awakening is very likely to respond to treatment with sclerotherapy. Most commonly, a burning quality to the discomfort that worsens with standing for long hours indicates a venous problem. Focal burning also may occur suddenly, producing a sensation of breakage or rupture. This burning may be the result of decreased breaking strength of already enlarged veins.[12] Tenderness is less likely to be a symptom unless superficial phlebitis is a factor. Other important clues are the relief or improvement of symptoms by the use of support hose or a worsening of symptoms during menses. Pain from telangiectasia, in our experience, is rarely referred to the knee joint or hip. The distribution of pain also may help in diagnosis; for example, pain from a venous source is likely to be located on the lateral to lateroposterior calf or thigh in the distribution of the lateral subdermic venous system varicosities.

Physical examination also is important in determining the source of pain. Obviously, if a patient points to a focal area of pain with an overlying telangiectatic web, the pain is likely to arise from this group (Figure 20-5). Associated reticular veins usually can be identified visually. We prefer the use of Doppler ultrasound to locate the primary source of reflux into the telangiectatic group. The method for using the Doppler probe to elicit reflux in varicosities has been described by Schultz-Ehrenburg.[24] For reticular veins, the method is identical. The patient should be examined while in a sitting or a standing position. With a series of manual compres-

Text continued on p. 401.

A

B

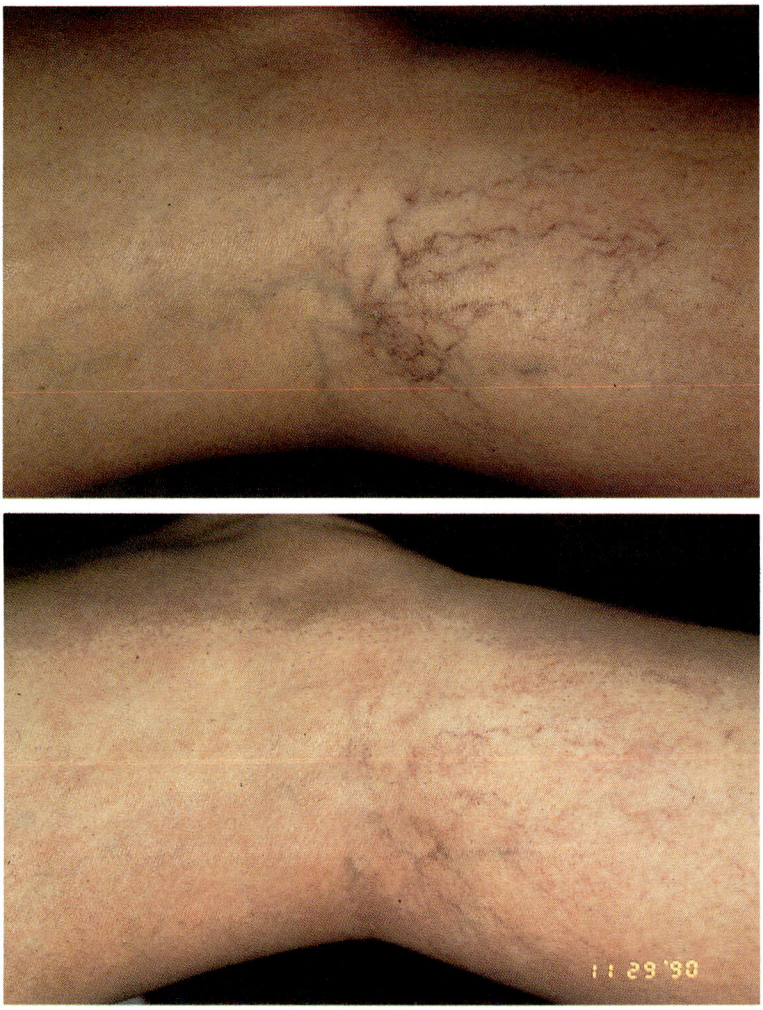

FIGURE 20-5. When a patient points out a focal area of pain with an overlying telangiectatic web, the pain is most likely to arise from this group. **A,** Focal burning pain associated with a telangiectatic web on the proximal lateroposterior calf. Several reticular veins were noted with two sites of reflux identified by Doppler ultrasound. Treatment consisted of 1 ml of 0.2% sodium tetradecyl sulfate (Sotradecol) injected into several points along the reticular veins with an additional injection of 0.5 ml of 0.1% Sotradecol into the telangiectatic web. **B,** Two months later almost complete cosmetic ablation was noted with complete resolution of the pain.

C

D

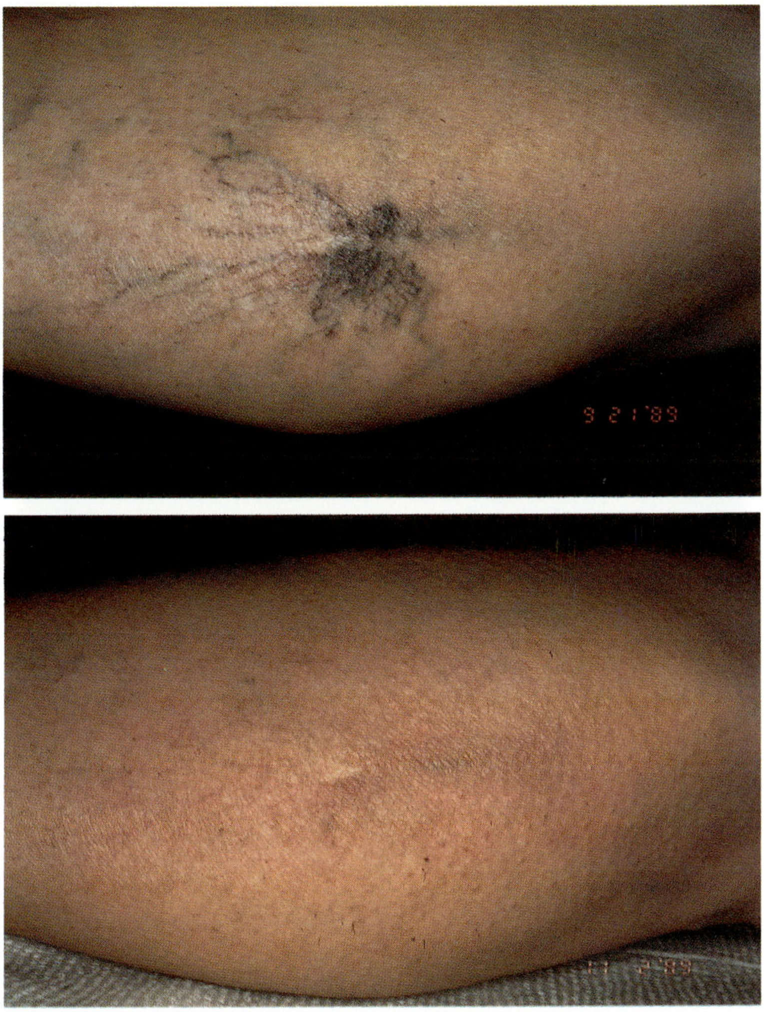

FIGURE 20-5, cont'd. C, Severe focal aching, burning, and night cramps were associated with a telangiectatic web occurring at the site of a previous ligation. A reticular vein (not easily visualized) was traced to the lateroposterior knee. Treatment consisted of 0.75 ml of hypertonic saline (23.4%) injected into the reticular vein with an additional 0.5 ml of hypertonic saline injected into the web. **D,** Painful symptoms resolved within 1 week. Within 6 weeks resolution of the dilated venules was seen.

Continued.

E

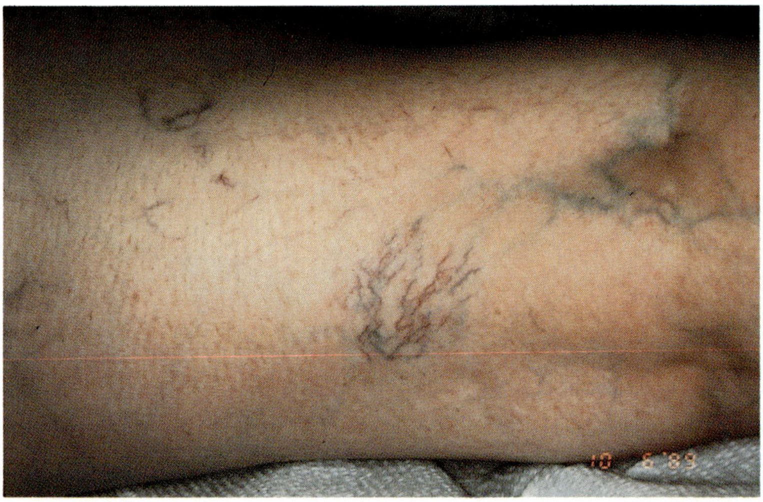

F

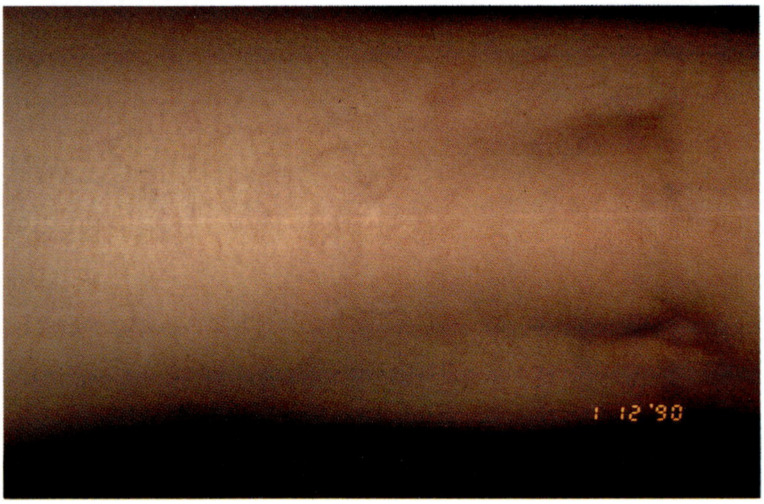

FIGURE 20-5, cont'd. E, Focal aching on the posterior thigh, which worsened with sitting for long periods, was associated with a lateral subdermic venous system reticular vein. Origin of reflux for this telangiectatic web was traced by Doppler ultrasound with distal compression release to a small perforator in the region of the fibular collateral ligament. Treatment consisted of injection of 0.5 ml of 1% polidocanol into the reticular vein and 0.5 ml of 0.5% polidocanol into the telangiectatic web. **F,** A second treatment was necessary to obtain resolution of pain and varicosities at 3 months.

sions and decompressions of the calf, the physician moves the Doppler probe over the reticular vein until the loudest flow signal is found. Thus a physiologic site of increased venous pressure into the telangiectasia can be documented and a cause for pain can be identified with greater certainty. The frequency with which reflux into a reticular vein is associated with a group of telangiectasias is quite high.[8,9] Occasionally a reflux signal is heard at the point of origin of a telangiectatic group without the visual identification of a reticular vein (Figure 20-6). Presumably the feeder vein is just below the surface, preventing its visualization.

A

B

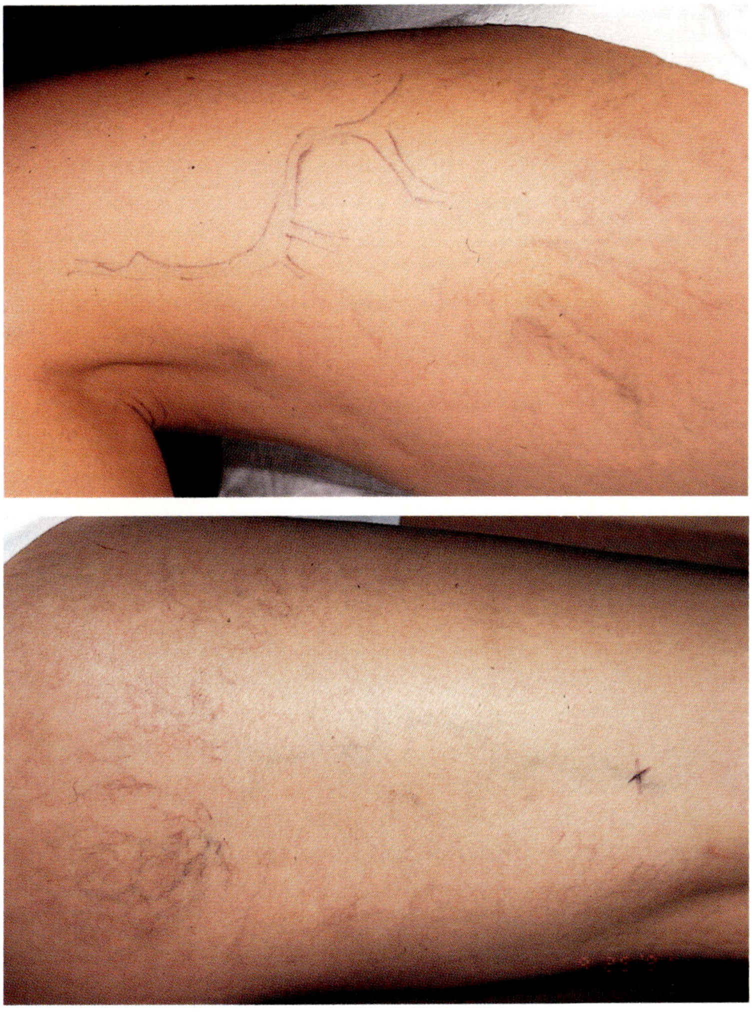

FIGURE 20-6. A, A subdermic reticular venous system (marked in pen) can be traced with 10 MHz Doppler ultrasound probe. **B,** A barely visible lateral venous system reticular vein associated with a bridge of telangiectasias on the thighs is easily identified by Doppler ultrasound. Loudest point of reflux, a good point to initiate injections, is marked with an X.

Certain occupations that involve long periods of standing carry an increased risk for developing painful telangiectasias. Examples include the work of beauticians, educators, nurses, clerks, assembly line workers, and many others. In our experience such workers complain of symptoms associated with telangiectasias, receive only slight relief from the use of support hose, and benefit a great deal from sclerotherapy.[2] Even when pain is not a problem with varicosities and telangiectasias, these conditions can be so psychologically disturbing to women that they will not wear shorts or bathing suits at all, thus eliminating major sources of recreation and exercise from their life-styles.[2]

TREATMENT PROTOCOLS

Painful Telangiectasias

The treatment of painful telangiectasias is identical to that of cosmetic telangiectasias except that particular attention is devoted to associated reticular veins. The basic principle of treatment, proceeding from the largest to the smallest varicosities, holds true. One should first inject the reticular veins, next inject the largest venulectases, and then proceed to the smallest telangiectasias.

As mentioned previously, the use of Doppler ultrasound helps to identify sources of reflux into telangiectatic groups. Often the Doppler reflux signal may be traced to its loudest point, and the injections can be initiated there. For example, a group of telangiectasias on the lateral thigh may have associated reticular veins that are part of a varicose lateral subdermic venous system; the loudest Doppler flow signal often can be traced to the area distal to the lateral femoral condyle. The injections would be initiated at this site and continued every 3 to 4 cm along the course of the reticular vein. Usually no more than 0.5 ml of sclerosing solution per injection site is necessary, although some longer reticular veins will require 1 ml of solution.

Occasionally the sclerosing solution is observed to enter the telangiectasia directly from the feeder vein; this occurrence may eliminate the need to inject the telangiectasia directly. Our experience also has shown the reverse situation; that is, when groups of telangiectasias are being injected, occasionally one may visualize sclerosing solution entering the feeder vein from injection through a telangiectasia. This occurrence was demonstrated in 20 patients in whom the flow of sclerosing solution from the telangiectasia into the reticular vein was documented by Doppler ultrasound.[8] In practical terms, the direction of valves in these veins should allow easy flow from smaller to larger veins. However, this method cannot be relied on for treatment of the reticular vein because the development of extravasation at the site of injection in the telangiectatic vein often prevents sufficient sclerosant volume or concentration to enter the larger reticular vein. Therefore the reticular vein would be inadequately treated, and recurrence of the telangiectasia would be more likely.

Based on our experience, injecting the telangiectasias directly is more successful than relying solely on sclerosing solution to reach the telangiectasia through reticular vein injection. In the process of flowing from reticular veins into telangiectatic veins, the sclerosing solution may be diluted, inactivated by blood proteins, or lost by leakage through damaged endothelium. The inactivation by binding to blood protein is theoretically possible if the elasticity of the venule was diminished during the process of becoming telangiectatic. The capacity of the venule to decrease in size may have been lost even with the elimination of an originating pressure source. When no clear feeder vessel is seen or identified by Doppler ultrasound, then the point at which the telangiectasias begin to branch out is the site at which injection should be begun. This approach saves time by decreasing the number of injection sites per telangiectatic group.

Reticular Veins

The first treatment session for reticular veins usually is limited to one or two sites in order to (1) observe the patient for any allergic reactions, (2) determine the patient's ability to tolerate the burning or cramping of a hypertonic solution, (3) judge the effectiveness of a particular concentration of sclerosing agent, and (4) observe any reactions to the tape used for compression. The patient returns in 4 to 6 weeks so that the test site can be compared with pretreatment photographs. At each follow-up session the patient is asked if the painful symptoms have decreased. When the symptoms have stopped, the physician can be confident that treatment has been successful even before visual improvement is recognized. Conversely, if visual improvement is noted but the symptoms have not improved, the source of reflux has not been eliminated and a recurrence in the treated area is highly likely.

Treatment of reticular veins is very similar to that of large varicose veins, although the concentration, strength, and volume of the sclerosing solution are decreased. Reticular veins are treated only after all sources of reflux from major varicosities have been treated by sclerotherapy and/or surgery. As previously mentioned, the hand-held Doppler probe also may be used as a guide to demonstrate reflux in the reticular veins and to locate those that require treatment.

While the patient is in a recumbent position, a 3 ml syringe with a 27- to 30-gauge needle, bent to an angle of 10 to 20 degrees, is inserted into the reticular vein. Since this vein usually is superficial and visibly blue, it does not require preliminary marking with a pen. When the sensation of piercing the vein is felt, the plunger is pulled back gently with the thumb of the dominant hand until blood is seen beginning to back up into the transparent plastic hub (this is possible even with a 30-gauge needle). If the wall of the reticular vein is very thin, the suction created by pulling back on the syringe may cause the wall to adhere to the needle bevel and prevent aspiration of blood. In this situation the needle can be moved gently forward and backward; if no resistance is felt, the vein probably has been cannulated, and the physician can proceed very cautiously with injection. We also have observed the reticular vein to shrink spasmodically and virtually disappear from view following an attempt at cannulation. When such shrinkage occurs, another injection site along the reticular vein must be sought. Cannulation of a reticular vein can be more difficult than a protuberant venulectasia or telangiectasia.

Usually the volume per injection site is no more than 0.5 ml, but the capacity of long reticular veins may even exceed 1 ml. The progress of the solution can be followed visually, and the injection can be stopped when the entire reticular vein has been cleared of blood and appears to be in contact with the sclerosing solution.

Sclerosing solutions and the concentrations that have been used include (1) 0.5% to 1% polidocanol (Aethoxysklerol; Kreussler & Co., Wiesbaden-Biebrich, Germany) (although not FDA-approved, polidocanol is a forgiving solution in fragile, thin-walled vessels); (2) 23.4% hypertonic saline; and (3) 0.2% to 0.5% sodium tetradecyl sulfate (Sotradecol; Wyeth-Ayerst Laboratories, Philadelphia, Pa.). Until the physician gains experience in cannulating reticular veins, cautious injection with the FDA-approved sclerosants cannot be overemphasized. A bruise usually will occur almost immediately, and resistance to injection will be felt when the reticular vein has not been cannulated properly.

Telangiectatic Veins

The injection method for treatment of telangiectasias has been described in Chapter 19 and by Goldman[25] and Duffy.[26] The concentrations of sclerosing solutions are reduced even further than for reticular veins: 0.25% to 0.5% polidocanol (not FDA-approved) (again, the most forgiving even when a bleb occurs at the injection site); 11.7% to 20% hypertonic saline; and 0.1% to 0.3% sodium tetradecyl sulfate. The injection technique requires a gentle, precise touch as one learns to appreciate the subtle sensation felt on entering the vessel or to recognize the appearance of needle bevel within the telangiectasia lumen. If these signs are not appreciated immediately, minimal withdrawal of the needle may allow the easy flow of sclerosing solution. A very sharp needle is critical for this fine touch, and the needle is changed often in order to minimize tearing the vessel. The use of 32- to 33-gauge needles is not advised because such needles dull quickly and are not disposable.

Injection of a tiny bolus of air (<0.05 cc) may be helpful to establish that the needle is within the vein as slight clearing 1 to 3 mm ahead of the bevel can be seen. Injection is performed *very slowly,* a small amount of sclerosant (0.1 to 0.5 ml or less) is used, and minimal or no pressure is applied to a 3 ml syringe to maintain filling of the veins for 10 to 15 seconds. Rapid flushing of the vessels with large volumes of sclerosant is not necessary for successful sclerotherapy. Particularly when a hypertonic solution is being used, injection of sclerosant is stopped when blanching in a radius of 2 cm has occurred or when 15 seconds have passed, thus minimizing cramping and burning. When painless detergent sclerosants are used (e.g., polidocanol or sodium tetradecyl sulfate), a small volume of the solution with a short interval (10 seconds) of blanching will minimize side effects such as telangiectatic matting.[27]

Occasionally no blanching occurs at the site of injection, and the sclerosing solution flows easily through the telangiectasia or can be seen flowing through adjacent telangiectasias or reticular veins several centimeters away from the injection site. In this situation the injection is stopped after 0.5 to 1 ml of sclerosant has been injected and gentle massage through immediate manual compression has been applied. Any vessel larger than approximately 0.5 mm or, more important, any vessel that protrudes above the surface of the skin benefits from compression. Cottonballs are secured over the injection sites with paper tape or Transpore tape (3M–Medical-Surgical Division, St. Paul, Minn.), and compression is subsequently maintained by the further application of Microfoam tape (3M–Medical-Surgical Division, St. Paul, Minn.) over the paper tape for 48 to 72 hours. Protuberant telangiectasias or telangiectasias associated with reticular veins also are treated for 2 weeks with graduated 30 to 40 mm Hg compression support hose after removal of the Microfoam tape. Patients are encouraged to walk and instructed not to restrict their activities (except for heavy weightlifting with the legs). Treatment intervals vary, but allowing 4 to 8 weeks between treatments of identical areas helps to minimize the total number of sessions.

REFERENCES

1. Pierce HE. Management of unsightly micro-varicosities. Am J Cosmet Surg 1:45-47, 1984.
2. Weiss RA, Weiss MA. Resolution of pain associated with varicose and telangiectatic leg veins after compression sclerotherapy. J Dermatol Surg Oncol 16:333-336, 1990.
3. Redisch W, Pelzer RH. Localized vascular dilatations of the human skin-capillary microscopy and related studies. Am Heart J 37:106-111, 1949.
4. Albanese AR, Albanese AM, Albanese EF. The lateral subdermic venous system of the legs. Vasc Surg 3:81-89, 1969.
5. De Faria JL, Moraes IN. Histopathology of the telangiectasias associated with varicose veins. Dermatologica 127:321-324, 1963.
6. Wokalek H, Vanscheidt W, Martay K, Leder O. Morphology and localization of sunburst varicosities: An electron microscopic and morphometric study. J Dermatol Surg Oncol 15:149-154, 1989.
7. Braverman IM, Keh-Yen A. Ultrastructure of the human dermal microcirculation. IV. Valve-containing collecting veins at the dermal-subcutaneous junction. J Invest Dermatol 81:438-444, 1983.
8. Weiss RA, Weiss MA. Doppler ultrasound findings in reticular veins of the thighs. J Dermatol Surg Oncol 18:62, 1992.
9. Tretbar LL. The origin of reflux in incompetent blue reticular/telangiectasia veins. In Davy A, Stemmer R, eds. Phlebologie '89. London: John Libbey Eurotext Ltd, 1989, pp 95-96.
10. Lofgren KA. Varicose veins: Their symptoms, complications, and management. Postgrad Med 65:131-139, 1979.
11. Maurel E, Azema C, Deloly J, Bouissou H. Collagen of the normal and varicose human saphenous vein: A biochemical study. Clin Chim Acta 193:27-38, 1990.
12. Psaila JV, Melhuish J. Viscoelastic properties and collagen content of the long saphenous vein in normal and varicose veins. Br J Surg 76:37-40, 1989.
13. Hochstetter F. Morphologisches Jahrbuch 17 Bd. 1891.
14. Goren G, Yellin AE. Primary varicose veins: Topographic and hemodynamic correlations. J Cardiovasc Surg 31:672-677, 1991.
15. Hirai M, Naiki K, Nakayama R. Prevalence and risk factors of varicose veins in Japanese women. Angiology 41:228-232, 1990.
16. Shields JL, Jansen GT. Therapy for superficial telangiectasias of the lower extremities. J Dermatol Surg Oncol 8:857-860, 1982.
17. Pierce HE. Management of unsightly micro-varicosities. Am J Cosmet Surg 1:45-47, 1984.
18. Tretbar LL. Spider angiomata: Treatment with sclerosant injections. J Kansas Med Soc 79:198-200, 1978.
19. Weiss MA, Weiss RA, Goldman MP. How minor varicosities cause leg pain. Contemp Obstet Gynecol 36:113-125, 1991.

20. McCausland AM, Holmes F, Trotter AD. Venous distensibility during the menstrual cycle. Am J Obstet Gynecol 86:640-645, 1963.
21. McPheeters HO. The value of estrogen therapy in the treatment of varicose veins complicating pregnancy. Lancet 69:2, 1949.
22. Widmer L. Peripheral venous disorders: Prevalence and sociomedical importance of observations in 4529 apparently healthy persons. Basel study III. Berne, Switzerland: Hans Huber, 1978.
23. Wilder CS. Prevalence of selected chronic circulatory conditions. Vital Health Stat 94:1-2, 1974.
24. Schultz-Ehrenburg U, Hubner H-J. Reflux Diagnosis with Doppler Ultrasound [monograph]. Stuttgart–New York: Schattauer, 1989, pp 5-10.
25. Goldman MP. Sclerotherapy: Treatment of Varicose and Telangiectatic Leg Veins. St. Louis: Mosby–Year Book, 1991, pp 307-315.
26. Duffy DM. Small vessel sclerotherapy: An overview. In Callen JP, Dahl MV, Golitz LE, et al., eds. Advances in Dermatology, vol 3. Chicago: Year Book, 1988, pp 221-242.
27. Ouvry PA, Davy A. The sclerotherapy of telangiectasia. Phlebologie 35:349-359, 1982.

Chapter 21

Techniques of Small Vessel Sclerotherapy*

David M. Duffy

What makes small vessels, 0.1 mm to 3 mm in diameter, so interesting is the diversity of their responses to treatment. Symmetrically distributed veins of identical size and color in the same patient can react quite differently to identical treatments. The exact outcome of sclerotherapy is only partially predictable because a large number of poorly understood host factors play a much more important role in treatment outcome than any combination or manipulation of treatment strategies. Small vessel sclerotherapy is an art, not a science, and many of the controversies regarding ideal treatment protocols are rooted in intrinsic variability, not controllable by changes in technique.

Ninety-eight percent of patients seeking treatment are females, most of whom describe the same problem in other family members.[1] These veins and arteries do not grow haphazardly. Their metabolic quiescence and proliferation are subject to complex and specific steps directed by peptide growth and inhibitory factors probably acting in concert with certain hormones to quickly orchestrate and then restrict the development of new vessels.

The word "varicose" means elevated, tortuous, and dilated. The varicose state can occur in both large and small "spider" veins (0.5 mm to 1.5 mm in diameter). Varicosity is an excellent marker of fragility, and small but convoluted vessels can be extraordinarily sensitive to treatment, responding to dilute sclerosants with sudden necrosis and thrombosis.

**Editor's note:* This chapter represents the extensive experience of one of the pioneer developers of sclerotherapy treatment of telangiectasia in the United States. Dr. Duffy's explanation of technique is both philosophical and informative. The chapter presents his unique viewpoint in a field in which there are few absolutes. The situations discussed here are certain to improve the interested physician's technique and stimulate better characterization of the lesions and blemishes of telangiectasia. Ultimately, this focus will refine treatment techniques and advance patient care.

GENERAL EFFECTS OF TREATMENT

Angiogenesis

Compared to tissue such as gastrointestinal mucosa, the cells that line the human vascular tree are relatively quiescent, with only two to three cells per 1000 undergoing mitosis. Endothelial cells are, however, poised to quickly initiate rapid proliferation, with entire cell populations turning over in 3 to 5 days after exposure to a variety of angiogenic stimuli. These stimuli, which include menstruation, ovulation, pregnancy, tissue trauma, and growth, also can occur in many pathologic states. Normally, vascular proliferation quickly stops when adequate new vessel growth has occurred. However, patients who seek treatment for large numbers of small vessels may have a genetically transmitted, abnormally sensitive response to minimal angiogenic stimuli producing many vessels with very little provocation (e.g., caused by tight clothes, crossed legs, or sclerotherapy). This exaggerated response also may be abnormally prolonged, intense, and exacerbated by the use of female hormones. The importance of these vascular dynamics centers on the fact that proliferative vessels can be, at least for a time, extraordinarily resistant to sclerotherapy yet appear clinically no different from vessels that will respond well to routine treatment schedules.

Clinically Inapparent Weakening

Previously treated vessels can look excactly as they did before treatment; however, they are, in fact, partially damaged and will be quickly destroyed by subsequent treatments. Conversely, vessels that have been treated repeatedly, particularly with low concentrations of sclerosants, and vessels that remain after multiple treatments often will resist extraordinarily high concentrations of sclerosants, concentrations that, in general, would destroy vessels of the same size and general characteristics if used for the first treatment. Accordingly, all descriptions of vessels should include a notation of their possible metabolic status, the relationship of this status to treatment history or other factors, and the impact of this proliferative state on the selection of sclerosants and the scheduling of treatment.

VESSEL CLASSIFICATION

As an aid in predicting treatment outcome, vessels are divided into two functional categories: proliferative and quiescent. Proliferative vessels, which respond to angiogenic stimuli with rapid endothelial cell turnover, are prototypically of recent onset (often following sclerotherapy or trauma) and are red in color and small in size (0.15 mm to 0.2 mm in diameter), although they can be any size. Quiescent vessels exhibit low cellular turnover times. These vessels, too, can come in all sizes, but they are usually >0.3 mm in diameter. In general, all vessels >1 mm can be considered quiescent. Quiescence is also the rule in vessels that are cyanotic to blue-green in color, occurring in patients whose history usually excludes exposure to angiogenic stimuli. Vessels are further typed on the basis of their response to sclerotherapy: type I (gradual response) and type II (sudden response). Vessels of both types and metabolic classes are subdivided morphologically on the basis of length of presence, size, color, location, and presence or absence of varicosity (elevation above surface, tortuosity, dilatation).

Type I Vessels: Slow Response to Sclerotherapy

Most vessels that respond with gradual fading following sclerotherapy vary in size between 0.15 mm and 0.5 mm in diameter. These small but metabolically inactive vessels and their attenuated remnants after treatment occur most frequently in patients less than 55 years of age and usually respond to repeated treatments with progressive diminution in size and lightening of color (fading). Hemosiderotic hyperpigmentation and thrombosis are most often noted at the larger end of this size spectrum (0.4 mm to 0.5 mm). The sudden and complete disappearance of these vessels after one treatment is occasionally noted. Small vessels that have undergone previous treatment can be weakened and suddenly destroyed by subsequent treatments, or they may become more resistant with repeated treatments, perhaps on the basis of treatment-induced fibrosis or mild hyperproliferation. Their true metabolic status is often clinically inapparent. Lability in terms of fast or slow response to treatment characterizes all vessels between 0.4 mm and 0.5 mm. The use of very high concentrations of sclerosants to treat these small vessels sometimes destroys them more quickly, but it often results in complications associated with rapid destruction, such as hyperpigmentation, thrombosis, and a probable increase in neovascularization (matting, visible neovascular proliferation, blush areas). All vessels from 0.15 mm to 2 mm usually are treated with between 0.25% and 0.75% POL or its equivalent. Lower concentrations are used (1) in patients of advanced age or easy bruisability, (2) when varicosity is present, or (3) in vessels between 0.6 mm and 2 mm. These factors suggest increased vascular fragility and mandate the use of lower concentrations of sclerosant.

Proliferative Vessels. These treatment-resistant vessels, which can be identical in size and color to their small quiescent counterparts, usually are <0.25 mm in diameter, rarely respond better to high concentrations of sclerosants, and will become quiescent and treatable over a variable period of time. Treatment with 0.75% POL or its equivalent is carried out by using modifications described later in this chapter.

Type II Vessels: Rapid Destruction/Varicose Pattern

Cyanotic at the smaller end of the spectrum (0.6 mm to approximately 1.5 mm in diameter), type II vessels become blue-green at approximately 2 mm. In this size range they can be presumed to be quiescent, although occasionally proliferative resistance may be noted. Sudden destruction and its sequelae (hemosiderotic hyperpigmentation, thrombosis, and occasional tissue necrosis) are common with these fragile vessels (Figure 21-1). A type II vessel, in communication with an incompetent saphenofemoral junction, may have been responsible for a pulmonary embolus that occurred in an elderly man after treatment (Figure 21-2). Vessels in this size range can be varicose or flat. When varicose, they are extraordinarily sensitive to treatment. All vessels between 0.6 mm and 2 mm are often quite delicate. A proliferative or resistant response to treatment is rare in vessels >0.6 mm.

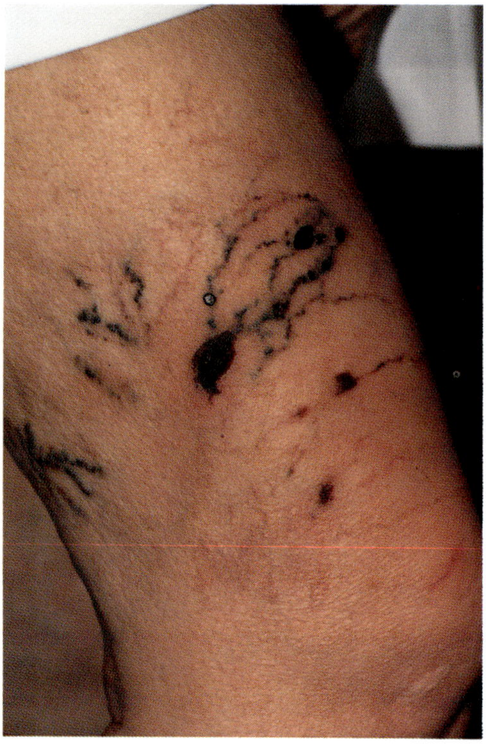

FIGURE 21-1. This elderly patient with veins between 0.5 and 1.5 mm was treated with 1% POL and developed severe tissue necrosis at injection sites.

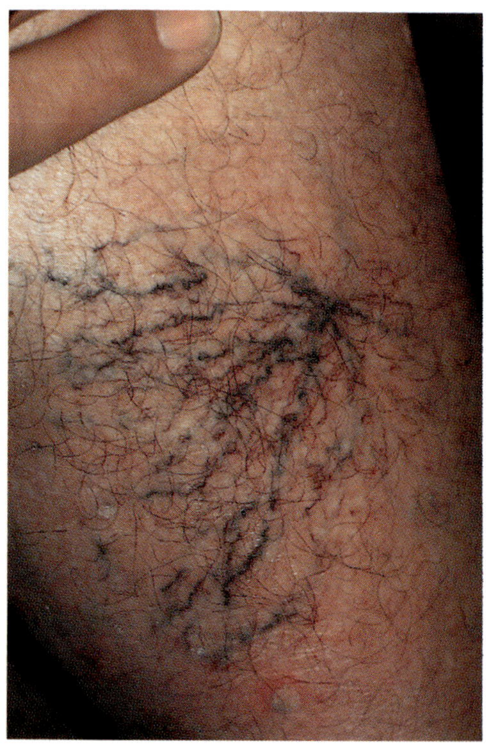

FIGURE 21-2. Sclerotherapy treatment of these 1 mm to 2 mm spider venules may have been partially responsible for a pulmonary embolus in this 73-year-old male who, at a later date, was found to have leukemia and a clotting disorder.

Type III: Fragile Vessels in Deep Vascular System

The presence of fragile vessels in the deep, and therefore invisible, circulation is one reason for using the lowest concentrations of sclerosants possible. Although the rate of treatment failures is higher with this approach, fewer disastrous results will be seen. Thrombosis can occur in type III vessels, often located far from the treated area and often in dependent sites, such as the ankles, where sclerosant pooling is likely to take place. Signs indicating that fragile vessels may be hidden beneath the surface are (1) the presence of masses of varicose vessels, both large and small, regularly seen in elderly patients with deep venous disease; (2) a history of spontaneous bleeding with minimal trauma; and (3) patients with symptoms such as swelling or aching (Figure 21-3). Patients with these risk factors are best evaluated for valvular incompetence, preferably with duplex scanning, but at the very least, with a hand-held Doppler instrument.

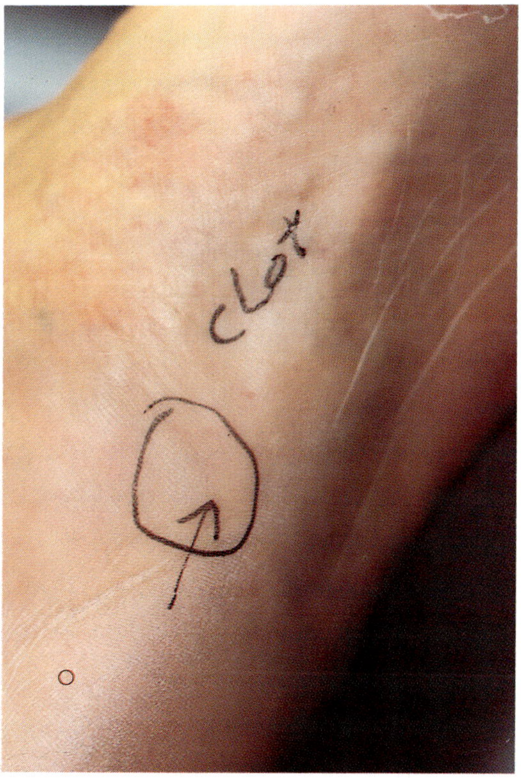

FIGURE 21-3. Thrombosis noted on the bottom of the foot following treatment of the leg. This vessel responded with sudden thrombosis. Several treatments were necessary for complete resolution.

A 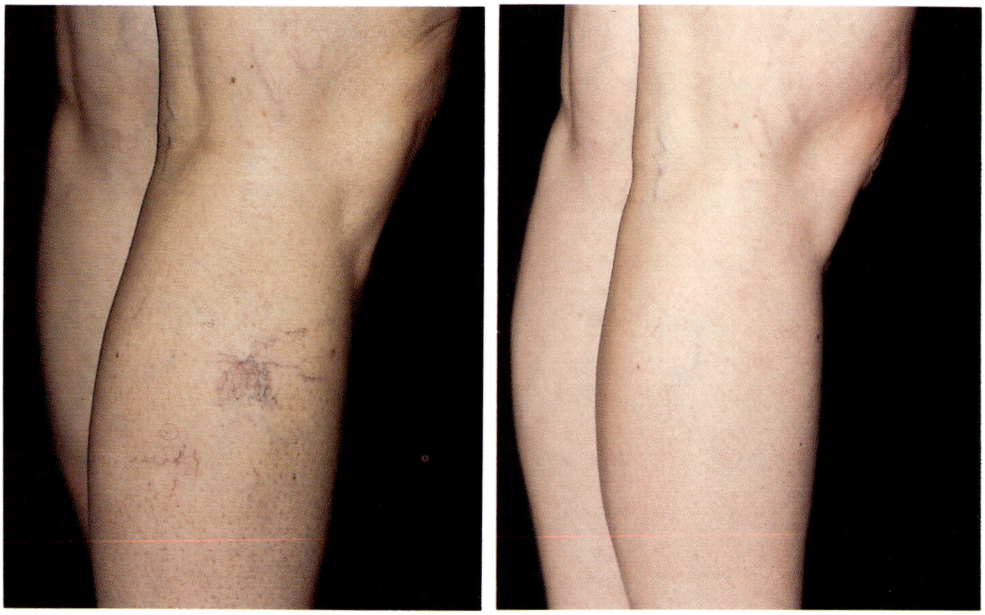 B

FIGURE 21-4. A, A mixture of vessels varying in size from 0.2 mm to slightly greater than 1 mm disappeared immediately after one treatment with 0.75% POL. B, Posttreatment appearance 2½ months later.

TREATMENT PROTOCOLS

Direct Injection

For the direct injection of vessels between 0.6 mm and 1.5 mm, solution strengths from 0.03% to 0.5% POL are used. All sclerosants, no matter how dilute, can produce sudden destruction or necrosis. The choice of concentrations is based on a clinical assessment of the individual patient's vascular fragility.

Indirect "Feeder" Injection

The injection of larger vessels as a substitute for or in association with the direct injection of smaller vessels has been advocated as a means of reducing complications (pigmentation, thrombosis, neovascularization, recurrence). For the treatment of "feeder" vessels >2.5 mm in size, 0.05% to 0.75% POL, 0.5 ml, is employed alone or in addition to direct injection (Figure 21-4).

TREATMENT SCHEDULE

The effects of sclerotherapy or other trauma leading to vascular proliferation and/or damage can be persistent in some patients and passing in others. In some patients, only one treatment will produce neovascularization, and repeated treatments will worsen the condition. In others, neovascularization occurs only after many treatments (or never); when it does occur, a wait of 3 to 6 months will render the vessel sensitive to repeated treatments (Figure 21-5).

A

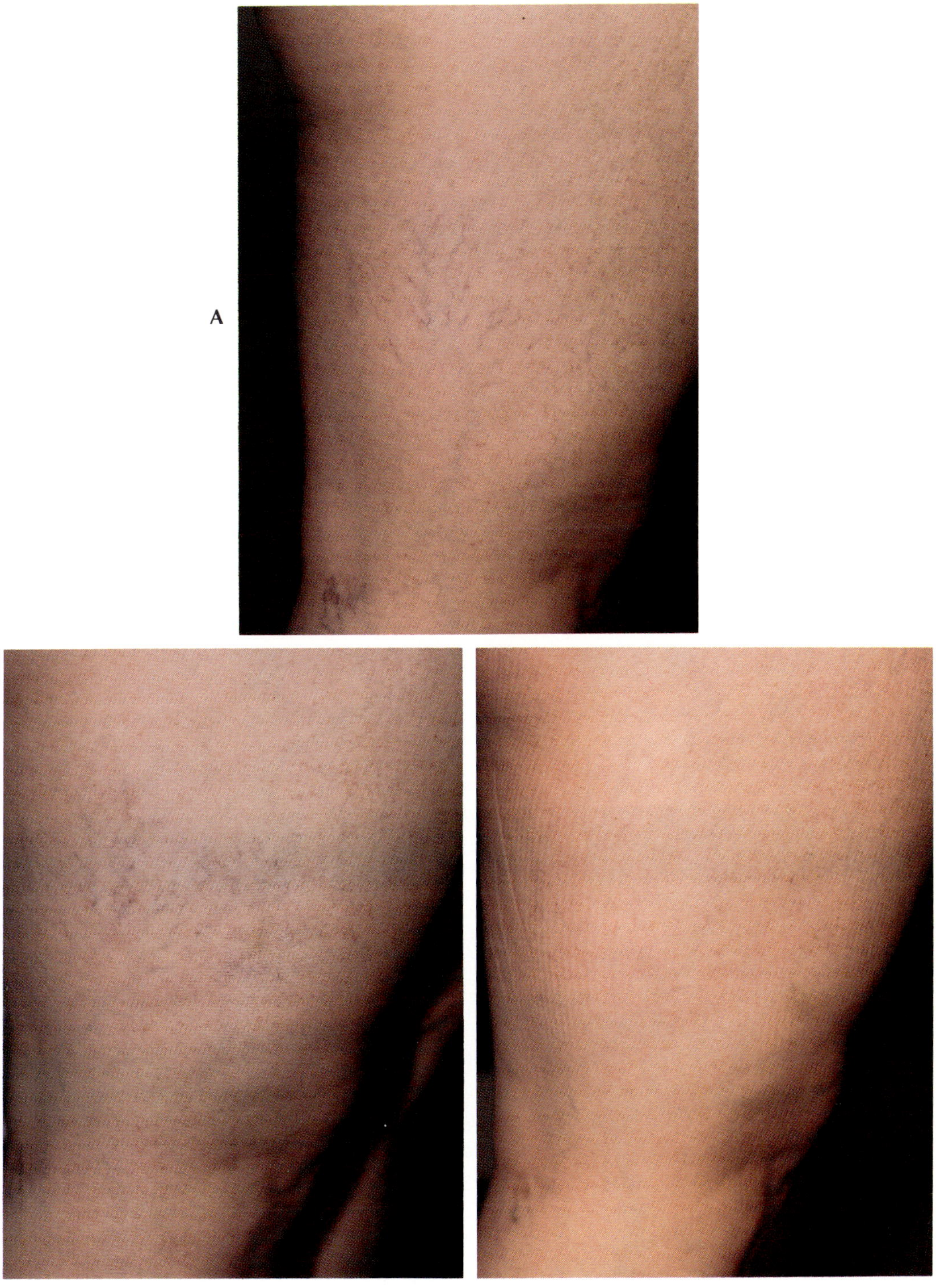

B C

FIGURE 21-5. **A,** Spider veins, 0.3 mm to 0.5 mm in size shown before treatment. **B,** One week after first treatment, neovascularization (matting) is observed. **C,** Neovascularization disappeared spontaneously within 2 months after the initial treatment.

Patients can be treated at 1- to 2-week intervals for three to five treatments. These treatments should be followed by a 3-month waiting period to assess neovascularization ("matting") before treatment is resumed. For patients who are not in a hurry, treatments at 6- to 8-week intervals, totaling no more than four or five, can be used to make the gradual fading process more effective and may reduce the total number of treatments necessary (Figure 21-6).

For spider veins, the same areas can be treated at 1- to 3-week intervals for a total of three to five treatments. In order to limit the volume of solution used in patients with extensive spider veins, new areas can be treated on the same day after a several-hour delay.

PATIENT EVALUATION

Pretreatment Guidelines

We ask patients not to shave the affected area for at least 48 hours before treatment because alcohol and dressings can irritate newly shaved skin. Alcohol is often applied to the skin in large quantities during treatment because it makes the skin transparent, which facilitates visualization of vessels, and acts as a cleansing agent. Many women use moisturizers on a regular basis, and the presence of these substances and the residue of moisturizer-containing soaps make the skin slippery and difficult to grasp. Accordingly, we ask patients to avoid using moisturizers for about 48 hours before treatment. Almost all our patients are females, and they are asked to bring shorts or culottes or to wear a full skirt, preferably an older garment, because bleeding may result from treatment.

Informed Consent

Patients fill out a thorough questionnaire to identify those factors that would place them at greater risk for complications: allergies, medications, symptoms, obesity, female hormones, significant systemic diseases (e.g., collagen vascular disease or diabetes), or history of significant venous disease. On the day of treatment, or sometimes by mail, we provide patients with a treatment brochure and a collection of about 40 photographs detailing the successes and failures of sclerotherapy. A written consent form, which informs patients of the risks of the procedure and permits their photographs to be used for educational purposes, must be signed by each patient. We inform patients both verbally and in writing of the FDA status of the sclerosants employed and the reasons for using them. The realities of sclerotherapy, for example, the possibility of complications and the fact that sclerotherapy is a treatment rather than a cure, are discussed with the patient. The discussions include the possibility of discomfort, the need for repeated treatments, the sometimes gradual nature of improvement, and the possibility of resistance to treatment or recurrence of disease. Everyone is told to expect some redness, bruising, pigmentation, or neovascular vessels. In addition, the occasional occurrence of more important complications (i.e., thrombophlebitis, allergies, deep venous thrombosis and its risk factors), the impact of the patient's age and general health, and the presence or absence of certain diseases in regard to treatment outcome are discussed. Patients also are warned about the possibility of ulcerations or scars. For many physicians

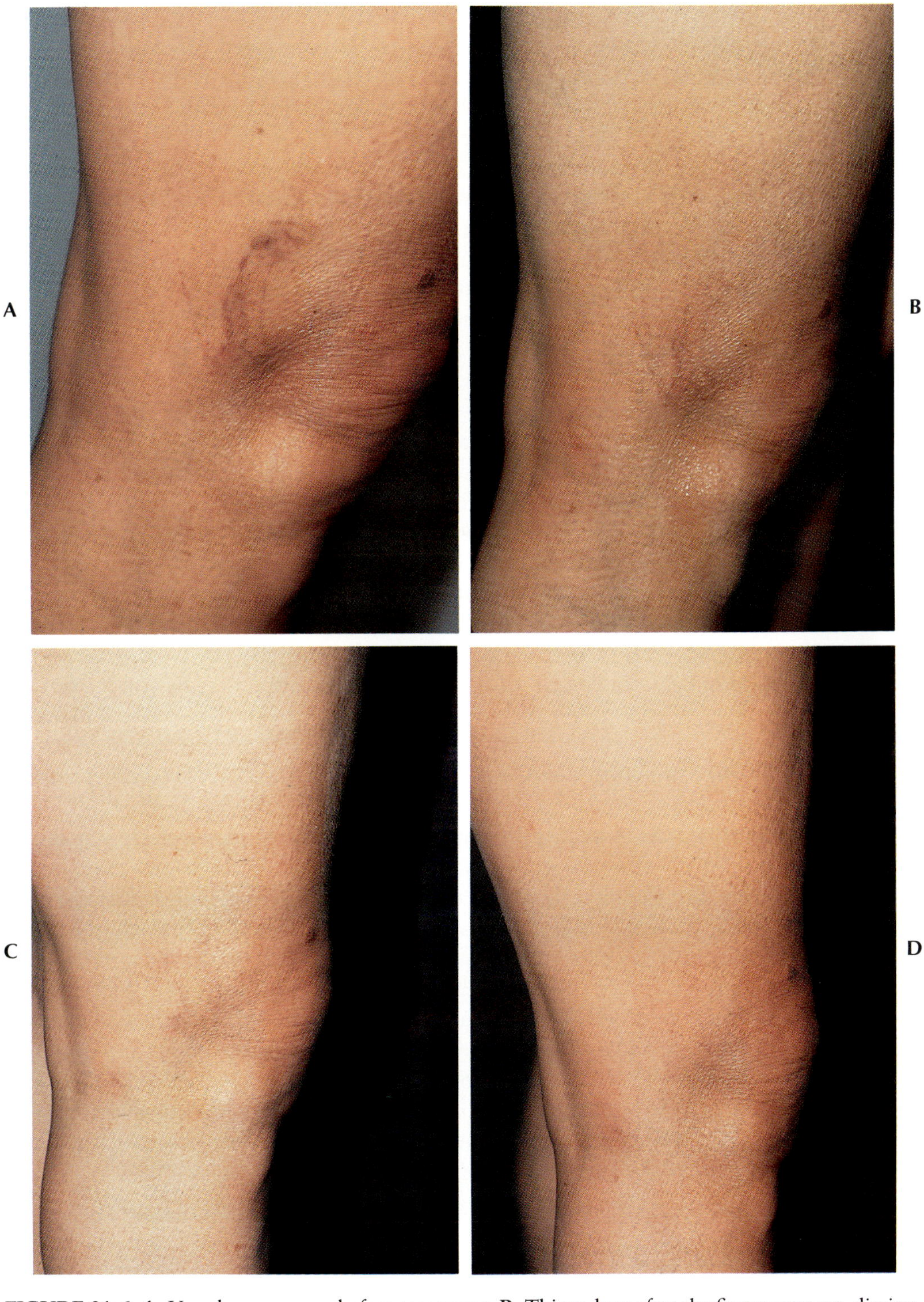

FIGURE 21-6. A, Vessel appearance before treatment. B, Thirty days after the first treatment, diminution of size and numbers of vessels can be seen. C, Three months after the second treatment, further clearing is noted. D, Almost complete disappearance of originally treated vessels is seen, but a small area of neovascularization (matting) also appears posterior to the treated area. At this point further treatment should be avoided for at least 3 to 6 months.

who perform this procedure, the problem is that the public and legal perception is that all ulcerations are caused by poor technique. Patients need to know that, even with a surgeon of great experience and excellent technique, ulcerations may occur and may be followed by scars, which are usually small and give the appearance of chickenpox.

The presence of arteriovenous malformations would seem to be related to the pathogenesis of these ulcers. However, the presence of such malformations has been reported only rarely in published studies.[2]

Patients are told that when injury occurs in individuals who do not develop spider vessels, the damage is quickly repaired and the vessels are precisely shut off so that too many new vessels do not emerge. However, patients who are prone to spider veins have a defective "switch" for shutting off vessel growth. New vessels may occur after a bruise, during pregnancy, after surgery, from a fall, from wearing tight hosiery, or as a consequence of treatment. We explain that for these patients multiple treatments might produce effects similar to those of multiple pregnancies, causing new vessel growth. For patients who sleep on their sides and have numerous vessels in the inner knees, we suggest placing a pillow between the knees.

It is important to tell patients that vessels either go away with little clots left behind or they fade, depending on their size and other factors. One way to avoid having unhappy patients is to tell them that the first four treatments are likely to be indicative of the results that can be expected. Some patients will experience ideal fading and excellent results. Others may have clotting early in the treatment phase. In patients with the type of vessels that fade, the remaining vessels (or those that appear after treatment) are often much more resistant to treatment, at least initially. Consequently, patients are encouraged to agree to a slow treatment approach, one that does not involve the compulsive treatment of every vessel. When larger vessels are treated, the patient may need a more extensive laboratory evaluation.

It is important to be honest with patients and to try to assess their particular risk factors for certain complications. Three common complications need to be discussed carefully and openly: (1) neovascularization, where it will occur and how difficult it will be to treat; (2) pigmentation; and (3) thrombi. Patients are routinely told that they will look worse before they look better, particularly if they have vessels that can be expected to resolve with pigmentation and thrombi. We have two protocols for testing type II vessels: (1) direct injection of ultralow concentrations of sclerosing solution (0.5 ml of 0.125% to 0.25% POL) into the spider veins in two sessions at 2-week intervals and (2) simultaneous injection of feeder vessels; in those >2.5 mm in size, with 0.5 ml of 0.5% or 0.75% POL or its equivalent. We then wait to assess the results. Although pigmentation and thrombi are transient, they can upset patients and have led to lawsuits.

Compression Therapy

The need for hosiery or compression dressings is assessed on an individual basis. Patients who need compression hosiery usually are fitted in advance of sclerotherapy. We encourage those who will require compression hosiery to wear it as much as possible before treatment to "break it in." We also provide instructions for hosiery care. In warmer climates patients who need compression treatment should be advised to wait until the winter months, when the cooler climate makes the process more comfortable.

With light hosiery (<20 mm Hg), most of the problems typically associated with heavier hosiery are minimized. The patient's arterial status is the primary concern. At the very least, possible symptoms of arterial insufficiency should be elicited and a brief check of arterial pulses should be performed before the hosiery fitting is done.

It is important to discuss foot problems before attempting to fit hosiery. Patients with bunions or other problems, particularly diabetes, are prone to various complications from wearing hosiery, for example, ulcerations and ischemia. Some individuals cannot tolerate short hosiery because it causes edema from obstruction of blood flow. In general, hosiery with open toes is the most comfortable type. Finally, for patients with a history of vaginal candidiasis, pantyhose should be avoided because it is occlusive and can provoke persistent infections.

Useful protocols. Compression therapy is generally used for any vessel over 0.5 mm that communicates with a larger varicose vein. Patients who are symptomatic (those with a history of edema, extreme fatigue, and visible large varicose veins) should undergo appropriate laboratory evaluation and be treated with compression schedules appropriate for their particular problem. In addition, small vessels may benefit from compression. Certain patients, particularly those with large numbers of small vessels (<2 mm) note improvement with the use of graduated compression hosiery. This group includes those whose work requires long periods of standing (e.g., nurses, flight attendants, grocery store checkers, and physicians). (Large vessels [>4 mm] and patients with valvular incompetence require special protocols and high compression.) Patients with small vessels do very well with 12 to 14 mm Hg graduated compression hosiery. Our routine for treating most patients with very small vessels (<1 mm) consists of injecting the vessels, applying bandages as necessary, and sending the patient home.

Personal experience. Over the years, for the purpose of comparison, we have routinely used compression on one leg of the patient (but not on the other) after treatment of small vessels. We have had several patients who received extraordinary benefits and rapid results from compression, but as time passed, we could not demonstrate that trend among the hundreds of patients in whom compression and noncompression therapy were followed. We also noted tremendous variability in terms of response to identical treatments. Accordingly, we generally reserve compression therapy for patients with large veins (>3 mm) or for symptomatic patients with small vessels.

Photographic Documentation

All patients are initially photographed, both at close range and at a distance, to demonstrate the nature and extent of vessels present before treatment. This is done for several reasons. First, patients commonly forget their pretreatment appearance and often are pleasantly surprised to see how much progress has been made. Second, photographs can help to correlate the specific effect of certain regimens on their vessels, which helps the sclerotherapist make decisions about sclerosant concentration, use of compression, and treatment frequency.

Precautions for Sclerotherapist

The sclerotherapist always should wear gloves during evaluation and when administering treatment. Although careful patient evaluation can help minimize the risks of certain contagious diseases, consideration should be given to the use of hepatitis vaccine, for example, to protect the sclerotherapist if he or she performs the procedure regularly and will continually be exposed to blood. Sharps containers always should be close at hand.

MATERIALS AND INSTRUMENTATION

Sclerosing Solutions

The choice of sclerosant is influenced by the needs of the patient, the availability and legal status of the agent, and the experience of the sclerotherapist. At this writing, in the United States only two drugs are approved for the treatment of varicose veins of any size involving the lower extremities: sodium morrhuate (approved in 1930) and sodium tetradecyl sulfate (approved in 1946). These agents are more toxic and no more efficacious for the treatment of small vessels than hypertonic saline or polidocanol (POL). POL soon will be sanctioned by the FDA for this purpose. In my practice, no solution stronger than 0.75% POL (or its equivalent 23.4% hypertonic saline or 0.25% Sotradecol) is routinely used for vessels <3 mm in size. The corresponding concentrations are all approximate. One sclerosant may work better than another on certain veins in certain individuals.

All sclerosants can produce pain, unwanted thrombosis (pulmonary emboli or deep venous thrombosis), necrosis, ulceration, and (with the exception of pure hypertonic saline) allergies.

The advantage of pure hypertonic saline is that it does not induce an allergic response. The disadvantages are that it is relatively uncomfortable to use and too weak for treatment of larger vessels. Ulcerations may occur with concentrations of sclerosants as low as 10% when the solution is injected intradermally in volumes >0.3 ml (unpublished data, 1990). This ulcerogenesis has the potential to cause severe tissue necrosis in the absence of almost perfect technique.

Sotradecol (sodium tetradecyl sulfate) has the advantages of FDA approval, a relatively low incidence of important complications compared to sodium morrhuate,[3] and relative painlessness compared to hypertonic saline. Using a volunteer, we determined that 0.33% Sotradecol, 0.5 ml in volume in the dermis, would not produce ulcers on contact but that the same volume of 1% solution would cause ulcers (unpublished data, 1990) (Figure 21-7).

POL, or dihydroxypolyethoxydodecane (Aethoxysklerol), is the most "fool-

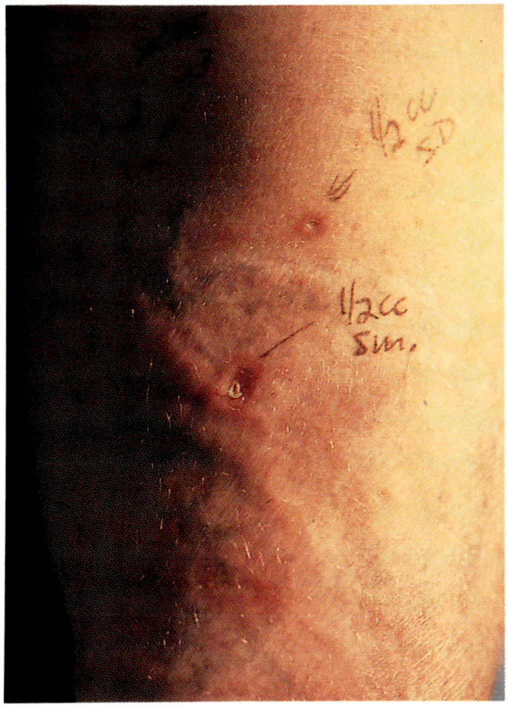

FIGURE 21-7. Ulceration associated with sclerotherapy. Upper ulcer, measuring approximately ¼ inch, resulted from 0.5 ml of 1% Sotradecol administered intradermally. Larger ulcer resulted from administration of 0.5 ml of 5% sodium morrhuate.

proof" of all available sclerosants. I received an injection of 0.5 ml of 3% POL directly into the middle dermis. Although ulcerations did not occur, mild hyperpigmentation occurred in the area where tiny cutaneous vessels were suddenly destroyed (Figure 21-8). However, all sclerosants can produce ulcers through other mechanisms. The rate of serious allergies and fatalities reported following the use of POL is lower than that reported for any other FDA-approved sclerosant.[4] In low concentrations POL is the most painless of all agents. It should not be used in patients being treated with disulfiram (Antabuse) because it contains alcohol.

For the treatment of small vessels, four concentrations of sclerosants are recommended: 0.75% POL; 0.5%, 0.25%, and 0.125% or equivalent concentrations of saline (23.4%; 15.6%, 7.8%, and 3.9%, respectively). Sotradecol is roughly three to four times as potent as POL on a percentage basis. Individual variability plays an enormous role in the treatment outcome, and it is difficult to absolutely equate one solution strength and type with another. The lowest concentrations are routinely used for fragile subsets of vessels, with a concomitant increase in treatment failures resulting. Moreover, in certain patients pigmentation and thrombosis will occur

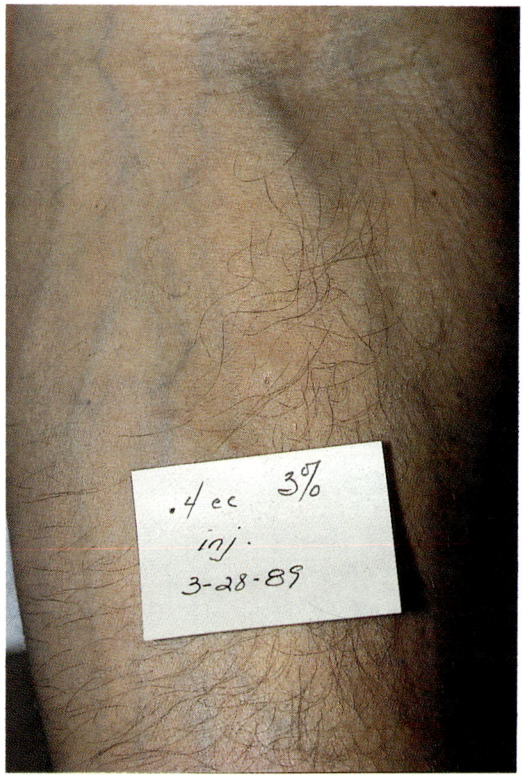

FIGURE 21-8. Appearance of skin of a volunteer who received 0.5 ml of 3% POL without tissue necrosis occurring.

even with very dilute solutions (0.03% POL or equivalent), which are roughly 18 times weaker than the same solution that can be used for vessels of an approximate size (Figure 21-9).

To summarize, all sclerosants work well. POL gets an "A" in terms of hypoallergenicity and extravasation safety; hypertonic saline, because it is hypoallergenic; and Sotradecol, for its potency in treating larger veins. For treatment of type I vessels, 0.75% POL or 23.4% hypertonic saline produce equivalent results. In patients with collagen vascular disease, those with serious underlying illness, or elderly patients with very frail skin, testing with ultralow concentrations in very small areas is done. Such patients are at greater risk for ulcers. Posttreatment proliferative type I (0.2 mm and smaller in size) are treated with 0.75% POL. Higher concentrations (up to 3% POL) have not produced better results in the treatment of neovascular vessels.

Syringes

Disposable 1 ml to 3 ml syringes (not Luer Lock) are recommended. The size of the syringe employed is a matter of individual preference. Physicians with larger

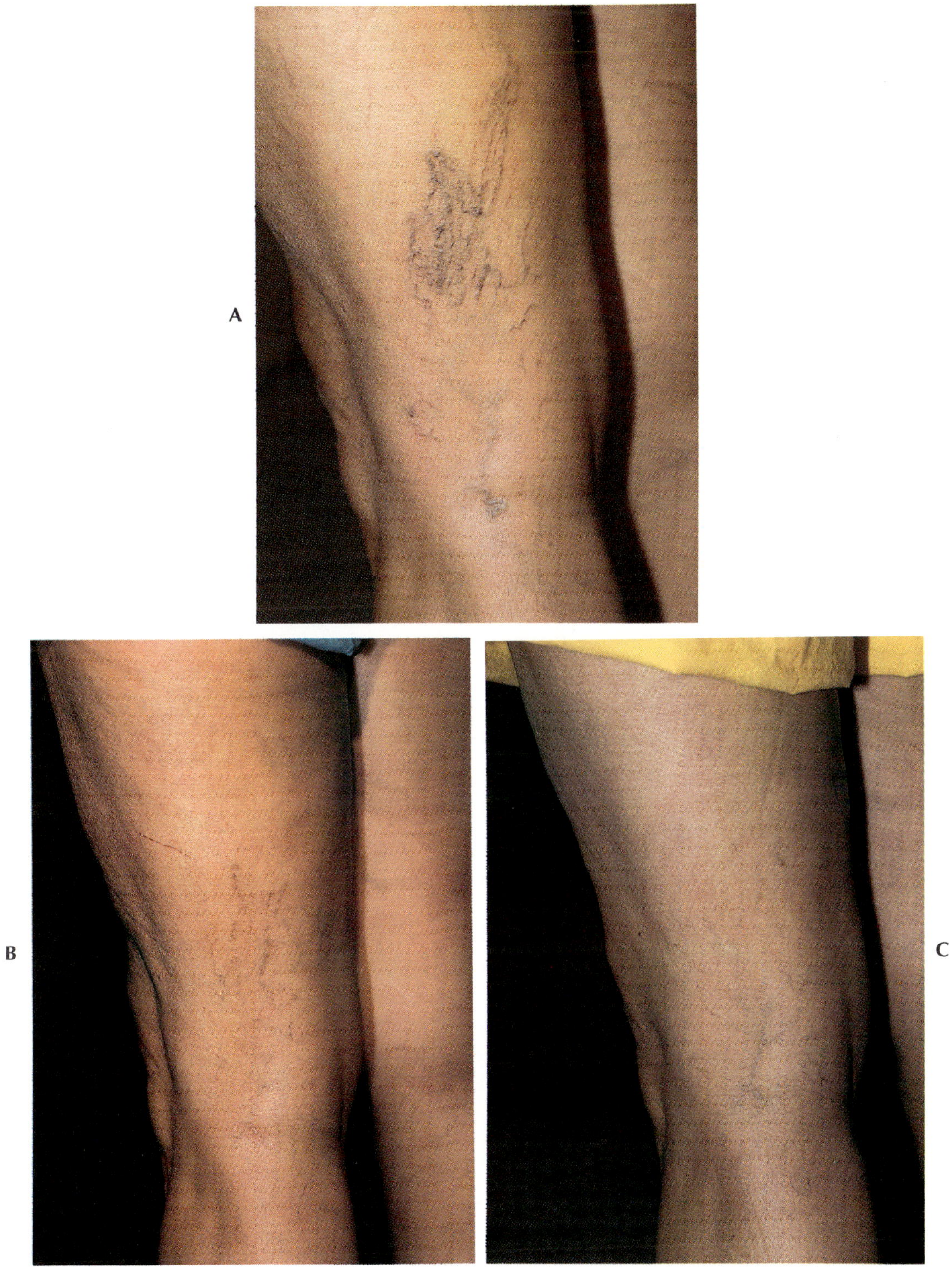

FIGURE 21-9. **A,** Pretreatment appearance of elevated, tortuous, and dilated spider varicosities measuring 0.5 mm to 1.5 mm on left posterior, lateral thigh. **B,** Pigmentation and a few thrombi were still present after two treatments at 2 months after initiation of treatment. **C,** Almost 2 years after treatment, a good residual result is noted with no apparent pigmentation. Since vessels of this type routinely undergo sudden destruction with transient pigmentation, patients must be warned of this effect.

hands sometimes like the delicacy and control afforded by the use of a 1 ml syringe, which is a great deal longer than a 3 ml syringe when full. In either size, a non-Luer Lock syringe is a better choice because it facilitates frequent needle changes. Moreover, the injection speed is greater with a 1 ml syringe because more pressure is generated with a 1 ml syringe than with a 3 ml syringe.

When the needle is put on the syringe, I place the bevel side up, positioned exactly 90 degrees to the T-handle. Routinely, the syringe is filled to only 2.5 ml so that the extension of the piston fits the operator's hand exactly. Beginners should experiment to find the exact volume piston extension and syringe that is best for their hand.

Hypodermic Needles

The best and most uniformly finished No. 30 needles seem to be 30-gauge ½-inch hypodermic needles, either Poly-Kote (metal hub needle with silicone-coated tribeveled point; distributed by Acuderm, Inc., Fort Lauderdale, Fla.) or Air-Tite (30-gauge ½-inch needle; distributed by AIR-TITE of Virginia, Inc., Virginia Beach, Va.). Needles smaller than 30 gauge are often nondisposable, dull, and unnecessary. A good, sharp No. 30 needle can be used easily to inject a vessel <0.15 mm in diameter.

One-half inch No. 30 needles, measuring 0.3 mm in diameter, are honed to an oblique bevel, which permits them to enter veins <0.1 mm in diameter. Needles longer than ½ inch are too flexible for easy use. A bend made in the needle with the bevel up (1) provides clearance for the fingers of the dominant hand between the patient's skin and the body of the syringe, (2) permits close approximation of the needle flat on the skin to minimize the angle of entry, and (3) places the tip of the needle and its bevel exactly where it can be seen. Before treatment is begun, the needle should be bent, with the angle varying according to the area being treated, and checked for patency by flushing a small amount of sclerosant through the needle tip. The piston is pulled back approximately ¼ inch to minimize air bubbles, which impair visibility. Finally, the skin is stretched, particularly in areas of high tissue mobility. Either the patient or an assistant can stretch the skin. Entry through the skin should be as close as possible to the vein in order to minimize the patient discomfort from "threading" of the needle. The vein should be entered with as narrow an angle between the needle and the skin as possible and with such little space under the needle that a piece of paper could be slid under it. Such an entry can be accomplished by exerting slight force downward on the tip of the needle to create a small dell in the skin.

Sharpness of needle. Needles are not necessarily perfect when they leave the manufacturing company. Flaws in the refinement process can create a needle tip that transmits a scratchy sensation. If this sensation is noted on the first injection, the needle should be discarded. If it happens often, another needle manufacturer should be chosen. About 1 in every 500 needles will lack a bevel completely. After multiple treatments, the needle tip becomes blunt and requires more force to penetrate the skin. When observed under the microscope, the needle tip is seen to be bent.

Frequent needle changes, often after every third to fifth injection, are the rule, particularly in areas where the skin is tough and rigid, such as the feet, knees, or ankles. The needle should be changed before injection of the inner thigh or the popliteal fossa, where tissue mobility or concavity makes the injection technique more awkward. In these areas it is sometimes worthwhile to do a test run to determine the degree of bend and the exact angle of entry.

Placement of needle. Ideally, only the tip and the bevel of the needle are placed in the vein. The needle lumen can be seen shadowed by the walls of the transparent vessel. The visual appearance of the needle, often associated with the sudden reflux of blood, is the most important factor in determining placement. Unlike larger thick-walled vessels (>3 mm), small vessels exhibit only slight tissue resistance upon entry. The amount of force exerted on the piston necessary to initiate sclerosant flow is only slightly less in these small vessels than the degree necessary to inject the skin itself.

Miscellaneous Materials

- ☐ Isopropyl alcohol, cottonballs, and a Petri dish need to be available. Cottonballs saturated with isopropyl alcohol can be kept in a Petri dish. The alcohol can be applied to treated areas to clarify the skin as an aid in deciding where to inject. Alternatively, a drop of sclerosant applied judiciously to a smaller area clarifies the skin and takes less time to apply.
- ☐ Microfoam surgical tape and Micropore 5 mm ½-inch tape (3M Medical-Surgical Division, St. Paul, Minn.), and cottonballs. Microfoam surgical tape is excellent for compression, but in areas where the skin flexes, particularly the popliteal fossa, we use Micropore tape beneath the Microfoam tape to minimize abrasion and the effects of occlusion.
- ☐ Cameras. Autofocus Nikon 2020, 4004, 5005, 6006, and 8008 cameras equipped with Nikon Speedlight 58-24 (with ASA 64 Kodachrome or Ektachrome film) are employed. All modern single-lens-reflex cameras use through-the-lenses flash systems, but autofocus lenses and flashes are used because the aperture and shutter speeds are more precise and controllable. I routinely use them in the manual focus mode, which permits faster focusing than autofocus and eliminates the tracking or hunting that occurs when the unsophisticated autofocus device cannot "decide" what small change in the contour of the skin represents the desired photo.
- ☐ Opticaid magnifiers with 2.5 power magnification or other similar magnifiers. These magnifiers have the advantages of lightness and ease of use (particularly with eyeglasses) but the disadvantage of the need for a closer working distance. The choice of magnification is an individual matter. It is best to try out various optical devices.
- ☐ Gauze pads (4 × 4 inch) and bandages.
- ☐ Timer. A timer can be set for the approximate time that injecting is to be continued because it is easy to lose track of time while concentrating on the work.

- ☐ Two overhead spotlights that converge on the treated area and are easy to move (even when one is sitting down injecting the veins). The presence of two lights permits the person injecting the veins to move his or her head in any direction without blocking light.
- ☐ Two stools with wheels. Such stools are the right height to permit the person doing the injection to sit comfortably with knees under the table and to move quickly when necessary.
- ☐ Power-operated surgical table.
- ☐ Peake's loupe magnifier. To measure vessels, I remove the clear plastic tube that contains a 0.1 mm reticle from its clumsy illumination device. This small plastic tube is extremely convenient to use with good surgical side lighting. I routinely wet the skin with alcohol first before applying the reticle. Another way to measure vessels is to place hypodermic needles of various sizes over the vein and use optical magnification.
- ☐ Patient information and consent forms.
- ☐ Graduated compression stockings (range, 12 mm Hg to 40 mm Hg), preferably with open toes.
- ☐ Band-Aids.
- ☐ Solu-Medrol, analeptics, Benadryl, cardiotonics, and normal saline in large 10 ml syringes attached to 25-gauge ½-inch needles for neutralization when extravasation of sclerosants occurs.

TECHNIQUE

Small vessels are always more superficial than they appear, and this misperception of their depth is complicated by the belief that the entire needle must be inserted into the vein to be effective, a concept fostered by training in drawing blood, in which the goal is to insert the entire needle into the vein. When small vessels are being injected, any attempt to insert more than the tip of the needle occludes the flow of sclerosant. The almost imperceptible "creep" of the needle generated by the friction of the forward motion of the piston in the syringe must be minimized by sustaining good tension away from the needle during the injection process and/or by applying firm downward force along the length of the needle to lock it into place.

Positioning of Patient and Initial Injection

For treatment of the relatively inaccessible lateroposterior thigh, the patient is placed in the prone position. The upper leg to be treated is flexed at the hip and knee, which angles the treated area up and away from the table and provides good accessibility for injection.

In most instances the patient is placed in a recumbent position or seated on a power-operated table that is high enough so that the person doing the injection can sit with his or her knees beneath the table. Two readily accessible lights are pointed exactly at the cluster of veins to be treated so that they sharply illuminate the tip of the needle without creating reflections. The ability to visualize the needle tip is what determines whether the injection is an easy or a difficult procedure. A No. 30 needle is bent between 10 and 30 degrees with the bevel positioned up. The syringe is held in the dominant hand between the index and middle fingers. The thumb, which is used to inject the solution, is on the piston before the injection sequence is begun. A few tenths of 1 ml of solution is injected to establish the patency of the needle. Then one to two thirds of the body of the needle is placed flat upon the skin with the bevel up. The vessel is entered, preferably with as little angle as possible. It must be remembered that the vessels are absolutely parallel to the skin. When the needle tip has been properly placed in the vein, it usually looks like a sliver. With continuous tissue tension applied, the sclerosant is slowly injected. Immediate blanching, confined to the vessel and its tributaries, can be seen. Ordinarily 0.25 ml to 0.5 ml of sclerosant is injected over 5 to 10 seconds. Our investigations suggest that tissue damage for the targeted vessels is maximal between 5 and 10 seconds if all the blood is displaced from the vein (unpublished data, 1984). Slow injections and small volumes minimize patient discomfort, extravasation, and damage to the deeper vasculature. Following injection, often to the patient's dismay, the treated veins refill with blood. The patient also should be warned to expect some swelling, elevation of the vessels, bruising, and urtication, all of which will subside rapidly. Urtication is common with the use of POL. Erythema, perivenular edema, and cramping are most common when hypertonic saline is the agent.

There is widespread agreement that the gentle injection of low volumes of low-concentration sclerosants that produce a small (<2 cm) blanch, will minimize the risk of several complications by reducing trauma to the treated areas and the surrounding normal vasculature. Conversely, rapid injection of highly concentrated sclerosants will maximize the risk of complications.

Patient Comfort and Injection Force

The patient should be told to expect a slight stinging sensation as the skin is penetrated. Many patients are frightened by needles, and a simple explanation that the needle being used is the size of a hair and the vessel to be treated is very close to the surface frequently will be comforting to such patients. Pain varies according to the type of sclerosant used and how fast it is being injected. Almost no pain results from using dilute POL or low concentrations (<0.5%) of Sotradecol. Some patients experience considerable discomfort from hypertonic saline. Sudden injection with air or sclerosant can produce distention and modest pain. Pain can be minimized through slow injection and using just enough sclerosant to fill the vessels in a radius of approximately 3 cm. Enough piston pressure should be maintained to keep that small area filled with solution for 5 to 10 seconds with almost no force.

The amount of force used to maintain the clearing of small vessels is generally about the same as that necessary to lightly seal an envelope. However, occasionally slightly more force will be needed to initiate flow, possibly because bits of skin are lodged in the needle lumen. Sometimes enough force is exerted to displace the needle from the vein, particularly when the air-block technique is used. In fragile vein subsets (varicose venules, 0.75 mm to 2 mm), excessive injection force may cause vessel rupture. In vessels <0.4 mm rupture probably will not occur.

Injections given very rapidly (i.e., when a great deal of force is used to inject or when a large needle is used) can push a bolus of sclerosant into deeper vessels. The possible results are vascular rupture, deep venous thrombosis, vascular compromise, and pulmonary emboli. If sclerosant seems to disappear into the deeper system during the injection of small vessels, it is best to stop the injection and begin injecting adjacent vessels in which sclerosant is seen flowing through highly visible, targeted superficial veins.

Air-Block Technique

If small amounts of air are used to precede the injection, this technique permits a preview for determining whether the needle is accurately positioned without subjecting the patient to the risk of extravasation. For larger vessels, using air to precede the injection has the advantage of stripping blood from the vessel walls, thus permitting sclerosant to contact endothelial tissue without dilution. For small vessels, however, the use of air does not prevent or modify the occurrence of complications or enhance the results. Instead, air blocks have several possible disadvantages when used for small vessels, including (1) sometimes requiring an awkward injection position, (2) frightening the patient with the sight of air going into the vein (although it is totally harmless), or (3) completely displacing the needle from the vein.

Methods of Increasing Tension

Without adequate tissue tension, the skin bunches up and accurate placement of the needle becomes impossible. During injection, tension can be created by the thumb and index finger of the nondominant hand, which pulls the skin away from the tip of the needle and stretches it laterally. The dominant hand can be useful in applying countertension. The lateral border or tip, the fifth finger, and the hypothenar eminence are used by experienced sclerotherapists to create balanced tension in concert with the nondominant hand. When the skin is slippery, 4 × 4-inch pads placed under either (or both) hand(s) can be useful to gain extra traction. In the event of great tissue mobility, particularly on the inner thighs, the patient or an assistant is asked to pull laterally around the area being treated while the person doing the injection pulls the skin directly away from the needle tip.

An excellent way to observe the effect of traction away from the needle during the injection sequence is to pull the skin directly away from the needle tip, with the needle held firmly in place through downward force. This method can be used to salvage an injection in which the needle has crept too deeply into the vein. With firm downward force on the needle, one can either pull the skin away from the needle tip or slowly pull the needle partially out of the vein.

Downward force with the needle has several useful applications. At the beginning of the injection, particularly on areas with thick musculature, such as the gastrocnemius, slight downward force applied while pressing the needle firmly against tightly stretched skin can minimize the angle of entry. After the injection has begun, downward force on the needle holds it in place and minimizes needle "creep," which results from piston friction.

There are at least two areas on the legs—knees and ankles—where rapidly thrusting the needle into the vein makes entry easier. This situation is particularly noticeable with small vessels (<0.2 mm). A sharp needle is easier to advance than a dull one. Therefore when increasing resistance is felt to the slow passage of a needle into the skin and vein, it is probably time to change needles.

Posttreatment Guidelines

For the treatment of small (<2 mm) type I vessels in young, ambulatory patients, very few postoperative instructions are necessary. Patients who play vigorous games of tennis are encouraged to avoid that activity for a day or two. Otherwise, their activities are unrestricted. For patients with type II vessels, particularly when they are widespread, postoperative care is a great deal more important. It includes alternating between elevating the legs as much as possible and vigorous walking. For patients with symptomatic vessels who have jobs that require prolonged periods of standing, we routinely advise them to take a couple of days off work and alternate vigorous walking with periods of leg elevation.

Patients are instructed to call the office if severe pain develops or if localized tenderness, swelling, scabs, blisters, or anything out of the ordinary is noted. The ordinary course of events is described in the treatment brochure given to the patient. Patients also are warned that certain areas are more prone to problems. Neovascularization is most common in treatment of the inner knees, ulcerations occur most commonly on the ankles, and thrombosis is the rule for vessels of a certain size.

TECHNIQUE MODIFICATIONS

Goldman and others have suggested that an excellent way to minimize excessive trauma and to reduce pigmentation, thrombosis, neovascularization, and recurrence is to inject the larger, blue-green reticular nonvaricose veins that are often seen in communication with smaller red vessels.[4,5] We have observed several problems in using this technique, a fact we determined by documenting the injection of 52 patients (unpublished data, 1991). Occasionally good results were obtained, particularly when the communication of the spider veins with the feeder vein was very slow. In these successfully treated patients, a metering out of dilute sclerosants probably occurs as the patient walks. Muscular movement pumps this dilute sclerosant into small vessels and produces an excellent outcome. The major problem encountered was the sudden destruction of the larger feeder vessels. Often these vessels were in the 1 mm to 2 mm range, and they would thrombose long before smaller spider veins (0.25 mm to 0.5 mm) showed any change. Conversely, when communication was rapid, we noted the same mechanism injecting the feeder vessels that we recognized injecting the smaller vessels themselves with the same concentrations. Neovascularization also occurred commonly after the treatment of larger vessels, particularly around the knees. We currently use a small volume of low-concentration sclerosant injected into communicating veins only if they are >2 mm; a more dilute concentration is used to directly inject the smaller vessels.

A

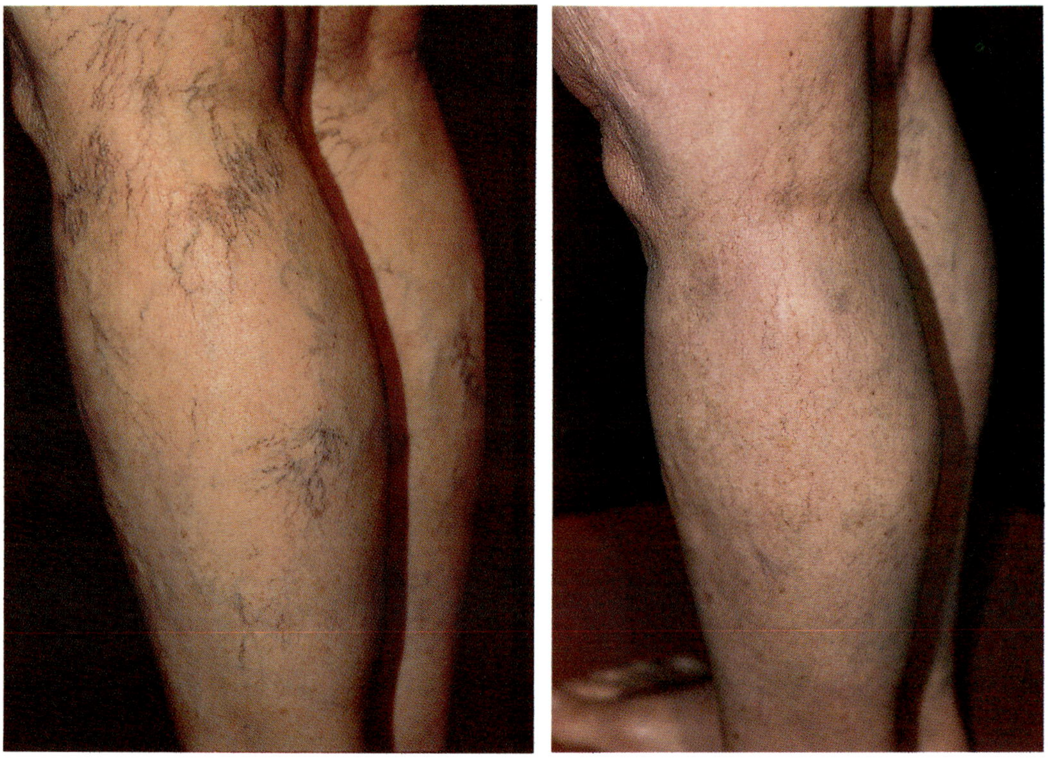

B

FIGURE 21-10. A, Pretreatment appearance of 0.5 mm to 1.5 mm spider veins on left lateral gastrocnemius and thigh. **B,** Complete disappearance without pigmentation is an unusual occurrence.

A

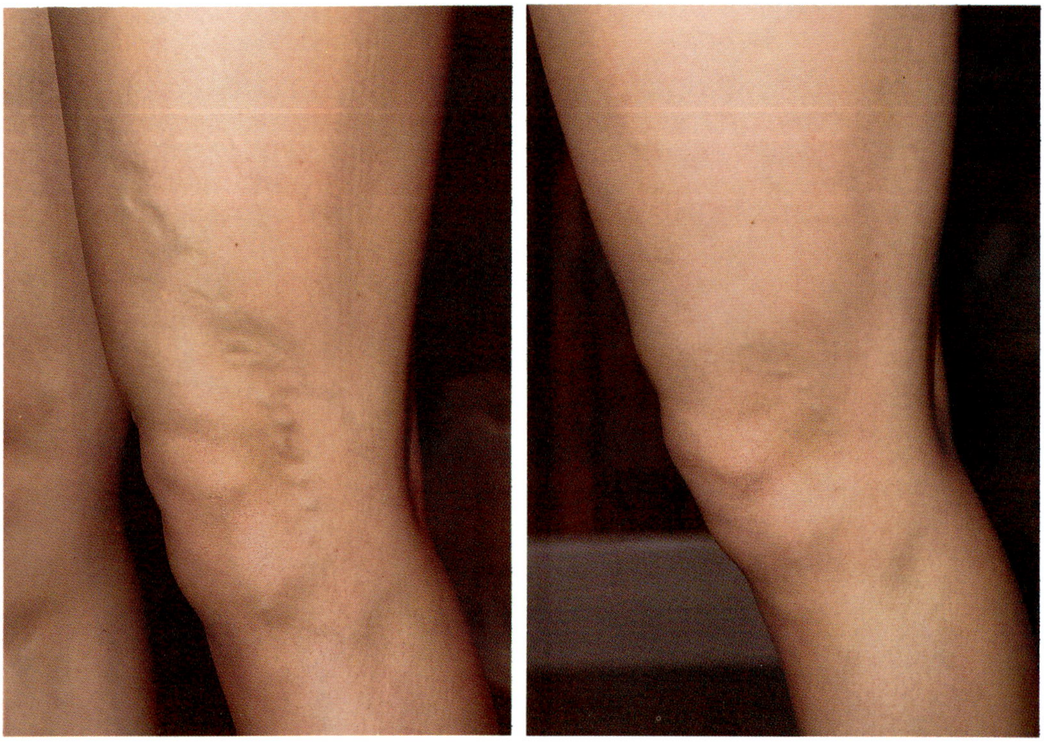

B

FIGURE 21-11. A, A 5 mm to 6 mm lateral saphenous varicosity before treatment. **B,** Prompt resolution without pigmentation is seen 2 months after a single treatment. Although extremely unusual, evolution of healing without pigmentation does occur, demonstrating the inherent variability in the treatment of veins.

SUMMARY

There are no absolutes in the treatment of small vessels. Variability in patients and experience with various solutions or treatment combinations are often better guides than fixed rules. The concept of a sclerosant causing trauma that induces exaggerated neovascularization and populations of resistant vessels makes an understanding of the complexity of treatment results a little easier. The treatment of small vessels is an excellent addition to the therapeutic armamentarium of those who are interested in learning the nuances of its technique (Figure 21-10). Large vessels can be treated successfully and symptoms can be resolved (Figure 21-11), perhaps in association with surgically oriented phlebologists and/or vascular surgeons.

REFERENCES

1. Duffy DM. Small vessel sclerotherapy: An overview. Adv Dermatol 3:221-242, 1988.
2. De Faria JL, Moraes IN. Histopathology of the telangiectasia associated with varicose veins. Dermatologica 127:321-329, 1963.
3. Imperiali G, Terruzi V, Spotti D, Minoli G. Heart failure as a side effect of polidocanol given for esophageal variceal sclerosis. Endoscopy 18:207, 1986.
4. Tretbar LL. Injection sclerotherapy for spider telangiectasias: A twenty-year experience with sodium tetradecyl sulfate. J Dermatol Surg Oncol 15:223-225, 1989.
5. Goldman MP. Sclerotherapy of varicose and telangiectatic leg veins. Case Log Use Newsletter 3(3):3-4, May/June 1990.

Index

Q

R

T